Physiology of the Heart

Second Edition

Physiology of the Heart

Second Edition

Arnold M. Katz, M.D.
Professor of Medicine
Head, Cardiology Division
University of Connecticut Health Center
Farmington, Connecticut

Raven Press   New York

Raven Press, Ltd., 1185 Avenue of the Americas, New York, New York 10036

Made in the United States of America

Library of Congress Cataloging-in-Publication Data

Katz, Arnold M.
    Physiology of the heart / Arnold M. Katz. — 2nd ed.
       p.   cm.
    Includes bibliographical references and index.
    ISBN 0-88167-838-4
    1. Heart—Physiology. 2. Heart—Pathophysiology. I. Title.
    [DNLM: 1. Biophysics. 2. Heart—physiology. WG 202 K19p]
    QP111.4.K38 1992
    612.1'7—dc20
    DNLM/DLC
    for Library of Congress   91-28788
                                                     CIP

9 8 7 6 5 4 3 2 1

To my father,
Louis N. Katz
1897–1973

Contents

Preface to the First Edition

Why write a textbook about the biophysical basis of cardiac function? Of what importance are the energetics and chemistry of myocardial contraction to anyone but a physical chemist or a biochemist? Why should electrical potentials at the surface of the myocardial cell concern those who are not basic electrophysiologists? The answers to all of these questions lie in the fact that *virtually every important physiological, pharmacological, or pathological change in cardiac function arises from alterations in the physical and chemical processes that are responsible for the heartbeat.*

Although it remains fashionable to consider the heart as a muscular pump, this organ is much more than a hollow viscus that provides mechanical energy to propel blood through the vasculature. It is an intricate biological machine that contains, within each cell, a complex of control and effector mechanisms. Both the strength of cardiac contraction and its electrical control are modulated by alterations in one or more of these cellular mechanisms, which are involved in the fundamental processes of excitability, excitation–contraction coupling, and contraction.

This text is written for medical students and graduate students in the biological sciences, and for the physician who would like to find a simplified exposition of our current understanding of the physiological and biophysical basis of cardiac function. Therefore, this book is intended to provide a synoptic view of our present knowledge in this rapidly expanding area. The major emphasis is on the relationships between the biochemical properties of individual constituents of the myocardial cell, the biophysics of cardiac muscle function, and the performance of the intact heart.

The task of relating these different aspects of cardiac function to each other has required much selectivity and, undoubtedly, an excess of simplification and speculation. There can be no doubt that much of this conceptual material will become invalid as our knowledge of cardiac function advances. This is, after all, the lesson taught to us by the history of science. The early neurophysiologists who tried to understand nerve conduction as the passage of fluid down hollow tubes were trying to explain physiological phenomena in terms of the limited biophysical knowledge of their time. With the development of an understanding of animal electricity, the focus in neurophysiology shifted to studies of the electrical properties of the nervous system, and attempts were made to explain phenomena such as neuron-to-neuron communication and memory in terms of electrical circuitry. More recently the enormous advances in our knowledge of chemical transmitters and the potential for information storage as newly synthesized macromolecules has cast doubt on many of the theories of the great neurophysiologists of the last century. Yet these were not unintelligent scientists. They were, however, required to interpret their observations within the framework of knowledge that existed during their lifetime. It would be presumptuous indeed for us now to assume that the evolution of new principles of science has ended. For this reason no apology is made for the misconceptions and faulty interpretation that will inevitably accompany the present attempt to organize our knowledge of cardiac function in terms of the broad principles that are understood today.

The only true "facts" in biology are the results of individual experiments carried out under controlled conditions by a carefully defined methodology. Yet it is not the purpose of this book to catalogue and discuss these biological "facts"; for this the reader is referred to the large number of reviews, symposia, multiauthored texts, and, most important, individual scientific papers. Instead, the present text attempts to identify and describe the unifying themes that connect different lines of investigation of the function of the heart and, in so doing, to set out interpretations of these biological "facts." The bibliographies to each chapter are intentionally brief and generally include one or more recent reviews to which the interested student may refer for more complete lists of references. In some cases "classic" articles are also cited.

Every effort has been made to keep this book simple—suitable for use as a text for graduate and undergraduate teaching. Achievement of this goal, however, requires the resolution, more or less arbitrarily as the case may require, of many serious conflicts, as well as the addition of speculative material to connect important biochemical, biophysical, physiological, and pathophysiological observations. It is the author's intention that these departures into the realm of speculation be clearly identified in the text. Yet the expert in these fields will undoubtedly be troubled by this attempt to provide a coherent and unified text. While the author is not laboring under the illusion that all of his interpretations will prove correct, it seems especially important to provide the student with an indication of the significance of the many biological "facts" describing the heart and its function rather than just to catalogue specific experimental findings. It is, after all, the pattern on the fabric that holds the interest of most of us, rather than the threads. For this reason, though with apologies to the protagonists of opposing viewpoints, the author has chosen the present format for this text.

Arnold M. Katz
Heidelberg, Germany
1976

Preface

Advances in our understanding of the normal and diseased heart have been rapid and dramatic since the first edition of *Physiology of the Heart* was published in 1977. This immense body of new information is important to the investigator who seeks to understand the causes of heart disease and to the health care professional who treats these patients.

A useful concept that may help the reader to organize the rapidly advancing knowledge of the physiology of the heart is that our focus in understanding the regulation of cardiac performance has shifted through three types of control that probably appeared sequentially during evolution. These three "paradigms," which are discussed in Chapter 14, are control by altered *organ physiology*, *cell biochemistry and biophysics*, and *gene expression* (Table 14.1). Regulation at the *organ* level, the most recent, could only operate in multicellular animals, where the heart is organized as a tissue. Regulation of *cell* function would have appeared earlier, when single-celled organisms became surrounded by a semipermeable membrane within which they could modify their internal environment. Even older is regulation by synthesis of altered *gene* products, which probably allowed primitive life forms, unable to control the milieu surrounding their genes, to adapt to a changing environment. Not only is regulation by altered gene expression the oldest control mechanism, but having had the longest time to evolve, it has become the most complex.

The first edition of *Physiology of the Heart* focused on the integration of *organ* physiology and *cell* biochemistry. This second edition adds new information about regulation by altered *gene* expression, for example the ability of one protein isoform to replace another to adapt the energy-starved myocardium to the chronic overload commonly seen in patients with heart failure. Other topics covered in much greater detail in this new edition include membrane structure, the signaling systems that mediate autonomic control, and the structures and behavior of ion channels.

This is essentially an entirely new text, although I have kept those strong parts of the first edition that remain useful and accurate. Throughout this revised edition I have made an effort to retain the clinical flavor that contributed to the success of the first edition.

This text can be considered in four sections: basic structure, metabolism, and energetics (Chapters 1–6); normal and abnormal contraction (Chapters 7–17); normal and abnormal electrical behavior (Chapters 18–23); and two integrated pathophysiological conditions: ischemic heart disease and heart failure (Chapters 24 and 25). While not formally designed as study units—all chapters are integrated with the other parts of the text—each of these four sections develops a different aspect of the flow of ideas between molecules and humans.

A number of major changes have been made in this new edition. The chapter in the first edition entitled "Valvular Heart Disease" has been omitted, and another, "Ionic and Pharmacological Actions on Cardiac Rate and Rhythm," has been incorporated into other chapters. The revision of the original chapter on "Excitation–Contraction Coupling" became so large that it had to be divided into three new chapters: "Excitation–Contraction Coupling: Calcium and Other Ion Fluxes Across the Plasma Membrane" (Chapter 10), "Excitation–Contraction Coupling: Calcium Fluxes Across the Sarcoplasmic Reticulum and Mitochondria" (Chapter 11), and "Receptors, Coupling Proteins, and Second Messengers" (Chapter 12). The chapters on arrhythmias have been reorganized as well as updated, arrhythmogenic mechanisms being discussed in "The Arrhythmias I: Introduction and Mechanisms" (Chapter 21). New chapters are: "Membrane Structure and Function" (Chapter 2), "Indices of Myocardial Contractility and Relaxation" (Chapter 17), and "Ion Channels of the Heart" (Chapter 18). The fields of study that encompass molecular biology of the heart are advancing so swiftly that concepts from this new discipline are included throughout the book, mainly in the chapters on "Regulation of Myocardial Contractility" (Chapter 14) and "Heart Failure" (Chapter 25).

About half of the illustrations are from the first edition; almost all of the rest are newly crafted to enhance the text. Citations of published works have been increased. Many references are still to vintage papers, a few over 50 years old, because they provide unmatched descriptions of fundamental concepts. Others are to more recent authoritative reviews. Citations of primary papers are often provided in areas that are advancing so rapidly that timely reviews are not available. Most references are provided as starting points for further reading, rather than to document the many statements in this text. Happily, Raven Press is publishing a series of updated reviews in the second edition of *The Heart and Cardiovascular System* (H. Fozzard, E. Haber, R. B. Jennings, A. M. Katz, and H. E. Morgan, editors) at the same time as this new edition of *Physiology of the Heart*. These two texts are, in many ways, complimentary.

I realize that my attempt to cover the broad range of topics form molecular biology to clinical cardiology is presumptuous; certainly I am not expert in all—or even most—of these fields. I have made every effort to provide accurate explanations, but it is inevitable that this text contains errors. I am somewhat reassured by a statement attributed to Dr. C. Sidney Burwell, who was Dean of Harvard Medical School in the early 1950s, who stated that half of what the faculty teaches to medical students is wrong, but the faculty does not know which half. A more conventional multiauthored book would have been more authoritative, but to have enlisted co-authors might have compromised my primary goal of providing lucid explanations of complex concepts using a single voice. This text is not intended as a reference book to be consulted to verify facts, but instead to explain and integrate.

This second edition of *Physiology of the Heart*, like the first edition, maintains a fluid, "user-friendly" presentation. It is intended to be read from cover to cover. I hope, therefore, that the reader can find both the time and a comfortable chair in which to read, to learn, and, hopefully, to appreciate the beauty that characterizes the physiology of the heart.

Arnold M. Katz
Farmington, Connecticut
Hanover, New Hampshire

Acknowledgments

Almost 20 years ago I began planning to co-author a textbook on cardiac physiology with my father, to whom this book is dedicated. Dad's death in 1973 made this impossible, but those who remember him will, I hope, recognize his forthright and lucid approach in this text. A few may even recognize the influence of his teachers, Carl J. Wiggers and A. V. Hill, whose wisdom was part of my early education.

The first edition was written while I was Philip J. and Harriet L. Goodhart Professor of Medicine (Cardiology) at the Mount Sinai School of Medicine of the City of New York. An award from the Alexander von Humboldt Stiftung, and the stimulating and serene environment provided by Professor Wilhelm Hasselbach during a sabbatical year at the Max-Planck-Institut-für Medizinische Forschung in Heidelberg, Germany, allowed me to write the first edition.

Clearly, this second edition is long overdue. I offer as an explanation, not an excuse, my responsibilities as a Cardiology Chief, which preempted what protected time I tried to set aside for this task.

Once again, a sabbatical leave made it possible to complete this second edition. For this I thank my colleagues at the University of Connecticut, who dealt with the many problems I left behind, and my old friend, Dr. Ellis Rolett, who arranged for me to have a quiet carrel *without a phone* in the Dana Medical Library at the Dartmouth Medical School. I am grateful to the staff of this library who patiently coped with my many needs and offered much help.

I apologize for the many broken promises to my publisher, friend, and former student Dr. Alan Edelson in meeting earlier deadlines. Many others at Raven Press encouraged me in preparing this revision, including Diana Schneider and Lisa Berger. I owe much to Georgia Willett, who, with many "Yikes" and an occasional "Oh bother," transformed my ideas into the new illustrations for the second edition. I also thank Lorraine Moseley, whose illustrations from the first edition appear in this update. I am greatly indebted to Joanne LaMothe, Cathy Zaza, and Priscilla Nash-Adler who shared in typing the first draft of this revision into my computer and provided many forms of assistance in this project.

I again acknowledge the kindness of Lea and Febiger, Philadelphia, who generously allowed me to quote, essentially verbatim, Professor Wiggers' classical description of the cardiac cycle; this appeared in his book *Physiology in Health and Disease*, now a collector's item. Several publishers and individuals who provided electronmicrophotographs, electrocardiograms, and other illustrations are acknowledged in the appropriate figure legends. Parts of the completed text were reviewed by Drs. Barbara Erhlich and Harold Strauss, who made corrections and clarified obscurities; these individuals are to be credited only with correct statements in this text—any errors are mine alone.

Acknowledgment is warmly given to the many students I have taught over the past 27 years, at Columbia University, The University of Chicago, The Mount Sinai School of Medicine, The University of Connecticut, and Dartmouth Medical School. These students were largely responsible for my writing this book. They have served as gentle but firm critics of my efforts and have contributed to the clarity of this text.

Last, but certainly not least, I thank my wife, Phyllis, and my children, Paul, Sarah, Amy, and Laura, who encouraged me and, on some occasions, badgered me to get on with this second edition.

Arnold M. Katz

1

Structure of the Heart and Cardiac Muscle

It has been shown by reason and experiment that blood by the beat of the ventricles flows through the lungs and heart and is pumped to the whole body . . . the blood in the animal body moves around in a circle continuously, and . . . the action or function of the heart is to accomplish this by pumping. This is the only reason for the motion and beat of the heart.

William Harvey
Exercitatio Anatomica de Moto Cordis et Sanquinis in Animalibus, 1628

The contractile activity of the muscular walls of the heart propels blood throughout the body, delivering nutrients to and removing wastes from each organ. The heart also provides for the transport of hormones, neurotransmitters, and other messengers between various regions of the body. These transport functions are made possible by the pumping action of the heart, which can be viewed simply as a hollow muscular pump provided with valves that moves blood "around in a circle continuously."

In both structure and function, cardiac muscle is more complex than skeletal muscle. Control of the contractile properties of the myocardium, for example, is quite different from the mechanisms that regulate contractile performance in skeletal muscle. In the latter, each fiber contracts in a virtually stereotyped manner when stimuli reach the muscle via motoneurons from the central nervous system. Each cardiac muscle cell, on the other hand, is provided with a complex control system that modulates the pumping of the heart to meet the constantly changing demands of the body. Furthermore, neither the initiation nor conduction of the signal that activates the heart involves nervous tissue. Instead, specialized heart muscle cells initiate an electrical signal, the action potential, which is then propagated throughout the heart by other myocardial cells that are specialized for conduction. This does not mean that the heart is not under nervous, or for that matter, humoral control, although it is true that the nerves supplying the heart play only a regulatory role, serving to increase or decrease various aspects of cardiac function.

1

GROSS STRUCTURE

The heart is divided into four pumping chambers: the *right* and *left atria* and the *right* and *left ventricles* (Fig. 1.1). Between the cavities of the atria and ventricles lie the *atrioventricular valves:* on the right the *tricuspid valve,* and on the left the *mitral* (bicuspid) *valve.* The *semilunar valves* lie between the outflow tracts of each ventricle and the great arteries into which each ventricle ejects blood: forward flow out of the right ventricle into the pulmonary artery is through the *pulmonic valve,* and between the left ventricle and aorta lies the *aortic valve.*

The overall designs of the semilunar and atrioventricular valves are quite different. Regurgitation of blood back into the ventricles through the aortic and pulmonary valves is prevented by thick, tendinous fibers in the margins of the valve cusps. In contrast, the free edges of the mitral and tricuspid valves are supported by fibrous cords (chordae tendineae) that arise from fingers of myocardium, the *papillary muscles,* which project from the inner walls of the ventricles into the cavities of the right and left ventricles. Several chordae tendineae arise from each papillary muscle, much as the many strands of a parachute arise from a sky diver's harness. Considerable variability is seen at the ends of the chordae tendineae that support the free margins of the atrioventricular valves (Becker and deWit, 1979).

> Laxity of the connective tissue supporting the atrioventricular valves often allows some backward movement of the valves into the atria when intraventricular pressure reaches its maximum—like turning a portion of the margin of a sky diver's parachute "inside out." In the mitral valve, this situation is one cause for "mitral valve prolapse

It is essential to recognize that the atrial myocardium is completely separated from that of the ventricles by a fibrous framework (the "cardiac skeleton") formed by the rings (annuli) of the four valves and surrounding connective tissue (Fig. 1.2). The *atrioventricular (AV) bundle,* which normally provides the *only* electrically conducting link between the atria and ventricles, penetrates this connective tissue "insulator" in a somewhat precarious location—between the annuli of the mitral, aortic, and tricuspid valves. Damage to this critical conducting structure by abnormalities in these valves explains the common appearance of atrioventricular (conduction) block (Chapter 22) when these valve structures are abnormal in both congenital and acquired heart disease.

The atria are thin-walled muscular chambers, the thinness of their walls being appropriate for the low pressures normally developed in the atrial cavities. The atrial walls are irregular in thickness, however, and contain "ridges" of myocardium, the *pectinate muscles* (Fig. 1.3). These structures, rather than specialized fiber tracts, probably account for rapidly conducting pathways (the so-called internodal tracts) found in the walls of the atria (Hayashi et al., 1982) (see Chapter 20). The ventricles, which develop much higher pressures than the atria, have thick muscular walls, especially the left ventricle, which has approximately three times the mass and twice the thickness of the right ventricle. The cavity of the left ventricle resembles an elongated cone in which both the inflow and outflow tracts are

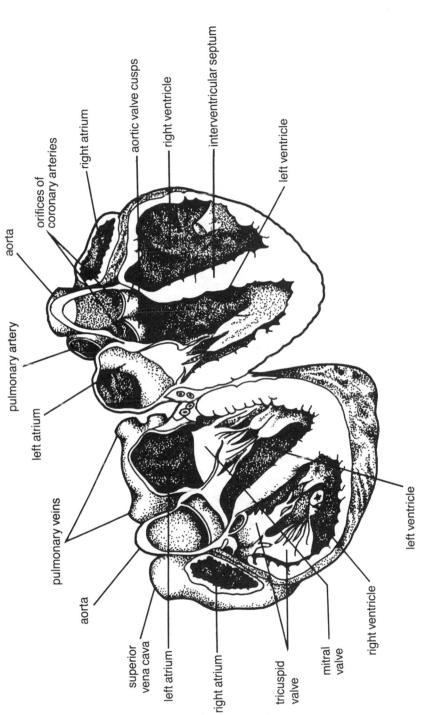

FIG. 1.1. The heart transected slightly anterior to its midline. Note the more elongated left ventricle, which has thicker walls than the right ventricle. (Modified from Berne and Levy: *Cardiovascular Physiology*, 1967, Mosby, St. Louis.)

aorta

orifices of coronary arteries

right atrium

aortic valve cusps

right ventricle

interventricular septum

left ventricle

pulmonary artery

left atrium

pulmonary veins

aorta

superior vena cava

left atrium

right atrium

tricuspid valve

mitral valve

right ventricle

left ventricle

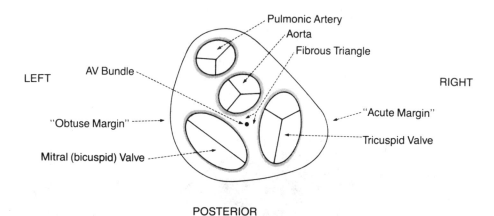

FIG. 1.2. Schematic diagram of the fibrous skeleton of the heart, viewed from above with the atria removed. The annuli fibrosi surrounding the mitral and tricuspid valves are thicker than those surrounding the pulmonic and aortic valves. The atrioventricular (AV) bundle crosses the fibrous skeleton through a trigone (the fibrous triangle), which is bounded by the annuli of the mitral, aortic, and tricuspid valves. The sketch also shows the more rounded shape of the left cardiac border (obtuse margin) than the right (acute margin), which is the basis for some nomenclature of the coronary arteries.

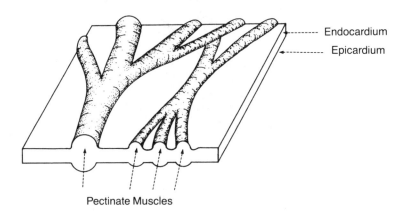

FIG. 1.3. Schematic drawing of a cross section of the atrial wall showing pectinate muscles, which lie on the endocardial (inner) side of the atrial wall.

adjacent to each other at the wider end of the left ventricular cavity (Fig. 1.4). The right ventricle, in contrast, is crescentic in cross section, and its inflow and outflow tracts are separated so that the right ventricular cavity forms a shallow U (Fig. 1.4). As described later (Chapter 16), this adaptation of form to function can be understood in terms of the different pressures developed by the two ventricles.

The inflow and outflow tracts of the left ventricle are separated by the anterior leaflet of the mitral valve, which is echocardiographically continuous with the posterior wall of the aorta. Opposite is the interventricular septum, which in echocardiographic views is continuous with the anterior wall of the aorta (Fig. 1.4). An exotic feature of the overall shape of the heart, which has contributed to the clinical nomenclature of the coronary arteries, is that when viewed from the apex, the margin of the left ventricle is rounded (forming an "obtuse" angle), whereas the margin of the right ventricle is rather sharp (forming an "acute" angle [Fig. 1.2]).

The depiction of the right and left ventricles as distinct structures (Fig. 1.4) should not be interpreted to mean that these two pumping chambers function independently. In fact, important interactions between the ventricles occur both in normal and diseased hearts (Bore and Santamore, 1981, Olson et al., 1983). Normally, the interventricular septum is functionally a part of the left ventricle, and moves toward the left ventricular free wall during systole. However, with chronic right ventricular overload, as occurs in pulmonary hypertension, the septum can move paradoxically as part of the right ventricle, away from the left ventricular cavity during systole.

ANTERIOR VIEW

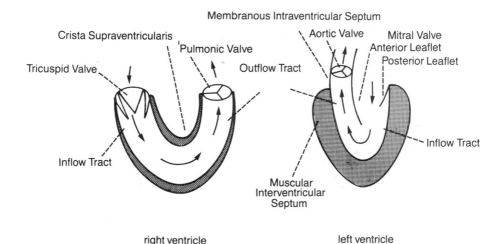

FIG. 1.4. Right and left ventricular chambers, showing the elongated right ventricular cavity, and the narrower, more conical, pumping chamber of the left ventricle.

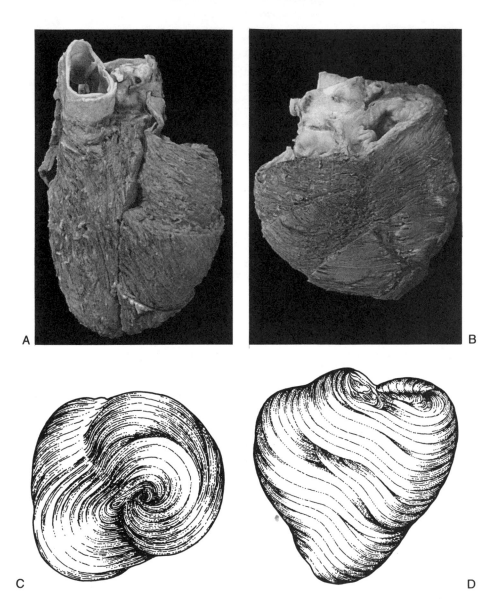

FIG. 1.5. Spiral musculature of the ventricular walls. **A:** Human heart viewed from the left and anteriorly. The right ventricle (*left*) and left ventricle (*right*) have been dissected to show differing fiber orientations at two depths. **B:** Posterior surface of the same specimen. **C** and **D:** Schematic drawing of heart viewed from the apex (C) and anteriorly (D). (A and B from Becker and Caruso, 1982 through the kindness of Prof. A. E. Becker.)

The inner surfaces of the atria and ventricles are covered with connective tissue, the *endocardium,* which also extends over the valves. The cell layer that lines the endocardium regulates transendocardial transport; these cells have also been suggested to produce chemical messengers (analogous to the endothelial-derived relaxing factor, or EDRF, produced by the vascular endothelium), and possibly also to serve as a sensor for changes in atrial and ventricular volume (Brutsaert, 1989).

The outer surface of the heart is covered by the *epicardium,* or *visceral pericardium,* which is continuous with the *parietal pericardium* at the base of the heart, where the great vessels enter and leave the heart. The pericardial cavity is therefore lined by a continuous layer of connective tissue that covers both the epicardial surface of the heart and the inner surface of the pericardial sac.

The *ventricular myocardium,* which lies between the epicardium and endocardium, consists of a series of overlapping sheets of muscle bundles (Fig. 1.5) that arise from the fibrous at the base of the heart. These sheets of myocardium follow spiral paths as they sweep from the base of the heart to its apex, and are sometimes called "bulbospiral" and "sinuspiral" muscles. The muscle fibers at the epicardial surface of the left ventricle tend to be oriented perpendicularly to the base-apex axis of the heart, whereas the muscle fibers at the endocardial surface are more circumferentially oriented (Fig. 1.6). Analysis of the patterns of contraction at different levels within the left ventricular wall support the view that the contracting ventricle resembles a series of concentric shells that, while thickening as they shorten, undergo only minor angular distortion (Fenton et al., 1978).

The anatomy of the system responsible for the generation and conduction of electrical impulses that activate the heart bears important relationships to the sequence of events occurring during each heart beat (The Cardiac Cycle, Chapter 15). Activation of the heart normally begins in pacemaker cells of the *sinoatrial (SA) node* (Fig. 1.7), which lies in the sulcus between the superior vena cava and the right atrium. These sinus pacemaker cells normally initiate the wave of depolarization that is propagated through the myocardium to excite all the rest of the heart; for this reason, the SA node is the normal cardiac pacemaker.

> The SA node is actually a band of specialized cells extending around the superior portion of the junction between the right atrium and superior vena cava, rather than a compact node. The anatomical dispersion of these pacemaker cells appears to be of considerable functional importance as variations in the heart's rate and rhythm can arise from complex interactions among a population of electrically coupled pacemaker cells with different frequencies of discharge (Michaels et al., 1987).

Because of the proximity of the SA node to the right atrium, the first structures to be depolarized in the normal activation sequence are the atria; first the right atrium, and shortly thereafter, the left atrium. After a delay, due to the slow passage of the wave of depolarization from atria to ventricles by way of slowly conducting cells in the *AV node,* the wave of electrical activation reaches the ventricles via the *AV bundle* (also called the *common bundle,* or *bundle of His*). The AV bundle bifurcates at the top of the interventricular septum; its divisions, the *right* and *left bundle branches,* depolarize the right and left ventricles, respectively (Chapter 20).

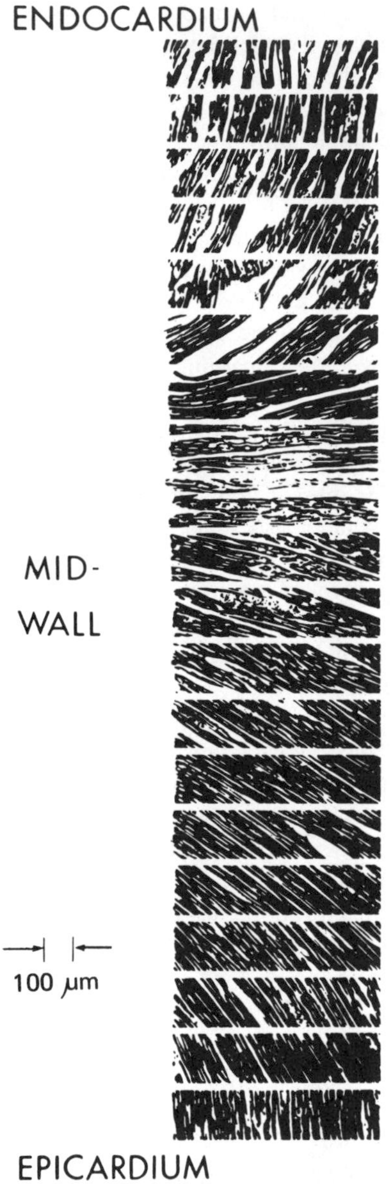

ENDOCARDIUM

MID-
WALL

100 μm

EPICARDIUM

FIG. 1.6. Reconstruction of the left ventricular wall, prepared from a series of microphotographs, showing changing fiber angles at different depths. Compare with Fig. 1.5 to obtain a concept of nonparallel forces generated during systole. (From Streeter et al., 1969, by permission of the American Heart Association.)

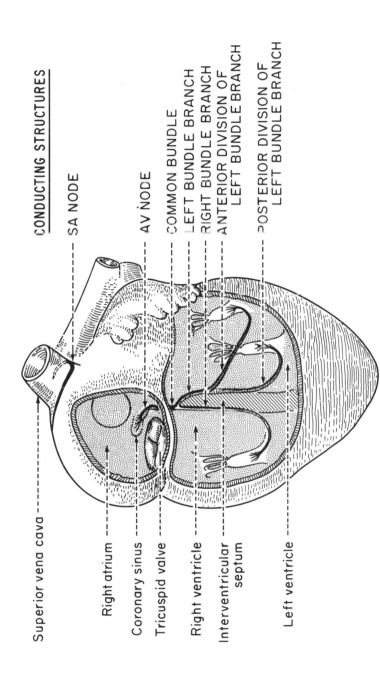

CONDUCTING STRUCTURES

SA NODE

AV NODE

COMMON BUNDLE
LEFT BUNDLE BRANCH
RIGHT BUNDLE BRANCH
ANTERIOR DIVISION OF
  LEFT BUNDLE BRANCH

POSTERIOR DIVISION OF
  LEFT BUNDLE BRANCH

Superior vena cava

Right atrium

Coronary sinus

Tricuspid valve

Right ventricle

Interventricular
septum

Left ventricle

FIG. 1.7. Conducting system of the human heart, showing anatomical features of the heart (labels at *left*) and the conducting structures (labels at *right*). (Modified from Benninghoff: *Lehrbuch der Anatomie des Menschen*, 1944, JF Lehmanns Verlag, Munich.)

A branch of the right bundle branch generally crosses the cavity of the right ventricle to reach the free wall of the right ventricle within a muscular bundle, the *moderator band,* which usually extends from the interventricular septum to the base of the anterior papillary muscle that supports the anterior leaflet of the tricuspid valve.

Ramifications of the bundle branches give rise to a subendocardial network of *Purkinje fibers;* these specialized conducting fibers transmit the electrical impulse to all portions of the ventricular myocardium. Electrocardiographers generally consider the left bundle branch as giving rise to two discrete divisions or fascicles (Fig. 1.7); however, the branching of the left bundle is extremely complex and variable (see Chapter 20). Additional details of the anatomy of the conduction system of the ventricles and the physiology of these activation processes are discussed in Chapter 20.

THE CORONARY CIRCULATION[1]

The blood supply of the heart arises from the *right* and *left coronary arteries* and their branches, which course over the epicardial surface of the heart (Fig. 1.8). The distribution of the coronary arteries bears a very important relationship to the various structures of the heart, and especially the individual components of the heart's conduction system. Cardiologists, notably coronary angiographers, consider the blood supply as arising from three vessels—the *right coronary artery* (RCA), and the two major branches of the *left coronary artery* (LCA): the *left anterior descending* (LAD) and the *circumflex* (CIRC).

Tracing first the course of the LCA, this vessel arises from the left posterior aortic sinus as a single trunk of variable length, the *left main coronary artery* and divides into its two important branches: the LAD and CIRC. The LAD courses down the anterior interventricular groove, where it gives rise to *septal perforating arteries,* usually three or four in number, that supply the anterior two-thirds of the interventricular septum. *Diagonal branches* of the LAD supply the anterior wall of the left ventricle, and small *right ventricular branches* provide blood to the anterior wall of the right ventricle. The LAD generally crosses the apex of the heart, turning upward toward the base to run a variable distance in the posterior interventricular groove. The CIRC courses to the left in the atrioventricular groove along the "obtuse margin" of the heart, giving rise to *obtuse marginal branches* that supply the lateral wall of the left ventricle. Continuing around the left ventricle to reach the posterior interventricular groove, the CIRC in most human hearts ends at or before the *crux of the heart,* where the plane of the interventricular septum crosses the plane of the atrioventricular groove. In a small minority of human hearts the CIRC continues as the *posterior descending branch* (PDA) that courses toward the apex in

---

[1]In spite of the author's distaste for abbreviations, to conserve space the major coronary arteries are abbreviated in this chapter as follows: RCA: right coronary artery, LCA: left coronary artery, LAD: left anterior descending, CIRC: circumflex, PDA: posterior descending.

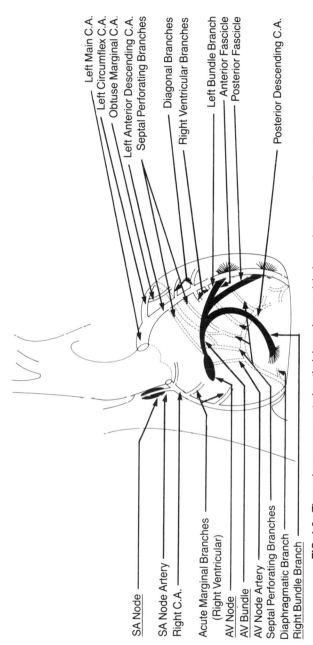

Left Main C.A.
Left Circumflex C.A.
Obtuse Marginal C.A.
Left Anterior Descending C.A.
Septal Perforating Branches

Diagonal Branches

Right Ventricular Branches

Left Bundle Branch
Anterior Fascicle
Posterior Fascicle

Posterior Descending C.A.

SA Node

SA Node Artery

Right C.A.

Acute Marginal Branches
(Right Ventricular)
AV Node
AV Bundle
AV Node Artery
Septal Perforating Branches
Diaphragmatic Branch
Right Bundle Branch

FIG. 1.8. The major coronary arteries, their branches, and their supply to the cardiac conduction system (underlined).

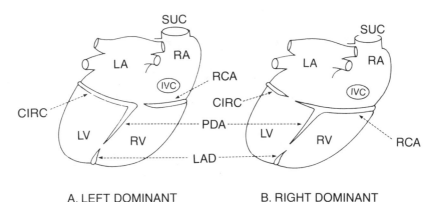

FIG. 1.9. Diagrammatic views of the posterior surfaces of the human heart showing left (A) and right dominant (B) patterns of coronary artery supply. In the left dominant pattern, the posterior descending artery (PDA) is supplied by the circumflex branch of the left coronary artery (CIRC). In the right dominant pattern, the posterior descending artery is supplied by the right coronary artery (RCA). Other abbreviations: LAD, left anterior descending coronary artery; LA, left atrium; RA, right atrium; LV, left ventricle; RV, right ventricle; SVC, superior vena cava; IVC, inferior vena cava.

the posterior interventricular groove (Fig. 1.9). When the PDA arises from the CIRC, the coronary circulation is designated as "left dominant."

The RCA, which is usually smaller in diameter than the left main, arises from the anterior aortic sinus. (The third aortic sinus, the right posterior, does not give rise to a coronary artery and so is often called the "noncoronary" sinus.) The RCA first runs toward the right in the atrioventricular groove, then crosses the acute margin of the heart to turn back to the left in the posterior atrioventricular groove. Throughout its course in the right atrioventricular groove, the RCA gives rise to *right ventricular* (or *acute marginal*) *branches* that supply the free wall of the right ventricle. In approximately 90% of human hearts, when the RCA reaches the crux of the heart, it turns toward the apex in the posterior interventricular groove as the PDA (Fig. 1.9) in a "right dominant" circulation. The *septal perforating branches* of the PDA, which supply blood to the posterior third of the interventricular septum, therefore generally arise from the RCA (approximately 90%), rather than from the CIRC (approximately 10%). As pointed out in Chapter 24, these relationships help to explain the variety of clinical syndromes encountered in patients who have experienced a heart attack, which is usually caused by the sudden occlusion of a coronary artery.

BLOOD SUPPLY OF THE CARDIAC CONDUCTION SYSTEM

An appreciation of the blood supply to the structures that initiate and conduct the electrical impulse that controls the heartbeat is essential to understanding the impact of coronary occlusion on the heart. Although the coronary circulation varies considerably from individual to individual (for example, see Fig. 1.9), certain generalizations are useful in understanding the locations of coronary artery occlusions in patients who experience disturbances of rate and rhythm after a heart attack (see Chapter 24).

The blood supply to the SA node is derived from an artery that runs through this structure, the *SA nodal artery,* which in slightly more than half of human hearts is a branch of the RCA. In the remainder, it is a branch of the CIRC. The AV node is usually supplied by the *AV nodal artery,* which is a branch of the PDA; therefore, the blood supply to this important structure is derived from a branch of the RCA in approximately 90% of human hearts, and from the CIRC, a branch of the LCA, in approximately 10%.

The AV bundle, including the proximal portions of both right and left bundle branches, has a dual blood supply. This critical structure is supplied by septal perforating branches that arise from both the LAD and PDA. This blood supply includes many *collateral vessels* (i.e., vessels that connect two arterial systems derived from different major arteries), so that damage to the AV bundle in the setting of a myocardial infarction implies severe and extensive occlusive disease of the coronary arteries (Chapter 24). The anterior division of the left bundle branch and midportion of the right bundle branch are supplied by septal perforating branches arising from the LAD, whereas the posterior division of the left bundle branch is supplied by septal perforators arising from the PDA.

BLOOD SUPPLY OF THE VENTRICULAR MYOCARDIUM

Nutrient blood flow reaches the myocardium by way of vessels that penetrate the walls of the ventricles (Fig. 1.10), so that the endocardial regions of the heart, especially of the left ventricle, are at "the end of the line" of coronary artery flow. This contributes to the susceptibility of the subendocardial regions of the left ventricle to a decrease in coronary flow. Because the coronary arteries penetrate the ventricular walls, delivery of blood to the endocardial regions of the left ventricle is also influenced by intramyocardial pressure, which during systole is higher than that in the coronary arteries. For this reason, virtually all nutrient coronary flow takes place during diastole.

The effects of intramyocardial pressure are especially significant in aortic stenosis, where intraventricular pressure, and so intramyocardial pressure, can be much higher than aortic and coronary perfusion pressures. The resulting restriction of nutrient coronary flow, especially to the endocardium, can produce symptoms of myocardial ischemia (angina pectoris), even in the absence of occlusive coronary artery disease.

Epicardial arteries can form extensive collaterals, especially in patients with severe coronary atherosclerosis (see Chapter 24). However, intercoronary collaterals are much less important at the level of the microcirculation; as a result, occlusion of a major epicardial artery will, in the absence of preexisting collaterals, cause an ischemic infarct whose borders are sharply demarcated from normal myocardium supplied by other, patent arteries (Factor et al., 1981).

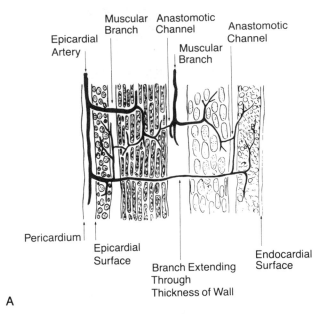

Epicardial Artery

Muscular Branch

Anastomotic Channel

Muscular Branch

Anastomotic Channel

Pericardium

Epicardial Surface

Branch Extending Through Thickness of Wall

Endocardial Surface

A

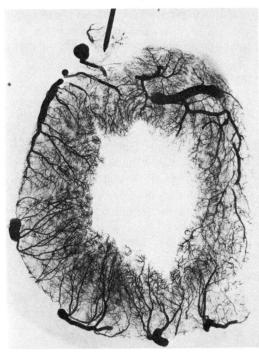

B

FIG. 1.10. A: Schematic diagram of the distribution of the coronary arteries that enter the myocardium from the epicardial surface (*left*) and reach the endocardium (*right*) after penetrating the various layers of muscle bundles. (Modified from Lowe T. E. Some principles governing the supply of blood to the myocardium in occlusive arterial disease: *Am Heart J,* 1941; 21:326–344. **B:** Postmortem angiogram showing blood supply in a thick section of the canine left ventricle. (From Schäper W, ed.: *The Pathophysiology of Myocardial Perfusion*, 1979, Elsevier/North Holland, Amsterdam, courtesy of Dr. B. Wüsten.)

The *left ventricular papillary muscles,* which support the mitral valve leaflets, are supplied by large, penetrating vessels (perforators) that must cross the full thickness of the left ventricular wall before entering the base of the papillary muscle. The anterolateral papillary muscle, which supports the anterior leaflet of the mitral valve, is supplied by branches from the CIRC. The posteromedial papillary muscle, which supports the posterior leaflet, receives its blood supply from the PDA, and thus from the RCA in about 90% of human hearts, and the CIRC (and so the LCA) in about 10%. A thin shell of the endocardial surface of the ventricles is nourished by blood entering from the ventricular cavities via *arterioluminal vessels.*

The venous effluent from the ventricles is collected in small intramyocardial veins that carry venous blood to larger veins that parallel the coronary arteries on the epicardial surface of the heart. A minor fraction of the venous drainage of the ventricular myocardium drains directly into the cavities of the right and left ventricles by way of *thebesian veins.* Most of the venous drainage of the left ventricle enters the *coronary sinus,* which runs alongside the CIRC in the atrioventricular groove on the inferior surface of the left ventricle and empties into the posterior wall of the right atrium. The ostium of the coronary sinus on the posterior wall of the right atrium serves as a landmark for the location of the atrioventricular node, which lies immediately above this opening. A small portion of the venous drainage of the left ventricle, and much of that derived from the right ventricle, reaches the right atrium and right ventricle by way of the *anterior cardiac veins.*

Fractal Anatomy of the Heart

The mathematical concept of *fractals,* which provides order to the complex—and seemingly random—geometry of biological structures can be applied to the heart (West and Goldberger, 1987). Several asymmetrical systems in the heart, including the chordae tendineae, the coronary blood vessels, and the branches of the interventricular conduction system, can be described in terms of fractal networks, as can the branching of blood vessels.

LYMPHATICS

The *lymphatics* of the heart, like the veins, parallel the coronary arteries. Although the lymphatic drainage of the heart is variable, most cardiac lymph drains via channels that cross the anterior surface of the pulmonary artery to reach a *pretracheal lymph node,* from which the lymphatic drainage of the heart is directed to the *cardiac lymph node* (situated between the superior vena cava and right innominate artery) ultimately to drain into the thoracic duct.

INNERVATION

The heart is *innervated* by both sympathetic and parasympathetic fibers (Norris and Randall, 1977). The former arise mainly from the fourth and fifth segments of the thoracic spinal cord and from synaptic connections in the cervical and thoracic cervical ganglia (stellate ganglia) and cardiac plexus. Postganglionic sympathetic fibers are distributed to all regions of the heart. Specialized sympathetic nerve endings have not been identified in the heart; instead, these nerves terminate in depressions in the sarcolemma of the cells they innervate.

> The sympathetic nerves that reach the heart via the right stellate ganglion appear to play a more important role in maintaining myocardial contractile force, and especially heart rate, than those arising in the left stellate ganglion (Schwartz et al., 1978). An imbalance of the heart's sympathetic innervation, in which outflow from the left stellate ganglion exceeds that from the right, plays a role in the genesis of certain cardiac arrhythmias (Schwartz, 1985).

The parasympathetic innervation of the heart originates in the dorsal efferent nuclei of the medulla oblongata. Parasympathetic fibers arising in these brainstem nuclei reach the heart via the cardiac branches of the vagus nerve, where they impinge on ganglion cells generally located within the heart. The parasympathetic innervation of the heart supplies mainly the SA and AV nodes and the atria. Parasympathetic fibers also innervate the ventricular blood vessels, and there is functional evidence for limited parasympathetic innervation of the ventricular myocardium.

Sympathetic fibers appear to traverse the ventricle within the epicardium before penetrating to the endocardium, whereas the parasympathetic innervation of the ventricles is distributed from their endocardial surface (Barber et al., 1984).

HISTOLOGY

The cavities of the atria and ventricles are lined by squamous endocardial cells, which also cover the surfaces of the values. Beneath the endocardium are layers of collagen and elastic fibers, and a rudimentary layer of smooth muscle. The muscle fibers of the *myocardium,* which make up the vast majority of the thickness of the heart's wall, are sandwiched between the endocardium and epicardium. The latter is a layer of cuboidal or squamous epithelium overlying a network of fibroelastic connective tissue that, as noted earlier, can also be viewed as the *visceral pericardium.*

Several cell types are found within the myocardium, all of which represent functionally specialized striated muscle cells (Fig. 1.11). Most important are the *working myocardial cells* of the atria and ventricles, which are specialized for contraction; the *Purkinje fibers,* which effect rapid conduction of the electrical impulse through the heart; and the *nodal cells* of the SA and AV nodes, which are responsible for pacemaker activity and atrioventricular conduction, respectively.

The cells of the *working myocardium* (Fig. 1.11A) stain darkly and are filled with cross-striated myofibers. The cells of the atria are smaller in diameter than those of the ventricles; both usually contain a single centrally located nucleus. The normal

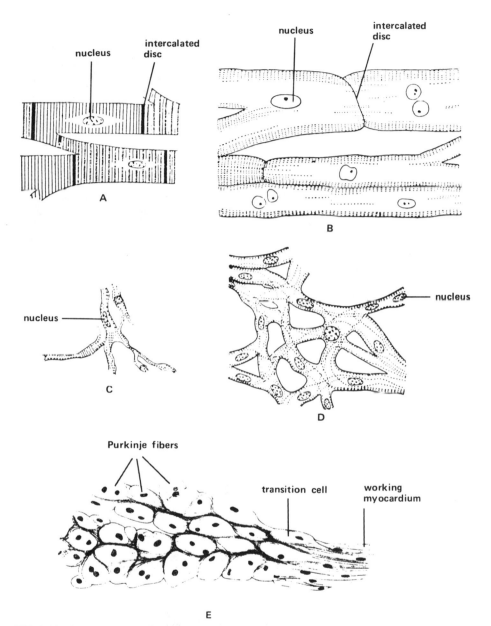

FIG. 1.11. Cells comprising the human heart. **A:** Working myocardial cell of the ventricle, show-ing intensely staining cross-striations, central nuclei, and intercalated discs. **B:** Purkinje fiber, showing large, faintly staining cells with sparse cross-striation. **C:** SA node. **D:** AV node. Both nodes have a network of small, sparsely cross-striated cells. **E:** Point of impingement of Purkinje fibers (*left*) on the working myocardium (*right*), showing transition cells. The scale for E is about half that of A–D. (Modified from Benninghoff: *Lehrbuch der Anatomie des Menschen*, 1944, JF Lehmanns Verlag, Munich.)

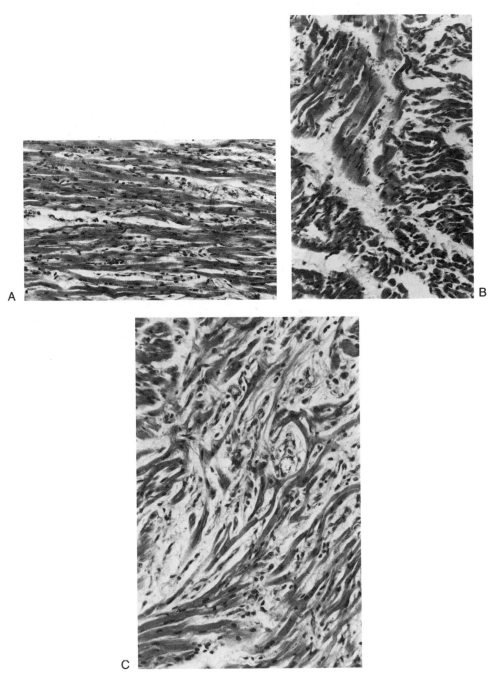

FIG. 1.12. Fiber orientation in the wall of the human ventricle in a single block of tissue cut in three planes **(A, B, C)** each at right angles to the other two. (From Becker AE, Caruso G: *Paediatric Cardiology*, 1981; 3:317, by permission of Churchill Livingstone.)

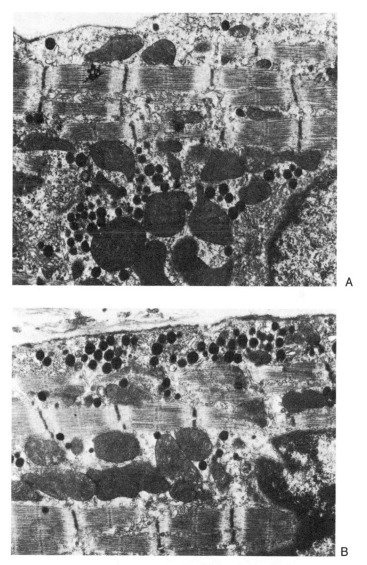

FIG. 1.13. Atrial "granules" in unstretched (A) and stretched (B) rat atrial myocytes. G, atrial specific granules; S, sarcolemma; N, nucleus. (From Agnoletti et al., 1989.)

histological appearance of the working myocardium is generally an orderly, parallel, arrangement of fibers, as shown in Fig. 1.12A. If one takes the block from which such a section was cut and turns it so that each of the planes is at right angles to that of Fig. 1.12A, the parallel orientation of the fibers is lost (Fig. 1.12B, C); instead, one sees a fiber "disarray" (Becker and Caruso, 1982). Exaggeration of this disarray is associated with certain disorders of myocardial structure and function, notably *hypertrophic cardiomyopathy* (Chapter 25).

The *Purkinje fibers* (Fig. 1.11B) are large, pale cells containing more glycogen and many fewer contractile filaments than the cells of the working myocardium (see also Fig. 1.15). The SA (Fig. 1.11C) and AV nodes (Fig. 1.11D) are made up of small, glycogen-rich *nodal cells,* which, like the Purkinje fibers, contain very few contractile filaments. Cells in the atria and ventricles that are intermediate in appearance between the Purkinje fibers and the ordinary working myocardial cells are often called *transition cells* (Fig. 1.11E).

Transition cells are found in the ventricle where the Purkinje network communicates with the myocardium; similar cells are scattered in the atria in patterns that may contribute to preferential atrial conduction pathways (the "internodal tracts," Chapter 20).

All of these myocardial cell types make up a branched network that early histologists thought represented a true anatomical syncytium. However, the *intercalated discs,* densely staining transverse bands that characteristically appear at right angles to the long axis of the cardiac myofibers, are now known to represent specialized cell-cell junctions, so that the myocardium is not a true anatomical syncytium. As the intercalated discs represent regions of low electrical resistance that provide preferential longitudinal electrical coupling between cells (Chapter 20). The heart can be considered to be a functional syncytium, even though it is not an anatomical syncytium.

The atrial myocardium has long been known to contain granules (Fig. 1.13); these have been known to contain biologically active "atriopeptides" which are natriuretic and diuretic, and also promote smooth muscle relaxation (Currie et al., 1984). These granules move to the periphery when the heart is stretched (Agnoletti et al., 1989). Thus, the heart is not just a pump; it is also an endocrine organ!

ULTRASTRUCTURE

The cells of the working myocardium (Fig. 1.14) contain large numbers of contractile proteins that are organized in myofibrils (Fig. 1.15). A large fraction of the cell volume is occupied by mitochondria, which regenerate ATP for use during contraction. Together, these structures occupy almost 85% of the myocardial cell volume (Table 1.1). Important membrane structures include the sarcolemma, which surrounds the cell, and two distinct intracellular membranes: the transverse tubular system (t-system) and the sarcoplasmic reticulum.

Nodal cells and the Purkinje fibers in the heart's conduction system have a rela-

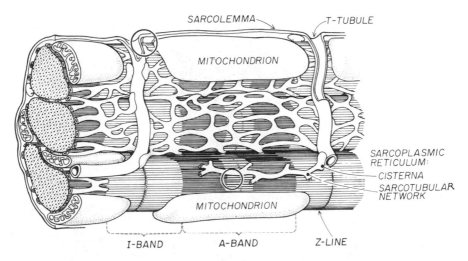

SARCOLEMMA

T-TUBULE

MITOCHONDRION

SARCOPLASMIC RETICULUM:
CISTERNA
SARCOTUBULAR NETWORK

MITOCHONDRION

I-BAND · · · A-BAND · · · Z-LINE

FIG. 1.14. Ultrastructure of the working myocardial cell. Contractile proteins are arranged in a regular array of thick and thin filaments (seen in cross section at the *left*). The A-band represents the region of the sarcomere occupied by the thick filaments into which thin filaments extend from either side. The I-band is the region of the sarcomere occupied only by thin filaments; these extend toward the center of the sarcomere from the Z-lines, which bisect each I-band. The sarcomere, the functional unit of the contractile apparatus, is defined as the region between a pair of Z-lines, and contains two half I-bands and one A-band. The sarcoplasmic reticulum, a membrane network that surrounds the contractile proteins, consists of the sarcotubular network at the center of the sarcomere, and the cisternae, which abut the t-tubules and the sarcolemma. The transverse tubular system (t-tubule) is lined by a membrane that is continuous with the sarcolemma, so that the lumen of the t-tubules carries the extracellular space toward the center of the mycardial cell. Mitochondria are shown in the central sarcomere and in cross section at the left. (From Katz AM: Congestive heart failure: Role of altered myocardial cellular control. *N Engl J Med*, 1975; 293:1184–1191.)

tively large amount of cytoplasm that contains many fewer mitochondria and myofibrils. Although varying from species to species, the Purkinje fibers, which from a biochemical standpoint are adapted more for anaerobic than oxidative metabolism have only about half the content of oxidative enzymes as the cells of the working myocardium, although contents of glycolytic enzymes are similar (Henry and Lowry, 1983). The fact that the contractile activity of the conduction tissue is much myocardium, although contents of glycolytic enzymes are similar (Henry and Lowry, 1983). The fact that the contratile activity of the conduction tissue is much less than that of the working myocardium is reflected in a low content of myofibrils; furthermore, the t-system of the Purkinje cells is less well developed, and in some species may be absent.

The myofibrils of the working myocardium, like those of mammalian skeletal muscle, are striated and exhibit a characteristic repeating pattern of light and dark transverse bands (Fig. 1.17). When viewed through crossed polarizing lenses, the more darkly staining bands rotate the polarized light and so are birefringent, or

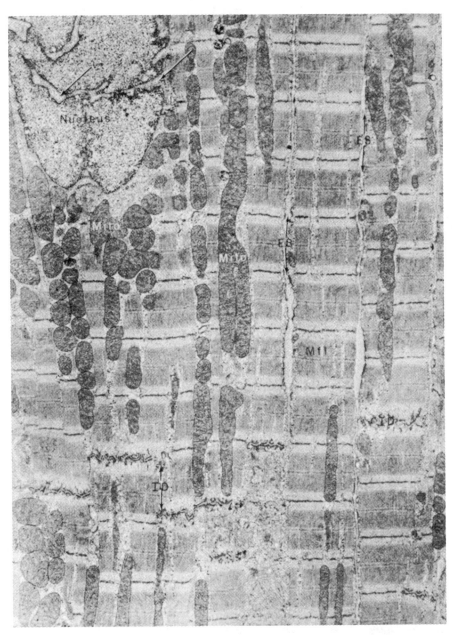

FIG. 1.15. Electron microphotograph of working myocardial cells of the cat ventricle, showing the nucleus (*arrows*, invagination of nuclear envelope), myofibrils (Mfl), and mitochondria (Mito). The latter occupy approximately 40% of the cell volume. The sarcolemma lies immediately adjacent to the extracellular space (ES) and merges with the intercalated discs (ID), which represent a specialized cell-cell junction. (From McNutt and Fawcett, 1974, courtesy of Wiley, New York.)

TABLE 1.1. *Morphology of a working myocardial cell
(rat left ventricle)*

Component	Percent of cell volume
Myofibrils	47
Mitochondria	36
Sarcoplasmic reticulum	3.5
Subsarcolemmal cisternae	0.35
Sarcotubular network	3.15
Nuclei	2
Other (mainly cytosol)	11.5

Modified from Page (1978).

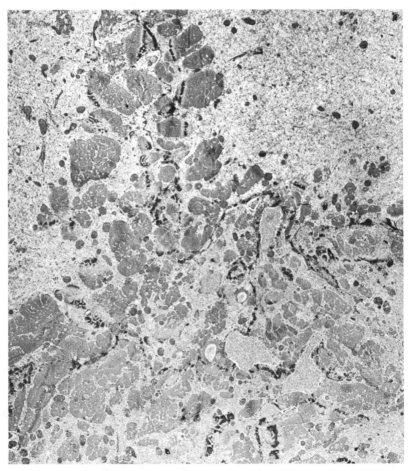

FIG. 1.16. Electron microphotograph of sheep Purkinje fibers; the field contains four cells that come together in the center of the picture. Note that most of the cell volume is made up of cytosol; a few mitochondria and small amounts of contractile material are present at the cell peripheries. Clefts between cells are narrow. (From Sommer and Dolber, 1982.)

anisotropic; hence their designation *A-bands.* This ability to rotate polarized light indicates that the A-bands contain a highly ordered parallel array of macromolecules. The more lightly staining of the striations are less birefringent and, because of their more isotropic nature, are named *I-bands.* Each I-band is bisected by a narrow, darkly staining *Z-line;* a broad, dense *M-band* is found in the center of the A-band.

The fundamental morphological unit of striated muscle is the *sarcomere,* which is defined as the region between two Z-lines. Each sarcomere thus consists of a central A-band plus the two adjacent half I-bands (Fig. 1.17).

The discovery of thick and thin filaments within the sarcomere, and the formulation of the sliding filament model of muscular contraction during the mid-1950s by H. E. Huxley and Hanson, represents one of the most elegant discoveries in the field of muscle research. These investigators demonstrated that the cross-striations of vertebrate skeletal muscle arise from the organization of the contractile proteins into thick and thin filaments. The thick filaments, which are composed largely of myosin, extend the length of the A-band to which they contribute both its darkly staining characteristics and high birefringence. The lightly staining half I-bands at either side of the A-band contain only thin filaments, which extend from their origin in the Z-lines into the A-band in the center of the sarcomere. The thin filaments which are composed largely of actin, also contain the regulatory proteins tropomyosin and troponin (Chapter 7).

In cross section the A-band contains a hexagonal array of thick filaments, each of which is surrounded by six thin filaments that lie at the trigonal points between adjacent thick filaments (Figs. 1.18, 1.19). In the I-band, which contains only thin filaments, the filament array is less orderly than in the A-band. In cross section, the M-band (at the center of the A-band) contains thick filaments held together in a

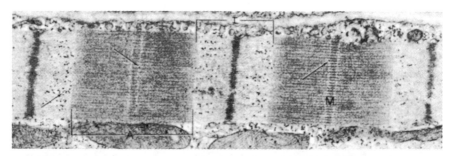

FIG. 1.17. Longitudinal section of a myofiber of cat atrial myocardium, showing the characteristic cross-striations. Closely arrayed thick filaments make up the A-band (A) in the center of which is a region of increased electron density, the M-band (M). Very thin filaments running transversely to the long axis of the myofiber are visible in the region of the M-band. The I-band (I) is made up of the thin filaments and is bisected by the Z-line. Glycogen granules are present in the cytoplasm and between the myofilaments (*arrows*), and mitochondria are seen below. (From McNutt and Fawcett (1974), courtesy of Wiley, New York.)

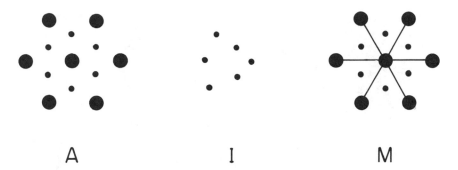

FIG. 1.18. Cross section of myofilaments at different levels of the sarcomere. A: The A-band, where thin filaments lie at the trigonal points in the hexagonal array of thick filaments. I: The I-band, where thick filaments are absent and the thin filaments are less ordered. M: The M-band in the center of the A-band, where thin radial filaments connect adjacent thick filaments.

hexagonal array of radial cross-links. The Z-lines, which define the limits of the sarcomere, are made up of interwoven ends of the thin filaments from the adjacent sarcomeres (Goldstein et al., 1977).

The sliding filament hypothesis of muscular contraction is based on the observation that as a muscle shortens, the lengths of both the thick and thin filaments remain constant. As sarcomere length decreases, the thin filaments are pulled into the thick filament lattice of the A-band; this causes the I-bands to narrow, whereas the A-band width remains constant (Chapter 8). This finding, initially predicted from x-ray diffraction studies by H. E. Huxley and subsequently confirmed by electron microscopic findings, effectively disproved the earlier view that muscular contraction was due to the folding of large macromolecules. According to the sliding filament hypothesis, the thin filaments are pulled toward the center of the sarcomere during contraction, by motion of *cross-bridges* that project from the thick filaments to establish links with adjacent thin filaments (Fig. 1.20). Cross-bridge motion, which can be viewed as like the rowing of the oars of a racing shell, sweeps the thin filaments toward the center of the sarcomere, thereby causing the muscle to contract. It should be pointed out that there remain adherents of other theories of muscular contraction in which cross-bridge motion need not represent the primary cause of tension development and shortening (Pollack, 1983).

At very short sarcomere lengths, the thin filaments from the two half I-bands at either side of the sarcomere can pass through the M-line, giving rise to a "double overlap." Double overlap between thick and thin filaments does not allow tension to be generated because both the thick and thin filaments have opposite polarities in the two halves of the sarcomere. For this reason, a thin filament penetrating the A-band from one side of the sarcomere cannot interact with the cross-bridges of the opposite half of the thick filament to develop tension and to shorten. Thus, in regions of double overlap, no tension-producing interactions occur between the por-

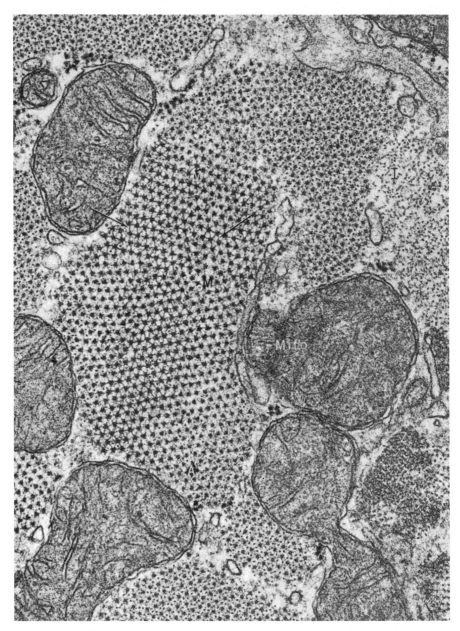

FIG. 1.19. Transverse section through a myofiber of cat right ventricular papillary muscle, showing mitochondria (Mito) and myofilaments cut at the level of the M-band (M), A-band (A), and I-band (I). *Arrows* point to the radial filaments between the thick filaments in the center of the A-band (compare with Fig. 1.15). Also shown is the Z-line (Z, *lower right*), which appears as a dense network. (From McNutt and Fawcett (1974), courtesy of Wiley, New York.)

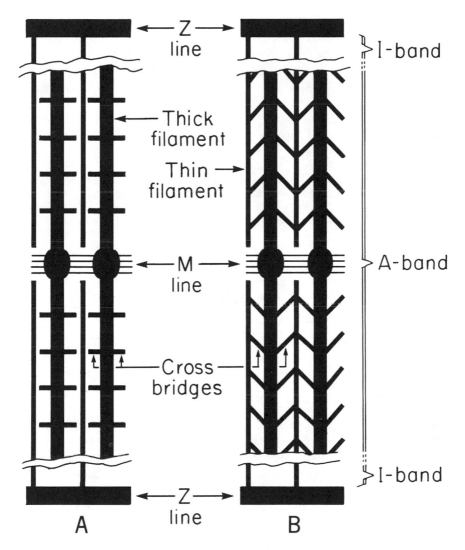

FIG. 1.20. A single sarcomere during diastole (A) and systole (B). This illustration, based on data from insect flight muscle, shows a shift in cross-bridge orientation that accompanies their attachment to the thin filaments. A similar shift in the heart during systole causes shortening and the development of tension. (Modified from Reedy: Cross-bridges and periods in insect flight muscle. *Am Zool*, 1967; 7:465–481.)

tion of the thin filament that crosses from one half of the sarcomere into the domain
of the other half of the thick filament.

The *mitochondria,* which are largely responsible for aerobic adenosine triphosphate (ATP) production directly in the myocardium (Chapter 5), are located immediately adjacent to the myofilaments (Fig. 1.15). The volume of the myocardial cell
occupied by the mitochondria is correlated with the rate of energy utilization, being
greatest in rapidly beating hearts and less in larger mammals with slower heart rates.
Mitochondria are complex structures that contain the enzymes responsible for oxidative phosphorylation (Chapter 5).

> The surface of the inner mitochondrial membrane is markedly increased by a series of
> infoldings, the *cristae,* whose electron microscopic configuration reflects the func-
> tional state of the mitochondria at the time the muscle is fixed for electron microscopy.
> In cells that are fixed under conditions that do not allow active oxidative phosphoryla-
> tion (e.g., low oxygen tension or low substrate concentration), the cristae appear as
> stacks of flat membrane sheets, whereas cells that are fixed when the mitochondria are
> actively performing oxidative phosphorylation contain cristae that are angulated and
> often form a network, the so-called energized configuration.

Phase contrast studies of living cardiac muscle show that the shape of the mitochondria is constantly changing; these dynamic structures appear not only to enlarge
and contrast, but also to branch and fuse with each other.

> Mitochondria, which contain their own DNA, can be viewed as microorganisms that,
> hundreds of millions of years ago, crept into the cells of our progenitors. In return for a
> moist, nutrient-filled environment, these symbiotic invaders provide our cells with a
> generous supply of ATP.

The myocardial cell is enclosed by the *sarcolemma* or *plasma membrane,* which
represents a barrier between the intracellular and extracellular spaces (Fig. 1.15).
Extensions of the extracellular space are brought into the central regions of the cell
by the *transverse tubular* or *t-system,* which opens freely to the extracellular space.
The t-system, which in the myocardium not only extends in a transverse direction,
can turn and run longitudinally between adjacent sarcomeres (Fig. 1.14). In mammalian cardiac muscle the t-system is much larger in diameter than in skeletal muscle, and the openings of the tubules through the sarcolemma into the extracellular
space are more clearly seen.

The sarcolemma and the membranes of the t-system represent barriers (Chapter
2) that delimit an intracellular environment which is different from that of the extracellular fluid. In addition, these membranes contain ion pumps that establish important chemical and charge differences between the intracellular and extracellular environments (Chapter 10), as well as a number of ion channels that effect transient
changes in membrane potential (Chapter 18). Enzymes, such as adenylyl cyclase,
which synthesizes adenosine 3', 5'-cyclic monophosphate (cyclic AMP), are also
present on the sarcolemma and possibly on the membranes of the t-system, as are
receptors and coupling proteins that respond to a variety of important hormones and
neurotransmitters (Chapter 12).

In addition to the sarcolemma and the membranes of the t-system, which separate the extracellular and intracellular spaces, intracellular membrane systems divide the cell interior into separate regions or "compartments" (Table 1.2). One of these is represented by the mitochondria, which have already been mentioned in terms of their ability to carry out aerobic energy production. The functional significance of the intramitochondrial compartment, which has an ionic composition different from the remainder of the cytosol, is related to the ability of the mitochondrial membrane to serve as an energy transducer. This membrane transduces the osmotic energy available when protons move along their electrochemical gradients into chemical energy that is trapped when ATP is synthesized (Chapter 5). Most other intracellular membranes, however, effect the opposite process, i.e., they utilize chemical energy derived from the hydrolysis of ATP for the active transport of substances, including ions, against an electrochemical gradient.

The *sarcoplasmic reticulum* is a specialized form of the endoplasmic reticulum, a system of intracellular membranes found in virtually every cell.

The endoplasmic reticulum in most cells of the body is comprised of two morphologically distinct membranes. In the *rough endoplasmic reticulum*, where the outer surface is studded with ribosomes, this membrane is involved primarily in protein synthesis. The *smooth endoplasmic reticulum*, which in nonmotile cells participates in such processes as lipid metabolism and drug detoxification, is structurally similar to the sarcoplasmic reticulum of muscle.

The vast majority of the cardiac sarcoplasmic reticulum lacks ribosomes and so is smooth in appearance; this smooth sarcoplasmic reticulum, which will be referred to simply as the *sarcoplasmic reticulum,* plays a major role in controlling the calcium concentration within myocardial cells (Chapter 11). The heart's sarcoplasmic reticulum consists of two regions. A network of intracellular tubules, the *sarcotubular network,* surrounds the bundles of contractile proteins (Figs. 1.14, 1.21), whereas other parts of the sarcoplasmic reticulum flatten to form specialized structures, the *subsarcolemmal cisternae,* where they come in contact with the sarcolemma and t-system (Figs. 1.14, 1.22). The term *subsarcolemmal cisternae* is to some extent a misnomer in that these structures are found adjacent to the mem-

TABLE 1.2. *Membrane areas in a working myocardial cell (rat left ventricle)*

Membrane	μm^3 Membrane area/μm^3 cell volume
Total sarcolemma	0.465
External sarcolemma	0.31
T-tubules	0.15
Nexus	0.005
Total sarcoplasmic reticulum	1.22
Subsarcolemmal cisternae	0.19
Sarcotubular network	1.03
Mitochondria	20

Modified from Page (1978).

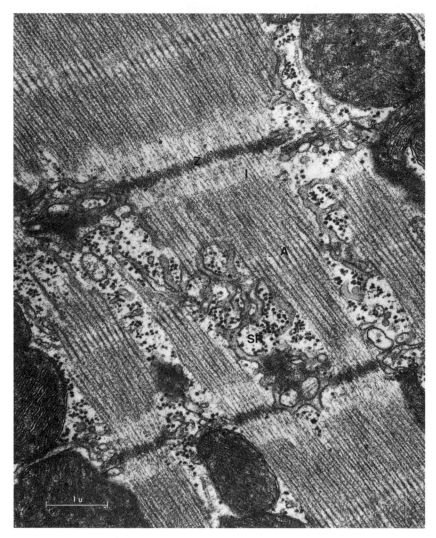

FIG. 1.21. Electron micrograph showing sarcotubular network (SR) of rat ventricular muscle in a "grazing" section over the sarcomeres (*center*). The dark granules near this structure are glycogen. Mito, mitochondria; A, A-band; I, I-band; Z, Z-line. The faint linear structure, composed of two parallel lines, crossing the sarcotubular network at the *lower right* probably represents a microtubule. Scale = 1 μm. (Courtesy of Mrs. Judy Upshaw-Earley and Dr. Ernest Page.)

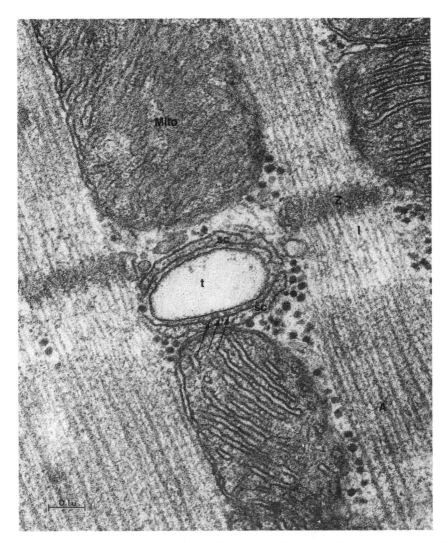

FIG. 1.22. Cross section of triad of rat ventricular muscle. The large central structure represents a portion of the transverse tubular system (t) surrounded by two subsarcolemmal cisternae (sc), each of which partially envelops the transverse tubule. The membrane of the subsarcolemmal cisternae fails to establish intimate contact with that of the t-tubule; instead, electron-dense "foot processes" lie between these two membranes (*arrows*). Mito, mitochondria; A, A-band; I, I-band; Z, Z-line. Scale = 0.1 μm. (Courtesy of Mrs. Judy Upshaw-Earley and Dr. Ernest Page.)

branes of the t-system as well as the sarcolemma; however, if one remembers that the composition of the fluid within the t-tubule is probably similar to that in the extracellular space, the subsarcolemmal cisternae can be considered to have similar functions in both locations.

The composite structure formed by the subsarcolemmal cisternae and the adjacent regions of the sarcolemma or t-tubule is called the *dyad* (Fig. 1.22), where the membranes of the sarcoplasmic reticulum approach those of either the sarcolemma or t-system. However, the two membranes neither fuse nor establish intimate contact; instead, a narrow space remains between these membranes that contain tetrameric structures called the foot proteins (Fig. 1.23). This space, and the foot proteins play an important role in releasing calcium from the sarcoplasmic reticulum, a key step in the process of "excitation-contraction coupling" that initiates contraction of the heart (Chapter 11).

Studies of the structure of the junctions between the t-tubule and sarcoplasmic reticulum in skeletal muscle show that the foot proteins bridge the gap between the t-tubules and the subsarcolemmal cisternae (Franzini-Armstrong and Nunzi, 1983). It is now clear that the foot proteins represent the calcium release channels through which this activator ion flows out of the sarcoplasmic reticulum into the cytosol (Chapter 11). As these proteins bind ryanodine, a plant alkaloid known to interact with the calcium release channels of muscle, this protein is also called the "ryanodine receptor"; furthermore, the ryanodine receptor forms tetrameric structures that are identical to the foot proteins.

Microtubules, hollow cylinders having an outer diameter of ~24 Å and an inner diameter of ~12Å are likely to play a role in intracellular transport and cell division. Cell rigidity is maintained by *intermediate filaments* made up of cytoskeletal proteins, in-

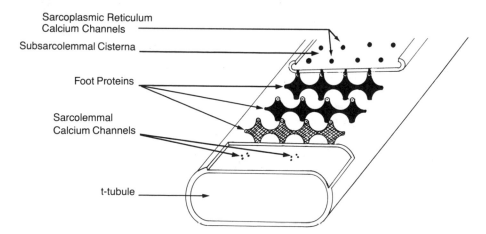

FIG. 1.23. Schematic diagram of a triad showing the foot proteins, now recognized to be the calcium channel through which this cation leaves the subsarcolemmal cisternae of the sarcoplasmic reticulum. The foot protein is a tetrameric structure that surrounds a central channel.

cluding *desmin*, *vimentin*, and *laminins*. Other proteins, similar to erythrocyte *spectrin*, *ankyrin*, and *band 4.1 protein*, along with actin, appear to provide structural support to the plasma membrane (Chapter 7).

The *intercalated disc* (Fig. 1.24), as already noted, represents a specialized cell-cell junction that provides both strong mechanical linkages between myocardial cells and a low resistance pathway that facilitates conduction of the cardiac impulse. Three types of specialized areas are found along the intercalated disc; *fascia ad-*

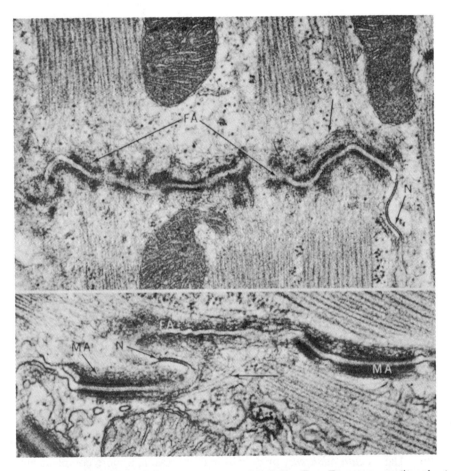

FIG. 1.24. Electron microphotographs of the intercalated disc. **Top:** Transverse section of cat ventricular myocardium, showing insertions of thin filaments into filamentous mats (*arrows*), which bind to the intercalated disc to form the fascia adherens (FA). This intracellular junction changes form at the *right* of the figure, where the two cells come into contact at a nexus, of gap junction (N). **Bottom:** Oblique section of intercalated disc in mouse ventricular myocardium, showing filaments (*arrow*) joining fascia adherens (FA) and a nexus (N). Two maculae adherens (MA), or desmosomes, are also shown. All of these structures represent specialized cell-cell junctions. (From McNutt and Fawcett (1974), courtesy of Wiley, New York.)

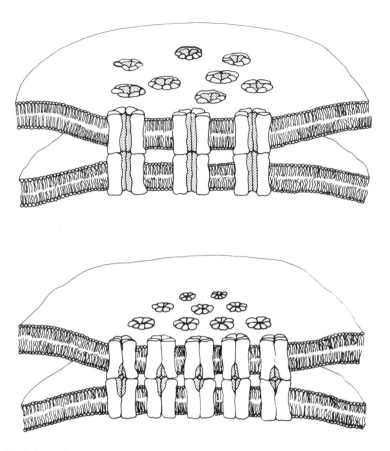

FIG. 1.25. Schematic model of the architecture of the gap junction in its open (coupled) state (*top*) and closed (uncoupled) state (*bottom*). (Modified from Peracchia C, Bernardini G: Gap junction structure and cell-to-cell coupling regulation: Is there a calmodulin involvement? *Fed Proc*, 1989; 43:2681–2691.)

herens, macula adherens, and *nexus.* The *fascia adherens,* which makes up most of the intercalated disc, is composed of the two plasma membranes of adjacent cells that parallel each other, separated by a distance of 200 to 300 Å. Extensions from the thin filaments of the myofibrils appear to bind tightly to the plasma membrane at either side of the fascia adherens in a manner similar to their interweaving at the Z-line. The *macula adherens,* or *desmosome,* represents a more complex, almost laminated structure made up of the two plasma membranes. The *nexus,* or *gap junction,* is a region of close contact between the plasma membranes of adjacent cells that is freely permeable to many ions. Ion channels present in the nexus (Fig. 1.25) account for the low electrical resistance of the intercalated disc (Chapter 18).

The intercalated discs in the cells of the SA and AV nodes contain fewer and smaller nexuses. This anatomic feature is of importance in understanding the high internal resistance that is partly responsible for the slow velocity with which electrical impulses propagate through these structures (see Chapter 21).

REFERENCES

Agnoletti G, Ferrari R, Slade AM, Severs NJ, Harris P. (1989). Stretch-induced centrifugal movement of atrial specific granules—a preparatory step in atrial naturetic peptide secretion. *J Mol Cell Cardiol* 21:235–239.

Barber MJ, Mueller TM, Davies BG, Zipes D. (1984). Phenol topically applied to canine left ventricular epicardium interrupts sympathetic but not vagal afferents. *Circ Res* 55:532–544.

Becker A-E, Caruso G. (1982). Myocardial disarray. A critical review. *Br Heart J* 47:527–538.

Becker A-E, deWit APM. (1979). Mitral valve apparatus. A spectrum of normality relevant to mitral valve prolapse. *Br Heart J* 42:680–689.

Bore A-A, Santamore WP. (1981). Ventricular inter-dependence. *Prog Cardiovasc Dis* 23:365–388.

Brutsaert DL. (1989). The endocardium. *Annu Rev Physiol* 51:263–273.

Currie DM, Cole BR, Siegel NR, Kok KF, Adams SP, Galluppi GR, Needleman P. (1984). Purification and sequence of bioactive atrial peptides (Atriopeptins). *Science* 223:67–69.

Factor SM, Okun EM, Kirk ES. (1981). The histological lateral border of acute canine myocardial infarction. A function of microcirculation. *Circ Res* 48:640–649.

Fenton TR, Cherry JM, Klassen GA. (1978). Transmural myocardial deformation in the canine left ventricular wall. *Am J Physiol* 235:H523–H530.

Franzini-Armstrong C, Nunzi G. (1983). Junctional feet and particles in the triads of a fast-twitch muscle fibre. *J Muscle Res Cell Motil* 4:233–252.

Goldstein MA, Schroeter JP, Sass RL. (1977). Optical diffraction of the Z lattice in canine cardiac muscle. *J Cell Biol* 75:818–836.

Hayashi H, Lux RL, Wyatt RF, Burgess MJ, Abildskov JA. (1982). Relation of canine atrial activation sequence to anatomical landmarks. *Am J Physiol* 242:H421–H428.

Henry CG, Lowry OH. (1983). Quantitative histochemistry of canine Purkinje fibers. *Am J Physiol* 245:H824–H829.

Michaels DC, Matyas EP, Jalife J. (1987). Mechanism of sinoatrial pacemaker synchronization: a new hypothesis. *Circ Res* 61:704–714.

Norris JE, Randall WC. (1977). Responses of the canine myocardium to stimulation of thoracic cardiac nerves. *Am J Physiol* 232:H485–H494.

Olsen CO, Tyson GS, Maier GW, Spratt JA, Davis JW, Rankin JS. (1983). Dynamic ventricular interaction in the conscious dog. *Circ Res* 52:85–104.

Page E. (1978). Quantitative ultrastructural analysis in cardiac membrane physiology. *Am J Physiol* 63:C147–C158.

Pollack GH. (1983). The cross-bridge theory. *Physiol Rev* 63:1049–1113.

Schwartz PJ. (1985). Idiopathic long-QT syndromes. Progress and questions. *Am Heart J* 109:399–411.

Schwartz PJ, Brown AM, Malliani A, Zanchetti A, eds. (1978). *Neural mechanisms in cardiac arrhythmias,* Perspectives in cardiovascular research, Vol 2. Katz AM, series ed. New York: Raven Press.

West BJ, Goldberger AL. (1987). Physiology in fractal dimensions. *Am Scientist* 75:354–365.

BIBLIOGRAPHY

Alberts B, Bray D, Lewis J, Raff M, Roberts K, Watson JD. (1989). *Molecular biology of the cell,* 2nd ed. New York: Garland.

Greenbaum RA, Ho SY, Gibson DG, Becker AE, Anderson RH. (1981). Left ventricular fibre architecture in man. *Br Heart J* 45:248–263.

Hawthorne EW, et al. (1969). Physiology Society symposium: dynamic geometry of the left ventricle. *Fed Proc* 28:1323–1367.

James TN. (1961). *Anatomy of the coronary arteries.* New York: P.B. Hoeber.

McNutt NS, Fawcett DW. (1974). Myocardial ultrastructure. In: Langer GA, Brady AJ, eds. *The mammalian myocardium,* New York: Wiley; 1–49.

Miller AJ. (1982). *Lymphatics of the heart.* New York: Raven Press.

Schäper W. (1979). *The pathophysiology of myocardial perfusion.* Amsterdam: Elsevier/North Holland.

Sommer JR, Dolber PC. (1982). Cardiac muscle: ultrastructure of its cells and bundles. In: de Carvalho AP, Hoffman BF, Lieberman M, eds. *Normal and abnormal conduction in the heart.* Mt. Kisco, NY: Futura.

Sommer JR, Johnson EA. (1979). Ultrastructure of cardiac muscle. In: Berne RM, Sperelakis N, Geiger JR, eds. *Handbook of physiology, section 2: The cardiovascular system,* vol 1, *The heart,* Bethesda, MD: American Physiology Society; 113–186.

Streeter DD, Spotnitz HM, Patel DP, Ross J Jr, Sonnenblick EH. (1969). Fiber orientation in the canine left ventricle during systole and diastole. *Circ Res* 24:339–347.

2

Membrane Structure and Function[1]

Membranes play a central role in controlling many of the critical electrical and chemical processes in the myocardial cell. This chapter, which describes the molecular architecture of biological membranes, provides a basis for understanding the functional properties of the heart's membranes and, in the last analysis, much of the physiological, pathophysiological, and pharmacological control of the heart described in this text.

THE MEMBRANE BARRIER AND PHOSPHOLIPID BILAYER

The simplest model of a membrane is a lipid sheet, or barrier, that impedes the passage of a variety of substances between the aqueous compartments (Fig. 2.1). In the heart, the sarcolemmal membrane separates the fluid within the cell (the cytosol) from the extracellular fluid, whereas other, internal, membranes divide various regions within cells. The sarcolemma is the plasma membrane, or plasmalemma, of a muscle cell (*sarc* being derived from the Greek word for muscle). By regulating the movements of ions and other molecules from one compartment to another, these membranes control both electrical and chemical processes in the heart.

Membrane lipids make up the barriers that limit the movement of a variety of substances, notably charged particles, between cell compartments and across the sarcolemma. Embedded within these lipid barriers are a variety of proteins that mediate almost all communications between the aqueous media on the two sides of the membrane. The membrane proteins carry out the highly regulated transport of a variety of ions, substrates, and other molecules from one side of the membrane barrier to the other, thereby serving most of the important transport and signaling functions of the membrane.

The basic structure of all biological membrane is the lipid bilayer (Fig. 2.2),

---

[1]This chapter is based on a chapter by the author, "Membrane Structure," that appeared in *The Heart and Cardiovascular System*, 2nd ed, Raven Press, New York, 1991.

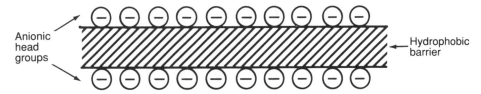

Anionic head groups

Hydrophobic barrier

FIG. 2.1. Simple view of a lipid bilayer as a barrier (*shaded*) lined by anionic charged groups.

which contains a hydrophobic core that is essentially impermeable to charged molecules. Charged head groups that line the two surfaces of this hydrophobic core allow the bilayer to interact with the aqueous media on the two sides of the membrane. The membrane bilayer is made up mainly of phospholipid molecules; most, but not all, membranes also contain cholesterol molecules that are deeply embedded in the bilayer, as shown in Fig. 2.2.

Different regions of the membrane bilayer have special physical properties. The head group regions are highly polar and admit both water and charged ions, whereas tightly packed regions immediately below the head groups may exclude the passage of larger substances. Most important from a physiological standpoint is the hydrophobic core, which is made up mainly of hydrocarbon fatty acyl chains that form a highly impermeable barrier to the passage of charged ions.

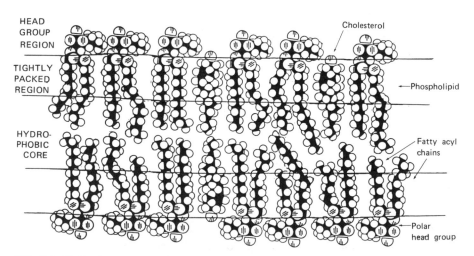

HEAD GROUP REGION

Cholesterol

TIGHTLY PACKED REGION

Phospholipid

HYDRO-PHOBIC CORE

Fatty acyl chains

Polar head group

FIG. 2.2. Stylized representation of a membrane bilayer containing phospholipids and cholesterol. Lining both surfaces of the bilayer are charged (polar, or hydrophilic) phospholipid "head groups," whereas the membrane interior is made up of the uncharged (apolar, or hydrophobic) fatty acyl chains of the membrane phospholipids and the hydrocarbon ring structures of cholesterol. This bilayer can be divided into a *head group region*, and *tightly packed region*, and a *hydrophobic core*.

Membrane Lipids

The lipids of the membrane bilayer are a heterogeneous mixture of molecules, most of which are *amphipathic* in that they contain both hydrophilic (polar) and hydrophobic (apolar) moieties. Each membane lipid generally contains a single hydrophilic "head group" and one or two hydrophobic fatty acyl "tails." The polar head groups of most membrane lipids contain charged phosphate groups; hence they are called "phospholipids." In mammalian membranes, the polar and apolar moieties are generally esterified to glycerol, a 3-carbon sugar that makes up the "backbone" of the abundant *glycerolipid* class of phospholipid molecules (Fig. 2.3). Phosphatidic acid, shown in Fig. 2.3, contains a hydrogen atom (H*) that can be replaced by choline, ethanolamine, serine, etc., to form the phospholipids listed in Table 2.1. Figure 2.3 also shows a lysophosphatide in which the 2-carbon of the glycerol is not esterfied to a fatty acid; such lysolipids, which tend to disrupt membrane bilayers (Lucy, 1970), normally make up only a small fraction of the membrane lipids.

Other lipid structures are also found in small amounts in biological membranes; these include sphingolipids and glycolipids. In the *sphingo-lipids*, the 3-carbon glycerol is not esterified to a fatty acid; such lysolipids, which tend to disrupt member of this class of lipids is *sphingosine*, which contains a single fatty acid linked to the serine (Fig. 2.4). *Ceramides* represent a group of sugar-containing membrane

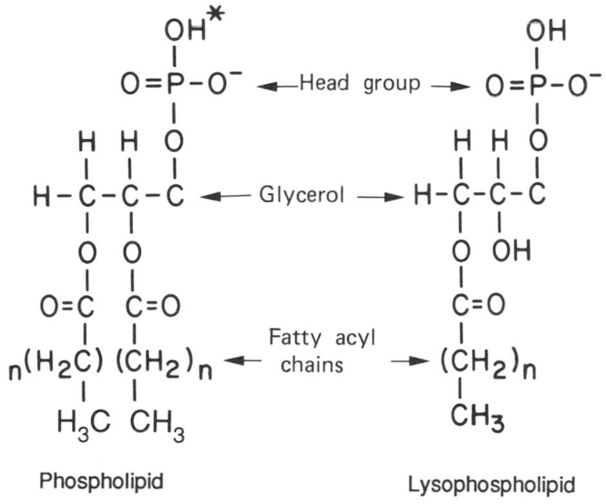

FIG. 2.3. Structure of a phospholipid, oriented so that the surface of the bilayer is at the *top* of the figure, showing the glycerol "backbone," a phosphatidic acid head group, and two fatty acyl chains. The numbering of the glycerol carbons (1-, 2-, 3-) is from *left* to *right*, so that the fatty acids are esterified to the 1- and 2-carbons and the head group is esterified to the 3-carbon. The hydrogen atom with an asterisk (H*) can be replaced by several compounds, listed in Table 2.1.

TABLE 2.1. *Nomenclature of membrane phospholipids*

Substituent on the phosphate (at H*)	Name of phospholipid	Abbreviation	Charge
Hydrogen	Phosphatidic acid		Anionic
Choline	Phosphatidylcholine	PC	Zwitterionic
Serine	Phosphatidylserine	PS	Anionic
Ethanolamine	Phosphatidylethanolamine	PE	Anionic
Glyerol[a]	Diphosphatidylglycerol (cardiolipin)	DPG	Anionic
Inositol	Phosphatidylinositol	PI	Anionic

[a]Diphosphatidylglycerols are formed when a glycerol molecule is esterified to the phosphatidic acid residues of two adjacent phospholipids that are "bridged" to form DPG.

lipids in which a second fatty acid has been esterified to the amino group of sphingosine. *Sphingomyelin* is a special ceramide in which phosphorylcholine is esterified to the hydroxyl group of the serine (Fig. 2.4).

> Although biological membranes are basically symmetrical, specific classes of lipids are often distributed asymmetrically. In the cardiac sarcolemma, for example, phosphatidylinositol, phosphatidylethanolamine, and phosphatidylserine are found mainly in the inner (cytosolic) leaflet of the bilayer, while much of the sphingomyelin is within the outer leaflet (Post et al., 1988).

Membrane *glycolipids* are generally made up of ceramides in which sugars, rather than phosphorylcholine, are esterified to the serine hydroxyl group (Fig. 2.4). Glycolipids built upon the glycerol backbone are found only rarely in animal mem-

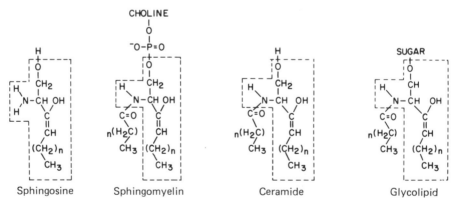

FIG. 2.4. Structure of sphingolipids oriented as in Fig. 2.3. The sphingosine "backbone" is enclosed within a *dashed line*. Unlike the glycerolipid shown at the left of Fig. 2.3, which has a glycerol backbone, the sphingolipids contain the 3-carbon amino acid serine. Both sphingomyelin and ceramides contain a second fatty acid linked to the amino group of sphingosine; the former also contains phosphorylcholine esterified to the serine hydroxyl group. As the choline group on sphingomyelin is positively charged, this phospholipid is a zwitterion. Glycolipids are formed when sugars are esterified to ceramide.

branes. Esterification of a single galactosyl residue to sphinogosine yields a *cere-broside*; much more complex *gangliosides* are formed when the esterified sugars are oligosaccharides containing neutral and amino sugars. The glycolipids, most of which are found on the external surface of the plasma membrane, contribute to a variety of cell-surface receptors and participate in cell-cell interactions, often serving as antigenic sites. Much like the plumage of a tropical bird, therefore, the membrane sugars are primarily involved in recognition.

> The extracellular surface of the plasma membrane is coated with a layer of mucopolysaccharides, called the *glycocalyx*. This coat probably serves mainly to strengthen the physical structure of the membrane. The glycocalyx contains a variety of sugars, including sialic acid, fructose, galactose, *N*-acetylgalactosamine, and *N*-acetylglucosamine.

A variety of fatty acids can be esterified to membrane phospholipids. Virtually all have an even number of carbon atoms, more than 80% being C_{16}, C_{18}, and C_{20} fatty acids. Mammalian membranes contain mainly palmitic and stearic acids (saturated C_{16} and C_{18} fatty acids), oleic, linoleic, and linolenic acids (unsaturated C_{18} fatty acids). Smaller amounts of longer chain fatty acids are found in sphingolipids. As discussed below, arachidonic acid (an unsaturated C_{20} fatty acid) is of special importance as the precursor of important messengers, as are lipids that contain the sugar inositol.

Dynamic Nature of Membrane Structures

Membranes can be viewed as two-dimensional fluids in which are dissolved a variety of functionally important membrane proteins. The fluidity of biological membranes, an important determinant of the mobility of proteins within the membrane bilayer, is determined to a large extent by the degree of unsaturation of its fatty acids. The fatty acyl chains within the hydrophobic core of the membrane bilayer can bend, forming angles that, in turn, are determined by the degree of unsaturation of the membrane fatty acids. Figure 2.5 shows some of the conformations that can be assumed by the hydrocarbon chain of an 18-carbon fatty acid. Each *cis double bond* in an unsaturated fatty acid creates an approximately 30° angle in the fatty acyl chain, as shown in Fig. 2.5A; *trans double bonds* produce a much smaller angle. The *single bonds* of the fatty acyl chain in a saturated fatty acid can assume a number of conformations; the lowest energy state being the *all trans* conformation shown in Fig. 2.5B. As there is only a small energy difference between this conformation and the *gauche* conformation shown for one of the single bonds in Fig. 2.5C, saturated fatty acids can also form "kinks." As shown in Fig. 2.5D, a pair of gauche conformations straightens the fatty acyl chain, thereby reducing the volume that it occupies in the membrane.

Saturated fatty acids tend to form crystalline "gel" structures in membranes because their hydrophobic chains can pack tightly within the core of the membrane. In contrast, the unsaturated fatty acids tend to create a two-dimensional "fluid" struc-

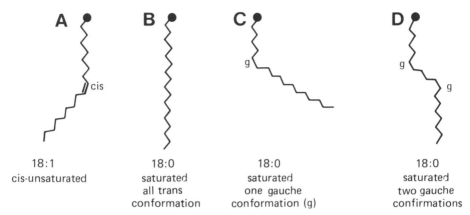

FIG. 2.5. Four conformations of 18-carbon fatty acids. The head group, depicted as a *solid circle*, is oriented toward the membrane surface. The fatty acyl chain in the core of the bilayer can exhibit many conformations. Shown are (A) the fatty acid which contains one cis double bond (oleic) and (B–D) no double bonds (stearic). In B, the fatty acyl chain contains all *trans* conformations, whereas C and D contain 1 and 2 *gauche* (g) conformations, respectively.

ture within the lipid bilayer in which membrane proteins can move more freely. Because biological membranes contain a mixture of saturated and unsaturated acids, they are in the fluid form at physiological temperatures. Changes in the fatty acid composition of a membrane can influence the behavior of intrinsic membrane proteins, which are generally more mobile in membranes that contain a high proportion of unsaturated fatty acids (see below). Cholesterol, which reduces membrane fluidity, has a dramatic ability to "stiffen" membranes. Thus, cholesterol plays a major role in maintaining the mechanical stability of animal plasma membranes, which unlike those of plant cells lack a rigid cell wall.

Animal plasma membranes contain approximately 20% cholesterol by weight, but the cholesterol contents of intracellular membranes such as the mitochondria and sarcoplasmic reticulum are much less, only about 5%.

Phospholipid Bilayers

Amphipathic lipid molecules, when purified and added to aqueous solutions, tend to form bilayers as shown in Fig. 2.6. As in the biological membranes, the hydrophobic fatty acyl chains form a sheet in the center of the bilayer, whereas the polar head groups that line the surface of the bilayer interact with the aqueous solutions on either side of the membrane.

The influence of fatty acyl chain conformation on the physical properties of membranes is shown in Fig. 2.7, which depicts small regions of bilayers made up of pure phospholipids containing either saturated (Figs. 2.7A,B) or cis-monounsaturated fatty acids (Fig. 2.7C). Because of the angles formed by cis double bonds, mem-

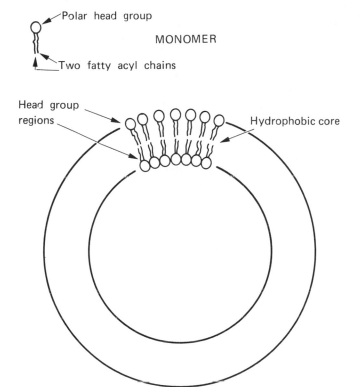

FIG. 2.6. Aggregation of a phospholipid, showing a monomer and the micelle created when high amphipathic lipid concentrations form bilayers in aqueous solution.

brane lipids that contain unsaturated fatty acids occupy more volume in the plane of the membrane than do those containing saturated fatty acids, When the temperature of a bilayer made from a single class of phospholipids is raised, the transition from the gel structure depicted in Fig. 2.7A to the fluid structure shown in Fig. 2.7B occurs at a specific temperature, the "phase transition temperature." Phase transitions involving an entire phospholipid bilayer do not occur in biological membranes, which are composed of a mixture of different phospholipids containing a variety of head groups and fatty acyl moieties. There is, however, evidence that biological membranes may contain "domains" that differ in their fluidity (Klausner et al., 1980).

Membrane structure is readily disordered by high concentrations of several naturally occurring amphipathic substances, such as fatty acids and their carnitine or coenzyme A derivatives (Chapter 5), and lysophosphatides. High concentrations of amphipathic drugs, when incorporated into membranes, can also increase membrane fluidity (Katz and Messineo, 1981).

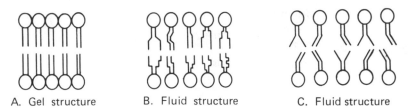

A. Gel structure　　B. Fluid structure　　C. Fluid structure

FIG. 2.7. Schematic diagram of different bilayer structures formed by pure phospholipids. A: *Gel structure* formed when the fatty acyl chains of a saturated fatty acid are all in the trans conformation. B: *Fluid structure* formed when the fatty acyl chains of a saturated fatty acid form gauche conformations. C: *Fluid structure* formed by the fatty acyl chains of a cis monounsaturated fatty acid.

The intoxicating effects of ethanol are likely to be due in part to its ability to increase membrane fluidity (Taraschi and Rubin, 1985), and it is possible that the puzzling correlation between reduction in serum cholesterol and violent death (Muldoon et al., 1990) may reflect behavioral changes caused by altered cholesterol content of brain membranes.

Lipolytic Enzymes

The myocardial cell contains several enzymes, called *phospholipases*, which can hydrolyze membrane lipids. In certain pathological settings, activation of some of these enzymes may contribute to membrane damage. Figure 2.8 shows the bonds hydrolyzed by some of these phospholipases. *Phospholipases A_1 and A_2* hydrolyze the ester bonds linking the fatty acids to the 1 and 2 positions of glycerol, respectively. (*Phospholipase B*, which hydrolyzes both of these ester bonds, probably represents a mixture of phospholipases A_1 and A_2.) *Phospholipase C* removes the phosphate head group and any attached groups (see Table 2.1) from the 3 position of the glycerol "backbone," whereas *phospholipase D* removes only the polar groups attached to the phosphate. The toxicity of many snake venoms is due to these phospholipases.

Lysophosphatides, which, along with a free fatty acid, are produced by the action of phospholipase A_2, are powerful detergents because they tend to assume a "wedge" shape in the membrane. Their appearance in the membranes of growing cells may play an important role in cell division (Lucy, 1970). When lysophosphates appear in the heart, they are probably hydrolyzed rapidly by *lysophospholipases*, and so tend not to accumulate in large quantities.

Membrane Lipids as Precursors for Intracellular Messengers

In recent years it has become apparent that the membrane phospholipids represent more than simply the building blocks of an inert barrier. It is now clear that bilayer

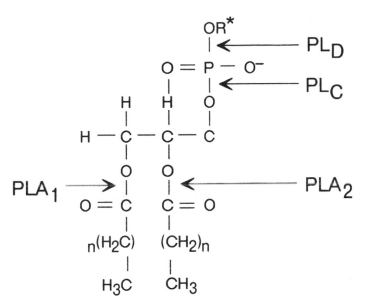

FIG. 2.8. Points of attack of phospholipases on a glycerolipid. Phospholipases A_1 and A_2 release the fatty acids esterified to the 1 and 2 positions on glycerol, respectively. When the latter is an arachidonic acid moiety, release of this fatty acid provides the substrate for production of prostaglandins, thromboxanes, and leukotrienes. Phospholipases C and D release the head groups from the 3 positions of the glycerol backbone. When R represents inositol, release of this product by phospholipase C provides the precursor for inositol phosphates. The diacylglycerol that remains bound within the membrane acts as an additional second messenger.

lipids also serve as substrates for the formation of important cellular messengers. One of these, arachidonic acid, represents the source of the *prostaglandins, thromboxanes,* and *leukotrienes,* a family of 20-carbon fatty acid derivatives that can generate a variety of biological responses (Holman, 1986). These substances are produced by enzymatic modification of arachidonic acid after this 20-carbon, unsaturated fatty acid is cleaved from its glycerol backbone by *phospholipase A_2* (Fig. 2.8).

Two additional intracellular messengers can be formed from membrane lipids when another lipolytic enzyme, a phosphoinositol-specific *phospholipase C,* is activated. This enzyme hydrolyzes the membrane lipid phosphatidylinositol 4,5-bisphosphate to form two second messengers, inositol 1,4,5-trisphosphate and diacylglycerol, each of which controls an intracellular signal transduction pathway (Berridge, 1989; Nishizuka, 1989 [Chapter 12]).

Transmembrane Potential and Surface Charge

In addition to separating environments having different chemical compositions, biological membranes have a high capacitance that allows them to separate regions having different electrical potential. This high capacitance is made possible by the insulating properties of the hydrophobic core of the membrane. The potential across the cardiac sarcolemma, for example, is generally 80 to 90 mV when the cell is at rest, changing in magnitude (and often polarity) when the cell is excited by the passage of an action potential over its surface (Chapter 19). Although absolute potential differences across biological membranes are small, the fact that they occur across a very thin surface gives rise to a large electrical potential gradient across a membrane. For example, a transmembrane potential of -90 mV (-90×10^{-3} V) across the cardiac sarcolemma, which is approximately 30 Å (30×10^{-8} cm) thick, gives a potential gradient of $-300,000$ V/cm (-90×10^{-3} V/30×10^{-8} cm)! If the membrane potential becomes $+30$ mV during depolarization, the potential gradient reverses to $+100,000$ V/cm, so that the *change* in transmembrane potential gradient is 400,000 V/cm. These considerations provide a basis for understanding how apparently small potential changes across a membrane can, in fact, provide powerful forces that induce molecular rearrangements in membrane proteins.

Because of the large numbers of phosphate groups in the head groups of membrane lipids, the membrane surface is negatively charged (Fig. 2.1). This creates a negative *surface charge* that attracts cations from the aqueous media to the surface of the membrane; the result is a gradual, rather than abrupt, potential change as one moves away from the membrane surface (Fig. 2.9). The cations at the bilayer surface are so strongly attracted to the negative head-group region of the membrane that they remain associated with the membrane surface within a "plane of shear" that separates the immobilized ions from those that are freely movable within the aqueous medium. The potential at the surface of this plane of shear is called the *zeta potential*.

When there is a potential difference between the aqueous media on the two sides of the membrane, the anionic charge on the surface of biological membranes influences the distribution of potential within the hydrophobic core of the membrane (McLaughlin and Harary, 1974) (Fig. 2.10). In a membrane that has no surface charge, any potential difference will be distributed uniformly across the hydrophobic core within the membrane (Fig. 2.10A). Anionic groups on the membrane surface, by contributing a negative surface charge, reduce the charge across the hydrophobic core as shown in Fig. 2.10B. When both aqueous media contain cations that tend to neutralize the anionic surface charge, the charge across the hydrophobic core of the membrane is increased at any overall transmembrane potential (Fig. 2.10C). This effect on charge distribution is especially marked for cations like Ca^{2+}, which bind tightly to the phosphate groups of membrane lipids.

The ability of cations, in particular Ca^{2+}, to increase the potential gradient across the membrane core for any given overall transmembrane potential difference is of considerable physiological importance. Thus, high concentrations of Ca^{2+} will increase the potential difference across the core of the membrane at any given potential between the aqueous solutions on the two sides of the membrane. For example, in the case of a transmembrane "voltage sensor" that opens a voltage-sensitive channel when the membrane is depolarized (see Chapter 18), elevation of the Ca^{2+} con-

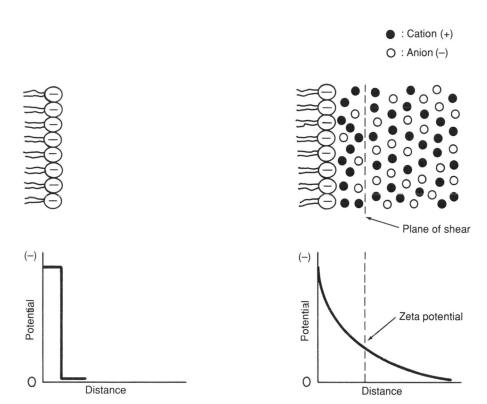

FIG. 2.9. Schematic representation of the electrical potential at the surface of a membrane composed of phospholipids with negatively charged head groups. In the absence of ions in the surrounding medium, the *surface charge* (potential at the membrane surface) falls sharply when an electrode is withdrawn from the membrane (A). If as is the case for biological membranes, the anionic head group region is in contact with an ionic medium, cations are attracted to the membrane surface, causing a more gradual fall in surface charge. Many of these cations remain associated with the membrane when it is moved relative to the surrounding aqueous medium. These immobilized ions are therefore to the left of a "plane of shear," to the right of which are the ions that are freely mobile within the aqueous medium. The potential at the plane of shear is the zeta potential.

centration on either side of the membrane will require a greater change in overall potential between the inside and outside of the cell to open the channel. This "stabilizing effect" explains the ability of elevated extracellular Ca^{2+} concentration to increase the extent of depolarization needed to initiate an action potential. Other substances that decrease the anionic surface charge on a membrane have a similar effect of impairing excitability, whereas an increase in anionic surface charge augments responses to membrane depolarization. This latter effect may explain, at least in part, the actions of messengers that induce phosphorylation of membrane proteins, and so incorporate anionic groups near the membrane surface (see Chapter 12).

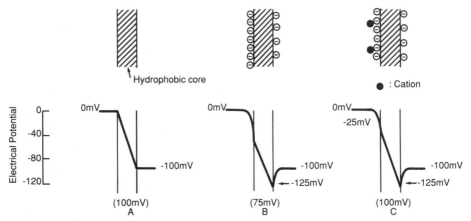

FIG. 2.10. Effect of surface charge and its modification on the electrical potential gradient within a membrane. Where there is no surface charge, a 100 mV potential difference across the hydrophobic core of a membrane will be uniformly distributed across a homogeneous core (A). When there are anionic head groups on both sides of the membrane, a portion of the potential difference will be distributed in the head group region so that the potential difference across the hydrophobic core is reduced (B), which assumes more anionic head groups on the outside than inside of the membrane. Neutralization of the charge on the anionic head groups will reduce the effect of the surface charge and thereby increase the potential difference across the hydrophobic core (C). (Numbers in parentheses represent the charge across the hydrophobic core of the membrane.)

MEMBRANE PROTEINS

Up to this point, our description of membrane structure has focused on the lipid bilayer, which serves the barrier function of the membrane. However, most biological membranes allow the passage of a variety of substances between the aqueous compartments on the two sides of the membrane. Some molecules cross the membrane by moving down their electrochemical gradients in a *passive* (downhill) manner that does not require the expenditure of energy. Other molecules, however, move across membranes by *active* (uphill) transport processes that require energy—for example, by way of active pumps. These essential transport functions, both active and passive, are mediated by the *membrane proteins*, a special class of proteins found in association with membranes.

Membrane proteins, some of which contain covalently bound lipid or carbohydrate (lipoproteins and glycoproteins, respectively), represent a highly diverse group of structural and functional entities that can make up more than half of the weight of a membrane. These proteins, which include antigens, receptors, enzymes, channels, and pumps, serve many of the key biological functions of membranes.

Several membrane proteins contribute structural stability to biological membranes. These *cytoskeletal proteins* have been characterized most completely in the erythrocyte, where the filamentous proteins *spectrin* (actually two distinct peptide chains: α and β spectrin) and *actin* are attached to the cytosolic surface of the bilayer by two other proteins: *ankyrin* and *band 4.1* (Bershadsky and Vasiliev, 1988; Lux et al., 1990; Sheetz, 1983). In muscle cells, these cytoskeletal proteins not only strengthen the phospholipid bilayer, but also play an essential role in transmitting the force developed by the contractile proteins down the length of the muscle from one cell to another (see also Chapter 1).

Membrane proteins can be adsorbed to the membrane surface, embedded in one leaflet of the bilayer, or can span the bilayer so as to make contact with the aqueous phases on either side of the membrane (Fig. 2.11). Proteins that are incorporated into one or both leaflets of the bilayer cannot easily be extracted from the membranes, and so are designated *intrinsic (or integral) membrane proteins*. Adsorbed proteins, sometimes designated *peripheral membrane proteins*, are more readily dissociated from the membrane; although they often play an important role in membrane function, they may also represent contaminants that become associated with membrane fractions during purification. The fluid nature of the membrane lipid bilayer allows intrinsic membrane proteins to move in the plane of the bilayer, so that membranes can be viewed as a collection of protein icebergs floating in a lipid sea.

The intrinsic membrane proteins represent a special class of polypeptides whose unique biophysical properties are readily understood in terms of the diverse physical regions found within the membrane bilayer. Although some portions of these proteins are in contact with the aqueous, hydrophilic, environment at either side of the membrane, other regions of the intrinsic membrane proteins must interact with the fatty acyl chains within the hydrophobic core of the membrane bilayer (Fig. 2.12). Those portions of the polypeptide chains of membrane proteins that pass through the hydrophobic core of the membrane are generally arranged as α-helices (Fig. 2.13) that contain large amounts of apolar amino acids, notably tryptophan, phenylalanine, tyrosine, leucine, valine, methionine, and alanine. These hydrophobic

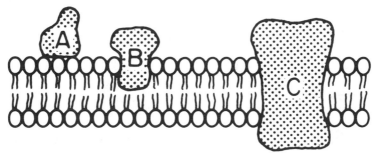

FIG. 2.11. Membrane proteins (*shaded*) can be adsorbed to the membrane surface (A), incorporated into one leaflet of the bilayer (B), or can span the bilayer (C). Both B and C represent intrinsic membrane proteins.

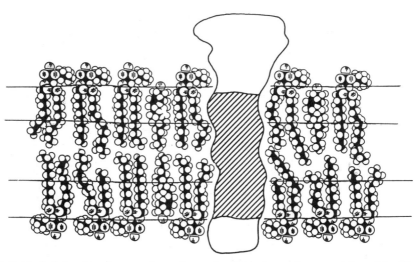

FIG. 2.12. Relationships between the surfaces of an intrinsic membrane protein and the bilayer. The hydrophobic (*shaded*) surface is seen to insert into the fatty acyl chain region of the bilayer, whereas the hydrophilic (*unshaded*) surfaces are in contact with the aqueous media at the two sides of the bilayer.

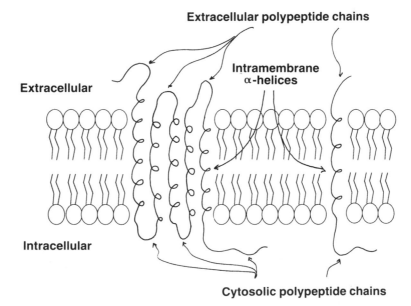

FIG. 2.13. Schematic diagram of two intrinsic membrane proteins showing the α-helices that span the membrane bilayer, and cytosolic and extracellular amino acid sequences on the two sides of the membrane.

amino acids stabilize the interaction of intrinsic membrane proteins with the hydrophobic core of the bilayer. Most functionally important membrane proteins, such as
ion channels (Chapter 18) and neurotransmitter receptor proteins (Chapter 12), contain several hydrophobic transmembrane helices.

When intrinsic membrane proteins are purifed and placed in an aqueous medium,
they are readily denatured because the polar environment cannot maintain the native
conformation of their hydrophobic regions. For this reason, membrane proteins are
generally stabilized in solutions containing *detergents*, which are small amphipathic
molecules that contain both a polar head group and a hydrophobic tail. The detergent molecules, by forming stable complexes with these proteins, are able to satisfy
the requirement that the hydrophobic surface of the membrane protein interact with
other hydrophobic groups (Fig. 2.14).

Interactions between membrane proteins and their surrounding phospholipids can
be of considerable functional significance. The lipids that surround the membrane
proteins are sometimes called the *boundary layer lipids* or *annulus*, but these terms
have led to some controversy because of early reports that certain lipid molecules
maintain prolonged contact with the proteins and did not exchange freely with the
remainder of the "bulk" membrane lipids. Although this concept of a long-lived

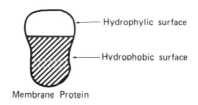

Membrane Protein

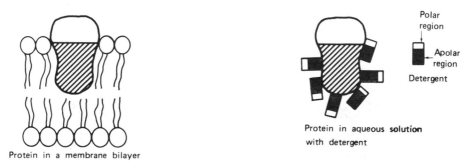

Protein in a membrane bilayer

Protein in aqueous solution
with detergent

FIG. 2.14. Schematic diagram showing the similarities between the interactions of a membrane
protein inserted into a bilayer (*below*, *left*) and those of the same protein dispersed in an
aqueous solution and stabilized by a detergent (*below*, *right*). As in Fig. 2.9, the hydrophobic
surface of the protein is *shaded*.

annulus is no longer tenable, the regions of hydrophobic interaction between membrane proteins and the surrounding membrane lipids may play an important role in some membrane activities (Rhodes et al., 1985).

Hypothetical examples of some hydrophobic interactions within the membrane bilayer that could influence membrane function are given in Figs. 2.15 and 2.16, which depict structures calculated on the basis of thermodynamic and packing considerations (Israelachvili, 1977). A membrane protein could influence the structure of the membrane lipids that surround its hydrophobic surface by associating with lipids containing fatty acids with longer (Fig. 2.15C) or shorter (Fig. 2.15D) hydrocarbon chains. Thermodynamic and packing characteristics of the interactions between membrane proteins and their surrounding lipids could contribute to protein-protein interactions within biological membranes, as depicted in Fig. 2.16. In the example shown in Fig. 2.16A, the most stable state of two membrane proteins that deform the bilayer is achieved by formation of a dimer. Association of proteins in opposite leaflets of the bilayer could occur as shown in Fig. 2.16B. It is possible that a change in transmembrane potential, or ligand-binding to a receptor, could cause conformational changes in membrane proteins that favor such interactions; however, such scenarios are entirely speculative.

DETERGENT EFFECTS

All drugs have potentially harmful side effects. For most useful drugs, the therapeutic effect occurs at a much lower concentration than that which produces undesirable side effects. In the case of membrane- active drugs, useful effects are generally achieved when the drug inactivates or blocks, or in some cases activates, a

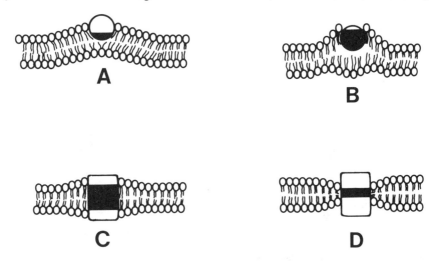

FIG. 2.15. Influence on bilayer structure of the extent of the hydrophobic surface of intrinsic membrane proteins inserted in one leaflet of the bilayer (A, B) and spanning the bilayer (C, D). The hydrophobic portion of the protein is *shaded*. (Modified from Israelachvili, 1977.)

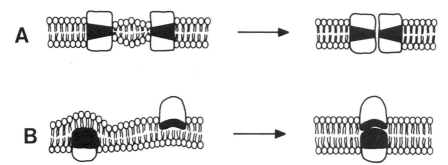

FIG. 2.16. Possible mechanism by which interactions between membrane proteins form stable oligomers. In A, two proteins with "mirror image" hydrophobic asymmetry that span the membrane (*left*) achieve the most stable conformation (*right*) by forming a dimer. In B, two proteins with different but complementary hydrophobic surfaces, each in one leaflet of the bilayer (*left*), form a stable dimer when they interact across the bilayer (*right*). Hydrophobic surfaces are *shaded*.

specific membrane function. Although most neurotransmitters and some drugs bind with high affinity to specific membrane "receptors," the majority of cardiac drugs, notably the antiarrhythmic agents, bind to their receptors with low specificity. Because less specific drug molecules often interact with other membrane proteins at the high concentrations needed to produce their desired effects, such drugs have low therapeutic/toxic ratios. Even less specific are the anesthetic agents, most of which probably do not bind to receptor sites, but instead modify membrane function when high drug concentrations become dissolved in the bulk lipids of the bilayer. These latter effects, sometimes called "local anesthetic," "nonspecific," or "membrane stabilizing" actions, are referred to here as *detergent effects.*

> These principles, and especially the function of detergents, are well known to salad makers. If one shakes a mixture of vinegar and oil, the mixture quickly separates because the water in the vinegar "seeks" water, and oil "seeks" oil. Such mixtures are readily stabilized by addition of egg yolk, which contains lecithin (a mixture of phosphatidylcholines) that acts as a detergent. By providing hydrophobic groups (the fatty acids) to interact with the oil, and polar groups (phosphate and choline) to interact with the (aqueous) vinegar, the egg yolk lecithin forms a stable mixture. With appropriate seasoning, this is of course mayonnaise. Soaps, made by our forebears by mixing ashes (alkali) and fat (lipid), also function as detergents because the mixture forms amphipathic molecules that are able to lift lipid "dirt" from our clothes or our bodies into water.

The simplest concept of a detergent effect, which is analogous to that produced by a common household dishwashing product, is the solubilization of membrane proteins by high concentrations of amphipathic molecules that contain both hydrophilic and hydrophobic regions (Fig. 2.17C). Detergent effects, however, are actually quite complex and depend on the relative concentrations of detergent and membrane lipids. At low concentrations, detergents become associated with membranes, in general by incorporation into the bilayer, where they modify its physical properties (Fig. 2.17A). Raising the detergent concentration causes greater amounts of the

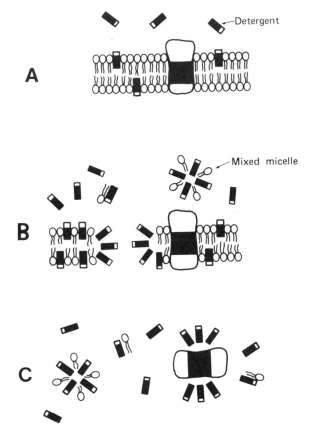

FIG. 2.17. Detergent effects on membranes. A: At low concentrations detergents insert into the membrane, where they can change the physical state of the phospholipid bilayer. B: Higher detergent concentrations "pull" membrane lipids out of the membrane, sometimes forming "mixed micelles" containing a mixture of the detergent and membrane lipids. C: Very high detergent concentrations can separate membrane proteins from membrane lipids.

detergent to become incorporated into the bilayer, where they tend to disrupt the membrane barrier (Fig. 2.17B). At still higher detergent concentrations, the membrane proteins become separated from the membrane lipids and the bilayer is disrupted (Fig. 2.17C). Both of these latter effects (membrane disruption and removal of membrane proteins) severely impair membrane function, and can cause cell death.

Anesthetic Effects on Membranes

The ability of some lipid-soluble drugs to induce sleep may arise from mechanisms such as that depicted in Fig. 2.17A, where incorporation of a small amount of an amphipathic compound in the membrane modifies the function of the ion channels that propagate the action potential. Several mechanisms have been proposed to explain these anesthetic effects. *Specific* interactions with membrane proteins, such as binding to sodium channels, may account for the clinical effects of some anesthetic agents (and, in the case of the heart, some antiarrhythmic drugs). However, the broad range of organic structures that produce these effects indicates that most anesthetics block excitation by nonspecific effects that arise after these drugs are incorporated into the membrane bilayer.

> The nonspecifity of the actions of anesthetic agents was shown at the beginning of this century, when a close parallel was found between the anesthetic potency of a wide variety of organic compounds and their solubility in olive oil. Recognition that the anesthetic potency of any "chemically indifferent" compound correlated with its lipid solubility (the Meyer-Overton law) led to the hypothesis that the anesthetic effect was due to the accumulation of the compound in the "lipoids of the cell." These "lipoids," of course, are now recognized to be the lipids of the membrane bilayer.

The presence of large amounts of an amphipathic drug in the bilayer can have a number of physical effects on membrane structure; these include *membrane expansion, interference with lateral phase separations*, and *calcium displacement*.

Membrane expansion can occur when a drug incorporated in the membrane bilayer causes the membrane to expand in a lateral direction (Fig. 2.18A), due both to the volume occupied by the drug and to its ability to disorder ("melt") the more ordered domains in the membrane (see below). A simplistic view of these consequences of membrane expansion is to imagine that the membrane channels become "compressed," as shown in Fig. 2.18A. Solvation of an anesthetic in the membrane bilayer could also cause the membrane to thicken, as may occur when a drug containing a large hydrophobic group is incorporated into a membrane as shown in Fig. 2.18B.

A modification of the membrane expansion model for anesthetic action is based on evidence that biological membranes contain "domains" in which different regions of the lipid bilayer can be found in either a gel or liquid state (Klausner et al., 1980), and that *lateral phase separations* between gel and fluid domains play an important role in the function of membrane proteins (Trudell, 1977). According to this model, opening of a channel increases the volume that it occupies in the lateral plane of the membrane. The increased volume occupied by the open state of the channel could be accommodated by ordering of the lipids at the points of "lateral phase separation" between the channel proteins and surrounding bilayer lipids, as shown in Fig. 2.19A,B. As incorporation of an anesthetic in the bilayer would tend to disorder the gel structure (see above), the drug could interfere with the ability of the lateral phase separations to accommodate the increased volume caused by channel opening, as shown in Fig. 2.19C,D. By inhibiting lateral phase separations, therefore, the drug could inhibit movements of the membrane channel proteins necessary for the generation of excitatory currents.

Anesthetic effects may also result from *displacement of Ca^{2+} ions* bound to the phosphate head groups of membrane lipids (Hauser and Dawson, 1968), especially

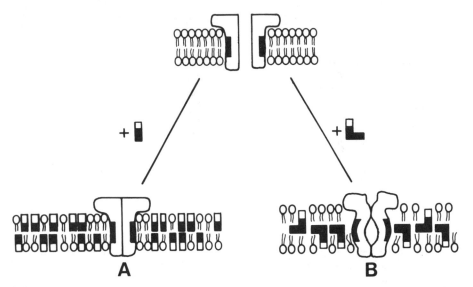

FIG. 2.18. Two models of the mechanism of anesthetic action caused by membrane expansion: (A) lateral expansion and (B) membrane thickening. The anesthetic molecules are depicted as *rectangles* (A) or *angles* (B), the hydrophobic portions being *darkly shaded*.

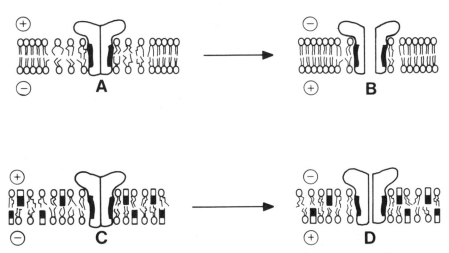

FIG. 2.19. Model of anesthetic action due to reduced ability of lateral phase separations to accommodate an increase in membrane volume caused by opening of an ion channel. (A, B): In the untreated membrane, depolarization (reversal of transmembrane potential) causes the channel proteins to move apart when the channel opens (B). The accompanying increase in channel volume is accommodated by tighter packing of the membrane lipids that undergo transition from a fluid to a gel structure at the lateral phase separation surrounding the channel proteins. (C, D): When an anesthetic drug inhibits formation of the gel sturcture at the lateral phase separation, the transmembrane potential change cannot open the channel, because the volume expansion needed to compensate for channel opening cannot be accommodated in the detergent-filled membrane (D).

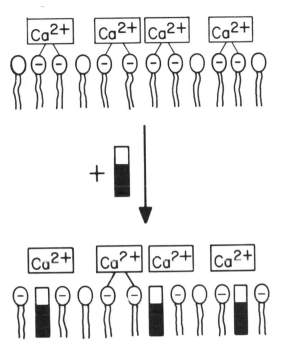

FIG. 2.20. Model of anesthetic action based on displacement of membrane-bound Ca^{2+}. Incorporation of anesthetic molecules (*half-shaded rectangles*) into the outer (extracellular) leaflet of the bilayer interferes with the coordination of divalent Ca^{2+} to anionic groups on two adjacent phospholipids.

at the extracellular surface of plasma membranes which is in contact with the high, millimolar, Ca^{2+} concentration of the extracellular fluid (Fig. 2.20). As each divalent Ca^{2+} coordinates with the anionic phosphate group of two adjacent membrane phospholipids, the interposition of an anesthetic molecule between a coordinating pair of membrane lipids could displace membrane-bound Ca^{2+}, thereby modifying surface charge so as to interfere with membrane activation (Fig. 2.10C).

Drug Effects on Membrane Proteins

It should be emphasized that not all postulated mechanisms for drug actions on membranes arise from the nonspecific detergent effects just described. Instead, most neurotransmitters, and some drugs and hormones, interact specifically with binding sites on one or another of the membrane proteins, rather than with the bulk membrane lipids. In this way, a highly selective membrane action of a chemical substance generally arises when that substance has a high affinity interaction with a single type of membrane protein, or protein complex, that participates in a single function.

The distinction between a nonspecific detergent action and a specific drug interaction with a unique class of membrane proteins is not always clear. For example,
commonly encountered drug side effects generally arise from interactions of the
drug with proteins other than their primary pharmacological targets. Lack of specificity is especially troublesome in the case of the antiarrhythmic agents, most of
which exert effects on more than one type of ion channel.

A number of models that aid in understanding drug actions on specific membrane
proteins have been proposed (Courtney, 1980; Hille, 1977; Hondeghem and Katzung, 1977 [Chapter 23]). One important controversy regarding the mechanism of
antiarrhythmic drug action is depicted schematically in Fig. 2.21, which shows two
different mechanisms that can explain the finding that drugs often tend to block an
ion channel when the latter is in its open state. In Fig. 2.21B the drug is shown to
bind to a hydrophilic surface within the channel that is exposed when the channel
opens; i.e., the drug can be said to bind in the "mouth" of the channel. An alternative explanation for the common finding that drugs have greater inhibitory effects
on open channels is shown in Fig. 2.21C, where a drug is seen to bind preferentially
to the conformation of the hydrophobic surface assumed when the the channel protein is in its open state.

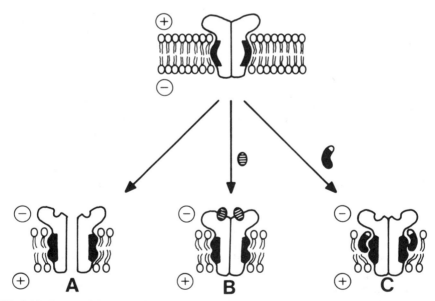

FIG. 2.21. The ability of a drug to block a voltage-dependent membrane channel selectively in
its open state can be explained by either of two different mechanisms: block of the open channel
by insertion of a drug into the "mouth" of the channel (B); or block of the channel when an
amphipathic drug inserts into the membrane bilayer and binds to a "new" hydrophobic conformation that the channel protein assumes when the channel is opened by membrane depolarization
(C). Normal channel opening caused by a change in transmembrane potential is shown in (A).

The ability of a number of cardiac drugs to partition into membrane lipids can explain several of their pharmacokinetic properties. For example, amiodarone, an antiarrhythmic drug with a remarkably long half-life that can extend for many months (hence the quip: "Amiodarone effects can last longer than some marriages") tends to partition more deeply into membrane bilayers than drugs with shorter biological half-lives (Herbette et al., 1988).

Use-Dependence of Drug Actions

The sensitivity of transmembrane currents to several drugs can be significantly influenced by the functional state of the channels that allow the ions to cross the membrane. For example, depolarization of the cardiac cell membrane markedly potentiates the ability of some drugs to "block" sodium channels; thus, a drug like quinidine is a much more potent inhibitor of the sodium current at a fast heart rate than when the heart rate is slow (Chapter 23). A currently popular interpretation of this well-documented phenomenon (sometimes called "use-dependence" because the effect of the drug is increased by prior "use" of the ion channel), is that depolarization alters the structure of the channel in a manner that increases its ability to bind to the drug. This ability of a drug to bind preferentially to a "depolarized" channel may occur because the drug binds within the "mouth" of the open channel, to a changed formation of the polar region of the channel protein, or to a changed conformation in the hydrophobic surface of the protein within the bilayer (Fig. 2.21). This and other influences of the state of a channel on its interactions with drugs is discussed further in Chapter 23.

DIFFERENT MECHANISMS OF MEMBRANE TRANSPORT

The regulated passage of a variety of substances across the membrane barrier is, of course, a critical function of all membranes. Although descriptions of the many different types of transport are beyond the scope of this chapter, it is useful at this point to distinguish between two fundamentally different types of membrane transport. The first is the regulated passage of single molecules through "channels" that can be highly ion-specific and which can open, inactivate, and close with rigidly defined properties (Chapter 18). Second, many larger molecules are transported in small "packets" when part of a membrane pinches off to form vesicles that carry these molecules, often bound to a receptor, through the cell.

The transport of small molecules across membranes is generally mediated by a variety of ion pumps, carriers, and channels that represent highly regulated intrinsic membrane proteins. In contrast, the ability of large molecules to cross membranes generally involves a quite different process, in which the macromolecules are surrounded by membrane vesicles that carry these substances between the interior of the cell and the extracellular space (Pastan and Willingham, 1985). The processes of *exocytosis*, by which substances manufactured in the cell are carried to the cell surface, mediate both the formation and repair of the plasma membrane, as well as the transport of large molecules made in the Golgi apparatus and subsequently secreted by the cell. With the exception of atrial natriuretic factor (see Chapter 1), secretory processes are of relatively little prominence in most muscle cells of the cardiovascular system.

The uptake of macromolecules into the cell (*endocytosis*), like exocytosis, involves the formation and intracellular movement of vesicles (Fig. 2.22). In the case of endocytosis, vesicles are formed from regions of plasma membrane that invaginate from the cell surface and surround the macromolecule to be transported into the cell. This type of transport is commonly initiated when a large molecule, such as a lipoprotein, binds to a specific receptor on the outer surface of the plasma mem-

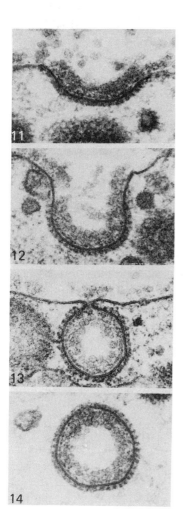

FIG. 2.22. Four stages in endocytosis, showing the probable sequence in steps from the coated pit (*top*) to the coated vesicle (*bottom*). The extracellular space is at the *top* of the upper three panels. (From Perry and Gilbert, 1979, with permission of the Company of Biologists Ltd.)

brane bilayer. The occupied receptor then stimulates invagination of the membrane adajcent to the immobilized macromolecule, which forms a *coated pit*. Coated pits generally appear as depressions in a region of the cell surface where the intracellular surface of the bilayer is lined by the protein *clathrin*. This protein remains attached to the membrane as it seals within the cell to form the *coated vesicle* that carries the macromolecule into the cell interior. The role of clathrin in these transport processes remains unclear; it is likely that this protein may form a basket-like structure around the coated vesicle, but the nature of the forces involved in the formation and transport of these membrane vesicles remains to be defined.

It should be emphasized that, although bulk transport mechanisms play little or no role in the physiological control of cardiac excitation or contraction, these processes are important in the movements of large molecules and a variety of messengers that bind to membrane receptors that are then transported through the cytosol, along with their membrane receptor, in a membrane vesicle.

REFERENCES

Berridge MJ. (1989). Inositol trisphosphate, calcium, lithium, and cell signalling. *JAMA* 262:1834–1841.

Bershadsky AD, Vasiliev JM. (1988). *Cytoskeleton*. New York: Plenum Press.

Courtney KR. (1980). Structure-activity relations for frequency-dependent sodium channel block in nerve by local anesthetics. *J Pharmacol Exp Ther* 213:114–119.

Hauser H, Dawson RMC. (1968). The displacement of calcium ions from phospholipid monolayers by pharmacologically active and other organic bases. *Biochem J* 109:909–916.

Herbette LG, Trumbore M, Chester DW, Katz AM. (1988). Possible molecular basis for the pharmacodynamics of three membrane active drugs: propranolol, nimodipine, amiodarone. *J Mol Cell Cardiol* 20:373–378.

Hille B. (1977). Local anesthetics: hydrophylic and hydrophobic pathways for the drug-receptor reaction. *J Gen Physiol* 69:497–515.

Holman RT. (1986). *Progress in lipid research*, Vol. 25: Essential fatty acids, prostaglandins and leukotrienes. Oxford: Pergamon Press.

Hondeghem IM, Katzung BG. (1977). Time and voltage-dependent interactions of antiarrhythmic drugs with cardiac sodium channels. *Biochim Biophys Acta* 472:373–398.

Israelachvili JN. (1977). Refinement of the fluid-mosaic model of membrane structure. *Biochim Biophys Acta* 469:221–225.

Katz AM, Messineo FC. (1981). Lipid-membrane interactions and the pathogenesis of ischemic damage in the myocardium. *Circ Res* 48:1–16.

Klausner RD, Kleinfeld AM, Hoover RL, Karnovsky MJ. (1980). Lipid domains in membranes. Evidence derived from structural perturbations induced by free fatty acids and lifetime heterogeneity analysis. *J Biol Chem* 255:1286–1295.

Lucy JA. (1970). The fusion of biological membranes. *Nature* 227:815–817.

Lux SE, John KM, Bennett V. (1990). Analysis of cDNA for human erythrocyte ankyrin indicates a repeated structure with homology to tissue-differentiation and cell-cycle control proteins. *Nature* 344:26–42.

McLaughlin S, Harary H. (1974). Phospholipid flip-flop and the distribution of surface charges in excitable membranes. *Biophys J* 14:200–208.

Muldoon MF, Manuck SB, Matthews KA. (1990). Lowering serum cholesterol concentrations and mortality: a quantitiative review of primary prevention trials. *Br Med J* 1990 (ii) 309–314.

Nishizuka Y. (1989). The family of protein kinase C for signal transduction. *JAMA* 262:1826–1833.

Pastan IH, Willingham MH. (1985). *Endocytosis*. New York: Pergamon Press.

Perry MM, Gilbert AB. (1979). Yolk transport in the follicle of the hen (Gallus domesticus); Lipoprotein-like particles at the periphery of the oocyte in the rapid growth phase. *J Cell Sci* 39:257–272.

Post JA, Langer GA, Op den Kamp JAF, Verkleij AJ. (1988). Phospholipid asymmetry in cardiac sarcolemma. Analysis of intact cells and "gas dissected" membrane. *Biochim Biophys Acta* 943:256–266.
Rhodes DG, Sarmiento JG, Herbette LG. (1985). Kinetics of binding of membrane-active drugs to receptor sites. Diffusion-limited rates for a membrane approach of 1,4-dihydropyridine calcium channel antagonists to their active site. *Mol Pharmacol* 27:621–623.
Sheetz MP. (1983). Membrane skeletal dynamics: role in modulation of red cell deformability, mobility of transmembrane proteins, and shape. *Semin Hematol* 20:175–188.
Taraschi TF, Rubin E. (1985). The effects of ethanol on the chemical and structural properties of biological membranes. *Lab Invest* 52:120–131.
Trudell JR. (1977). A unitary theory of anesthesia based on lateral phase separations in nerve membranes. *Anesthesiology* 46:5–10.

BIBLIOGRAPHY

Alberts B, Bray D, Lewis J, Raff M, Roberts K, Watson JD. (1989). *Molecular biology of the cell*, 2nd ed. New York: Garland; 276–340 (Chapter 6: The plasma membrane).
Finean JB, Coleman R, Michell RH. (1978). *Membranes and their cellular functions*. Oxford: Blackwell.
Helenius A, Simons K. (1975). Solubilization of membranes by detergents. *Biochim Biophys Acta* 415:29–79.
Jain MK, Wagner RC. (1980). *Introduction to biological membranes*. New York: Wiley-Interscience.
Luttgau HC, Glitsch H. (1976). Membrane physiology of nerve and muscle fibers. *Fortschr Zool* 24:1–132.
Quinn PJ. (1976). *The molecular biology of cellular membranes*. Baltimore: University Park Press.
Robertson RN. (1983). *The lively membranes*. Cambridge: Cambridge University Press.
Seeman P. (1972). The membrane action of anesthetics and tranquilizers. *Pharmacol Rev* 24:583–655.

3

Energetics of Muscle

The pumping action of the heart results from the contractile activity of its muscular walls, so that for the ventricles to eject blood under pressure into the aorta and pulmonary artery the individual muscle fibers must shorten under load. The product of force times distance, which represents the *work* performed by each element of the myocardium, is a measure of the mechanical energy liberated during systole. According to the first law of thermodynamics, energy cannot be created *de novo*, so the mechanical energy that appears during the muscular work of the ventricular walls must be matched by the disappearance of energy elsewhere. In the case of the heart, this energy is lost by utilization of the energy contained in a variety of chemical compounds. Thus like all muscles, the heart can be regarded as a *mechanochemical transducer* in that during contraction chemical energy is transformed into mechanical energy. This chapter examines the overall patterns of the chemical processes responsible for energy production in the heart and their relationship to both the liberation of mechanical energy and the physiological constraints under which the mammalian heart is required to function.

If a strand of muscle is isolated in a closed, insulated box and arranged so that it lifts a load when stimulated (Fig. 3.1), two kinds of energy appear after stimulation: *mechanical energy*, which is equal to the product of the load and the distance shortened, and *heat*. According to the first law of thermodynamics, the sum of all energies in a closed system must remain constant, so that the appearance of energy (as work and as heat) must be matched by the disappearance of energy elsewhere. As already indicated, a loss of *chemical* (or internal) *energy* accompanies muscular contraction, so it is both theoretically and experimentally possible to measure changes in the chemical composition of contracting muscle.

In thermodynamic terminology the change in internal energy during muscle contraction can be defined as $- \Delta E$, which is equal to E_2 (the chemical energy at the end of the contraction) minus E_1 (the chemical energy at the beginning of contraction). One can therefore describe the net change in chemical energy during contraction by the following equation:

$$- \Delta E = E_2 - E_1.$$ [3.1]

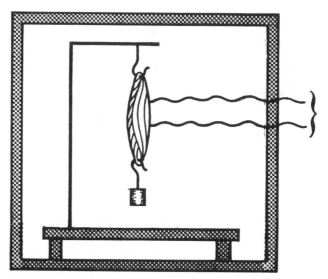

FIG. 3.1. A muscle within an insulated box, the only communication with the outside environment being the two stimulating wires. Delivery of a minute amount of electrical energy causes the muscle to contract. The accompanying appearance of energy, as work and heat, must be matched by the disappearance of chemical energy within the muscle because the sum of the energies within the box must remain constant.

The change in external energy, which in a closed system is also ΔE, is the sum of energies liberated as heat (q) and as work ($-W$).[1] Thus the net change in external energy during muscular contraction can be described by the equation:

$$\Delta E = q - W. \qquad [3.2]$$

With the use of modern recording and analytical methods, it is possible to measure all the parameters in Eq. 3.1 and 3.2. The terms E_2 and E_1 can be evaluated by chemical determination of the concentrations of key metabolic compounds at the beginning and end of the contractile cycle. The net changes in these concentrations are then multiplied by the enthalpy changes (ΔH) in the chemical reactions to approximate the free energy made available. These enthalpy changes, which represent the heat produced or absorbed during the individual chemical reactions, provide a useful index of the energy changes accompanying each reaction. The relationship between ΔE and ΔH is given by the equation:

$$\Delta E = \Delta H + P\Delta V \qquad [3.3]$$

where P is the pressure at which the reaction takes place and ΔV is the change in volume that accompanies the reaction. Because muscular contraction takes place with little or no volume change, it can be taken that $\Delta E \cong \Delta H$.

More precise estimates for E_2 and E_1 require knowledge of the free energy changes

---

[1]The use of the negative sign for the work term ($-W$) is a convention of thermodynamics that can be confusing if the reader is not warned that the conventions of muscle physiology reverse this sign (Chapter 6).

(ΔG) which accompany each chemical reaction. The relationship between ΔH and ΔG is given by the equation:

$$\Delta H = \Delta G + T\Delta S \qquad [3.4]$$

where T is the absolute temperature and ΔS the entropy change, a measurement directly proportional to the "disorder" or randomness of the system at the beginning and end of the reaction. Because of the difficulties in measuring these entropy changes, it is most convenient to relate the change in internal energy ($-\Delta E$) to the enthalpy change ($-\Delta H$), although this evaluation of $-\Delta E$ clearly requires that certain assumptions be made regarding the relationship between changes in metabolite concentration and the energy made available.

Accurate measurements of heat liberation *(q)* in active muscle have been made possible by the use of the *thermopile*, which is a series of *thermocouples*. Each thermocouple represents a pair of junctions between two dissimilar metals, in which the appearance of a temperature gradient generates a small electrical potential. Finally, the liberation of energy as work ($-W$) can be calculated by multiplying the force, or load, by the distance over which the muscle shortens. In Chapter 6 we examine Eq. 3.2 to define more precisely the characteristics of energy liberation, and as work and heat; Chapters 4 and 5 focus on the reactions that provide the chemical energy for contraction, i.e., those encompassed by Eq. 3.1.

PROVISION OF CHEMICAL ENERGY FOR MUSCULAR CONTRACTION

It is appropriate here to review how our present understanding grew concerning the provision of chemical energy for muscular contraction; this historical evolution not only facilitates an understanding of this important topic but illustrates some of the pitfalls encountered in scientific investigation. The early observations by Fletcher and Hopkins in 1907 that lactic acid was produced in muscle that went into rigor after death, and the subsequent demonstration that this lactic acid came from glycogen metabolism, led Myerhof during the 1920s to examine the relationship between lactic acid formation and muscular work. Experiments carried out under anaerobic conditions, in which oxidation of lactic acid was blocked, showed that the amount of carbohydrate metabolized was proportional to the work done during muscular contraction. This led to the view that glycolysis, measured as lactic acid formation from glycogen, was directly coupled to muscular contraction by a reaction that could be described as:

Glycogen $\rightarrow$ lactic acid + mechanical energy.

This attractive formulation, which was consistent with and explained a large body of experimental data, collapsed with the publication of a single, but well-documented observation: that exposure of muscle to iodoacetic acid could stop lactic acid production under conditions where the ability to contract was preserved. Lundsgaard, who reported this observation in 1930, found that in the presence of iodoacetic acid, which inhibits glycolysis, muscular work could take place under conditions where neither glycogen was metabolized nor lactic acid produced. It was soon found, instead, that liberation of mechanical energy by the muscle was accompanied by the breakdown of phosphocreatine, a labile compound containing creatine and phosphoric acid. At this time, Eggleton and Eggleton showed that during muscular contraction the decrease in phosphocreatine content was proportional to the work done. It thus seemed reasonable to postulate that energy was provided for muscular contraction by the breakdown of phosphocreatine to creatine and inorganic phosphate (P_i) according to the reaction:

$$\text{Phosphocreatine} \rightarrow \text{creatine} + P_i + \text{mechanical energy.}$$

The energy derived from the metabolism of glycogen to form lactic acid was recognized, therefore, not to provide energy directly to the contractile machinery, but instead to provide for the resynthesis of phosphocreatine from creatine and P_i.

The view that phosphocreatine was the direct source of energy for muscular contraction lasted only a few years. Another substance, discovered independently by Lohman and by Fiske and Subbarow, was found to be synthesized during glycolysis and to release energy on hydrolysis. This substance, the adenine nucleotide adenosine triphosphate (ATP,), was found to be necessary for the hydrolysis of phosphocreatine in that cell-free extracts were unable to catalyze the breakdown of phosphocreatine to form creatine and P_i, and thus to liberate energy, unless adenine nucleotides were present. This function of the adenine nucleotides could be shown to reflect their ability to transfer P_1, and thus chemical energy, from phosphocreatine to a number of energy-consuming reactions. The role of the phosphocreatine therefore is to phosphorylate adenosine diphosphate (ADP) to form ATP, which then can be hydrolyzed to yield ADP, P_i, and energy. The overall reactions that describe the adenine nucleotide requirement for phosphocreatine breakdown can be written:

$$\text{Phosphocreatine} + \text{ADP} \rightleftharpoons \text{creatine} + \text{ATP}$$
$$\text{ATP} \rightarrow \text{ADP} + P_i.$$

These equations explain the finding that phosphocreatine is not itself hydrolyzed to creatine unless adenine nucleotides are present.

Since they were discovered, the adenine nucleotides have been found to participate in a number of chemical reactions within the cell. In these reactions ADP accepts chemical energy by incorporating P_i to form a high-energy bond in ATP, whereas ATP is able to donate chemical energy through the hydrolysis of this phosphate bond. This function of ATP has been likened by A. Szent-Györgyi to that of money, ATP being the "chemical currency" of the cell. Thus, like money, ATP can be obtained (synthesized) in exchange for the energy derived from a number of different chemical processes (e.g., the metabolism of fats and carbohydrates); and like money, ATP can be used for a variety of energy-consuming processes (e.g., muscular contraction, biosynthesis, membrane transport). In the process of muscular contraction, therefore, ATP is viewed as carrying the chemical energy from phosphocreatine stores, which in this context serve as a reserve of "ready cash." In addition, the energy obtained from intermediary metabolism must first be converted to ATP to provide for the performance of mechanical work by the muscle.

Although ATP has been thought since the mid-1930s to provide the energy for muscular contraction, it was not until the early 1960s that a decrease in ATP concentration could be shown to accompany muscular contraction. Prior to that time, it had been impossible to inhibit selectively the transfer of phosphate from phosphocreatine to ADP, so that all that could be detected to accompany muscular work was a decrease in phosphocreatine. It was not until 1962 that Davies found that fluorodinitrobenzene (Sanger's reagent, an early tool of the protein chemist) could be used to poison specifically the enzyme creatine phosphokinase, which catalyzes the transfer of P_i from phosphocreatine to ADP. This finding made it possible to demonstrate a proportionality between ATP hydrolysis and muscular work:

$$ATP \rightarrow ADP + P_i + \text{mechanical energy}.$$

Our situation today is different, however, from that of our scientific forebears—who had earlier demonstrated the proportionality between lactic acid production from glycogen, and later phosphocreatine breakdown and the liberation of mechanical energy—because the direct participation of ATP in the chemical processes responsible for contraction has now been shown experimentally (Chapter 7).

GENERATION OF CHEMICAL ENERGY FOR CONTRACTION

The metabolic pathways by which ATP is regenerated are not the same in all types of muscle. With functional specialization, different muscle types have been found to employ different pathways of energy production; and as we shall see, this biochemical specialization is closely related to the functional needs of the individual muscles. In considering these differences, it will be more illuminating if we examine first the physiological requirements of different muscle types and then consider the biochemical specializations and their functional significance. A useful approach is to compare the life habits of two long-eared mammals, the rabbit and the hare[2] (Fig. 3.2).

In Europe the *rabbit* lives in a burrow from which it ventures only short distances in search of food and adventure. Such animals rely on a sprint to their burrow in order to escape predators, for it is in their ability to accelerate and run rapidly for short distances that they survive in nature. Although the rabbit is thus an excellent sprinter, it is a poor distance runner as can be attested to by anyone who has allowed a rabbit to escape in the laboratory. Many species of European *hare*, on the other hand, have no burrow but range widely in their habitat. Such hares are excellent distance runners, relying on their staying power to escape pursuers—indeed the coursing of hares has been known since antiquity.

---

[2]The description in the next paragraph is valid for the European rabbit and hare but not their American counterparts as was first pointed out to the author by a cardiology fellow from Texas.

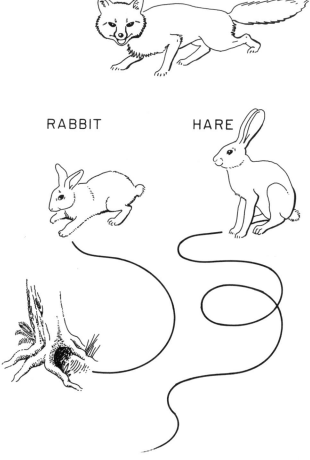

FIG. 3.2. Ecological adaptations of the rabbit and hare. When confronted with danger, such as an encounter with a fox, the rabbit tries to escape by a sprint to its burrow, whereas the hare tries to outrun and outlast the pursuing fox.

Early in this century it became clear to scientists, although this information must already have been well known to hunters and cooks, that the muscles used for locomotion by rabbits and hares differ grossly in appearance. Those in the rabbit are pale pink, almost white in color, whereas the back and leg muscles of the hare are deep red. Similar differences in muscle color are found in other vertebrate species; i.e., "white" is generally found where the muscle is called on for short bursts of intense activity, and "red" is present in muscles where activity is sustained. In common culinary experience, for example, the chicken breast, which powers wings that are used only intermittently, is white meat, whereas the dark meat of the chicken leg represents a muscle that is used for the more continuous activity of walking. In birds capable of sustained flight, on the other hand, the breast muscles are "red" (e.g., the dark meat of duck or goose breast).

In the following discussion we focus on these two "extremes" of muscle specialization: red and white. Intermediate fiber types exist, and there are exceptions to the general patterns described below, but for the sake of clarity these are not considered further in this attempt to describe the means by which nature can adapt biochemical specialization to meet the physiological needs of the organism.

BIOCHEMICAL DIFFERENCES BETWEEN RED AND WHITE MUSCLE

In *red muscle* (Table 3.1), which is specialized for sustained activity without rest periods, it is essential that the rate of energy production not exceed that of energy utilization. In these muscles therefore, ATP is produced in large quantities by the efficient pathways of oxidative metabolism. The red color of these muscles is due largely to a high myoglobin content, which serves to facilitate the diffusion of oxygen through the muscle fibers. The most important substrates for aerobic energy production are lipids, although carbohydrates including lactate are oxidized when delivered in appropriate concentrations via the arterial blood supply (Chapter 5). Red muscles are capable of carrying out anaerobic glycolysis (Chapter 4) and have some high-energy phosphate (phosphocreatine) reserves, but these are of lesser functional significance in that neither can provide the large amounts of ATP needed for sustained contraction. Thus if oxygen lack halts aerobic ATP production (e.g., when blood flow is interrupted, or under conditions of anoxia), the phosphocreatine stores are quickly exhausted. Acceleration of glycolysis can provide only a very limited increase in the rate of ATP production. Furthermore, under anaerobic conditions the increased production of lactate is accompanied by hydrogen ion liberation, so that a state of intracellular acidosis develops which inhibits key regulatory enzymes that control the rate of glycolysis. For this reason accelerated glycolysis is not only limited in its ability to generate ATP under anaerobic conditions, it is also transient and cannot be sustained, especially when the anaerobic state results from interrupted blood flow to the muscle (Chapter 24).

TABLE 3.1. *Biochemical differences between red and white muscle*

Biochemical characteristic	Red muscle	White muscle
Pathways of energy production	Aerobic	Anaerobic
Substrates	Lipid, carbohydrate	Carbohydrate
Metabolites	CO_2, H_2O	Lactic acid
Glycolytic enzymes	Sparse	Abundant
Mitochondria	Abundant	Sparse
Phosphocreatine stores	Minor	Significant
Dependence on oxygen	Marked	Little
Intrinsic ATPase of contractile proteins	Low	High

The apparent luxury of a high rate of ATP production in red muscle is not without cost to the muscle. The price that such a muscle must pay is threefold: First, the muscle becomes absolutely dependent on an uninterrupted supply of oxygen without which ATP cannot be generated for contraction. Second, these muscles must contain large numbers of bulky mitochondria that occupy space otherwise available for the contractile machinery. This, as we shall see (Chapter 10), makes the muscle intrinsically weaker. The third price for this biochemical specialization is that the intrinsic rate of ATP hydrolysis by the contractile proteins is generally lower than that of the contractile proteins of white muscle. This low intrinsic rate of chemical energy utilization aids in maintaining a balance between energy utilization and energy production. Although not all red muscles contain low ATPase contractile proteins, where this adaptation is found the intrinsic speed of shortening is reduced and muscular contractility is lessened (Chapter 8).

In *white muscle* (Table 3.1), where specialization is for brief but intense activity, periods of rest allow the rate of energy expenditure to exceed temporarily that of energy production. Thus there is no need for these muscles to be provided with the highly efficient but bulky mitochondria that carry out oxidative metabolism. Instead, the volume of muscle otherwise needed for mitochondria is occupied by contractile proteins, thereby adding to the strength of the muscle. During their brief bursts of activity, white muscles utilize primarily energy stored as phosphocreatine and the limited supply of energy available from anaerobic glycolysis. The lactate produced during activity is oxidized largely during the periods of rest, either within the muscle or in the liver to which lactate is transported by the circulation. This delayed requirement for oxidative metabolism of lactate represents an "oxygen debt," in that anaerobic glycolysis during the period of contraction leaves behind a quantity of this metabolite, which must subsequently be oxidized to CO_2 and water by aerobic processes. Freed of the need to balance the rates of energy production and energy utilization during normal activity, most white muscles contain contractile proteins that have a high intrinsic rate of ATP hydrolysis. This specialization, as we shall see later (Chapter 9), permits these muscles to achieve a high velocity of shortening, so that these white muscles are properly called "fast" muscles. This specialization is clearly in accord with the functional requirement for speed (in the rabbit, for example, to facilitate escape to the burrow).

Returning to the physiological—and ecological—consequences of these biochemical differences, we can see how the rabbit escapes pursuit by a rapid dash to its burrow (the "jackrabbit" start), which utilizes a limited supply of energy stored as phosphocreatine and derived from anaerobic glycolysis. If far from the burrow, the rabbit soon tires because the phosphocreatine stores are quickly depleted and lactic acid accumulation causes the muscle cells to become acidotic, thereby arresting anaerobic glycolysis. If it reaches the safety of its burrow, the rabbit must rest in order to replenish its phosphocreatine reserves and to repay the "oxygen debt" by oxidation of lactate. The hare, on the other hand, relies on its staying power to elude pursuit. It can run long distances because during activity its red muscle regenerates ATP at the same rate at which it is being consumed. The muscle of the hare, however, requires a continuing supply of oxygen and substrate that must be delivered via the bloodstream. Furthermore, the running muscles of the hare are both slower and weaker than those of the rabbit owing to the lower intrinsic ATPase of the contractile proteins and the large volume of muscle occupied by the mitochondria. In this context it is clear that the myocardium functions like, and so has biochemical properties similar to those of, red muscle. These differences between white and red muscle were summarized concisely by Mommaerts, who said that white muscle operates on a "twitch now, pay later" basis, whereas the modus operandi of red muscle is "pay as you go."

> With few exceptions, human skeletal muscles are of a mixed type and contain three types of fibers. These are *slow oxidative*, which are similar to the red muscles described above, *fast glycolytic*, which are like white muscle (although they are pink in color), and *fast oxidative-glycolytic*, which have high ATPase contractile proteins but also contain numerous mitochondria and therefore are able to produce ATP by oxidative reactions.

It is well documented that physical training can alter the biochemical characteristics of individual muscle fibers, notably to increase the content of oxidative enzymes and mitochondria. Although individuals who successfully participate in endurance training tend to have a large fraction of muscle fibers with low myosin adenosine triphosphatase (ATPase) activity, this may be a result of self-selection; that is, athletes with a high proportion of slow muscle fibers tend to do well as marathon runners. Training itself may have some capacity to alter the relative proportions of high and low myosin ATPase fibers in skeletal muscle (Simoneau et al., 1985); however, the more important effects of training appear to be to modify capillary supply and the activities of enzymes involved in energy production (Ingjer, 1979; Tesch et al., 1985).

> A skeletal muscle abnormality that is of importance to the cardiologist is seen in patients with chronic heart failure, in whom troublesome symptoms of weakness and fatigue are due in large part to a skeletal muscle myopathy (Massie et al., 1988). This myopathy, which cannot be attributed simply to reduced perfusion and oxygen delivery to the skeletal muscle, is characterized by increased glycolytic metabolism and impaired oxidative metabolism. As these patients often improve dramatically when they increase their level of exercise, the "skeletal muscle myopathy of heart failure" may represent, in part, a form of disuse atrophy.

MUSCULAR EFFICIENCY

The term *efficiency* has many meanings, the most precise of which is that used in thermodynamics: that fraction of the free energy change associated with the chemical reactions that take place during a cycle of contraction and relaxation that appears as mechanical work. *Thermodynamic efficiency* therefore equals $W \div -\Delta G$. Because the many chemical reactions that take place during the contractile cycle are incompletely described and because the free energy changes of most individual reactions are not precisely known, a rigorous definition of thermodynamic efficiency cannot be achieved. Instead it is customary to measure the ratio between useful work and the enthalpy change that accompanies the chemical reactions which occur during contraction. Expressed in this way, *mechanical efficiency* equals $W \div -\Delta H$. In the heart, which derives its energy almost entirely by oxidative metabolism, enthalpy changes can be closely approximated by measuring the oxygen consumption. This is true because even though the amount of heat energy liberated per gram of fat oxidized ($\sim$9 kcal) is more than twice that per gram of either carbohydrate or protein ($\sim$4 kcal), the enthalpies when expressed per liter of oxygen consumed are quite similar (fat 4.69 kcal, carbohydrate 5.05 kcal, protein 4.60 kcal). This follows because more oxygen is needed to metabolize a gram of fat than a gram of either carbohydrate or protein. Regardless of the substrate being oxidized, therefore, the enthalpies of the metabolic reactions responsible for ATP production can be estimated quite well from measurements of oxygen consumption. This fact permits cardiovascular physiologists to estimate the mechanical efficiency of the heart from the ratio between useful work performed and oxygen consumed. The proportion of the energy that does not appear as useful work (i.e., that contributing to the "inefficiency" of the muscle) is liberated largely as heat (Eq. 3.2) or contributes to "internal work" (Chapter 15).

Studies of different skeletal muscles have shown that the efficiency with which a muscle performs a given type of work is determined in part by the intrinsic rate of ATP hydrolysis by the contractile proteins. The amount of energy utilized by a fast white muscle when shortening rapidly in the face of a light load is less than that of a slow red muscle, which has contractile proteins that hydrolyze ATP at a slower intrinsic rate (Table 3.1). Conversely, tension is maintained at lesser energy cost by a slow red muscle than by a fast white muscle. Thus rapidly contracting muscles, in which the contractile proteins have a high intrinsic rate of ATP hydrolysis, work most efficiently when shortening rapidly against light loads, whereas more slowly contracting muscles, with contractile proteins that have low intrinsic rates of ATP hydrolysis, function at highest efficiency when developing tension. These differences may be significant in the adaptive response of the myocardium to sustained hemodynamic overloading (Chapters 14 and 25).

Actual values for the efficiency of muscular contraction, as would be expected from the preceding discussion, depend on whether one is considering mechanical or thermodynamic efficiency. Based on measurements of external work and oxygen consumption in the working heart, mechanical efficiency ranges up to 20 to 25%. In skeletal muscle—in which a decline in high-energy phosphate, or ATP levels, can be used to calculate the denominator in the expression $W \div -\Delta H$ for mechanical efficiency—values of efficiency up to 40% can be recorded. As up to 25% of the total energy consumed during muscular activity is used not for the contractile process itself but for the release and reuptake of activator calcium (Chapter 11), the true mechanical efficiency of the contractile process is significantly higher (over 50%). The thermodynamic efficiency of the contractile process itself is probably much higher because the hydrolysis of the high-energy phosphate bond of ATP is accompanied by the release of a hydrogen ion. Neutralization of this proton by the buffer systems of the muscle liberates energy that, while it probably does not contribute to the energy available to the contractile proteins, has a significant enthalpy. As a result, almost 40% of the energy available from ATP hydrolysis can be utilized when this neutralization takes place. Thus if the energy for muscular contraction comes only from the remainder of the energy available from ATP hydrolysis, the true thermodynamic efficiency of muscle may be higher than 90%, a value which compares favorably with those of man-made machines, e.g., the gasoline engine with an efficiency of only approximately 30%.

REFERENCES

Ingjer F. (1979). Effects of endurance training on muscle fibre ATP-ase activity, capillary supply and mitochondrial content in man. *J Physiol (Lond)* 294:419–432.

Massie BM, Conway M, Rajagopalan B, Yonge R, Frostick S, Ledingham J, Sleight P, Radda G. (1988). Skeletal muscle metabolism during exercise under ischemic conditions in congestive heart failure. Evidence for abnormalties unrelated to blood flow. *Circulation* 78:320–326.

Simoneau J-A, Lortie G, Boula MR, Marcotte M, Thibault M-C, Bouchard C. (1985). Human skeletal muscle fiber type alteration with high-intensity intermittent training. *Eur J Appl Physiol* 54:250–253.

Tesch PA, Wright JE, Vogel JA, Daniels WL, Sharp DS, Sjödin B. (1985). The influence of muscle metabolic characteristics on physical performance. *Eur J Appl Physiol* 54:237–243.

BIBLIOGRAPHY

Alpert NR, Mulieri LL, Hasenfuss G. (1991). Myocardial chemo-mechanical energy transduction. In: Fozzard H, Haber E, Katz A, Jennings R, Morgan HE, eds. *The heart and cardiovascular system*, 2nd ed. New York: Raven Press: in press.

Curtin NA, Woldedge RC. (1978). Energy changes and muscular contraction. *Physiol Rev* 58:690–761.

Gibbs CL. (1974). Cardiac energetics. *Physiol Rev* 58:174–254.

Symposium. (1982). Chemical energy balance in amphibian and mammalian skeletal muscle. 41:147–184.

4

Anaerobic and
Aerobic Glycolysis

Adenosine triphosphate (ATP) is generated in the myocardium by two distinct, but linked, metabolic processes: glycolysis and oxidative phosphorylation. Although the latter normally represents the major energy-producing reaction in the heart, glycolysis also provides substrates essential for aerobic metabolism. In the hypoxic or ischemic heart, where aerobic ATP production is not possible, accelerated glycolysis can help to compensate, albeit briefly, for the cessation of aerobic metabolism. This chapter focuses on the overall scheme of glycolysis, and especially on its control. Many individual steps in this series of reactions are not described, nor are structural formulae written for most of the metabolites, this material being readily available in standard textbooks of biochemistry.

Although the control of glycolysis is extremely complex, an interesting overall pattern of regulation emerges from among the details of these reactions (see also Chapter 5): three distinct types of regulatory influences can modify the glycolytic rate. The first, exemplified by the mechanisms controlling the interconversions between glucose and glycogen, is *humoral*. Hormones and neurotransmitters, for example epinephrine, that increase energy utilization during cardiac contraction also promote the breakdown of glycogen into glucose. This humoral control allows the same signal that increases the work of the heart to provide additional substrate for energy production. A second type of control—seen in the key glycolytic reaction catalyzed by phosphofructokinase—is exerted by factors related to the *energy requirements of the cell*; in this reaction, overall glycolytic rate is accelerated when high-energy phosphates are depleted, and inhibited when ATP concentrations are high. The third type of control, seen with the enzyme glyceraldehyde-3-phosphate dehydrogenase, permits the rate of glycolysis to respond to changes in the *supply of essential coenzymes for oxidation*. This response to the redox state of the myocardial cell slows glycolysis after prolonged hypoxia or ischemia, when excessive reliance on anaerobic energy production has exhausted the supply of oxidized coenzymes. Control by reduced coenzymes also appears to be critical in regulating the rate of oxidative metabolism (Chapter 5).

The initial metabolic reactions of glycolysis, which provide for the entry of glucose and glycogen, are under *humoral control*; those toward the middle of these pathways are regulated mainly by *energy requirements*, whereas the latter steps in this pathway respond to the supply of oxidized *coenzymes* essential for substrate oxidation. In terms of the monetary analogy cited in Chapter 3, these control mechanisms are like those which regulate the flow of capital through a bank account. Expenditures are determined first by the wish to spend (hormones and neurotransmitters), second by the balance in the account (high-energy phosphates), and ultimately by the earning capacity (supply of oxidized coenzymes). Although this monetary analogy is helpful in understanding the principles by which energy production is regulated in the myocardial cells, it is an oversimplification; for example, most enzymatic reactions of energy production in the heart are subject to more than one of these control mechanisms.

In the 40 years since the author first learned of glycolysis, our appreciation of the complexity of its regulation has exploded like a Roman candle. In the 1950s I memorized a reaction sequence not unlike that shown in Fig. 4.1, learning that each step was catalyzed by an enzyme whose function was mainly to lower energy barriers, which allowed each reaction to proceed at a reasonable rate. By the 1970s, when the first edition of this book was written, it had become apparent that many of these enzymes were, in fact, highly regulated catalytic proteins. Emphasis at that time was on the compounds that regulated catalytic rate, and on the phosphorylations and dephosphorylations of many of the glycolytic enzymes. At the present time we are seeking to understand glycolytic regulation in terms of complex protein-protein, and protein-substrate interactions, many of which are influenced by a multiplicity of hierarchical phosphorylation and dephosphorylation reactions. Furthermore, it is also becoming clear that the subunits of many key enzymes are members of isoform families, and that the cell, like a fastidious diner at a three-star restaurant, selects and synthesizes specific enzyme isoforms that best suit the tastes (needs) of the moment. One can only wonder what is coming next!

ACYL PHOSPHATES AND PHOSPHOESTERS

The phosphorylation reactions involved in the regulation of many of the metabolic reactions discussed in this chapter differ markedly from the phosphorylations that activate proteins, notably in energy metabolism, contraction and the ion pumps, where high-energy phosphate bonds are formed and hydrolyzed. In the latter (e.g., the high-energy phosphate bonds in ATP, phosphocreatine, the "activated" states of myosin, and the energized ion pumps of the sarcoplasmic reticulum and Na-K-ATPase) phosphate is linked to a carboxyl group through a high-energy *acyl phosphate bond*:

$$\begin{matrix} O \\ \| \\ R-C-O\sim P. \end{matrix}$$

In contrast, in the regulatory phosphorylations, phosphate is bound to enzymes and other regulatory proteins (e.g., glycogen synthetase, phosphorylase, troponin I,

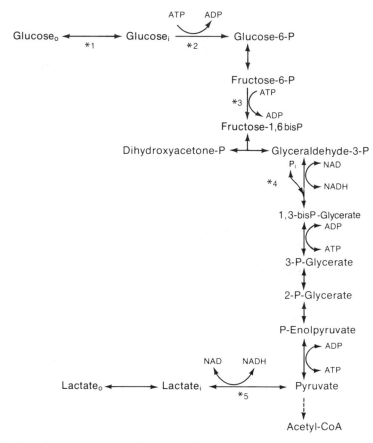

FIG. 4.1. Overall reaction scheme of glycolysis. Major control points are (*1) glucose transport; (*2) the hexokinase reaction (glucose phosphorylation); (*3) the phosphofructokinase reaction (fructose-6-phosphate phosphorylation); (*4) the glyceraldehyde-3-phosphate dehydrogenase reaction (glyceraldehyde-3-phosphate oxidation); (*5) the lactate dehydrogenase reaction (pyruvate reduction); and (*6) the pyruvate dehydrogenase reaction (formation of acetyl-CoA). Adenosine triphosphate (ATP) is utilized at two steps at the beginning of the scheme, whereas 2 moles of ATP are generated at each of two steps toward the end of the scheme, giving a net yield of 2 moles of ATP per mole of glucose. (Two moles of ATP are produced per mole of glucose at each of the reactions involving 3-carbon metabolites, whereas only 1 mole of ATP is needed to phosphorylate each mole of the 6-carbon sugars.) Glycolysis involves a single oxidative step, where nicotinamide-adenine dinucleotide (NAD) is reduced to NADH. Under anaerobic conditions, NADH can be oxidized to NAD at the step where pyruvate is reduced to lactate.

and phospholamban) in the form of *phosphoester bonds* with the hydroxyl groups of serine or threonine:

$$R-CH_2-O-P.$$

Phosphoesters are not high-energy bonds and cannot participate in energy transfer.

Enzymes that form regulatory phosphoester bonds are called *protein kinases*, and are generally named according to the messengers that cause their activation: *ade-*

nosine 3', 5'-cyclic monophosphate (cyclic AMP)-dependent protein kinase (protein kinase A), calcium, calmodulin-dependent protein kinase, and *protein kinase C* (so named because it is activated by lipids cleaved by a lipolytic enzyme: phospholipase C).

THE GLYCOLYTIC PATHWAY

The major glycolytic pathway of the heart is outlined in Fig. 4.1. In the overall reaction, one molecule of glucose is broken down to form two molecules of pyruvate under aerobic conditions, and two molecules of lactate when the heart is forced to function in the absence of a continuing supply of oxygen. Although a total of 4 moles of ATP is synthesized in the later reactions of glycolysis, *net* ATP synthesis is only 2 moles because the myocardial cell must "invest" 2 moles of ATP to phosphorylate each 6-carbon sugar. Thus, although 4 moles of ATP are recovered through the metabolism of each of two 3-carbon glucose fragments (dihydroxyacetone phosphate and glyceraldehyde-3-phosphate), the net yield is 2 moles of ATP per 6-carbon sugar.

The initial investment of phosphate-bond energy, which may seem wasteful to the cell, serves two purposes. First, the fact that glycolysis occurs through the action of soluble enzymes on soluble substrates in the cytosol requires that neither leak out of the cell in appreciable amounts. The glycolytic enzymes are large proteins that do not pass readily through the sarcolemma, but the permeability properties of the cell membrane do not prevent loss of uncharged 3- and 6-carbon sugars. As phosphorylation of these glycolytic intermediates converts the permeant, nonpolar sugars into negatively charged ions to which the sarcolemma is impermeable, the investment of phosphate-bond energy reduces the tendency of the glycolytic intermediates to leak out of the cell. The second function of phosphorylation of glycolytic intermediates is to "prime" intramolecular forces that allow additional high-energy phosphate bonds to be formed later in this sequence.

The glycolytic pathway contains one oxidative step (*4 in Fig. 4.1), in which glyceraldehyde-3-phosphate is oxidized in a reaction that incorporates inorganic phosphate into the molecule to form 1,3-bisphosphoglycerate. This step requires that the oxidized coenzyme NAD[1] (nicotinamide-adenine dinucleotide) be reduced to NADH, so that if this reaction is to proceed, a steady supply of oxidized NAD is needed. This requires that the reduced NADH be reoxidized in order for glycolysis to continue. Reoxidation of NADH to NAD normally takes place by aerobic reactions in the mitochondria (Chapter 5). When the heart functions under anaerobic conditions, as during ischemia, limited oxidation of NADH can take place through coupling to the reduction of pyruvate to lactate, a reaction that leads to the formation of large quantities of lactate.

---

[1]NAD is protonated, but for simplicity NAD rather than NAD$^+$ is used in this text.

Aerobic Versus Anaerobic Glycolysis

When the glycolytic pathway shown in Fig. 4.1 proceeds in the absence of oxygen, and pyruvate is converted to lactate, the process is called *anaerobic glycolysis*. In the presence of oxygen, on the other hand, *aerobic glycolysis* produces acetyl-coenzyme A (acetyl-CoA). The energy yields of these two types of glycolysis differ markedly.

Normally, under aerobic conditions, the pyruvate produced by aerobic glycolysis is converted to acetyl-CoA, a 2-carbon fragment that is subsequently oxidized in the tricarboxylic acid cycle (see Chapter 5). The NADH formed during aerobic glycolysis is also oxidized in the mitochondria, which generates large quantities of ATP. During anaerobic glycolysis, however, the oxidation of NADH that accompanies conversion of pyruvate to lactate provides no energy for cell function. Thus, even though anaerobic glycolysis is able to provide limited amounts of ATP, the breakdown of carbohydrate to lactate by the reactions shown in Fig. 4.1 is far from optimal in generating ATP using the energy potentially available in the glucose molecule.

> In mammalian tissues, the excess lactate produced by anaerobic glycolysis can be harmful. On the other hand, when yeast and a variety of bacteria metabolize under anaerobic conditions, they utilize their excess reducing equivalents to form ethanol, a substance that has pleasant as well as harmful effects in man, and is clearly of no small economic importance.

CONTROL OF GLYCOLYSIS

The glycolytic pathway is controlled primarily by four enzymes and by the transport of glucose into the cell; these steps are marked by an asterisk in Fig. 4.1. Each of these control points is governed by a complex mechanism of regulation.

Glucose Transport

The entry of glucose into the myocardial cell (*1 in Fig. 4.1) is carrier mediated but does not require energy as the sugar moves from a region of high concentration outside the cell to one of lower concentration in the cytosol. In this process, the combination of glucose with a glucose-carrier facilitates its diffusion across the sarcolemma, allowing this substrate to gain rapid entry into the cell.

The carrier-mediated transport of glucose into the cell can be accelerated by a number of factors, including insulin and epinephrine. The fact that glucose transport is promoted by epinephrine contributes to the ability of this neurotransmitter to accelerate glycolytic rate; the resulting increase in energy production complements the actions of epinephrine to accelerate energy utilization when it increases both contractile strength (Chapter 14) and heart rate (Chapter 23). Glucose transport is also stimulated in the hypoxic myocardium, which increases the availability of this substrate for anaerobic glycolysis under conditions where oxidative metabolism is inhibited.

Hexokinase

The enzyme *hexokinase* catalyzes glucose phosphorylation (*2 in Fig. 4.1), in a reaction that, as already pointed out, requires the investment of one molecule of ATP per molecule of glucose. Changes in the intracellular levels of glucose-6-phosphate, and to a lesser extent ATP, adenosine diphosphate (ADP), adenosine monophosphate (AMP), and P_i, play an important role in regulating the rate of hexokinase-catalyzed glucose phosphorylation. Most important of these control mechanisms is that mediated by glucose-6- phosphate, which at high concentrations inhibits the ability of hexokinase to catalyze glucose phosphorylation. Control of the hexokinase reaction by glucose-6-phosphate also helps to match glucose phosphorylation rate to the rate at which glucose-6-phosphate is consumed in subsequent glycolytic reactions (Fig. 4.1). This inhibition is not due simply to the operation of the law of mass action (i.e., by increasing the reverse of the hexokinase reaction; Fig. 4.1) because this reaction is essentially irreversible. More importantly, high concentrations of glucose-6-phosphate, a reaction product, modify the structure of the hexokinase molecule so as to exert allosteric effects that reduce the ability of hexokinase to phosphorylate glucose.

The ability of glucose-6-phosphate to inhibit hexokinase is modulated by changing concentrations of other phosphate compounds in the cell: ATP, ADP, AMP, and P_i. The high-energy compound ATP promotes the inhibitory effect of glucose-6-phosphate on hexokinase, whereas the products of ATP utilization (ADP, AMP, and P_i) blunt this inhibition and so accelerate glucose phosphorylation. In this way, the rate of the hexokinase reaction is regulated by the availability of phosphate-bond energy in the cell. These effects are due to *amplification* of the controlling influence of glucose-6-phosphate on this enzyme, much as an amplifying electronic circuit increases the strength of an electromagnetic signal. The process of amplification is described later, when regulation of the step catalyzed by phosphofructokinase is discussed.

Control by high-energy phosphates is important when the work of the heart is suddenly increased, which causes ATP levels to fall and increases those of ADP, AMP, and P_i. Thus, the ability of high-energy phosphate compounds to modify the hexokinase reaction accelerates glucose phosphorylation when ATP levels fall and the concentrations of the products of ATP hydrolysis are increased.

Phosphofructokinase

The most important point of control of the glycolytic pathway in the well-oxygenated heart is at the step where *phosphofructokinase* catalyzes the formation of fructose-1, 6- bisphosphate (*3 in Fig. 4.1). The phosphofructokinase reaction influences the rate of the preceding steps in glycolysis mainly through its ability to control the degradation of glucose-6-phosphate, which as we have seen is a major regulator of the hexokinase reaction. This key rate-limiting step in glycolysis, which like that catalyzed by hexokinase is virtually irreversible, also determines the production of the subsequent glycolytic intermediates.

> Interconversions between fructose-6-phosphate and fructose-1, 6-bisphosphate would, if both reactions were to proceed simultaneously, represent a *futile* (or *substrate*) *cycle* in which ATP is first incorporated into fructose-6-phosphate and then degraded, yielding heat but no useful energy. The fact that futile cycles do not usually occur reflects the close control exerted by the allosteric regulation of key enzymes. An exception is seen in some unusual settings; for example the bumblebee appears to use the "waste heat" from this futile cycle on cold days to warm her thoracic muscles in preparation for flight (Clark et al., 1973).

A number of substances exert important regulatory effects on phosphofructokinase (Table 4.1), largely by influencing allosteric interactions between the four $\sim$80,000 kD subunits of this tetrameric enzyme. Although the tetramer represents the smallest active oligomer of phosphofructokinase, these oligomers can form huge aggregates with molecular weights exceeding 1,000,000.

Both *high-* and *low-energy phosphate compounds* modulate the catalytic activity of this enzyme (Table 4.1). As is the case for the hexokinase reaction, the former are inhibitory and the latter stimulatory. As a result, phosphofructokinase activity is increased in the hearts of patients following a coronary artery occlusion. In this situation, where high-energy phosphates are depleted, marked acceleration of glycolysis during the initial response to ischemia can be attributed to the increased cellular concentrations of ADP, P_i, and, most important, AMP, and to the declining concentration of ATP and phosphocreatine (Chapter 24).

Another important activator of phosphofructokinase activity is fructose 2,6- bisphosphate, which is produced from fructose-6-phosphate in a reaction catalyzed by *6-phosphofructo-2-kinase*. This reaction parallels that catalyzed by phosphofruc-

TABLE 4.1. *Regulation of phosphofructose activity in the heart*

Humoral	
Cyclic AMP	Stimulation
Mediated by fructose 2,6-bisphosphate stimulation	
Calcium	Stimulation
Phosphate compounds	
ATP	Inhibition
ADP	Stimulation
AMP	Stimulation
P_i	Stimulation
Phosphenolpyruvate	Inhibition
Metabolic integration	
Citrate	Inhibition
Ammonia	Stimulation
H^+	Inhibition

tokinase, which according to this terminology, would be "6-phosphofructo-1-kinase."

Regulation of 6-phosphofructo-2-kinase activity by cyclic AMP allows β-adrenergic agonists to stimulate the phosphofructose reaction. This occurs when 6-phosphofructo-2-kinase is phosphorylated by protein kinase A, which by increasing the formation of fructose 2,6-bisphosphate, activates phosphofructokinase.

Regulation by fructose 2,6-bisphosphate is highly tissue specific; in the liver, 6-phosphofructo-2-kinase is inhibited by cyclic AMP, the second messenger produced when the cell is stimulated by epinephrine (Pilkis et al., 1982). In contrast, the cardiac enzyme is activated by cyclic AMP (Kitamura et al., 1988). This important difference is readily understood in terms of the different functions of the heart and liver: the heart uses glucose for contraction, whereas the liver synthesizes glucose for other organs of the body. During exercise, for example, epinephrine promotes gluconeogenesis in the hepatocyte, and glycogen breakdown in the myocardium (Clark and Patten, 1984).

Production of fructose 2,6-bisphosphate by the cyclic AMP–sensitive enzyme 6-phosphofructo-2-kinase represents an important mechanism that mediates the *humoral control* of phosphofructokinase, in which epinephrine stimulates this enzyme, albeit indirectly, in the heart. β-adrenergic agonists may also stimulate the phosphofructokinase reaction through the increased intracellular Ca^{2+} concentration that accompanies the inotropic response.

Citrate, an intermediate of the tricarboxylic acid cycle (see Chapter 5) has an important action to inhibit phosphofructokinase. This aspect of the control of phosphofructokinase activity allows increased aerobic metabolism, which produces citrate, to slow glycolysis. This inhibitory effect of citrate thus plays an essential role in integrating glycolytic rate with that of oxidative metabolism.

Regulation of glycolytic rate by the phosphofructokinase reaction contributes to the integration between glycolysis and oxidative metabolism called the *Pasteur effect*. Described in 1861 when Louis Pasteur examined the production of alcohol during yeast fermentation, this effect reflects the ability of oxygen to inhibit carbohydrate uptake and metabolism. The Pasteur effect occurs when anaerobic glycolysis is slowed at the step catalyzed by phosphofructokinase by inhibitory effects of the ATP and citrate produced during active oxidative metabolism.

Acidosis exerts a powerful inhibitory effect on phosphofructokinase; this inhibition contributes to the eventual slowing of glycolysis that follows its transient acceleration in the ischemic myocardium (see also Chapter 24). The ability of ammonium ion to stimulate phosphofructokinase may represent a part of a mechanism that provides substrates for the trapping of NH_4^+ in the cell.

Amplification

One feature of the mechanisms by which glycolytic flux is regulated by phosphofructokinase warrants some elaboration. This mechanism, called *amplification*, allows enzymatic reactions to be tightly regulated while avoiding large changes in substrate concentration. For example, in a first-order reaction that does not show amplication, more than an 80-fold increase in substrate concentration would be needed to increase enzyme activity from 10 to 90% of its maximum. (This value is readily calculated from classic saturation kinetics.) The existence of cooperative (allosteric) interactions between the enzyme and its substrate can obviate the need for such large fluctuations in substrate concentration. For example, if there were four cooperative binding sites for a substrate, an increase in activity from 10 to 90% of maximal activity would require an approximately fourfold, rather than a ninefold increase in substrate concentration. Such changes in the concentrations of a substrate like ATP would, however, be detrimental to cellular energetics because, from a thermodynamic standpoint, the free energy made available by ATP hydrolysis decreases when ATP concentration falls and ADP rises. (A fourfold decrease in ATP concentration with a concomitant increase in ADP concentration would reduce the energy released during ATP hydrolysis by approximately one-third.) It is probably for this reason that our cells have evolved elaborate mechanisms to amplify the effects of changing ATP concentration that allow a variety of cellular systems, including phosphofructokinase, to respond to very small changes in ATP concentration.

Amplification in the control of phosphofructokinase reaction is achieved by an interplay between ATP, ADP, and AMP in which ATP inhibits the enzyme, and the products of ATP hydrolysis counteract these inhibitory effects. To understand this interplay, it is essential to recognize that the concentrations of ATP, ADP, and AMP are maintained in equilibrium by the enzyme *adenylate kinase* (myokinase), which catalyzes the reaction:

$$ATP + AMP \leftrightarrow 2ADP.$$

The equilibrium constant for this enzyme maintains AMP concentration at an extremely low level, which allows the heart to respond to net breakdown of ATP with little change in the concentration of ATP and its first hydrolytic product, ADP. At the physiological ATP/ADP ratio of approximately 9:1, assuming total adenine nucleotide concentration to be 5 mM, the equilibrium constant for adenylate kinase would maintain ATP concentration at 4.48 mM, ADP at 0.5 mM, and AMP at 0.02 mM.

> Maintenance of a low AMP concentration is also important because it is rapidly deaminated to form inosine; were this to occur in the heart, the adenine nucleotide pool (ATP, ADP, AMP) would soon be depleted. In fact, when excessive ATP hydrolysis does take place—in the ischemic heart—the resulting depletion of adenine nucleotides takes several days to be replenished by *de novo* adenine synthesis (Chapter 24).

According to the equilibrium constant for adenylate kinase, a 13% fall in ATP concentration, to 3.89 mM, would at equilibrium, double ADP concentration to 1.0 mM and increase AMP concentration more than fivefold, to 0.11 mM. These proportionately large increases in AMP and ADP concentrations amplify the slight change in ATP concentration severalfold. These changes, which can be initiated by marked acceleration of high-energy phosphate utilization, would stimulate glycolysis at the step catalyzed by phosphofructokinase by an allosteric effect of de-creased ATP concentration that is amplified by the more marked increases in ADP and AMP concentrations. The advantages of this amplification are clear; the cell is able to call effectively for the rapid regeneration of high-energy phosphates, while avoiding both a large fall in ATP concentration, which would reduce the free energy released by ATP hydrolysis, and an increase in AMP, which could deplete adenine nucleotides.

Glyceraldehyde-3 Phosphate Dehydrogenase

Oxidation of glyceraldehyde-3-phosphate and the resulting formation of 1,3-bis-phosphoglycerate (*4 in Fig. 4.1) couples an oxidative reaction, in which NAD is reduced to NADH + H$^+$, (Fig. 4.1) to the formation of a second high-energy phosphate bond in the 3-carbon sugar. This reaction, which is catalyzed by *glyceraldehyde-3-phosphate dehydrogenase*, is not of major importance in regulating glycolysis in the aerobic heart, where the phosphofructokinase reaction is rate limiting. However, when the heart is performing high levels of work, and especially under conditions of hypoxia or ischemia, a fall in ATP concentration and rises of ADP, AMP, and P$_i$ levels strongly activate phosphofructokinase. Under these conditions, control of overall glycolytic rate shifts to later reactions in the glycolytic pathway, notably that catalyzed by glyceraldehyde-3-phosphate dehydrogenase. This enzyme is regulated largely by product inhibition, being extremely sensitive to the inhibitory effects of 1,3-bisphosphoglycerate and NADH; thus, when the heart becomes unable to oxidize NADH, as occurs under anaerobic conditions, accumulation of reduced NADH slows glycolysis. In this way regulation of glycolysis in the anaerobic heart shifts to a different step, and involves different metabolites than those which control the rate-limiting phosphofructokinase reaction in the well-oxygenated heart.

Looked at another way, the control of glycolytic rate changes drastically when oxygen demands greatly exceed oxygen delivery. Under conditions of low cardiac work, and when there is an abundant supply of oxygen, glycolysis is regulated mainly by high-energy phosphate compounds at the step catalyzed by phosphofructokinase, which accelerates glycolysis when ATP is consumed more rapidly than it is being generated. When ATP consumption is drastically increased, or under anaerobic conditions, glycolytic flux at the step catalyzed by phosphofructokinase becomes accelerated and is no longer rate limiting; instead, regulation of glycolysis shifts to the later step catalyzed by glyceraldehyde-3-phosphate dehydrogenase which, unlike phosphofructokinase, is regulated mainly by factors related to the redox state of the cell, notably the level of reduced NADH. For this reason, glycolytic control in the ischemic heart (Chapter 24) shifts from a step that is governed by energy needs (*3 in Fig. 4.1) to one in which control is exerted by the ability of the cell to oxidize substrates and coenzymes (*4 in Fig. 4.1).

Pyruvate Kinase

In some tissues, *pyruvate kinase*, which catalyzes the formation of pyruvate and ATP from phosphoenolpyruvate and ADP—the step in which net ATP synthesis occurs—is of considerable regulatory importance. In the heart, however, this enzyme plays little role in metabolic control.

Lactate Dehydrogenase

Anaerobic glycolysis, which by definition occurs in the absence of oxygen, ends when lactate is produced from pyruvate. In contrast, aerobic glycolysis, the normal glycolytic mechanism in the heart, does not lead to lactate formation; instead, pyruvate is converted to acetyl-CoA, which is then degraded to CO_2 and H_2O (see below).

The reaction in which pyruvate is reduced to lactate (*5 in Fig. 4.1) provides the anaerobic heart with a limited capacity to regenerate oxidized NAD for the glyceraldehyde-3-phosphate dehydrogenase reaction (see above). This reaction is catalyzed by the enzyme *lactate dehydrogenase*. In white skeletal muscles, which depend mainly on anaerobic glycolysis for energy production (Chapter 3), lactate dehydrogenase is of major importance in providing NAD for the earlier steps in glycolysis. However, in the well-oxygenated heart, NAD is regenerated from NADH by the mitochondria (Chapter 5).

Lactate dehydrogenase is a tetramer made up of two types of 35,000 dalton subunit: M (found mainly in skeletal muscle), and H (found mainly in the heart). All five possible combinations can be found: H_4, H_3M, H_2M_2, HM_3, and M_4. Differences in the fate of pyruvate among different muscle types are reflected in the lactate dehydrogenase isoforms found in cardiac and skeletal muscle. In skeletal muscles that depend mainly on glycolysis for their energy supply (Table 3.1), the M subunits of lactate dehydrogenase have a high affinity for pyruvate, so that pyruvate is preferentially reduced to lactate. In the myocardium, on the other hand, the H subunits have a low affinity for pyruvate; as a result, pyruvate is not normally reduced to lactate unless, as in the ischemic heart, pyruvate levels become very high. Instead, in the well-oxygenated heart, pyruvate is converted by pyruvate dehydrogenase to acetyl-CoA, a 2-carbon fragment that is subsequently oxidized in the tricarboxylic acid cycle (see below). Although the reaction catalyzed by lactate dehydrogenase plays a little role in determining the metabolic fate of pyruvate in the normal myocardium, lactate production can be viewed as a "safety valve" that allows some NAD to be regenerated for anaerobic glycolysis.

GLYCOGEN FORMATION AND BREAKDOWN

Glycogen represents a storage form of glucose that can be readily mobilized by the heart. Its synthesis and breakdown do not occur by forward and reverse fluxes through a single series of reactions; but instead involve two separate pathways, each of which is controlled by a highly regulated enzyme (Fig. 4.2). The enzymes that control glycogen formation (*glycogen synthetase*) and glycogen breakdown (*phosphorylase*) both exist physiologically in active and inactive forms. Interconversions between these different forms of the enzymes are regulated by a fascinating, reciprocating, series of reactions that are under hormonal control.

As noted at the beginning of this chapter, three types of regulatory mechanism control glycolytic rate. The first, humoral control, has been seen to regulate glucose transport and thus the entry of substrate into the glycolytic pathway. The second, control by the availability of high-energy phosphate, is manifest most strikingly by the enzyme phosphofructokinase, which in the normal heart is the rate-limiting glycolytic enzyme. The third, regulation by the ability of the cell to reoxidize reduced coenzymes, is seen in the control exerted by glyceraldehyde-3-phosphate dehydrogenase, an enzyme that can become rate limiting when oxygen is in short supply. The first of these mechanisms—control by circulating hormones and neurotransmitters—also plays a major role in determining the rate of glycogen formation and breakdown, although regulation by high-energy phosphates is also significant.

The transfer of glucose units to glycogen involves two reactions (Fig. 4.2), one of which utilizes the nucleotide *uridine* to activate the glucose subunits. The first, in which uridine diphosphoglucose (UDPG) is formed by the condensation of glucose-1-phosphate with uridine triphosphate (UTP), is not rate limiting, but instead uses the phosphate-bond energy of UTP to activate glucose-1-phosphate. The second reaction, addition of the activated sugar to glycogen and release of uridine diphosphate (UDP) is rate limiting.

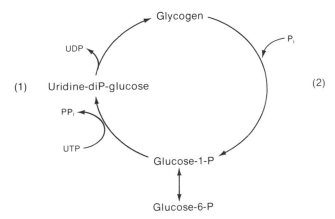

FIG. 4.2. Pathways of glycogen synthesis (*left*, reading upward) differ from those of glycogenolysis (*right*, reading downward). Glycogen synthesis is controlled mainly by glycogen synthetase, which catalyzes reaction 1. Glycogenolysis is regulated by phosphorylase, which catalyzes reaction 2.

Glycogen Synthetase and Glycogen Formation

Glycogen synthesis is controlled by the catalytic activity of *glycogen synthetase*, a highly regulated tetrameric enzyme made up of 90,000 dalton subunits. Glycogen synthetase can exist in two major forms whose interconversions are controlled by phosphorylation reactions that are, in turn, hormonally regulated.

The *a* (dephospho-) form of glycogen synthetase, which is the more active form of the enzyme, is converted to the less active *b* (phospho) form when the heart is stimulated by β-adrenergic agonists like epinephrine, which increase cellular levels of cyclic AMP. Cyclic AMP accelerates the reaction shown in Fig. 4.3A, in which a *cyclic AMP–dependent protein kinase* tranfers the terminal phosphate of ATP to form a phosphoester bond in glycogen synthetase. The protein kinase A that catalyzes the phosphorylation of glycogen synthetase is itself controlled by the level of cyclic AMP within the cell.

When cyclic AMP stimulates the phosphorylation of glycogen synthetase *a*, the less active glycogen synthetase *b* is formed. This reaction thus allows sympathetic stimulation, which increases cyclic AMP production, to "turn off" glycogen synthesis at the same time that the sympathetic nervous system increases cardiac energy utilization, as occurs during exercise.

Glycogen formation can be returned to its high, basal rate by the enzyme *synthetase phosphatase*, which dephosphorylates glycogen synthetase *b* to form dephosphorylated glycogen synthetase *a* (Fig. 4.3B). The latter is independent of control by several regulatory substances, most important of which is glucose-6-phosphate, which promotes the full catalytic activity of the phosphorylated glycogen synthetase *b*. Glucose-6-phosphate controls glycogen synthetase *b* activity through its ability to reverse inhibitory effects of many substrates and metabolites normally found in the myocardium. Dephosphorylation of the inactive glycogen synthetase *b* to form a more active glycogen synthetase *a* is, therefore, not a true

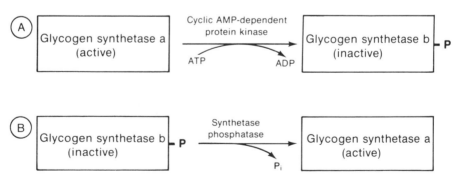

FIG. 4.3. Phosphorylation (A) and dephosphorylation (B) reactions that modulate glycogen synthetase activity. A: Phosphorylation by a cyclic AMP–dependent protein kinase converts the active, dephosphorylated glycogen synthetase *a* to the inactive, phosphorylated glycogen synthetase *b*. B: Dephosphorylation by synthetase phosphatase converts the inactive, phosphorylated glycogen synthetase *b* to the active, dephosphorylated glycogen synthetase *a*.

"activation" of the enzyme; instead, dephosphorylation of glycogen synthetase *b* accelerates glycogen synthesis by freeing the enzyme from the inhibitory effects of regulatory influences within the cell. Conversely, the physiological slowing of glycogen synthesis occurs when phosphorylation by protein kinase A converts the enzyme to its more highly regulated *b* form, in which the enzyme is resensitized to these inhibitory effects.

Glycogen synthetase contains multiple sites for phosphorylation, and can be phosphorylated by at least ten types of protein kinase, including protein kinase A, calcium, calmodulin–dependent protein kinases, and phosphorylase kinase (Cohen, 1986) Indeed, very few protein kinases lack the ability to phosphorylate this highly receptive enzyme! The hospitality of glycogen synthetase is also manifest in the ability of several phosphatases to dephosphorylate its *b* form.

It should be noted that not all phosphorylations significantly inactivate this enzyme; in general, secondary phosphorylations have greater effects than initial phosphorylations, suggesting that they proceed in a hierarchical fashion (Roach, 1990). The remarkable susceptibility of glycogen synthetase to modification by multiple phosphorylation reactions probably provides a "fine-tuning" that allows this enzyme to respond to a variety of physiological interventions.

Phosphorylase and Glycogen Breakdown

The enzyme *phosphorylase* is largely responsible for controlling the breakdown of glycogen to form glucose-1-phosphate (reaction 2 in Fig. 4.2.) Like glycogen synthetase, phosphorylase exists in phosphorylated and dephosphorylated forms (Fig. 4.4); however, in contrast to the two forms of glycogen synthetase, the phos-

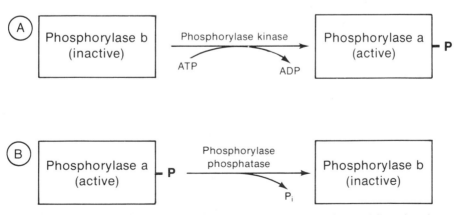

FIG. 4.4. Phosphorylation (A) and dephosphorylation (B) reactions that modulate phosphorylase activity. A: Phosphorylation by phosphorylase kinase, a calcium-calmodulin–dependent protein kinase, converts the inactive, dephosphorylated phosphorylase *b* to the active, phosphorylated phosphorylase *a*. B: Dephosphorylation by phosphorylase phosphatase converts the active, phosphorylated phosphorylase *a* to the inactive, dephosphorylated phosphorylase *b*.

phorylated phosphorylase *a* is the active enzyme, whereas the dephosphorylated phosphorylase *b* is a less active, regulated, form of the enzyme. The interconversions of phosphorylase by protein kinase A are basically similar to those of glycogen synthetase, but control of the phosphorylating enzymes differs (see below).

Phosphorylase *b*, like the less active glycogen synthetase *b*, is not really inactive. Instead, phosphorylase *b* activity is less than that of phosphorylase *a* because the high concentrations of glucose-6-phosphate and ATP normally present in the cell inhibit the full expression of its activity. Thus, hormonal regulation of both glycogen synthetase and phosphorylase does not convert an inactive enzyme to an active enzyme, or vice versa; rather, phosphorylation and dephosphorylation of these enzymes alters their sensitivity to control by other cell metabolites. In the case of glycogen synthetase, phosphorylation increases inhibitory control, whereas phosphorylation of phosphorylase causes inhibitory control to be reduced.

> Phosphorylase, like many of the enzymes already discussed in this chapter, is an oligomeric protein. In skeletal muscle, phosphorylase *a* is a tetramer of nearly identical subunits and phosphorylase *b* is a dimer. In the heart, however, both phosphorylase *a* and *b* are dimers.

Phosphorylase b kinase, the enzyme that catalyzes the phosphorylation of phosphorylase *b*, is a calcium, calmodulin–dependent protein kinase. As a result, the activity of phosphorylase kinase, and thus the conversion of phosphorylase *b* to phosphorylase *a*, is regulated by cytosolic Ca^{2+} levels. At the low Ca^{2+} concentrations found in the resting myocardium (~ 0.1 μM), phosphorylase kinase is inhibited, so that phosphorylase is largely in the dephospho- form (phosphorylase *b*). Phosphorylase kinase activity is markedly increased at Ca^{2+} concentrations above 1 μM, as occur when the heart contracts. The physiological consequences of the control of this enzyme by calcium, which are readily demonstrated in studies of the enzyme *in vitro*, are probably related to glycogen mobilization during periods of active cardiac work, when average cytosolic Ca^{2+} levels are high.

Phosphorylase *b* kinase is a protein complex containing four different subunits; the largest can be present as either of at least two isoforms. Another subunit binds to calcium, and is quite similar to calmodulin. This enzyme also contains multiple sites for phosphorylations that can be catalyzed by a number of protein kinases, including those activated by cyclic AMP. Although phosphorylase kinase is not *directly* controlled by cyclic AMP, this second messenger has an important *indirect* effect that is mediated by phosphorylation of yet another enzyme, *phosphorylase kinase kinase*, which increases the activity of this enzyme. This effect is described below, when the overall actions of cyclic AMP on glycogen metabolism are summarized.

Interplay Between Glycogen Synthetase and Phosphorylase

The effects of protein phosphorylation and dephosphorylation on the enzymes responsible for glycogen synthesis and breakdown provide a reciprocating system by which hormones and neurotransmitters that promote cyclic AMP production in the heart are able to control the net flux of glucose-1-phosphate into and out of intracellular glycogen stores (Fig. 4.2). Cyclic AMP–induced phosphorylation of these enzymes both inhibits glycogen synthesis (Fig. 4.3) and stimulates glycogen breakdown (Fig. 4.4), whereas their dephosphorylation has opposite effects (Figs. 4.3 and 4.4) that shift the balance toward glycogen synthesis (Fig. 4.5). Before describing Fig. 4.5, however, it is useful to compare and contrast the control exerted by cyclic AMP on glycogen synthesis with that exerted on glycogen breakdown.

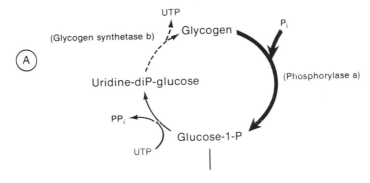

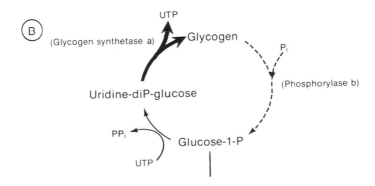

FIG. 4.5. Interlocking control of glycogen formation and breakdown by phosphorylation-dephosphorylation of the regulatory enzymes glycogen synthetase and phosphorylase. A: When both enzymes are phosphorylated, glycogen synthetase is in the inactive *b* form, and phosphorylase is in the active *a* form. Hence, glycogen synthesis is inhibited and glycogen breakdown accelerated. B: When both enzymes are dephosphorylated, glycogen synthetase is in the active *a* form and phosphorylase is in the inactive *b* form. Hence, glycogen synthesis is accelerated and glycogen breakdown inhibited.

In the case of glycogen synthetase, cyclic AMP is *directly* involved in the conversion of the dephosphorylated (active) form of the enzyme to the phosphorylated (inactive) form (Fig. 4.3). This control results when cyclic AMP activates a protein kinase that catalyzes the phosphorylation of glycogen synthetase. In contrast, conversion of the dephosphorylated (inactive) form of phosphorylase into the phosphorylated (active) form is not *directly* dependent on cyclic AMP; instead, an *indirect* mechanism explains the ability of cyclic AMP to regulate phosphorylase *b* phosphorylation, and thus the rate of glycogen breakdown. This indirect control by cyclic AMP is exerted through its direct stimulation of the phosphorylation of yet another enzyme: *phosphorylase kinase*.

Phosphorylase kinase, like glycogen synthetase and phosphorylase, can exist in phosphorylated and dephosphorylated forms (Fig. 4.6). Cyclic AMP promotes the phosphorylation of phosphorylase kinase by activating *phosphorylase kinase kinase*, another cyclic AMP–dependent protein kinase that converts the inactive dephospho- form of phosphorylase kinase to the active phospho- form (Fig. 4.6). The active phosphorylase kinase is inactivated when it is dephosphorylated by a phosphatase called *phosphorylase kinase phosphatase*.

In the last analysis, therefore, *both glycogen synthesis and breakdown are controlled by cyclic AMP*. This hormonal control favors glycogen breakdown when cardiac energy utilization is stimulated by the sympathetic neurotransmitters, as during exercise. The only essential difference between the control of glycogen synthesis and glycogen breakdown is the specific point in the "cascade" of enzymatic reactions at which the cyclic AMP–dependent phosphorylation occurs (Fig. 4.7).

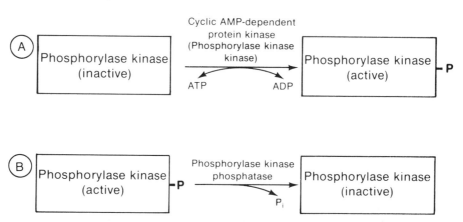

FIG. 4.6. Phosphorylation (A) and dephosphorylation (B) reactions that control the activity of phosphorylase kinase. A: Phosphorylation by a cyclic AMP–dependent protein kinase (phosphorylase kinase kinase) converts the inactive, dephosphorylated form of phosphorylase to the active, phosphorylated form. B: Dephosphorylation by phosphorylase kinase phosphatase converts the active, phosphorylated phosphorylase kinase to the inactive, dephosphorylated form.

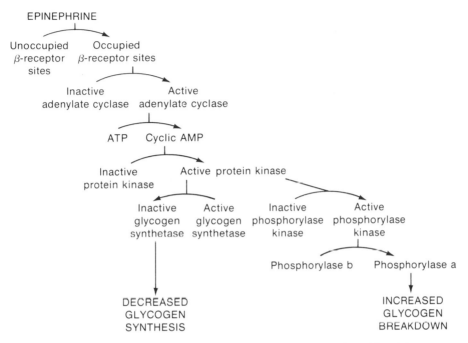

FIG. 4.7. Cascade of reactions that allows rates of glycogen synthesis and breakdown to respond to a β-adrenergic agonist (e.g., epinephrine). The reactions in this cascade mediate a decrease in glycogen synthesis and an increase in glycogen breakdown in response to humoral influence that increases cyclic AMP production. The earlier steps in this cascade—those leading to cyclic AMP formation—are discussed in Chapter 12.

The earlier portions of the cascade introduced in Fig. 4.7 are discussed more extensively in Chapter 12. At this point attention should be directed to two major features of the control of glycogen synthesis and breakdown: first, that a complex cascade of chemical reactions mediates the action of cyclic AMP on glycogen metabolism (Fig. 4.7); and second, that glycogen synthesis and glycogen breakdown are subject to a reciprocating control that allows β-adrenergic stimulation to promote reactions that stimulate glycogen breakdown and inhibit glycogen synthesis (Fig. 4.5).

"Debranching" Enzymes

Glycogen is a highly branched polysaccharide, but phosphorylase cannot catalyze the removal of glucose residues near the many branch points of this polymer. Thus, the latter must be removed by "debranching" enzymes. Although molecular defects in these enzymes contribute to certain rare glycogen storage diseases, the debranching enzymes do not appear to be rate limiting for glycogen breakdown in the normal heart.

Aerobic Glycolysis

In the well-oxygenated heart, glycolysis is an aerobic process. Whereas the end product of anaerobic glycolysis is lactate (see above), that of aerobic glycolysis is acetyl-CoA, a 2-carbon fragment that can be oxidized within the mitochondria (*6 in Fig. 4.1). The 2-carbon fragments that enter the tricarboxylic acid cycle are not free acetate, but a complex with coenzyme A, abbreviated CoA-SH because the coenzyme contains a sulfhydryl group. In the complex between acetate and CoA-SH, acetate is attached to the sulfhydryl group of CoA by a high-energy thioester bond, much as the γ-phosphate group is attached to ATP by a high-energy phospho-ester bond. CoA "activates" acetate; that is, its energy is transferred to the acetyl-CoA complex so as to facilitate its reactivity in the subsequent reactions of aerobic metabolism. Formation of acetyl-CoA, both from carbohydrates during aerobic gly-colysis and from the β-oxidation of fatty acids (Chapter 5), takes place in the mito-chondria. The reactions that generate the 2-carbon fragments that are subsequently oxidized within the mitochondria, represent another major site at which energy production in the heart can be regulated.

Pyruvate Dehydrogenase

The formation of acetyl-CoA from pyruvate during aerobic glycolysis is cata-lyzed by a highly regulated enzyme complex called *pyruvate dehydrogenase*. (PDH) The overall reaction catalyzed by this enzyme involves the decarboxylation of pyruvate, activation of the resulting 2-carbon fragment by the formation of a complex first with thiamine pyrophosphate (TPP) and then with lipoic acid, and finally replacement of the lipoic acid with CoA to yield acetyl-CoA (Fig. 4.8). A "side" reaction oxidizes the reduced SH·SH lipoic acid (dihydrolipoic acid), formed during the overall reaction, to restore the (S·S) lipoic acid required for this reaction. One reaction in this sequence is not reversible: that of pyruvate decarboxylation.

The series of reactions in which pyruvate is converted to acetyl-CoA is catalyzed by a huge multienzyme complex. It is rather difficult to grasp the intricacy of this enzyme, which has been estimated to contain upward of 150 subunits having an aggregate molecular weight of 8,500,000 (Reed and Yeaman, 1986). The PDH complex contains three component enzymes that catalyze the linked reaction se-quence shown in Fig. 4.9. The first enzyme is a *dehydrogenase* that decarboxylates pyruvate at a step in which TPP is incorporated into the 2-carbon fragment formed when CO_2 is liberated from pyruvate; this dehydrogenase also replaces the sub-strate-bound TPP with lipoic acid.

Beriberi heart disease, a rare nutritional cardiomyopathy caused by thiamine defi-ciency (in the United States seen mainly in alcoholics) weakens the myocardium by depriving this key oxidative reaction of TPP. The hemodynamic picture in this condi-tion is dominated by high output failure, which is due to vasodilatation that results from the effects of thiamine deficiency on skeletal muscle.

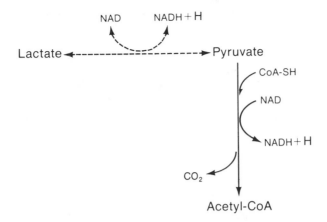

FIG. 4.8. Overall reaction that leads to the production of a 2-carbon fragment as the final step in aerobic glycolysis. Decarboxylation of pyruvate leads to formation of acetyl-CoA, the 2-carbon fragment that is subsequently oxidized in the tricarboxylic acid.

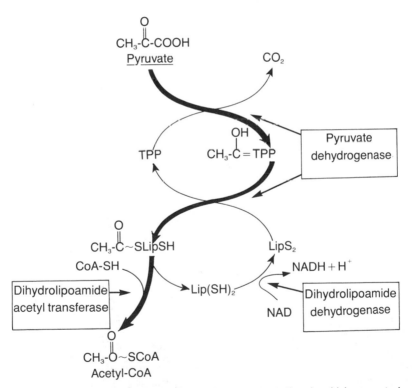

FIG. 4.9. Major reactions in the pyruvate dehydrogenase reaction, in which pyruvate is converted to acetyl-CoA (*heavy lines*) by three component enzymes (pyruvate dehydrogenase, dihydrolipoamide acetyltransferase, and dihydrolipoamide dehydrogenase). Lipoic acid in the oxidized form, (S·S)-lipoic acid, is reduced to (SH·SH) lipoic acid and so must be reoxidized to allow the overall reaction to continue.

The second component enzyme of PDH is a *dihydrolipoamide acetyltransferase*, which replaces the substrate-bound lipoic acid with CoA. Finally, a flavoprotein *dihydrolipoamide dehydrogenase* catalyzes the reoxygenation of dihydrolipoic acid in a reaction where NAD is reduced to NADH.

Regulation of PDH activity involves interactions among its many subunits, as well as with the substrates and cofactors. The overall reaction involves, and so can be influenced by, CoA-SH, lipoic acid, TPP, and NAD. In addition, the PDH reaction is subject to physiological control by changing Ca^{2+} and Mg^{2+} concentrations. Like glycogen synthetase, PDH contains multiple phosphorylation sites. The protein kinase that controls PDH phosphorylation, which is an integral part of the PDH complex, is not regulated by cyclic AMP, but is activated by the reaction products (NADH and acetyl-CoA) and inhibited by the substrates (pyruvate, coenzyme A, and NAD) and ADP (Table 4.2). This key enzyme, and so acetyl-CoA formation, is inactivated by phosphorylation of the enzyme, and reactivated by dephosphorylation, as summarized in Table 4.2.

Acetyl-CoA formation by the PDH reaction is inhibited directly by acetyl-CoA and NADH, the products of the PDH reaction, and indirectly by phosphorylation of the enzyme. In the heart, PDH phosphorylation and dephosphorylation, rather than product inhibition, appear to provide the most important regulation of this enzyme (Fig. 4.10). Phosphorylation of the pyrvuate dehydrogenase complex totally inactivates the enzyme, which unlike glycogen synthetase and phosphorylase, is not subject to allosteric regulation. In view of the total inhibition of PDH by phosphorylation, it is not surprising that both its phosphorylation and dephosphorylation are extensively regulated.

Phosphorylation of PDH is catalyzed by yet another enzyme, *pyruvate dehydrogenase kinase*. The latter is influenced by calcium, which by a rather convoluted mechanism (see below), allows the increased cytosolic Ca^{2+} concentration that ac-

TABLE 4.2. *Regulation of pyruvate dehydrogenase*

Direct: (effects on pyruvate dehydrogenase itself)	
Acetyl-CoA	Inhibition[a]
NADH	Inhibition
Indirect: (phosphorylation by pyruvate dehydrogenase kinase)	
Acetyl-CoA	Inhibition (by stimulating phosphorylation)
NADH	Inhibition (by stimulating phosphorylation)
ADP	Stimulation (by inhibiting phosphorylation)
Pyruvate	Stimulation (by inhibiting phosphorylation)
Thiamine diphosphate	Stimulation (by inhibiting phosphorylation)
Indirect: (dephosphorylation by pyruvate dehydrogenase phosphatase)	
Calcium	Stimulation (by stimulating dephosphorylation)
InsP$_3$[b]	Stimulation (probably calcium mediated, see above)
NAD	Inhibition (by inhibiting dephosphorylation)
NADH	Stimulation (by stimulating dephosphorylation)
Citrate	Inhibition (by inhibiting dephosphorylation)

[a]Effects listed are on the overall pyruvate dehydrogenase reaction.
[b]InsP$_3$: Inositol 1,4,5-trisphosphate.

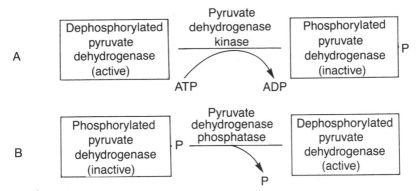

FIG. 4.10. Phosphorylation (A) and dephosphorylation (B) reactions that modulate pyruvate dehydrogenase activity. A: Phosphorylation by pyruvate dehydrogenase kinase converts the active, dephosphorylated pyruvate dehydrogenase to the inactive phosphorylated enzyme. B: Dephosphorylation by pyruvate dehydrogenase phosphatase converts the inactive enzyme to the active, dephosphorylated pyruvate dehydrogenase.

companies an increase in myocardial contractility to increase the flux of substrates through the reaction catalyzed by PDH (Bünger and Permanetter, 1984). The phosphorylation reaction that inactivates PDH is promoted by NADH which inhibits pyruvate dehydrogenase kinase; this effect is reversed by NAD. Thus, NADH (a reaction product) inhibits this enzyme indirectly.

The *pyruvate dehydrogenase phosphatase* that reactivates PDH also plays a key role in regulating acetyl-CoA formation. This enzyme is inhibited by NADH. In the ischemic heart, therefore, when NADH accumulates, formation of acetyl-CoA from pyruvate is inhibited. Instead, lactate is produced in an anaerobic reaction that, as pointed out earlier, leads to the formation of additional NAD. Pyruvate dehydrogenase phosphatase is also inhibited by citrate; the ability of this tricarboxylic acid cycle intermediate to inhibit the glycolytic production of 2-carbon fragments allows active fatty acid oxidation, which also produces acetyl-CoA in reactions that regenerate much larger amounts of ATP (Chapter 5), to inhibit carbohydrate metabolism. This represents an important mechanism for the integration of carbohydrate and lipid metabolism.

In addition to the indirect—but highly important—control by phosphorylation and dephosphorylation, active (dephosphorylated) PDH is inhibited by acetyl-CoA and NADH; the inhibitory effects of these reaction products are competitive with the stimulatory effects of the corresponding substrates: coenzyme A and NAD. Thus, acetyl- CoA formation is regulated by the ratios acetyl-CoA/coenzyme A and NADH/NAD.

The complexity of the enzyme complex that governs this step in carbohydrate metabolism can be understood when it is recognized that the metabolic fate of pyruvate stands at the crossroads between anaerobic and aerobic metabolism. Pyruvate can be converted to lactate (Fig. 4.1), thereby regenerating oxidized NAD for anaerobic glycolysis, as in the ischemic heart (see Chapter 24); whereas in the well-oxygenated heart, PDH favors the oxidative metabolism of pyruvate by forming the activated 2-carbon fragment, acetyl-CoA (Fig. 4.8).

Pyruvate, which is an α-keto acid, can be readily transaminated to form the amino acid alanine. Conversely, amino acids are able to enter the metabolic pathways of energy production by transamination of alanine to form pyruvate. Thus, the PDH reaction also contributes to the limited capacity of the heart to use amino acids as a source of energy.

As noted in the first edition, the existence of multiple, interacting control mechanisms at this important step in intermediary metabolism is in accord with the general rule that the more critical the reaction, the more checks and balances are provided by nature. The operation of this rule is apparent throughout this text. Nature is neither simple nor an adherent of the famous precept of William of Ockham, who during the early 14th century wrote: "Essentials ought not to be multiplied" ("Ockham's razor"). The survival of our complex biological machinery in the hostile natural environment is attributable to the great wisdom of nature, which provides layer upon layer of checks and balances for the protection of every important regulatory process that governs our bodily function. The words of Stephen Hales, written in 1733, seem especially appropriate in this regard: "So curiously are we wrought, so fearfully and wonderfully are we made."

REFERENCES

Bünger R, Permanetter B. (1984). Parallel stimulation by Ca^{2+} of inotropism and pyruvate dehydrogenase in perfused heart. *Am J Physiol* 247:C45–C52.

Clark MG, Bloxham DP, Holland PC, Lardy HA. (1973). Estimation of the fructose diphosphate- phosphofructokinase substrate cycle in the flight muscles of *Bombus affinis*. *Biochem J* 134:589–597.

Clark MG, Patten GS. (1984). Adrenergic control of phosphofructokinase and glycolysis. *Curr Top Cell Regul* 23:127–176.

Cohen P. (1986). Muscle glycogen synthetase. In: Boyer PD, Krebs EC. *The enzymes*, vol 17. 462–497.

Kitamura K, Kangawa K, Matsuo H, Uyeda K. (1988) Phosphorylation of myocardial fructose-6-phosphate, 2-kinase: Fructose-2, 6-bisphosphatase by cAMP-dependent protein kinase and protein kinase C. Activation by phosphorylation and amino acid sequences of the phosphorylation sites. *J Biol Chem* 263:16796–16801.

Pilkis SJ, El-Maghrabi MR, McGrane M, Pilkis J, Claus TH. (1982). Regulation by glucagon of hepatic pyruvate kinase, 6-phosphofructo-1-kinase, and fructose-1,6-bisphosphatase. *Fed Proc* 41:2623–2628.

Reed LJ, Yeaman SJ. (1986). Pyruvate dehydrogenase. In: Boyer PD, Krebs EC. *The enzymes*, vol 17. Orlando: The Academic Press; 77–95.

Roach, P.J., and Larner, J. (1977) Covalent phosphorylation in the regulation of glycogen synthetase activity. *Mol Cell Biochem* 15:179–200.

BIBLIOGRAPHY

Chock PB, Stadtman ER. (1977). Superiority of interconvertible enzyme cascades in metabolic regulation: analysis of multicyclic systems. *Proc Natl Acad Sci USA* 74:2766–2770.

Dunway GA. (1983). A review of animal phosophofructokinase isozymes with an emphasis on their physiological role. *Mol Cell Biochem* 52:75–91.

Kobayshi K, Neely JR. (1979). Control of the maximum rates of glycolysis in rat cardiac muscle. *Circ Res* 44:166–175.

Madsen NB. (1986). Glycogen phosphorylase. In: Boyer PD, Krebs EC. *The enzymes*, vol 17. Orlando: The Academic Press; 366–394.

Neely JR, Morgan HE. (1974). Relationship between carbohydrate and lipid metabolism and the energy balance of heart muscle. *Annu Rev Physiol* 31:413–459.

Newsholme EA. (1971–1972). The regulation of phosphofructokinase in muscle. *Cardiology* 56:22–34.

Nimmo HG, Cohen P. (1977). Hormonal control of protein phosphorylation. *Adv Cyclic Nucl Res* 8:145–266.

Pickett-Gies CA, Walsh DA. (1986). Phosphorylase kinase. In: Boyer PD, Krebs EC. *The enzymes*, vol 17. 396–459.

Randle PJ. (1981). Phosphorylation-dephosphorylation cycles and the regulation of fuel selection in mammals. *Curr Top Cell Regul* 18:107–128.

Stadtman ER, Chock PB. (1977). Superiority of interconvertible enzyme cascades in metabolic regulation: analysis of monocyclic systems. *Proc Natl Acad Sci USA* 74:2761–2765.

Stryer L. (1989). *Biochemistry*, 3d ed. New York: WH Freeman.

Wildenthal K, Morgan HE, Opie LH, Srere PA. (1976). Regulation of cardiac metabolism (symposium). *Circ Res* 38 (Suppl 1):I1–I160.

5

Oxidative Metabolism

The concluding sentences in the preceding chapter on the principles of glycolytic control serve equally well to introduce our discussion of oxidative metabolism, the most important of the energy-producing processes in the heart. Oxidative phosphorylation is, however, quite different from glycolysis, the latter being, from an evolutionary standpoint, more primitive. Whereas glycolysis is catalyzed by soluble cytosolic enzymes, oxidative metabolism takes place mainly within specialized membrane structures, the *mitochondria*. This itself increases the complexity of oxidative metabolism because all of the substrates, metabolites, and cofactors must cross the membrane that separates two aqueous compartments within the cell—the *cytosol* and the *mitochondrial matrix*. This membrane barrier maintains concentration (or more precisely, activity) gradients between the cytosol and mitochondrial matrix that enable this membrane to modulate energy transfer and the formation of high-energy phosphate compounds.

Variations in the catalytic properties of individual enzymes, which give rise to complex and interwoven control mechanisms, also participate in the regulation of oxidative metabolism. However, oxidative metabolism differs fundamentally from glycolysis in that most oxidative enzymes are bound to the mitochondrial membrane in highly ordered structures that facilitate enzyme-membrane and enzyme-enzyme interactions in the integrated control of oxidative energy production.

> Mitochondria contain a small amount of DNA that resembles the genetic material of small bacterial viruses, rather than that of mammalian cell nuclei. This indicates that the mitochondria represent welcome guests within our cells, into which they wandered hundreds of millions of years ago to establish a symbiotic relationship with animal tissues, providing large quantities of chemical energy in return for a warm, moist, compositionally satisfying environment. The mitochondrial membrane plays a major role in the communications between the "symbiote" and the "host."

Both carbohydrates and fats can be oxidized in the mitochondria; some amino acids are also oxidized by the heart, although protein metabolism normally contributes little to normal cardiac energy production. Fats and carbohydrates enter the final reactions of oxidative metabolism as acetylcoenzyme A (acetyl-CoA), an activated 2-carbon fragment that can be broken down to form CO_2 and H_2O. The conversion of carbohydrates to acetyl-CoA is described in Chapter 4. The following section describes the processes by which this 2-carbon fragment is derived from fats.

FATTY ACID METABOLISM

Fats, as are well known to hikers, can be viewed as "concentrated energy." Whereas carbohydrate and protein oxidation yields 4 calories/gm substrate, fats yield 9 calories/gm. Fats are transported in the blood from the gut to the heart mainly as triglycerides and free fatty acids (FFA); the latter represent the major source of lipid for myocardial energy production. The triglycerides represent complexes of fatty acids that are esterified to the 3-carbon sugar glycerol (see Chapter 2). Free fatty acids are "free" only in that they are not bound as esters [hence the older terms: nonesterified fatty acids (NEFA) and unesterified fatty acids (UFA)]; FFAs are in fact bound to the plasma proteins, mainly to albumin.

Oxidation of trigylcerides requires that the esterified fatty acids first be cleaved from the gylcerol backbone, after which they are taken up by the cells of the myocardium. Once inside the cell, the fatty acids are "activated" and transported into the mitochondria where they are oxidized to form acetyl-CoA according to the overall scheme shown in Fig. 5.1.

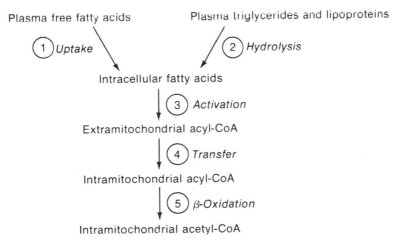

FIG. 5.1. Overall scheme of fatty acid metabolism. Long-chain fatty acids are prepared for oxidation within the cell through five key reactions: (1) uptake of plasma free fatty acids; (2) hydrolysis of plasma triglycerides and lipoproteins that delivers free fatty acids to the heart; (3) activation of fatty acids by binding to CoA; (4) transfer of activated fatty acids (acyl-CoA) from the cytosol to the mitochondrial matrix; and (5) β-oxidation to yield the 2-carbon fragment acetyl-CoA.

Hydrolysis of Phospholipids

Circulating triglycerides and phospholipids cannot be taken up by the myocardium without prior hydrolysis of the ester bonds linking the fatty acids to glycerol. The capillary endothelium contains an enzyme, *lipoprotein lipase*, that releases free fatty acids from triglycerides. Control of fatty acid release has been studied most extensively in adipose tissue, which contains a hormone-sensitive *triglyceride lipase* whose activity is increased by a phosphorylation reaction that is probably catalyzed by a cyclic AMP–dependent protein kinase (Steinberg, 1977). In the heart, the release of fatty acids from triglycerides also appears to be accelerated by β-adrenergic agonists. Thus, as in glycolysis (Chapter 4), the entry of lipid into the pathways of energy production is under *humoral* control.

Uptake of Free Fatty Acids by the Cell

Fatty acids that reach the heart as FFA must cross two barriers before entering the cell: the capillary endothelium and the cardiac sarcolemma. The most important of these barriers is the capillary endothelium (Rose and Goresky, 1977). Fatty acid uptake by the heart appears to be due to passive diffusion, possibly involving fatty acid carrier proteins in the sarcolemma (Abumrad et al., 1981); thus, high plasma FFA concentrations increase fatty acid uptake by the law of mass action. Accelerated fatty acid oxidation in the working heart, by reducing cytoplasmic fatty acid concentration, also favors uptake of these lipid substrates into the cell (see below).

Fatty Acid Activation and Transport into the Mitochondria

Fatty acid activation, like the phosphorylation of glucose (Chapter 4), requires that energy be "invested" to form a high-energy complex; in fat metabolism, energy derived from adenosine triphosphate (ATP) is used to form an activated complex with coenzyme A (CoA). The resulting fatty acyl esters, *acyl-CoA* (which are analogous to *acetyl-CoA*) do not cross the mitochondrial inner membrane; instead, fatty acyl-CoA is readily converted in the cytosol to *acyl-carnitine* derivatives that are able to enter the mitochondria. In this rather complex manner, fats are prepared for transport into the mitochondrial matrix, where they are subsequently oxidized.

Fatty Acid Activation

The formation of acyl-CoA requires that the high-energy bond of ATP be transferred to form a high-energy fatty acyl adenylate complex in the following reaction, which is catalyzed by an *acyl-CoA synthetase*:

$$\text{Fatty acid} + \text{ATP} \leftrightarrow \text{Fatty acid} \sim \text{AMP} + PP_i.$$

Coenzyme A then replaces the adenosine monophosphate (AMP) that is bound to the activated fatty acid, liberating acyl-CoA according to the reaction:

$$\text{Fatty acid} \sim \text{AMP} + \text{CoA} - \text{SH} \leftrightarrow \text{Acyl} - \text{CoA} + \text{AMP}.$$

The overall process of fatty acid activation can thus be written:

$$\underset{\text{Fatty acid}}{CH_3-(CH_2)_n-COOH} + ATP + \underset{\text{Reduced CoA}}{CoA-SH} \leftrightarrow \underset{\text{Acyl CoA}}{CH_3 (CH_2)_n- \overset{\overset{\text{O}}{\|}}{C} -SCoA} + AMP + PP_i.$$

Formation of acyl-CoA, which contains a high-energy thioester bond, requires that *two* high-energy bonds in ATP be hydrolyzed because each pyrophosphate (PP_i) formed in this reaction is subsequently hydrolyzed by a *pyrophosphatase* to form two molecules of inorganic phosphate. For this reason, this overall reaction is irreversible.

The rate of fatty acid activation is controlled largely by the concentrations of the reactants depicted above (Hochachka et al., 1977). Because a major portion of the activated acyl-CoA is generated by enzymes on the outer side of the mitochondrial membrane, fatty acid oxidation is also determined by the highly regulated transfer of the activated fatty acids into the mitochondrial matrix (see below).

Transfer of Acyl-CoA

Because long-chain fatty acyl-CoA molecules do not readily cross the mitochondrial inner membrane, activated fatty acids enter the mitochondria as *acyl-carnitine*. Carnitine is a 7-carbon organic acid that, after replacing the coenzyme A esterified to fatty acyl moieties serves as a "carrier" in an exchange-diffusion reaction in which acyl-coenzyme A is exchanged for carnitine according to the following three reactions:

$$\text{Acyl-CoA}_o + \text{carnitine} \rightarrow \text{acyl-carnitine}_o + \text{CoA-SH}$$

$$\text{Acyl-carnitine}_o \rightarrow \text{acyl-carnitine}_i$$

$$\text{Acyl-carnitine}_i + \text{CoA-SH} \rightarrow \text{acyl-CoA}_i + \text{carnitine}$$

where acyl-CoA_o and acyl-carnitine_o are the activated fatty acids outside the mitochondrial matrix and acyl-CoA_i and acyl-carnitine_i the activated fatty acid within the mitochondria.

The concentration of carnitine in the cytosol is ~200 times more than that of coenzyme A, whereas there is ~20 times more coenzyme A than carnitine in the mitochondrial matrix. Thus, fatty acyl-carnitine levels in the cytosol are higher than in the mitochondria, whereas most fatty acyl-CoA is within the mitochondria.

The transfer of fatty acids into the mitochondria requires the participation of two membrane-bound enzymes called carnitine acyltransferases. *Carnitine acyltrans-*

ferase I, located on the cytosolic (outer) side of the inner mitochondrial membrane, transfers acyl-carnitine to the matrix of the mitochondria, whereas *carnitine acyl-transferase II*, on the inner side of this membrane, reconverts the intramito-chondrial acyl-carnitine to carnitine and acyl-CoA. Carnitine formed by the latter reaction is then transported back into the cytosol where it exchanges for more acyl-CoA. The rate of this process, like that of fatty acid activation, is determined largely by the concentrations of the reactants.

> The carnitine acyltransferases play an important, albeit indirect role in the regulation of fatty acid entry into the myocardial cell. When cardiac energy demands are high and rapid oxidative metabolism reduces intramitochondrial levels of acetyl-CoA (see be-low), the conversion of acyl carnitines to acyl-CoA in the mitochondria is accelerated. This liberates carnitine that crosses back to the cytosol and accepts more acyl groups, thereby increasing cytosolic levels of coenzyme A. The increased availability of coen-zyme A in the cytosol, by accelerating acyl-CoA formation, lowers cytosolic free fatty acid concentration which, in turn, promotes fatty acid diffusion into the cell (Hochachka et al., 1977). In effect, therefore, the rapid return of carnitine to the cytosol from the mitochondrial matrix during periods of accelerated fatty acid oxida-tion increases fatty acid entry and activation in the cytosol.

β-Oxidation

Fatty acids enter the tricarboxylic acid cycle, the major oxidative pathway of the myocardium, as acetyl-CoA, which is generated by the stepwise breakdown of long-chain fatty acyl chains. Although anaerobic glycolysis provides an alternative pathway that can generate small amounts of ATP from carbohydrates under anaer-obic conditions (Chapter 4), fatty acid metabolism is absolutely dependent on a continuing supply of oxygen. As oxidative metabolism cannot proceed when coro-nary flow is interrupted, no ATP can be generated from fats in the ischemic heart.

Acetyl-CoA is produced from long-chain fatty acyl-CoA within the mitochondria by a series of reactions which, because the fatty acyl chain is progressively short-ened, can be viewed as a shrinking "spiral." Each "turn" of the spiral releases a 2-carbon fragment from the fatty acid according to the overall reaction shown in Fig. 5.2, which involves four steps that are catalyzed by different enzymes and involve several cofactors, including CoA, flavin adenine dinucleotide (FAD) and NAD (Fig. 5.3). Each cycle begins with an oxidation that forms enoyl-CoA, an activated unsaturated fatty acyl intermediate. After hydration, another oxidation, and addition of CoA, a thiolytic step shortens the fatty acid by 2-carbons by liberat-ing acetyl-CoA. The shortened fatty acid is then able to reenter another turn of the cycle, a process that continues until the fatty acid has been converted entirely to acetyl-CoA. The four sequential reactions that lead to the production of acetyl-CoA (Fig. 5.3) are very tightly coupled to each other, so that the concentrations of the fatty acyl intermediates arc normally very low. The energy that becomes available in the two oxidative steps of β-oxidation is trapped in the reduced coenzymes $FADH_2$ and NADH; these generate ATP when they are subsequently oxidized in the mitochondria (see below).

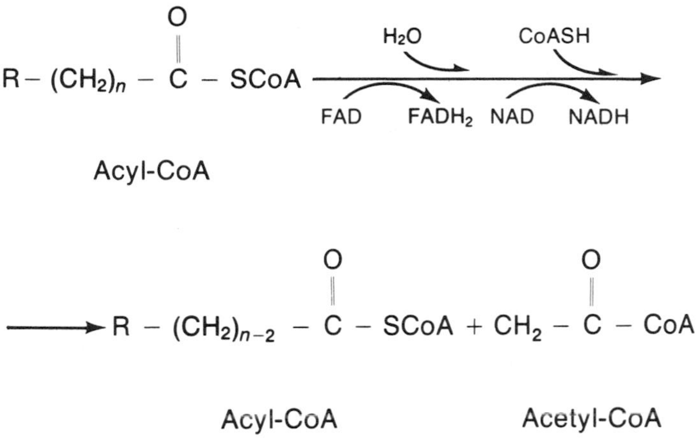

$$R - (CH_2)_n - \overset{\overset{\displaystyle O}{\|}}{C} - SCoA \xrightarrow[\substack{FAD \quad FADH_2}]{\substack{H_2O \qquad CoASH}} {}_{NAD \quad NADH}$$

Acyl-CoA

$$\longrightarrow R - (CH_2)_{n-2} - \overset{\overset{\displaystyle O}{\|}}{C} - SCoA + CH_2 - \overset{\overset{\displaystyle O}{\|}}{C} - CoA$$

Acyl-CoA   Acetyl-CoA

FIG. 5.2. Overall reaction of β-oxidation by which activated fatty acids (acyl-CoA) are broken down to form the 2-carbon fragment acetyl-CoA.

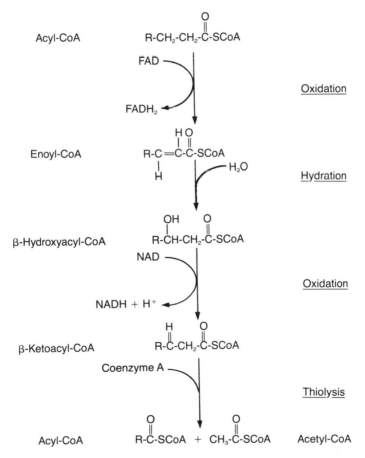

FIG. 5.3. Each cycle in the stepwise breakdown of long-chain fatty acids by β-oxidation involves four steps, two of oxidation, one of hydration, and one of thiolysis.

The rate of β-oxidation is much faster than that of fatty acid activation and transfer, so that the overall rate of fatty acid oxidation in the well-oxygenated heart is normally governed by the reactions responsible for fatty acid entry into the mitochondria.

The dependence of β-oxidation on the availability of oxidized NAD and FAD is reminiscent of the glyceraldehyde-3-phosphate dehydrogenase reaction in glycolysis (Chapter 4). Thus, fat metabolism, like glucose metabolism, is inhibited when the interior of the cell becomes reduced. As the oxidized FAD needed for β-oxidation also participates in the oxidation of succinate in the tricarboxylic acid cycle, conversion of FAD to $FADH_2$ during rapid succinate oxidation can inhibit β-oxidation. This dual role of FAD allows increased carbohydrate flux through the tricarboxylic acid cycle to inhibit fatty acid oxidation.

Fatty Acid Synthesis

Myocardial cells have a limited capacity to synthesize a reserve of lipid, although large amounts of fat can be stored in the epicardium. Fatty acid synthesis provides for the storage of substrate; and like lactate production, can generate limited amounts of NAD.

Fatty acid synthesis is catalyzed by two enzymes. The first, *acetyl-CoA carboxylase*, uses energy derived from ATP to form the activated intermediate malonyl-CoA from acetyl-CoA and bicarbonate. *Fatty acid synthetase*, the second, catalyzes the formation of palmitic acid from acetyl-CoA and seven molecules of malonyl-CoA in a reaction that generates 14 molecules of NADH from NAD, and releases seven molecules of CO_2. Fatty acid synthesis is more highly regulated than β-oxidation, and is controlled by allosteric interactions among a number of key metabolites (e.g., citrate). Like glycogen formation, fatty acid synthesis is influenced by complex phosphorylation-dephosphorylation reactions (Kim et al., 1989).

The overall pattern of fatty acid synthesis and breakdown also resembles glycogen formation and breakdown in that both proceed by different pathways. These are integrated largely by malonyl-CoA, the major product of the first step in fatty acid synthesis, which controls the transfer of fatty acids into the mitochondria by an action on carnitine acyltransferase.

Fatty acid synthesis may play a limited role in regenerating oxidized coenzymes in the ischemic heart, as lipid droplets appear in the tissues immediately surrounding the infarcted myocardium. However, production of oxidized NAD by the fatty acid synthetase reaction is probably of little importance to the vast majority of ischemic cells in the hearts of patients following a coronary occlusion.

OXIDATION OF ACETYLCOENZYME A BY THE TRICARBOXYLIC ACID CYCLE

As pointed out in Chapter 3, high-energy phosphate production in the heart must be regulated so that ATP is generated at the same rate that it is being utilized. Thus,

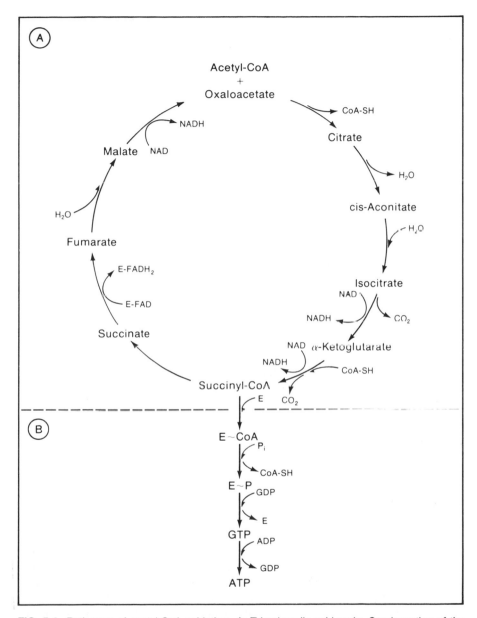

FIG. 5.4. Pathways of acetyl-CoA oxidation. A: Tricarboxylic acid cycle. Condensation of the 2-carbon fragment acetyl-CoA with the 4-carbon organic acid oxaloacetate (*top*) yields a 6-carbon organic acid (citrate). The latter, after isomerization to isocitrate, is oxidized and decarboxylated. The resulting 5-carbon organic acid (α-ketoglutarate) is oxidized and decarboxylated in a reaction that yields succinyl-CoA. Oxaloacetate is regenerated after succinyl-CoA undergoes two steps of oxidation and one of hydration. B: Substrate-level phosphorylation. Each mole of enzyme-bound CoA released from succinyl-CoA provides for generation of a single mode of ATP by substrate-level phosphorylation.

the metabolic reactions in the myocardium must allow increased energy utilization by the contractile machinery to signal an increased rate of high-energy phosphate production. Many of the metabolic controls already discussed illustrate the way in which energy utilization and energy production are integrated, for example, the ability of a fall in ATP concentration and rises in adenosine diphosphate (ADP) and P_i concentrations to stimulate the phosphofructokinase reaction (Chapter 4). The mechanisms controlling the tricarboxylic acid cycle provide further examples of this important regulation by high-energy phosphate levels.

The oxidation of acetyl-CoA to form CO_2 and H_2O occurs by a cyclic series of reactions, the *tricarboxylic acid* (or *Krebs*) *cycle*, which are catalyzed by enzymes that are free within the intramitochondrial matrix, and not bound to the mitochondrial membrane. The reactions of the tricarboxylic acid cycle, shown in Fig. 5.4, begin with the condensation of the 2-carbon fragment, acetyl-CoA, with a 4-carbon organic acid, oxaloacetate, to form citrate, a 6-carbon organic acid. Following configurational rearrangements that convert citrate to *cis*-aconitate, the 6-carbon organic acid is converted to isocitrate, which is then oxidized and decarboxylated to form α-ketoglutaric acid. The latter, a 5-carbon organic acid, is then oxidized and decarboxylated to form the activated 4-carbon organic acid succinyl-CoA.

The formation of succinyl-CoA from α-ketoglutarate requires coenzyme A, which forms a high-energy ester bond like that in acetyl-CoA. This high-energy bond is then transferred to the enzyme *succinyl CoA synthetase* (E), to form E~CoA (Fig. 5.4B). Phosphate then replaces CoA to form a high-energy phosphorylated intermediate, E~P. The high-energy phosphate bond is then transferred to GDP to form GTP, and subsequently from GTP to ADP, thereby forming ATP. The reactions shown in Fig. 5.4B, represent the only point in the tricarboxylic acid cycle where a high-energy phosphate bond is formed directly by *substrate-level phosphorylation*. As discussed later in this chapter, a far greater amount of ATP is formed when NADH and $FADH_2$ are oxidized by *respiratory chain-linked phosphorylation*.

The tricarboxylic acid continues when succinate produced in the reactions described in the preceding paragraph is oxidized by *succinyl dehydrogenase* (also called succinate-Q reductase or E-FAD, Fig. 5.4A), an iron sulfate flavoprotein enzyme that contains bound FAD. This E-FAD complex is reduced to E-$FADH_2$ when succinate is reduced to fumarate. After water is added to fumarate to form malate, the latter is oxidized by the conversion of NAD to NADH in a reaction that, by regenerating oxaloacetate, completes the tricarboxylic acid cycle.

The overall reaction of the tricarboxylic acid cycle (Fig. 5.5), as already noted, forms one high-energy phosphate bond per 2-carbon fragment by substrate-level phosphorylation. A much larger portion of the chemical energy released by the oxidation of acetyl-CoA is trapped in the reduced coenzymes generated in four oxidation reactions, three of which yield NADH and the other enzyme-bound $FADH_2$. It is apparent, therefore, that oxidative ATP production must involve yet another process; this is respiratory chain-linked phosphorylation, which is described later in this chapter.

Acetyl-CoA + 2H$_2$O + 3NAD + FAD + ADP + P$_1$ →

2CO$_2$ + Coenzyme A + 3NADH + FADH$_2$ + ATP

FIG. 5.5. Overall reaction of the tricarboxylic acid cycle.

Turnover of the tricarboxylic acid cycle is regulated in part by the availability of acetyl-CoA (see above), and in part by the supply of oxidized NAD and FAD (see below). The first step in the cycle, condensation of oxaloacetate and acetyl-CoA to form citrate, is also a key point of regulation. In addition to responding to changing levels of both of these precursors, citrate synthesis is inhibited by an allosteric effect of ATP. Conversely, as noted at many points in this and the preceding chapters, citrate is an important regulator of many other reactions.

The oxaloacetate level in the mitochondria is determined by the redox state in the mitochondria. The influence of this control can be seen in Fig. 5.4A, where the final step in the tricarboxylic acid cycle, the oxidation of malate to oxaloacetate, is coupled to the reduction of NAD to NADH. The NADH/NAD ratio, which reflects the redox state of the mitochondrial matrix, thus determines the oxaloacetate level because the NADH/NAD ratio is proportional to the oxaloacetate/malate ratio through the equilibrium:

malate + NAD ↔ oxaloacetate + NADH.

Thus, when the mitochondria become reduced, as occurs in the hypoxic or ischemic heart, the increased NADH/NAD ratio slows the tricarboxylic acid cycle by decreasing the amount of oxaloacetate available for condensation with acetyl-CoA. Conversely, a shift of the coenzymes to a more oxidized state (low NADH and high NAD), by increasing oxaloacetate levels, accelerates acetyl-CoA utilization.

Many additional reactions influence the turnover of the tricarboxylic acid cycle. The most important of these is catalyzed by *isocitrate dehydrogenase*, a large enzyme containing four subunits that controls the production of α-ketoglutarate from isocitrate. Much like phosphofructokinase in the regulation of glycolysis, isocitrate dehydrogenase is stimulated by ADP and inhibited by ATP (Rushbrook and Harvey, 1978); thus, a fall in the high energy phosphate levels within the cell (in the case of isocitrate dehydrogenase, within the mitochondria) accelerates the tricarboxylic acid cycle. This ability of high-energy phosphate levels to regulate the tricarboxylic acid cycle allows acetyl-CoA oxidation to be accelerated by an increase in the energy requirements of the cell, i.e., when ATP levels fall and ADP accumulates. The overall reaction catalyzed by isocitrate dehydrogenase is also promoted by Ca^{2+} and NAD, and inhibited by NADH (Gabriel and Plaut, 1984).

The NADH/NAD ratio controls the next step in the tricarboxylic acid cycle, which is catalyzed by α-*ketoglutarate dehydrogenase*, a multienzyme complex similar in some ways to pyruvate dehydrogenase. This enzyme, which requires lipoic acid, thiamine pyrophosphate (TPP), and CoA, is inhibited by its products: NADH and succinyl-CoA. The production of succinyl-CoA is inhibited in the anaerobic heart because of this effect of NADH.

The ability of increased energy utilization to stimulate the tricarboxylic acid cycle reflects the ability of ADP and P_i to enhance, and ATP to inhibit, α-ketoglutarate oxidation. An increase in cellular Ca^{2+}, as occurs when myocardial contractility is increased, may also modulate the tricarboxylic acid cycle by stimulating the oxidation of α-ketoglutarate to succinyl-CoA. The oxidation of α-ketoglutarate may also be important in regulating the metabolism of amino acids, which can be oxidized after transamination reactions that involve α-ketoglutarate (see below).

The many regulatory mechanisms summarized above allow the rate of acetyl-CoA oxidation in the mitochondria to respond to the changing energy requirements of the heart, the availability of oxidized coenzymes, and the supply of substrate.

TRANSPORT OF REDUCED NADH FROM CYTOSOL TO MITOCHONDRIA: THE MALATE-ASPARTATE CYCLE

The reduced NADH formed during oxidation of the acetyl-CoA derived from fats and carbohydrates gains ready access to the enzymes of the respiratory chain because all of these reactions occur within the mitochondria. When NADH is produced during glycolysis, however, the coenzyme is reduced in the cytosol and so must be returned to the mitochondria before it can be reoxidized. Conversely, during normal aerobic metabolism virtually all of the NAD essential for glycolysis in the cytosol is regenerated within the mitochondria; but because the mitochondrial inner membrane is not permeable to this coenzyme, the essential exchange of NADH produced in the cytosol for NAD produced in the mitochondria cannot take place by simple diffusion. Instead, NADH transfer into the mitochondria in exchange for NAD is effected by a special membrane transport mechanism, the *malate-aspartate cycle*.

In a number of tissues, notably the liver, the exchange of NAD and NADH across the inner mitochondrial membrane is effected by a "shuttle" that involves glycerol phosphate and dihydroxyacetone phosphate. This shuttle does not exchange the coenzyme, but instead transfers reducing equivalents across this membrane utilizing these glycolytic intermediates. In the heart a more complex malate-aspartate cycle exchanges reducing equivalents across the mitochondrial membrane. This cycle involves not only oxidation and reduction reactions, but also transaminations; i.e., the transfer of amino groups between the organic acids produced during carbohydrate metabolism and amino acids (Fig. 5.6).

Operation of the malate-aspartate cycle is most easily understood by considering first the transfer of reducing equivalents across the mitrochondrial membrane, which is a relatively simple process, and then by examining the additional reactions necessary to restore the two metabolic pools at either side of the mitochondrial membrane—the cytosol and the mitochondrial matrix—to their original states.

The reaction that in effect "transfers" NADH across the mitochondrial membrane is labeled 1 in Fig. 5.6. The reduced NADH formed in the cytosol during glycolysis is oxidized to NAD by the coupled reduction of oxaloacetate to malate (1a in Fig.

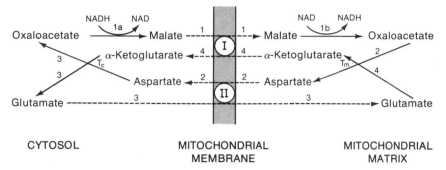

CYTOSOL   MITOCHONDRIAL   MITOCHONDRIAL
                            MEMBRANE   MATRIX

FIG. 5.6. Malate-aspartate cycle. This complex series of reactions proceeds by the following sequence: (1) reduction of oxaloacetate in the cytosol and transfer of the 4-carbon acid malate into the mitochondrial matrix by a membrane carrier (I). This step leads to oxidation of NADH in the cytosol (1a), and subsequent oxidation of malate leads to reduction of NAD in the mitochondria (1b). (2) Oxaloacetate, the 4-carbon acid that has appeared in the mitochondrial matrix during reaction 1b, is transferred back to the cytosol as the 4-carbon amino acid aspartate by a second membrane carrier (II) following a transamination (T_m) with mitochondrial glutamate. (3) Oxaloacetate is regenerated in the cytosol by transamination of aspartate with α-ketoglutarate (T_c). This reaction leads to formation of glutamate, which is subsequently transferred to the mitochondrial matrix in exchange for aspartate (produced during reaction 2) by membrane carrier II. (4) The glutamate transferred to the mitochondrial matrix is converted to α-ketoglutarate by transamination with oxaloacetate (T_m) as described in reaction 2. The α-ketoglutarate so produced moves back to the cytosol to replace that utilized in reaction 3, the transport being effected by membrane carrier I in exchange for the malate initially transported to the mitochondrial matrix (reaction 1).

5.6). Malate is then transported into the mitochondria by a specific membrane carrier (I in Fig. 5.6). Once inside the mitochondria, malate is oxidized by NAD to produce oxaloacetate and reduced by NADH (1b in Fig. 5.6). The net effect of this reaction is the same as if NADH from the cytosol were exchanged for NAD in the mitochondria: in the cytosol NADH has been oxidized to NAD, whereas NAD has been reduced to NADH in the mitochondria. In this manner, therefore, the cytosol is resupplied with oxidized NAD for further glycolysis, while at the same time the mitochondria obtain NADH that can serve as a substrate for the energy-yielding processes of oxidative phosphorylation. This "transfer" of NADH from cytosol to mitochondria, however, leaves the cytosol depleted of oxaloacetate, which has appeared within the mitochondria. Thus to complete the malate-aspartate cycle, additional reactions are needed to return the excess oxaloacetate from the mitochondria to the cytosol.

The simple transfer of oxaloacetate from cardiac mitochondria to cytosol is prevented by the impermeability of the inner mitochondrial membrane to this organic acid and the absence of an oxaloacetate carrier. Instead of moving directly back to the cytosol as oxaloacetate, therefore, this 4-carbon organic acid is first transaminated in the mitochondrial matrix (Tm) to form aspartate, a 4-carbon amino acid for which a carrier does exist in the mitochondrial membrane (II in Fig. 5.6). This carrier-mediated transfer of aspartate (2 in Fig. 5.6) does not, however, restore the two cell compartments to their original state. If anything, these two compartments are even more different than they were at the start of the process because amino groups have now been carried by aspartate from the mitochondrial matrix to the cytosol. The initial composition of these compartments must therefore be restored by two additional reactions, each of which provide substrates for cotransport by the two membrane carriers already mentioned. The first of these additional reactions (3 in Fig. 5.6) occurs when α-ketoglutarate, a 5-carbon organic acid in the cytosolic compartment, is transaminated with the amino groups carried into this compartment by aspartate (Tc). This reaction transfers the amino groups of aspartate to α-keto-glutarate, forming glutamate, a 5-carbon amino acid that returns to the mitochondrial matrix by carrier II (which is also the carrier of the 4-carbon amino acid aspartate that was transported to the cytosol). At the same time, the transaminase reaction Tc (Fig. 5.6) converts the cytosolic aspartate to oxaloacetate, thereby restoring the initial level of this 4-carbon organic acid in the cytosol.

The malate-aspartate cycle is completed when glutamate, which enters the mitochondrial matrix from the cytosol, is transaminated with oxaloacetate to form α-ketoglutarate in the mitochondrial matrix (Tm in Fig. 5.6). This final step—which both replenishes the α-ketoglutarate utilized in the step labeled 3 in Fig. 5.6 and supplies the amino groups for the initial transamination labeled Tm in Fig. 5.6—is made possible by the transfer of amino groups within the mitochondria from glutamate to oxaloacetate. (This transamination, you recall, provided the mechanism by which a 4-carbon acid was returned from the mitochondrial matrix to the cytosol as aspartate.) In Fig. 5.6 this final step is depicted by the reactions labeled 4, which include the second half of the transamination within the mitochondrial matrix, just described, and the transfer of α-ketoglutarate back to the cytosol. This final reaction is coupled to the transfer of malate into the mitochondrial matrix by the carrier labeled I, which was involved in the initial transfer of reducing equivalents into the mitochondria.

The complex series of reactions shown in Fig. 5.6 represents nothing more than a means to "move" NADH from the cytosol to the mitochondrial matrix for subsequent oxidation, and to "move" NAD back to the cytosol so as to allow glycolysis to proceed. The complexity of this transfer (why do the mitochondria not simply have a carrier that can transfer NADH in return for NAD?) again illustrates the nonadherence of the myocardium to the precepts of Ockham's razor. Yet this complexity is not without its advantages to the cell, for it provides yet another means by which metabolism can be controlled and by which the many individual catalytic reactions that are responsible for energy production in the heart can be integrated.

A number of features of the malate-aspartate cycle integrate the rates of anaerobic and aerobic energy production. In addition to regulating the transport of reducing equivalents across the inner mitochondrial membrane, this cycle influences the flux of substrates through the tricarboxylic cycle by modulating the concentrations of oxaloacetate and α-ketoglutarate within the mitochondria. (Recall that both of these are intermediates of the tricarboxylic acid cycle; see Fig. 5.4.)

The malate-aspartate cycle is also important under anaerobic conditions where inability of the mitochondria to oxidize oxaloacetate increases the concentration of this 4-carbon acid within the cytosol (reactions 2 and 3 in Fig. 5.6). Once in the cytosol, oxaloacetate can be reduced to malate (reaction 1a) thereby regenerating oxidized NAD, which in the ischemic heart becomes critical for the production of ATP by anaerobic glycolysis.

Movements of other substances by way of this cycle provide additional means of "communication" between the mitochondrial matrix and the cytosol. Citrate, which has an important regulatory influence on glycolytic rate (Chapter 4) cannot move across the mitochondrial membrane by simple diffusion; instead, this 6-carbon organic acid is converted in the mitochondrial matrix to α-ketoglutarate, which is readily transferred across the mitochondrial membrane by carrier I (Fig. 5.6) to the cytosol where the α-ketoglutarate is reconverted to citrate. The latter reactions, and their control by the malate-aspartate cycle, may be important in allowing citrate to control glycolytic rate as the glutamate-aspartate carrier (carrier II in Fig. 5.6) is energy dependent and thus sensitive to changes in cellular energy metabolism.

TRANSAMINATION

Measurements of transaminases released into the blood by necrotic heart muscle have for almost 40 years played an important role in the diagnosis of acute myocardial infarction. Although vital in linking amino acid metabolism with that of fat and carbohydrates, these enzymes play only a minor role in the overall production of ATP in the heart. Two transamination reactions in the malate-aspartate cycle partic ipate in the "transfer" of NAD and NADH across the inner mitochondrial membrane, but these transaminations, which involve 4- and 5-carbon compounds, play only an indirect role in energy production in the heart. Transaminations involving the 3-carbon compounds pyruvate and alanine are of limited importance in providing substrate for cardiac energy production, especially in the anoxic or ischemic heart. The transamination between pyruvate and glutamate (Fig. 5.7) which causes alanine to accumulate under anaerobic conditions, may slow the formation of lactate—an inhibitor of glycolysis—when cessation of oxidative metabolism causes pyruvate to accumulate (Taegtmeyer et al., 1977).

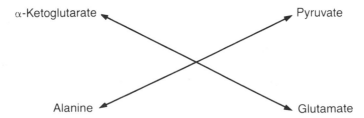

FIG. 5.7. Transamination reactions involving 3-carbon (alanine and pyruvate) and 4-carbon (α-ketoglutarate and glutamate) acids.

ADENINE NUCLEOTIDE TRANSFER

The impermeability of the mitochondrial inner membrane to adenine nucleotides mandates another reaction that, like the malate-aspartate cycle, effects the "transfer" of ATP and ADP between the cytosol and mitochondrial matrix. This exchange, which involves a carrier that couples the flux of ATP in one direction across the inner mitochondrial membrane to the flux of ADP in the opposite direction, is mediated by *ATP-ADP translocase*, a dimer of 30,000 dalton subunits, that can bind either ATP or ADP. Because ATP has three negative charges, whereas ADP has only two, the positive potential at the outer surface of the mitochondrial inner membrane (see below) favors ATP transfer out of, and ADP transfer into, the mitochondria.

POSSIBLE ROLE OF CREATINE AND PHOSPHOCREATINE AS "ENERGY SHUTTLES"

Although diffusion is an inherently rapid process, its ability to effect bulk transport depends on the overall concentrations of the molecules that are diffusing. The high content of ATP in the myocardial cell (which expressed as an average concentration is ~5 mM) poses little difficulty to the rapid diffusion of ATP from the mitochondria, where it is produced, to the various energy-consuming sites in the cytosol where it is consumed. It is more difficult, however, for simple diffusion to explain the return of ADP to the mitochondria because ADP content is low, only about 0.6 mmoles/kg wet weight. Estimated cytosolic ADP concentrations, as low as 0.02 mM, may be too low for diffusion to effect the rapid return of ADP to the mitochondria for rephosphorylation.

A fascinating mechanism to explain the rapid movement of ADP to the mitochondria is that creatine, and not ADP, is returned to the mitochondria for rephosphorylation (Jacobus, 1985). According to this hypothesis, phosphocreatine is not simply a high-energy reserve (Chapter 3), but is also instrumental in shuttling high-energy phosphate to the energy-utilizing systems of the cytosol. Because cytosolic creatine and phosphocreatine concentrations are high, their diffusion readily provides for the rapid bulk transport of both high-energy phosphate (as phosphocreatine) and phosphorylatable substrate (as creatine) between the mitochondria and the cytosol (Fig. 5.8).

It has been proposed that the high-energy phosphate that crosses the mitochondrial inner membrane as ATP is transferred to phosphocreatine, which then diffuses through the cytosol to be reconverted to ATP in reactions that are catalyzed by *cytosolic creatine phosphokinases* located near energy-utilizing cytosolic adenosine triphosphatases (ATPases) (for example, the contractile proteins and sarcoplasmic reticulum). Creatine, one product of this reaction, rather than ADP, thus represents the depleted high-energy phosphate carrier in the cytosol that is returned to the mitochondria for rephosphorylation. When this creatine diffuses back to the

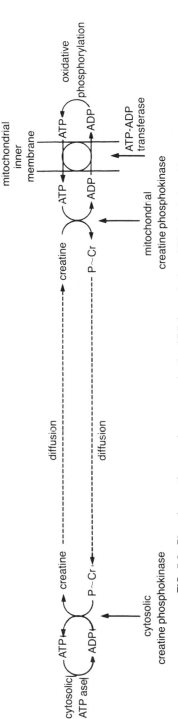

FIG. 5.8. Phosphocreatine-creatine energy shuttle. ADP formed when ATP is hydrolyzed by a cytosolic ATPase (*left*) gains a high-energy phosphate from phosphocreatine, which is converted to creatine by a cytosolic creatine phosphokinase. The creatine produced by this reaction rapidly diffuses to the mitochondria where it is rephosphorylated by ATP that enters the cytosol from the mitochondria (*right*) in a reaction that is catalyzed by a mitochondrial creatine phosphokinase. This reaction generates ADP at the surface of the mitochondria, which enters the mitochondrial matrix via the ATP-ADP transferase in exchange for ATP. The ADP that enters the mitochondria is then rephosphorylated by oxidative phosphorylation to form ATP.

mitochondria, it serves as a high-energy phosphate acceptor for ATP produced by the mitochondria in a transfer catalyzed by a *mitochondrial creatine phosphokinase*, which liberates ADP immediately outside the mitochondria. This ADP then reenters the mitochondria via the ATP-ADP transferase to be rephosphorylated by oxidative phosphorylation.

> Additional evidence for the importance of this "shuttle" comes from the finding that ADP bound to the contractile proteins can be rephosphorylated in hyperpermeable myocardial cells in which free ATP levels are very low (McClellan et al., 1983). The existence of this shuttle also explains the frequent finding that creatine phosphokinase enzymes copurify with mitochondria and many energy-consuming systems.

OXIDATIVE PHOSPHORYLATION

In the heart, the major reactions of aerobic ATP production do not occur in glycolysis, in fatty acid oxidation, or in the tricarboxylic acid cycle. Although limited *substrate-level phosphorylation* does occur in the heart, virtually all of the ATP that is generated by aerobic metabolism is obtained by *respiratory chain-linked phosphorylation*, or oxidative phosphorylation. These reactions are catalyzed by the enzymes of the respiratory chain, which are tightly bound to the mitochondrial inner membrane. A proton gradient across this membrane is now recognized as the key to oxidative energy transduction.

The substrates that provide the energy for regeneration of ATP by respiratory chain-linked phosphorylations are NADH and $FADH_2$, the reduced coenzymes produced by the oxidation of carbohydrates and fatty acids (see above). To understand how much energy is contained in these substrates, the reader should recall the explosive reaction that occurs when molecular hydrogen is ignited in an oxygen-containing environment. Oxidative phosphorylation simply provides a mechanism to "trap" this energy by regenerating the high-energy phosphate bonds of ATP.

Electrons or Reducing Equivalents

The reactions of the respiratory chain can be looked on either as the transfer of electrons, or the transfer of reducing equivalents. Thus, the overall reaction of oxidative phosphorylation can be viewed as the transfer of hydrogen from NADH and $FADH_2$ to oxygen (the positive charge on NAD is included in the following equations):

$$NADH + H^+ + \frac{1}{2} O_2 \leftrightarrow NAD^+ + H_2O$$

(reduced)   (oxidized)

and

$$FADH_2 + \frac{1}{2} O_2 \quad \leftrightarrow \quad FAD + H_2O$$

(reduced)   (oxidized)

However, it is more useful to consider these reactions in terms of electron fluxes.

The relationship between the transfer of hydrogen (i.e., reducing equivalents) and electron transfer is readily understood if one views each hydrogen atom (H) as a hydrogen ion (H^+) plus an electron ($e-$). In order to describe the function of the respiratory chain in terms of electron transport, NADH becomes $[(NAD-e)^- + H^+]$, and FADH, $[(FAD-2e)^{2-} + 2H^+]$, so that the overall reactions described above are:

$$[(NAD-e)^- + 2H^+] + \frac{1}{2}O_2 \leftrightarrow NAD^+ + 2H_2O$$

(reduced)   (oxidized)

and

$$[(FAD-2e)^{2-} + 2H^+] + \frac{1}{2}O_2 \leftrightarrow FAD + 2H_2O.$$

(reduced)   (oxidized)

Oxidative phosphorylation, therefore, occurs when the electrons carried by the reduced coenzymes $[(NAD-e)^-$ and $(FAD-2e)^-]$ are transferred to molecular oxygen.

Electrons are highly reactive, and were they to "escape" within the cell, could cause considerable damage by generating *free radicals* (Chapter 24). In the mitochondria of the well-oxygenated heart, negatively charged free radicals do not accumulate because the reactions of oxidative phosphorylation transfer the reactive electrons smoothly to oxygen, leading to the production of water. Disruption of these reactions, however, can lead to the appearance of highly toxic, negatively charged oxygen free radicals.

The oxidative reactions of carbohydrate and fatty acid metabolism produce the electrons that, when they pass through the respiratory chain, provide the energy required to regenerate ATP. Thus, the oxidations described in Chapter 4 and the preceding sections of this chapter can be viewed simply as the removal of electrons (accompanied by protons) from carbohydrates and fats. The electrons are then passed through the coenzymes and iron atoms in the respiratory chain, eventually reaching molecular oxygen (Fig. 5.9), where they are transferred to oxygen. The protons then combine with this negatively charged oxygen to form H_2O.

Electron Transfer Through the Respiratory Chain

The successive transfer of electons by the enzymes of the respiratory chain occurs through a series of tightly linked steps of oxidation and reduction. Starting with reduced NAD, the series of reactions can be depicted as shown in Fig. 5.9. The electrons "carried" in NAD and FAD (and coenzyme Q, or ubiquinone) are included in complex organic ring structures according to the general reactions:

$$= N^+- \quad + \quad e^- \quad \leftrightarrow \quad -N-$$

(reduced)   (oxidized)

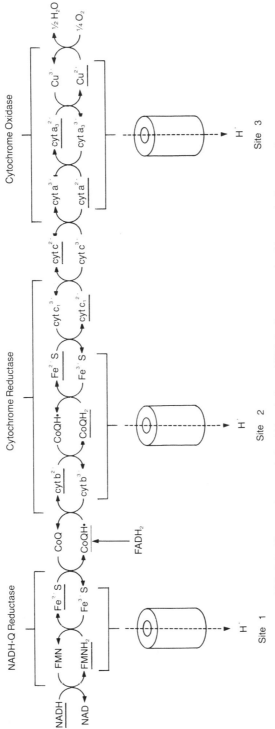

FIG. 5.9. The respiratory chain. Abbreviations: FMN, flavin mononucleotide prosthetic group of NADH-Q reductase; FeS, iron sulfate prosthetic group of *NADH-Q reductase*; CoQ, oxidized coenzyme Q (ubiquinone); *CoQH·*, semiquinone free radical; CoQH₂, reduced CoQ (ubiquinol); cyt, cytochrome; Cu, copper contained in cyt a₃. Reduced states of the respiratory chain components are underlined. The three enzyme complexes are named above the respiratory chain, and the three proton translocations are shown below. Note that reduced FADH₂ enters the chain after the first of the proton translocation steps through a redox step that is catalyzed by *succinate Q reductase*. FADH₂ is also produced by β-oxidation. The overall sequence starts when an electron is removed from NADH (which can be viewed as [NAD-e⁻ +H⁺]) and ends when this electron is combined with molecular oxygen.

and

$$= O \quad + \quad e^- \quad \leftrightarrow \quad -O^-.$$
$$\text{(reduced)} \qquad\qquad\qquad \text{(oxidized)}$$

As noted above, these structures protect the cell contents from attack by the highly reactive electrons. A similar principle applies when the electrons carried by the cytochromes reduce the ferric iron of the heme rings according to the general reaction:

$$Fe^{3+} \quad + \quad e^- \quad \leftrightarrow \quad Fe^{2+}.$$
$$\text{(reduced)} \qquad\qquad\qquad \text{(oxidized)}$$

The prosthetic groups and coenzymes of the respiratory chain shown in Fig. 5.9 are grouped in three large protein complexes, all of which span the mitochondrial inner membrane. Each traps the energy released as electrons pass through the enzyme complex to pump protons (H^+) across the mitochondrial inner membrane, much as water flowing down a waterwheel can lift a heavy object. This proton gradient is then coupled to high-energy phosphate regeneration (see below).

The first of the enzyme complexes of the respiratory chain is *NADH-Q reductase* (or *NADH-dehydrogenase*) which has a molecular weight of ~800,000 and contains about 25 peptides, flavin mononucleotide (FMN), and several iron sulfate clusters (FeS) that participate directly in electron flux. The coenzyme Q that couples NADH-Q reductase to the next of these enzyme complexes also accepts electrons from the FADH$_2$ formed by the oxidation of succinate (Fig. 5.4) and by β-oxidation (Fig. 5.2). The "late" entry of electrons from FADH$_2$, is catalyzed by *succinate-Q reductase* (or succinyl-CoA reductase, see above), which transfers the electrons from succinyl-CoA to coenzyme Q after the first proton translocation (Fig. 5.9).

The second enzyme complex in the respiratory chain, the *ubiquinol-cytochrome c reductase complex* (also called *cytochrome reductase*, or b-c$_1$ complex) is composed of at least eight proteins that are aggregated in a dimeric structure with a molecular weight of approximately 500,000. In addition to the heme iron atoms of two cytochromes (b and c), cytochrome reductase contains an FeS protein. The *cytochrome c oxidase complex* (or *cytochrome a,a$_3$*), the third enzyme complex, like NADH-Q reductase and ubiquinone-cytochrome c reductase, is an intrinsic membrane protein that can pump protons across the mitochondrial inner membrane. Cytochrome oxidase contains cytochromes a and a$_3$ and two copper atoms in a protein complex consisting of at least eight peptides in monomers of ~300,000 molecular weight.

Each of the three proton translocations that occur in the respiratory chains (Fig. 5.9) provides chemiosmotic energy that is subsequently trapped when 2 moles of ATP are regenerated (see below). Overall, therefore, 6 moles of ATP are produced per mole of NADH. In the case of the FADH$_2$ (the "late entry" produced in carbohydrate metabolism by succinate oxidation, and in β-oxidation), one of these sites is bypassed, so that each mole of FADH$_2$ leads to the production of 4 moles of ATP.

MECHANISM OF OXIDATIVE PHOSPHORYLATION

Attempts to define the molecular mechanism of oxidative phosphorylation have an interesting history that illustrates the pitfalls of extrapolating from one process to another. Much as the early students of nerve transmission looked to hydraulic and electrical systems to explain the passage of an impulse down a nerve (see Preface), the pioneers in the field of oxidative phosphorylation searched for a phosphorylated intermediate that, like the sugar-phosphates in glycolysis, contained a high-energy phosphate bond that could donate its energy to ADP to form ATP by a substrate-level phosphorylation. It is now clear, however, that respiratory chain-linked phosphorylation occurs by a different mechanism: the transfer of energy to ADP from a proton electrochemical gradient across the mitochondrial membrane.

The proton electrochemical gradient across the mitochondrial membrane is generated when the flow of electrons through the respiratory chain (Fig. 5.9) is used to pump protons "uphill" out of the mitochondrial matrix (Fig. 5.10). The "polarity" of this proton gradient generates an electronegative environment within the mitochondria (Fig. 5.10) that provides the proton-motive force that is "tapped" to provide energy for the synthesis of ATP from ADP and P_i.

In many ways, oxidative phosphorylation resembles the reverse reaction of an ion pump, which of course uses the energy of ATP for active ion transport. In the mitochondria, however, energy generated during the downhill flux of protons is coupled to the phosphorylation of ADP to form ATP, rather than the other way around.

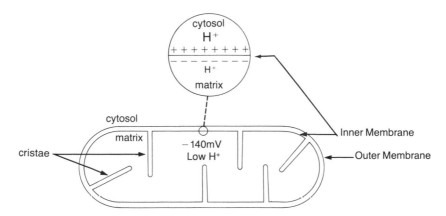

FIG. 5.10. The electrochemical gradient across the mitochondrial inner membrane, generated by proton translocation out of the mitochondria, consists of two components: a proton concentration gradient and electronegativity within the mitochondrial matrix.

ATP Synthetase

The proton-motive force created by the respiratory chain synthesizes ATP in reactions that are catalyzed by yet another membrane spanning, multimeric enzyme complex. This complex, *ATP synthetase*, projects from the surface of the mitochondrial inner membrane into the matrix in structures once called "membrane particles" (Fig. 5.11). ATP synthesis from ADP and P_i, that is, transduction of the electrochemical energy of the proton gradient into the chemical-bond energy found in the phosphate bonds of ATP, appears to involve at least two steps. The first occurs when proton translocation "energizes" ATP synthetase, which is followed by a subsequent step in which this energy is transferred to a high-energy bond between ADP and P_i.

> The reactions coupling ATP synthesis to proton fluxes can be run in reverse when ATP hydrolysis pumps protons uphill, against their concentration gradient. Normally, of course, ATP synthetase does not function as a proton pump, because another system (the respiratory chain) rather than ATP hydrolysis creates the ion gradient.

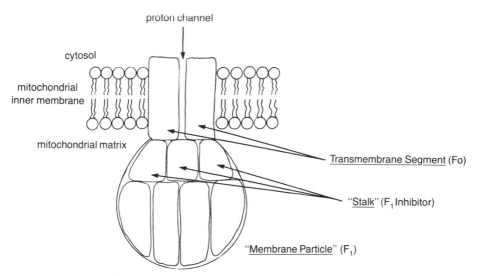

FIG. 5.11. ATP synthetase consists of intramembrane particles that project into the mitochondrial matrix. This complex transduces downhill proton flux into the mitochondria, which takes place through a channel in the transmembrane hydrophobic segment within the membrane (F_o), to generate high-energy phosphate bonds of ATP. The latter part of this reaction is mediated by the proteins of the "membrane particle" (F_i) that also contains a site that hydrolyzes ATP.

Calcium Fluxes Across the Mitochondria

Mitochondria are able to transport calcium both into and out of their matrix, but compared to the rapid proton movements that occur during oxidative phosphorylation, these calcium fluxes are extremely slow. Calcium uptake into the mitochondria is an energy-requiring process that can utilize either the negative intramitochondrial potential generated by the respiratory chain or an ATP-dependent calcium pump to concentrate this cation within the matrix.

Calcium overloading of myocardial cells can cause the mitochondria to take up so much calcium that insoluble calcium-phosphate precipitates appear within the mitochondrial matrix. This dissipates the proton electrochemical gradient across the mitochondrial inner membrane, and so "uncouples" oxidative phosphorylation in that electron transport through the respiratory chain no longer leads to the phosphorylation of ADP. This effect may be of importance in the ischemic heart where the mitochondria become filled with calcium (Chapter 24).

> The mitochondrial calcium pump was once thought to contribute to the removal of activator Ca^{2+} from the cytosol that causes the heart to relax. It is now generally agreed, however, that mitochondrial calcium uptake is too slow, and the Ca^{2+}-affinity of the mitochondrial calcium pump too low, for this energy-requiring process to play a role in the relaxation of the normal heart. However, under pathological conditions associated with cytosolic calcium overloading, mitochondrial calcium uptake may help the heart to relax.

ENERGY BALANCES

The generation of ATP during the metabolic processes described in this chapter, and in Chapter 4, results from two general types of reaction. The first, *substrate-level phosphorylation*, occurs when the substrate itself contains a high-energy phosphate bond that is transferred to ADP, yielding ATP. [In the case of succinyl-CoA oxidation, the inital transfer is to guanosine diphosphate (GDP).] Much more important from a quantitative standpoint is *respiratory chain-linked phosphorylation*, in which the high-energy phosphate bonds are formed during oxidative phosphorylation.

The net synthesis of ATP by *anaerobic* glycolysis, where the NADH produced by the oxidation of glyceraldehyde-3-phosphate is oxidized to NAD when pyruvate is reduced to lactate (Fig. 4.1), produces a net of only 2 moles of ATP per mole of glucose entirely by substrate-level phosphorylation (Table 5.1). During *aerobic* glycolysis, where NADH is oxidized to NAD, respiratory chain-linked phosphorylation of the electrons carried in NADH regenerates additional ATP. Glycolysis yields 2 moles of triose per mole of glucose, and metabolism of each mole of triose, in turn, generates one mole of NADH, so that during glyceraldehyde-3-phosphate oxidation, a total of 2 moles of NADH per mole of glucose are produced. Had these 2 moles of NADH been generated inside the mitochondria, they would have provided for the formation of a total of 6 moles of ATP. However, because glycolysis occurs

TABLE 5.1. *Energy balances: Net ATP generated (moles ATP/mole of glucose)*

Reaction	Substrate-level phosphorylation	Respiratory chain-linked phosphorylation	Total
Anaerobic			
Anaerobic glycolysis			
Glucose → lactate	2	0	2
Aerobic			
Aerobic glycolysis			
Glucose → pyruvate	2	0	
2 NADH → 2 NAD	0	4	
Total	2	4	6
Pyruvate oxidation			
2 pyruvate → 2 acetyl-CoA + CO_2	0	0	
2 NADH → 2 NAD	0	6	
Total	0	6	6
Acetate oxidation			
2 Acetyl-CoA → 4 CO_2	2	0	
6 NADH → 6 NAD	0	18	
2 $FADH_2$ → 2 FAD	0	4	
Total	2	22	24
Glucose oxidation (Total)			
Glucose → 6 CO_2	4	32	36

in the cytosol, this NADH first must be transported into the mitochondria by way of the malate-aspartate shuttle, a process that requires the expenditure of energy. For this reason, only 2 moles of ATP are recovered per mole of NADH generated in the cytosol. Aerobic glycolysis thus adds 4 moles of respiratory chain-linked ATP produced per mole of glucose to the net of 2 moles of substrate level ATP production, giving a total of 6 moles of ATP generated per mole of glucose (Table 5.1).

The aerobic metabolism of the pyruvate produced during glycolysis yields additional ATP because oxidation of pyruvate to acetyl-CoA, which occurs within the mitochondria, is accompanied by the reduction of NAD to form NADH (Fig. 4.9). Oxidation of this NADH through respiratory chain-linked phosphorylation provides an additional 3 moles of ATP per mole of pyruvate. As each glucose molecule yields two of pyruvate, this reaction generates 6 moles of ATP per mole of glucose (Table 5.1).

The oxidation of each mole of acetyl-CoA in the tricarboxylic acid cycle yields an additional 3 moles of NADH and one of enzyme-bound $FADH_2$ (Fig. 5.4A). Each mole of NADH (formed by the oxidation of isocitrate, α-ketoglutarate, and malate) yields 3 moles of ATP, so that NADH oxidation in the tricarboxylic acid cycle yields a total of 9 moles of ATP per mole of acetyl-CoA. Oxidation of each mole of E-$FADH_2$, the "late entry" formed during succinyl-CoA oxidation, yields only 2 moles of ATP, giving a total of 11 moles of ATP per each mole of acetyl-CoA. In addition to the ATP produced by respiratory chain-linked phosphorylation, a single mole of ATP is produced by the substrate-level phosphorylation that occurs when succinyl-CoA is oxidized (Fig. 5.4B). Oxidation of each mole of acetyl-CoA therefore provides 12 moles of ATP, 11 by respiratory chain-linked phosphorylation and 1 by substrate level phosphorylation. As 2 moles of acetyl-CoA are formed from each mole of glucose, a total of 24 moles of ATP are formed by the oxidation of both of the 2-carbon fragments derived from glucose (Table 5.1). Adding to this total the 6 moles of ATP generated by aerobic glycolysis and the 6 moles generated as the result of pyruvate oxidation allows aerobic metabolism to regenerate a total of 36 moles of ATP per mole of glucose.

The "balance sheet" presented in Table 5.1 shows that of the 36 moles of ATP that can be produced by the metabolism of a single mole of glucose, all but two require that the heart be provided with oxygen. For this reason, anoxia or ischemia halts the production of almost 95% of the ATP potentially available from glucose metabolism. As oxygen lack also inhibits completely the oxidation of fatty acids, which normally are a more important energy source for the heart than carbohydrates, the devastating effects of ischemia on cardiac function are readily apparent.

CONTROL OF OXIDATIVE PHOSPHORYLATION

Our understanding of the mechanisms that control the rate of oxidative phosphorylation have recently been advanced by nuclear magnetic resonance data that provide accurate measurements of substrate and high-energy phosphate levels in the living heart. Earlier studies of isolated mitochondria had suggested that the rate of ATP production was determined mainly by the availability of ADP, a mechanism called *acceptor control*. However, this explanation is no longer tenable as changes in ADP and P_i levels observed in the living heart are too small to account for marked changes in the rate of oxidative phosphorylation (Balaban, 1990). A role for changing oxygen tension in the physiological regulation of this important process can be excluded because of the remarkably low oxygen tensions needed for oxidative phosphorylation, which has a Michaelis constant (K_m) for oxygen of less than $1\mu M$. Thus, under all but the most extreme conditions of hypoxia, the high oxygen affinity of the mitochondria can maintain a normal rate of oxidative phosphorylation.

It now appears, instead, that oxidative phosphorylation is normally regulated mainly by the redox state of the heart, notably by the availability of NADH and $FADH_2$. However, substrate delivery, the availability of ADP and P_i, and possibly intracellular Ca^{2+} levels may also contribute to the regulation of this key mechanism for cardiac energy production. Because oxidative phosphorylation in the heart is so rapid, and its affinity for oxygen so great, when coronary artery occlusion interrupts the heart's blood supply, the ischemic cells quickly deplete the limited stores of oxygen (Chapter 24) until, within minutes, it runs out. Thus, when a myocardial cell is deprived of its blood supply, oxidative metabolism ceases rapidly, like a light bulb connected to an on-off switch, rather than to a dimmer.

The mechanisms that regulate oxidative phosphorylation probably shift under different conditions. Normally, in the aerobic heart, where oxygen and ATP levels

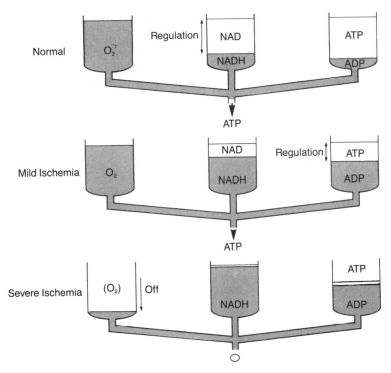

FIG. 5.12. Shifts in the mechanisms that regulate oxidative phosphorylation under normal conditions, and mild and severe ischemia. *Normal:* Under normal conditions supplies of O_2 are plentiful, and while ADP levels are low, oxidative phosphorylation is probably limited by the availability of NADH. When energy demands are increased, NADH is generated more rapidly than it can be oxidized; the resulting increased levels of NADH (and $FADH_2$) probably provide the most important regulatory mechanism in the well-oxygenated heart. *Mild ischemia:* When mild hypoxia decreases energy production, NADH levels rise, ATP levels fall modestly, and ADP levels increase. Under these conditions, regulation of oxidative phosphorylation may shift to control by ADP, rather than NADH. *Severe ischemia:* Under conditions of severe ischemia, lack of O_2 prevents reoxidation of NAD by the respiratory chain enzymes, ATP production virtually ceases, and ADP accumulates. The rate of oxidative phosphorylation is probably limited by the supply of O_2.

are high and ADP levels are low but stable, NADH concentrations are probably rate limiting. When the heart becomes mildly ischemic, as in patients with angina pectoris (Chapter 24), ADP accumulates and NADH increases; under these conditions, the elevated ADP levels may, through acceptor control, become important in regulating the rate of oxidative phosphorylation (Fig. 5.12). In severe ischemia, as in the patient with a myocardial infarction, NADH and $FADH_2$ accumulate and so cease to control the rate of oxidation; even though ADP accumulates, this too plays no role in regulation. Instead, O_2 supply becomes rate limiting (Fig. 5.12); but because of the heart's limited oxygen stores, aerobic metabolism soon ceases and the ischemic myocardial cells begin to die.

COMPARTMENTATION OF ATP IN THE HEART

The *content* (moles/unit weight) of ATP in the myocardium is about 5 mmoles/kg wet weight, so that if ATP were to be uniformly distributed in the cell, its *concentration* (moles/unit volume) would be slightly more than 5mM. However, the average ATP content that is readily measured in a frozen, pulverized tissue sample, cannot provide an accurate measurement of its concentration at critical ATPase sites. Calculations of adenine nucleotide concentrations based on the equilibrium constant of cytosolic creatine phosphokinase and observed rates of mitochondrial respiration indicate that there are large gradients for ATP, ADP, and especially adenosine monophosphate (AMP) between the cytosol and mitochondrial matrix (Illingworth et al., 1975).

For almost 20 years, evidence has accumulated that suggests that the ATP produced by glycolysis is, in some way, of special importance to the function of a variety of ion pumps and other membrane functions during ischemia (Owen et al., 1990; Weiss and Lamp, 1987). Although no membrane barrier has been identified that defines an anatomical "compartment" for this so-called glycolytic ATP, there is considerable evidence that ATP generated by glycolysis is, in some way, special. Perhaps the glycolytic enzymes that readily copurify with a variety of membrane preparations *in vitro* are able to generate ATP near sites at which it is consumed.

INTEGRATION OF GLYCOLYSIS AND RESPIRATION

The integration of fat and carbohydrate metabolism is of great importance in determining the substrates used for ATP production by the heart. Normally the heart resembles an omnivore in that it can derive energy from either carbohydrates or lipids. Lipids are the preferred substrate, so that when the well-oxygenated heart is presented with an adequate supply of fatty acids, glycogen and glycose breakdown are inhibited. This suppression of carbohydrate metabolism when fatty acids are oxidized reflects the effective integration of the rates of lipid and glycolytic metabolism.

The aerobic heart normally extracts lactate from the coronary arterial blood, so that lactate is oxidized by the myocardium under aerobic conditions. In the hypoxic or ischemic heart, however, large quantities of lactate appear in the coronary venous effluent because lactate cannot be oxidized, and this metabolite is produced as a by-product of anaerobic glycolysis. When the heart returns to aerobic conditions, the cessation of lactate production is accompanied by a shift from carbohydrate metabolism to fatty acid oxidation; together these represent an expression of the *Pasteur effect*, which is the inhibition of anaerobic glycolysis when oxidative metabolism becomes activated.

Lipid and carbohydrate metabolism are integrated at several of the metabolic steps described in this and the preceding chapter. The NADH/NAD ratio plays an important role in the regulation of *pyruvate metabolism*. Under aerobic conditions, where NAD is the predominant form of this coenzyme, pyruvate oxidation to acetyl-CoA is favored at the expense of its reduction to lactate (Fig. 4.9). At this control point, the oxidized NAD produced by the mitochondria of the well-oxygenated heart inhibits lactate production almost completely. Energy production from lipid oxidation also inhibits *glycogen breakdown*, due to allosteric inhibition of phosphorylase *b* activity (the predominant form of this enzyme in the heart under basal conditions) by the high levels of ATP, and the low levels of AMP and P_i.

Glucose utilization is inhibited at several steps when fatty acid metabolism is activated. Fatty acids inhibit *glucose transport* into the cell, and *glucose phosphorylation* by hexokinase is inhibited by the glucose-6-phosphate that accumulates when the phosphofructokinase reaction is inhibited by high ATP and low ADP and P_i levels, *Fructose-6-phosphate phosphorylation* is slowed when phosphofructokinase activity is inhibited by the rise in the ATP/ADP ratio that results from rapid ATP production during active lipid metabolism. *Citrate*, another important inhibitor of phosphofructokinase, is produced in the mitochondria when acetyl-CoA generated by β-oxidation accelerates the tricarboxylic acid cycle. At the same time, "transport" of citrate to the cytosol via the malate-aspartate cycle slows glycolysis by inhibiting phosphofructokinase. Inhibition of *pyruvate oxidation* by high concentrations of NADH and acetyl-CoA produced during fatty acid oxidation also reduces carbohydrate metabolism when the heart is rapidly oxidizing fats.

Another substance that integrates fat and carbohydrate metabolism is the coenzyme FAD, which is required both for the tricarboxylic acid cycle and for the β-oxidation of fatty acids. In the case of regulation by FAD, however, the inhibition may be of fat metabolism by carbohydrate metabolism, rather than the other way around. Fat and carbohydrate metabolism are also integrated by the tricarboxylic acid intermediate succinyl-CoA, which is generated by the metabolism of acetyl-CoA produced during aerobic glycolysis. When succinyl-CoA accumulates, a large proportion of the available FAD becomes enzyme-bound and so unable to participate in lipid oxidation (Fig. 5.2).

Overall, these complex interrelationships between lipid and carbohydrate metabolism allow the myocardium to reduce the rate of energy production from glycogen and glucose when there is an abundant supply of fats and oxygen.

"Energy-Wasting" in Lipid Metabolism

It is well established that the oxygen consumed by the heart in performing a given level of work is increased when high concentrations of fatty acids are delivered to the myocardium. The "inefficiency" of lipid metabolism may be functionally significant when coronary flow is limited, so that in the hypoxic or ischemic heart high fatty acid concentrations can impair cardiac performance. The mechanism responsible for this effect, which appears to be potentiated by β-adrenergic agonists, may be related to an effect of fatty acids to uncouple oxidative phosphorylation or to promote triglyceride formation (Vik-Mo and Mjos, 1981). High fatty acid concentrations also have detrimental effects on membranes, due to their detergent effects (Chapter 2), that may contribute to ischemic damage (Chapter 24).

OVERVIEW OF ENERGY PRODUCTION IN THE HEART

The complexity of the metabolic pathways that supply chemical energy for cardiac contraction illustrates the estraordinary extent to which cellular regulation has developed in the myocardium. These many reactions reflect many different principles of control, including *substrate availability, product inhibition*, and dependence on a variety of *cofactors* such as the substrates for phosphorylation and coenzymes for oxidation or reduction. Control of specific enzymes is also affected by *allosteric effects*, which regulate metabolic rate through changes in enzyme conformation that can increase of decrease catalytic activity. *Hormones* and *neurotransmitters* modulate the rates of enzymatic reactions by special types of allosteric regulation, notably enzyme phosphorylation through the cascade of reactions involving cyclic AMP and calcium (Fig. 4.7). Changes in *membrane transport* participate in the control of intermediary metabolism: at the sarcolemma by regulating substrate availability, and at the mitochondrial membrane by modulating the malate-aspartate cycle, adenine nucleotide transfer, and oxidative phosphorylation itself. Together these mechanisms "fine-tune" the pathways of energy production in the heart so as to optimize substrate-utilization to meet the specific needs existing at any moment. More importantly, these complex regulatory mechanisms help to fulfill the requirement that ATP be produced at a rate exactly equal to that at which it is being consumed, a mandatory condition for the uninterrupted beating of the heart in the intact animal (Chapter 3).

As noted at the beginning of Chapter 4, three general types of control govern the rate of energy production in the heart; each occupies a more or less defined "place" in these complex mechanisms of regulation. The first is *humoral*, which serves mainly to regulate the entry of substrates, both carbohydrate and fat, into the pathways of intermediary metabolism. This control allows circulating hormones and neurotransmitters, notably the β-adrenergic agonists, to provide additional substrate for energy production at the same time they increase the rate of energy utilization in the heart (see Chapters 12 and 14). Second, there is a control that responds to the cellular requirement for *high-energy phosphates*, which helps to match the rate of ATP production with that of ATP utilization. In the normal heart, these mechanisms allow cellular levels of high-energy phosphates to remain virtually constant in spite of marked changes in cardiac work. This regulation not only avoids problems that would arise if the rate of energy production were to fall behind that of energy utilization, but by maintaining a high ATP/ADP ratio, also maximizes the free energy of ATP hydrolysis. Finally, there is control by the *redox state* of the coenzymes essential for the critical oxidative steps of substrate metabolism, and probably also for the overall rate of oxidative phsophorylation in the well-oxygenated heart. Redox control also integrates oxidative and anaerobic metabolism, whereas integration of lipid and carbohydrate metabolism probably involves the operation of all these different regulatory mechanisms.

Together these control mechanisms maintain an almost constant level of ATP within the normal myocardium, while at the same time allowing the heart to make optimal use of the substrates delivered to it in the coronary arterial blood. Some effects of disordered cardiac function on these regulatory systems have already been mentioned; their functional significance is described later when the effects of ischemia (Chapter 24) and hemodynamic overloading (Chapter 25) are considered in detail.

REFERENCES

Abumrad NA, Perkins RC, Park JH, Park CR. (1981). Mechanism of long chain fatty acid permeation in the isolated adipocyte. *J Biol Chem* 256:9183–9191.

Balaban RS. (1990). Regulation of oxidative phosphorylation in the mammalian cell. *Am J Physiol* 258:C377–C389.

Gabriel JL, Plaut GWE. (1984). Inhibition of bovine heart NAD-specific isocitrate dehydrogenase by reduced pyridine nucleotides: modulation of inhibition by ADP, NAD$^+$, Ca^{2+}, citrate, and isocitrate. *Biochemistry* 23:2772–2778.

Hochachka PW, Neely JR, Driedzic WR. (1977). Integration of lipid utilization with Krebs cycle activity in muscle. *Fed Proc* 36:2009–2014.

Idell-Wenger JA, Grotyohann LW, Neely JR. (1982). Regulation of fatty acid utilization in heart. Role of the carnitine-acetyl-CoA transferase and carnitine-acetylcarnitine translocase system. *J Mol Cell Cardiol* 14:413–417.

Illingworth JA, Ford WCB, Kobayashi K, Williamson JR. (1975). Regulation of myocardial energy metabolism. *Recent Adv Stud Card Struct Metab* 8:271–290.

Jacobus WE. (1985). Respiratory control and the integration of heart high-energy phosphate metabolism by mitochondrial creatine kinase. *Annu Rev Physiol* 47:707–725.

Kim K-I, Lopez-Casillas F, Bai DH, Luo X, Pape ME. (1989). Role of reversible phosphorylation of acetyl-CoA carboxylase in long chain fatty acid synthesis. *FASEB J* 3:2250–2256.

Lech JJ, Jesmak GJ, Calvert DN. (1977). Effects of drugs and hormones on lipolysis in heart. *Fed Proc* 36:2000–2008.

McClellan G, Weisberg A, Winegrad S. (1983). Energy transport from mitochondria to myofibril by a creatine phosphate shuttle in cardiac cells. *Am J Physiol* 245:C423–C427.

Owen P, Dennis S, Opie LH. (1990). Glucose flux regulates the onset of ischemic contracture in globally underperfused rat hearts. *Circ Res* 66:344–354.

Rose CP, Goresky CA. (1977). Constraints on the uptake of labelled palmitate by the heart. The barriers at the capillary and sarcolemmal surfaces and the control of intracellular sequestration. *Circ Res* 41:534–545.

Rushbrook JI, Harvey RA. (1978). Nicotinamide adenine nucleotide dependent isocitrate dehydrogenase from beef heart: subunit heterogeneity and enzyme dissociation. *Biochemistry* 17:5339–5346.

Steinberg D. (1977). Interconvertible enzymes in adipose tissue regulated by cyclic AMP-dependent protein kinase. *Adv Cyclic Nucl Res* 7:157–198.

Taegtmeyer H, Peterson MB, Ragever VV, Ferguson AG, Lesch M. (1977). *De novo* alanine synthesis in isolated oxygen-deprived rabbit myocardium. *J Biol Chem* 252:5010–5018.

Vik-Mo H, Mjos OD. (1981). Influence of free fatty acids on myocardial oxygen consumption and ischemic injury. *Am J Cardiol* 48:361–365.

Weiss JN, Lamp SL (1987). Glycolysis preferentially inhibits ATP-sensitive K$^+$ channels in isolated guinea pig cardiac myocytes. *Science* 238:67–69.

BIBLIOGRAPHY

Boyer PD, Chance B, Ernster L, Mitchell P, Racker E, Slater EC. (1977). Oxidative phosphorylation and photophosphorylation. *Annu Rev Biochem* 67:955–1026.

Crass MF III. (1977). Regulation of triglyceride metabolism in the isotopically prelabeled perfused heart. *Fed Proc* 36:1995–1999.

Eckel RH. (1989). Lipoprotein lipase. A multifunctional enzyme relevant to common metabolic diseases. *N Engl J Med* 320:1060–1068.

Fain JN. (1982). Regulation of lipid metabolism by cyclic nucleotides. In: Kebabian JW, Nathanson JA, eds. *Handbook of experimental pharmacology*, vol 58/II. Berlin: Springer-Verlag; 89–150.

Lehninger AL. (1971). *Bioenergetics*, 2nd ed. Menlo Park, CA: W.A. Benjamin. (See also Bibliography to Chapter 3.)

Safer B. (1975). The metabolic significance of the malate-aspartate cycle in the heart. *Circ Res* 37:527–533.

Scarpa A. (1979). Transport across mitochondrial membranes. In: *Membrane transport in biology*. Giebisch G, Tosteson DC, Ussing HH, eds. Berlin: Springer-Verlag, 263–355.

Strålfors P, Olsson H, Belfrage P. (1987). Hormone-sensitive lipase. In: Boyer PD, Krebs EC. *The enzymes*, vol 18. Orlando: The Academic Press; 147–177.

6

Energy Utilization
(Work and Heat)

Elucidation of the relationship between the conditions under which a muscle works and its energy expenditure, as work and as heat, represents one of the more fascinating chapters in the history of biology. The understanding of the link between the *mechanical* expression of the metabolic activity of muscle and the *chemical* processes responsible for contraction, has made an important contribution to our knowledge of the chemistry of muscular contraction. As the processes that consume energy during contraction are tightly integrated with those of energy production (Chapters 4 and 5), there is a close coupling between muscular work, on the one hand, and muscle chemistry on the other.

When adenosine triphosphate (ATP) is consumed by the contractile machinery during the performance of external work, the internal energy content of a muscle becomes reduced (Chapter 3). This disappearance of internal energy, of course, constitutes only half of the energy change in the active muscle:

Net energy change = disappearance of internal (chemical) energy.

The other half of this equation is:

Net energy change = appearance of external energy (work and heat).

It is this second part of the energy equation, the performance of work and the appearance of heat, that completes the description of a muscle as a mechanochemical transducer.

The external energies of muscle are complex and include the useful work performed by the muscle, the product of tension and shortening, and the external energy that appears as heat. Although the heat produced by a muscle is not entirely "waste"—shivering, for example, can maintain body temperature in cold environments—the conversion of chemical energy to heat inevitably reduces muscular efficiency and so lessens the capacity of the muscle to do useful work (see Eq. 3.2). The heat produced by a muscle, therefore, defines the efficiency, or more precisely the inefficiency, of the contractile process.

Studies of the dependence of heat production on muscle loading conditions have provided remarkably detailed insights into the chemistry of the contractile process. This chapter describes the influence of loading on the mechanical and energetic behavior of a relatively simple skeletal muscle, the frog sartorius. Although the energetics of this amphibian muscle are much simpler than those of the myocardium, these classic relationships have provided a basis for understanding the chemistry and regulation of the contractile processes of the heart.

PRELOAD AND AFTERLOAD

At the outset it is essential to define two terms: *preload* and *afterload,* which describe two ways in which a muscle "sees" a load; these differ only in the time during the contraction when the muscle becomes influenced by the load (Fig. 6.1). Although mainly of theoretical interest in terms of skeletal muscle function, the concepts of preload and afterload are of considerable practical importance in the management of patients with diseased hearts.

A *preload* can be viewed as a weight that stretches a muscle before it is stimulated to contract; in contrast, an *afterload* is not apparent to the muscle when it is in a resting state, but is encountered only after the muscle has started to contract. In the case of a muscle suspended above a table, for example, an afterload rests on a support and so does not influence the muscle until *after* contraction begins (Fig. 6.1).

The loading conditions of the heart are such that its ventricles are both preloaded and afterloaded (Chapter 15). The venous return to the heart during diastole constitutes a preload that dilates the resting ventricle, whereas the blood under pressure in the great vessels (the aorta and pulmonary artery) represents an afterload that is not encountered until the ventricle has developed a significant fraction of its systolic pressure.

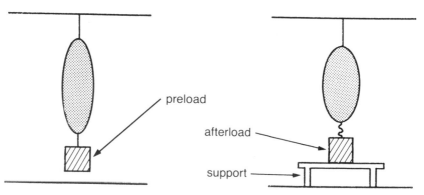

FIG. 6.1. Difference between preload and afterload. The preload stretches the resting muscle (*left*), whereas the afterload is supported so that it is not "felt" by the muscle until it has begun to contract (*right*).

DEPENDENCE OF WORK (MECHANICAL ENERGY LIBERATION) ON LOAD

Loading conditions are a key determinant of the work that can be performed by a contracting muscle. A simple basis for understanding the relationship between load and the performance of muscular work is illustrated by the properties of a spring (Fig. 6.2). Let us assume that when this spring is stretched 10 cm, it develops a tension equivalent to 10 g (Table. 6.1), and that as the spring is stretched, the force it develops is linearly proportional to the increase in length (i.e., the spring obeys Hooke's law). For each centimeter of lengthening, therefore, tension increases by 1 g. Conversely, if the 10-g load is decreased in 1-g steps, the spring shortens by 1 cm for each gram removed from the load. Thus, if a series of lesser weights is placed on the spring stretched 10 cm by a 10-g weight (column *a* in Table 6.1), the values for shortening in column *b* of Table 6.1 are obtained. The work done when the stretched spring is allowed to shorten is readily calculated by multiplying the weight on the spring (the force, expressed in grams in column *a*) by the distance shortened (column *b*); this gives the work performed at each load (column *c*), which is shown in Fig. 6.3 as a work-load relationship. Because work equals force times distance, when the load (P) is equal to the tension developed by the stretched spring (P_o), work is zero because the spring does not shorten. Work is also zero when P = 0, as no force is generated during shortening. Work performance is maximal at intermediate levels of both load and shortening (Table 6.1).

Work-load curves such as that in Fig. 6.3 are also produced by active muscle, although as we shall see, this relationship provides little information as to the process responsible for muscular contraction. Early physiologists, who recognized that work-load relationships for muscle resemble that shown in Fig. 6.3, postulated that during activity the muscle exists in a state analogous to a stretched spring. As a result, the "new elastic body" theory of muscular contraction was formulated. Although now known to be incorrect, this theory is presented in some detail at this point because recognition of its fundamental errors provides a basis for understand-

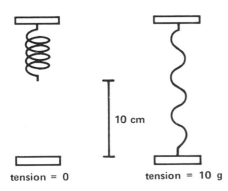

tension = 0

10 cm

tension = 10 g

FIG. 6.2. If a spring that obeys Hooke's law is stretched by a 10-g load and lengthens 10 cm, then for each gram of load removed from the stretched spring (*right*) the spring shortens by 1 cm. When the final load is zero, the spring shortens 10 cm (*left*). If this spring in its stretched state is presented with a series of lighter loads (less than 10 g), the relationship between load and work shown in Table 6.1 and Fig. 6.3 is generated.

TABLE 6.1. *Relationship between shortening and work performed by a stretched spring*

(a) Load (g)	(b) Shortening (cm)	(c) Work (g × cm)
10	0	0
9	1	9
8	2	16
7	3	21
6	4	24
5	5	25
4	6	24
3	7	21
2	8	16
1	9	9
0	10	0

ing the significance of the experiments carried out by Wallace Fenn during the early 1920s. Fenn's experiments, which decisively proved the new elastic body theory of muscular contraction to be wrong and led to the definition of the *Fenn effect,* are of central importance to our modern understanding of muscular contraction.

NEW ELASTIC BODY THEORY OF MUSCULAR CONTRACTION

Experiments such as that shown in Fig. 6.3 suggested that the transition from rest to activity in a muscle resulted from the appearance of new cross-links within the contractile machinery. These new cross-links, which would require chemical energy for their formation, were postulated to give the muscle a new set of spring-like characteristics, i.e., the muscle became a "new elastic body."

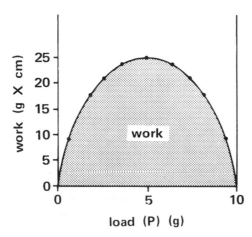

FIG. 6.3. Work-load curve of the spring in Fig. 6.2. Starting with the spring in its stretched state, presentation of the series of lighter loads indicated on the *abscissa* allows the spring to perform the amount of work indicated on the *ordinate*. The work of the spring is calculated simply as the product of load × distance shortened (Table 6.1).

According to the new elastic body theory of muscular contraction, the transition from rest to activity in a muscle is analogous to that in a spring that, at a constant length, assumes new elastic characteristics so as to increase its capacity to generate tension. Such a transition could occur, for example, by formation of chemical bonds along the chains of a polymer (Fig. 6.4). Although stretching of the resting muscle (Fig. 6.4, left) leads to the development of only a small amount of tension (resting tension), during activity much higher tensions develop because of the formation of new elastic cross-links (Fig. 6.4, right). These cause the muscle to assume the new characteristics of a stretched spring, as depicted in Fig. 6.2.

The new elastic body theory predicts that a fixed amount of chemical energy is delivered to the contractile machinery to effect this transition to the new elasticity; as a result, *a constant amount of energy should be released in each contraction regardless of the conditions under which the muscle contracts*. This added energy can be released as work and heat, so that because the work-load curve (Fig. 6.3) defines the load-dependence of work, the load-dependence of energy release as heat would be as shown in Fig. 6.5. At high loads, where $P = P_o$, all of the energy added during the transition from rest to activity should appear as heat because no work is done. Similarly, this added energy should appear solely as heat during contraction of the unloaded muscle, where $P = 0$. The release of work energy, as in the spring (Fig. 6.3), would be maximal at intermediate loads, where energy liberation as heat should be minimal. A key prediction of this model is that total energy release, as work and heat, would be independent of load as the amount of extra energy is determined solely by the new elasticity.

This postulated mechanism of muscular contraction, which was generally accepted until 1923, had to be abandoned with the fundamental discovery by Fenn that *the liberation of energy by contracting muscle is not constant but is influenced by the amount of work done*.

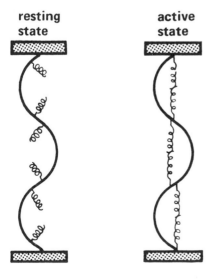

resting state

active state

FIG. 6.4. The new elastic body theory of muscle contraction states that transition of a muscle from its resting state (*left*) to its active state (*right*) can be depicted as the acquisition of new "spring-like" characteristics. This theory carried predictions as to muscle energetics, most important of which is that a constant amount of energy is added in the transition from rest to activity.

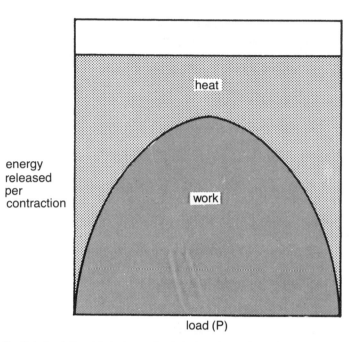

FIG. 6.5. Predicted relationship between load during shortening (*P*) and the total energy released during contraction of a muscle that operates according to the new elastic body theory. If a
fixed amount of energy is added to the muscle during the transition from resting to the active
state (Fig. 6.4), the energy released per contraction—as work plus heat—(*ordinate*) is the same
regardless of load (*abscissa*). Because the work-load curve of the muscle is similar to that depicted for the spring in Fig. 6.3, heat production is predicted to decrease at intermediate loads so
as to maintain energy release per contraction at a constant level.

FENN EFFECT

Fenn's decisive contribution to our understanding of the relationship between
work and total energy release in muscle (Fenn, 1923) is shown in Fig. 6.6. This
discovery was that the total energy released in muscular contraction, as work and
heat, is not constant, but varies in proportion to the work performed. Figure 6.6 thus
demonstrates that the energy available to active muscle is not predetermined at the
time of activation, but instead is influenced by the conditions under which contraction takes place. In simple terms, the Fenn effect states that *as muscle does more
work, more energy is liberated*. In this way a muscle is like an automobile, rather
than a new elastic body, in that the performance of additional work (as when the
automobile pulls a trailer) causes more energy to be utilized by the contractile machinery (reduced gas mileage).

The existence of the Fenn effect was confirmed in a different way during the early
1960s by Mommaerts and by Carlson, who determined the change in the *internal*
energy, measured as a decrease in high-energy phosphate compounds in contracting

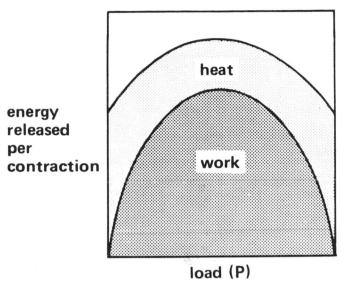

FIG. 6.6. Observed relationship between load during shortening (*P*) and total energy released during contraction of frog sartorius. The total energy released is variable and parallels the total work performed. The ability of a muscle to increase total energy release when performing a greater amount of work constitutes the Fenn effect.

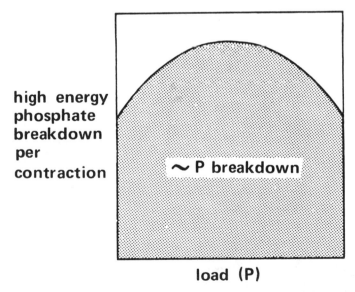

FIG. 6.7. Observed relationship between load during shortening (*P*) and high-energy phosphate breakdown per contraction. An increased amount of chemical energy is used when the muscle shortens at an intermediate load and so is performing a larger amount of work than at heavy or light loads (Fig. 6.3). These data provide an independent demonstration of the Fenn effect shown in Fig. 6.6.

muscle. They found that at intermediate loads, where the highest levels of work were performed, the utilization of high-energy compounds was maximal (Fig. 6.7).

> It is an historical curiosity that the Fenn effect was first documented in cardiac muscle almost a decade before Fenn carried out his classic experiments in skeletal muscle (Evans and Matsuoka, 1914–1915). Cardiac oxygen consumption, which is a valid index of internal energy release by the heart (Chapter 3), was found to increase when the work of the heart was increased. These observations, which had been overlooked by most muscle physiologists of the time, are noted in Fenn's classical paper.

As noted in Chapter 15, the relationship between load and total energy release in the heart differs from that in skeletal muscle; this is not a violation of the Fenn effect, but reflects the influence of the complex architecture of the myocardium (Chapter 1) on its energetics.

FORCE-VELOCITY RELATIONSHIP

The force-velocity relationship, which defines the influence of load on the velocity of muscle shortening, provides additional evidence that a contracting muscle does not behave like a stretched spring (a new elastic body). The correct shape of the curve relating load and shortening velocity was first shown clearly by Fenn and Marsh in 1935. Prior to that time contracting muscle was modeled as an elastic element that shortened in parallel with a viscous element (Fig. 6.8). If the viscous element had the characteristics of a Newtonian viscosity, then according to the new elastic body theory, shortening velocity should increase in a linear manner as load is decreased (curve A, Fig. 6.9). Fenn and Marsh found instead that the force-velocity relationship was hyperbolic (curve B, Fig. 6.9). Although this hyperbolic relationship could be explained within the context of the new elastic body theory by assum-

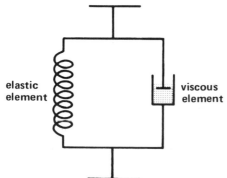

elastic
element

viscous
element

FIG. 6.8. Representation of an active muscle showing an elastic element (depicted at *left* as a spring) and a viscous element (depicted at *right* as a "dashpot").

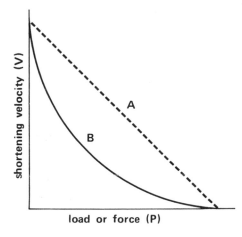

FIG. 6.9. Force-velocity relationship predicted from the model shown in Fig. 6.8 when the elastic element obeys Hooke's law and the viscous element has Newtonian characteristics (A). This predicted relationship differs from the hyperbolic force-velocity relationship actually found for frog sartorius muscle by Fenn and Marsh (B).

ing non-Newtonian characteristics for the viscous element of muscle, *it is now clear that the hyperbolic force-velocity curve of muscle is, instead, an expression of fundamental characteristics of the contractile machinery of muscle.*

The relationship between the energetics of muscular contraction and the characteristics of the contractile machinery was greatly clarified by the classic experiments carried out in 1938 by Hill. These experiments demonstrated, among other things, that the hyperbolic force-velocity curve shown in Fig. 6.9 could be predicted from measurements of the influence of load on the rate of energy liberation as work and heat.

HEAT LIBERATION BY ACTIVE MUSCLE

The accurate measurement of muscle heat was of central importance in the evolution of our understanding of the processes responsible for muscular contraction. This difficult subject can be simplified to some extent by dismissing from this discussion two of the three general classes of muscle heat (Table 6.2 and Fig. 6.10). One of these, *maintenance (or resting) heat,* the slow liberation of heat by resting muscle, is unrelated to contraction and so can be dismissed in the following discussion as representing a "background" heat.

When the muscle is stimulated and contracts, additional heat is liberated. This *activity-related heat* consists of *initial heat* and *recovery heat. Initial heat* is liberated during contraction, whereas *recovery heat* appears after the end of contraction. Recovery heat is related primarily to those processes that return the chemical state of muscle to that which existed before the contraction. In skeletal muscle, recovery heat is largely aerobic and appears to be related primarily to the oxidation of lactate

TABLE 6.2. *Energy liberated by muscle*

Heat	
Maintenance, or Resting heat	Maintenance of ion gradients, protein synthesis
Activity related heat	Excitation, contraction, relaxation, recovery
Initial heat	Excitation, contraction, and relaxation
Tension-independent heat	Sarcolemmal depolarization and repolarization, sarcoplasmic reticulum Ca-release and uptake, Ca binding to troponin, thin filament rearrangement
Activation heat	Tension-independent heat liberated to initiate contraction
Tension-dependent heat	Cross-bridge cycling of contractile proteins
Shortening heat	Muscle shortening, myosin-actin interactions
Tension-time heat	Cross-bridge turnover during tension development
Recovery heat	ATP resynthesis by mitochondria during recovery; includes potential energy returned as heat when muscle relaxes while still bearing a load
Work	
External work	Load (force) times distance (shortening)
Internal work (degraded to heat)	Cross-bridge turnover during tension (f[P,t] above), stretching of series elasticity, internal viscosity

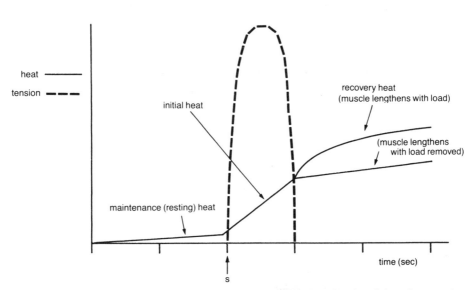

FIG. 6.10. Time course of heat liberation by an active muscle (*solid line*) and, for reference, the time course of tension developed by the muscle (*dashed line*). Maintenance heat is liberated by the resting muscle. Initial heat is liberated during contraction, and recovery heat is liberated during and immediately after relaxation. Note that recovery heat is considerably greater when the muscle is allowed to lengthen under loaded conditions than when the load is removed from the muscle prior to relaxation. s, time of stimulation.

produced during activity (Chapters 4 and 5). In the heart, on the other hand, recovery heat is related to ATP resynthesis in the mitochondria.

> The assumption that resynthesis of ATP (and reversal of other metabolic changes that occur during contraction) occurs only after a muscle has relaxed is, of course, an oversimplification. Tight coupling between the reactions involved in energy production (Chapters 4 and 5) means that many of these "recovery" processes actually begin at virtually the same time that contraction begins to consume ATP.
>
> A large additional quantity of recovery heat is liberated when a muscle is allowed to relax while still bearing a weight (Fig. 6.10). As this extra component of the recovery heat disappears if the load is removed from the muscle at the end of contraction, it can be seen to arise from dissipation of the potential energy of the lifted weight as it stretches the relaxing muscle.

Although of significance in the economy of muscle in the living animal, recovery heat, along with maintenance heat, is not directly related to the contractile process. Therefore recovery heat is also ignored in the following discussion.

The third form of muscle heat, which for historical reasons is called *initial heat,* is the extra heat (extra in that it exceeds maintenance heat) liberated during contraction (Fig. 6.10). The appearance of initial heat precedes and accompanies the onset of shortening and tension generation; it continues during the depolarization and repolarization of the sarcolemma, the release and reuptake of activator calcium by the sarcoplasmic reticulum, and the binding and removal of calcium to troponin.

If experiments are designed so as to prevent the contractile proteins from interacting, no mechanical work can be done. Under these conditions, the initial heat, which is generated by the processes of excitation-contraction coupling (Chapters 10 and 11), is called the *activation heat.* The total *tension-independent heat* released during a full cycle of contraction and relaxation consists of the activation heat plus the heat liberated by the processes that relax the muscle. A much larger component of initial heat is generated by the interactions of the activated contractile proteins; this is the *tension-dependent heat.*

The following section describes how measurements of initial heat permitted Hill to predict the hyperbolic shape of the force-velocity curve and to describe the chemistry of muscular contraction even before the discovery of actin and the adenosine triphosphatase (ATPase) activity of myosin.

LIBERATION OF INITIAL HEAT IN AN ISOMETRIC CONTRACTION

At the start of an *isometric contraction*—in which the ends of the muscle are fixed so that the muscle can neither shorten nor perform external work—two components of initial heat are seen (Fig. 6.11). The first, which appears immediately after stimulation of the muscle (s in Fig. 6.11) is the *activation heat* (A in Fig. 6.11). When tetanic tension is maintained during an isometric contraction, slow cycling of actin-myosin interactions gives rise to *tension-time heat* (see below).

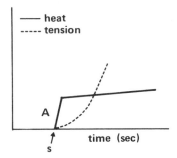

FIG. 6.11. Time course of initial heat liberation by a muscle contracting under isometric conditions (*solid line*) and, for reference, the time course of initial tension development (*dashed line*). The quantity of heat (A) liberated immediately after stimulation (s) is the activation heat.

Activation Heat

Activation heat is manifest as a brief burst of heat, most of which appears before the development of significant tension at the ends of the muscle. The major source of activation heat is probably the release of calcium from the sarcoplasmic reticulum, a region of high Ca^{2+} concentration, into the cytosol, where Ca^{2+} concentration is much lower. Some of the potential energy stored in the Ca^{2+} concentration gradient appears as heat (Rall, 1982). Calcium binding to troponin and the resulting rearrangement of the proteins of the thin filament that initiate contraction are also exothermic processes (Potter et al., 1977). Other changes occurring at the time of activation, notably the ion fluxes responsible for propagation of the action potential, generate much less heat. Thus, calcium release from the sarcoplasmic reticulum, its binding to troponin, and the structural rearrangements in the thin filament that are set in motion by this reaction, give rise to most of the activation heat. The reuptake of calcium by the sarcoplasmic reticulum along with thin filament changes that occur after calcium dissociates from troponin, which occur later during relaxation, also contribute to the initial heat; however, in the following discussion of the heat liberated at the onset of contraction, this component of the initial heat is not considered further.

LIBERATION OF INITIAL HEAT IN AN ISOMETRIC CONTRACTION

The liberation of energy during the development of an isometric contraction can be described by the following equation:

$$\Delta E = A + W_i, \qquad [6.1]$$

where the change in external energy (ΔE) is equal to the activation heat (A) plus the internal work that takes place in the isometrically contracting muscle (W_i). The appearance of a "work" term, (W_i), in the isometric contraction reflects the fact that even when the ends of a muscle are fixed, a small amount of internal work is done by the contractile elements because of slight shape changes in the muscle and stretching of the "series elasticity" (Chapter 9). The internal work, W_i in Eq. 6.1, as well as the small amount of heat liberated when tension is sustained, are discussed later in this chapter, using the term $f(P,t)$ as defined by Mommaerts (1969).

The conventions used in Eq. 6.1 are those of muscle physiology (Chapter 3). When stated in thermodynamic terms, Eq. 6.1 becomes

$$\Delta E = Q - W, \tag{6.2}$$

where Q is the activation heat and W the internal work.

LIBERATION OF INITIAL HEAT IN AN ISOTONIC CONTRACTION

The energetics of an *isotonic contraction,* where a muscle shortens, are more complex than when the muscle contracts under isometric conditions, because two additional forms of energy are released during shortening. The first is the energy made available as work when a loaded muscle is allowed to shorten. The second is an additional component of initial heat that appears when a muscle shortens: the *shortening heat.*

Shortening Heat

In 1938, Hill found that a quantity of extra heat (ax in Fig. 6.12) is liberated when an active muscle is allowed to shorten. This *shortening heat* is independent of the load but is determined only by the distance that the muscle shortens. If a muscle is presented with a series of loads, but constrained so that it can shorten only 1 cm, both the rate and amount of shortening heat can be measured as a function of the load on the muscle as it shortens over this constant distance (Fig. 6.12). When Hill allowed the muscle to shorten 1 cm against a light load (curve 1 in Fig. 6.12), the *total amount* of heat liberated (ax) was the same as that which appeared when the muscle shortened the same distance in the more heavily loaded contraction (curve 2

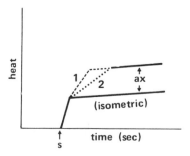

FIG. 6.12. Time course of initial heat liberation by a muscle allowed to shorten a constant distance while lifting a light load (*dashed line*, 1) or a heavy load (*dotted line*, 2). For reference, the time course of initial heat liberation by an isometrically contracting muscle (Fig. 6.11) is also shown. Although the *rate* of heat liberation subsequent to activation heat is slower when the muscle shortens while bearing a heavier load, the *total amount* of heat liberated during shortening (ax) is independent of load. s, time of stimulation.

in Fig. 6.12). However, as noted below, the *rate* of heat liberation was load dependent. When the distance the muscle shortens was increased, the liberation of shortening heat increased proportionately with the extent of shortening (Fig. 6.13).

The molecular reactions that generate shortening heat are related to the detachment and reformation of bonds linking the thick and thin filaments, which in turn arise from the chemical changes in the myosin cross-bridges as they proceed through their cycle, as described in Chapter 8. Although Hill found the total *amount* of extra heat associated with a given degree of shortening is independent of load (Fig. 6.12), the *rate* at which this heat was liberated decreases as the load is increased; this is apparent when the slopes of the dotted lines 1 and 2 in Fig. 6.12 are compared.

Hill introduced the term *a,* which is a constant that characterizes each given type of muscle, to define the amount of heat liberated for each centimeter of shortening. This constant has the dimensions of a force, so that if *x* is the distance the muscle shortens, the total amount of heat liberated during shortening is equal to *a* times *x*; that is,

$$\text{Shortening heat} = ax. \qquad [6.3]$$

It must be remembered, however, that even though the *amount* of shortening heat is independent of load, and depends only on the distance shortened, the *rate* at which the shortening heat appears is inversely related to the load on the muscle. As we have already seen (Fig. 6.9), the speed with which the load is lifted in an isotonic contraction is also inversely proportional to load. As a result, *the rate of energy*

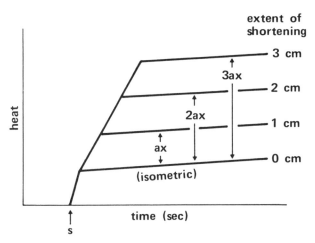

FIG. 6.13. Liberation of initial heat by a muscle allowed to shorten to various lengths while lifting a constant load. The shortening heat (*ax*) increases in proportion to the distance shortened (given as centimeters). Thus, a muscle shortening 2 cm liberates twice as much shortening heat (*2ax*) as a muscle shortening 1 cm (*ax*), whereas the muscle shortening 3 cm liberates a shortening heat of 3ax. s, time of stimulation.

liberation, both as work and as heat, decreases at heavier loads. These important relationships are described later in this chapter.

The energy balance in an isotonic contraction was defined in 1938 by Hill as:

$$E = A + W + ax \qquad [6.4]$$

where A is the activation heat (Eq. 6.1), W is the external work done (internal work is ignored in this formulation), and ax is the shortening heat. Viewed in thermo-dynamic terms (Eq. 6.2), the right side of Eq. 6.4 can be divided into two portions. The first, corresponding to Q in Eq. 6.2, contains the heat terms A and ax; the second, W, corresponds to work that can be expressed as Px, the load P times the distance shortened x (see Eq. 6.7 below).

Tension-Time Heat

The formulations in Eqs. 6.1 and 6.4 were revised during the mid-1960s when greater precision in the measurement of heat liberation became possible. These later studies showed that both activation heat (A) and the heat of shortening (ax) increased at higher loads. A simple interpretation of these findings was offered by Mommaerts (1969), who separated activation heat into two components: A and $f(P,t)$. The first component, A, is the true activation heat that results from the processes involved in excitation, excitation-contraction coupling, and activation of the contractile machinery (Table 6.2), whereas the second term, $f(P,t)$, represents heat liberated as a function of the tension on the muscle (P) and the length of time (t) the tension is maintained. This tension-time heat, which arises from the slow cycling of actin-attached myosin cross-bridges (see Chapter 8) that is independent of changing sarcomere length, is related in part to internal work. If this is included in Eq. 6.1, the equation for an isometric contraction becomes:

$$E = A + W_i + f(P,t). \qquad [6.5]$$

For an isotonic contraction, the term $f(P,t)$ can be included in Eq. 6.4 to give:

$$E = A + W + ax + f(P,t). \qquad [6.6]$$

The heat described by the term $f(P,t)$ is important to an understanding of the energetic consequences of the altered myosin ATPase activity seen in hearts subjected to sustained hemodynamic overloading, in aging, and in various endocrine abnormalities, conditions that can lead to synthesis of a low ATPase myosin isoform (Chapter 14). Although reducing maximal muscle shortening velocity, this alteration in gene expression improves muscle economy by decreasing the amount of energy wasted as tension-time heat [$f(P,t)$]. This improved efficiency is especially important when the heart contracts against an abnormally increased load, as occurs in heart failure (Chapter 25).

For simplicity in our subsequent discussions of the energetics of muscle, the tension-time heat, $f(P,t)$, is omitted. This simplification, although introducing a small error, helps to clarify important relationships between force, velocity, the rate of extra energy liberation, and the chemistry of the contractile proteins.

THE HILL EQUATION

Often called the "characteristic equation of muscle," the Hill equation defines the energetics of muscular contraction in a manner that predicts several key features of the chemistry of the contractile proteins. This remarkable equation, therefore, provides a conceptual link between the mechanical expression of the activity of the contractile machinery—as work and as heat—and the chemical processes that are responsible for contraction.

The Hill equation is derived from analysis of the "extra energy" liberated as work and as heat during muscle contraction. In a muscle that lifts the load P a distance equal to x, *the extra energy liberated as work* is P times x. *The extra energy liberated as heat* is a times x, i.e., the shortening heat (Eq. 6.4). Thus:

$$\text{Extra energy} = (Px) + (ax) = (P + a)x. \qquad [6.7]$$

$$\text{(work) (heat)} \qquad \text{(total energy)}$$

As noted above, activation heat (A in Eq. 6.4) has been omitted from Eq. 6.7 because it is not related to work performance, appearing before the muscle begins to shorten (Fig. 6.11). For simplicity, the $f(P,t)$ term has also been omitted, so that the quantity $(P + a)x$ represents the total amount of extra energy liberated by a muscle shortening under isotonic conditions.

The rate at which this extra energy is liberated is obtained by differentiating the quantity $(P + a)x$ with respect to time, so that:

$$\text{Rate of extra energy liberation} = (P + a)dx/dt. \qquad [6.8]$$

Because $dx/dt + \text{velocity } (v)$, the rate of extra energy liberation is $(P + a)v$; thus, Eq. 6.8 can be rewritten:

$$\text{Rate of extra energy liberation} = (P + a)v. \qquad [6.9]$$

The importance of Eq. 6.9 was made clear by Hill's experimental finding that the rate of extra energy liberation in a contracting muscle is an inverse, linear function of load (Fig. 6.14). In an isometrically contracting muscle, where $P = P_o$, the rate of extra energy liberation is zero because there is neither shortening heat (ax) nor work (Px), due to the fact that the distance shortened (x) is zero. In an unloaded, freely shortening muscle, where $P = 0$, even though no work is done, the rate of extra energy release is maximal (Fig. 6.14). At intermediate loads, Hill found a direct linear proportionality between the rate of extra energy liberation and the difference between the maximal load the muscle can lift (P_o) and the actual load on the muscle (P). As a result, the rate of extra energy release is directly proportional to $P_o - P$. Stated simply, this means that the smaller the load (P), the greater the rate of extra energy release during shortening.

Using a constant of proportionality (b), Hill was able to equate the rate of extra energy release [$(P + a)v$] to load (expressed as $P_o - P$):

$$(P + a)v = b(P_o - P). \qquad [6.10]$$

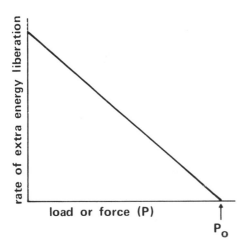

FIG. 6.14. Relationship between load (P) and the rate of extra energy liberation (as work plus heat) by an isotonically contracting muscle. This inverse relationship between load and the rate of energy liberation led Hill to conclude that the active points in muscle could exist in two states. In one of these, the active points maintain tension but do not participate in energy liberation (where $P = P_o$, the maximal tension the muscle can develop). In the other state, the active points rapidly liberate energy (where $P = 0$), but as the load is zero they cannot maintain tension.

Equation 6.10 can be rearranged algebraically so as to put all of the constants (a, b, P_o) on the right. The results is the famous Hill equation:

$$(P + a)(v + b) = (P_o + a)b. \qquad [6.11]$$

The beauty (and significance) of Eq. 6.11 lies in the fact that, because all the terms on the right are constants, the Hill equation assumes the form: x times $y = constant$, the general equation for a hyperbola. Thus, when Hill's data for the rate of extra energy liberation are plotted as a force-velocity relationship, it describes a hyperbolic curve (Fig. 6.15). Remarkably, this curve, which is based on measurements of heat and work and *not* direct measurement of muscle shortening velocity, was found by Hill to be identical to that obtained a few years earlier by Fenn and Marsh (Fig. 6.9), who directly measured the dependence of muscle shortening velocity on load!

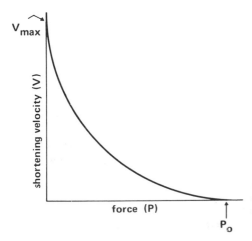

FIG. 6.15. Hyperbolic force-velocity relationship predicted from the Hill equation (Eq. 6.11). This curve is similar to that observed in studies of muscle mechanics (Fig. 6.9).

Significance of the Hill Equation

The reader who has patiently toiled through the concepts (and algebra) described above is entitled to ask how these features of muscular contraction—energetics, heat production, velocity, etc.—contribute to an understanding of the physiology of the heart. This question is answered at this point in general terms, which it is hoped will clarify the nature of the link between physiology and chemistry. After this topic is discussed more fully from a biochemical standpoint in Chapter 8, we return to the subject in Chapter 9 so as to define more precisely the relationship between the mechanics of muscular contraction and the chemical events that underlie this process.

It is fitting to quote directly from Hill's 1938 report in order to define the significance of Eq. 6.11. After examining this relationship, and especially data such as those in Fig. 6.14, Hill stated very eloquently how these experiments provided an insight into the chemistry of the working muscle:

> The control exercised by the tension P existing in the muscle at any moment, on the rate of its energy expenditure at that moment, may be due to some such mechanisms as the following. Imagine that the chemical transformations associated with the state of activity in muscle occur by combination at, or by the catalytic effect of, or perhaps by passage through, certain active points in the molecular machinery, the number of which is determined by the tension existing in the muscle at the moment. We can imagine that when the force in the muscle is high the affinities of more of these points are being satisfied by the attractions they exert on one another, and that fewer of them are available to take part in chemical transformation. When the tension is low the affinities of less of these points are being satisfied by mutual attraction, and more of them are exposed to chemical reaction. The rate at which chemical transformation would occur, and therefore, at which energy would be liberated, would be directly proportional to the number of exposed affinities or catalytic groups, and so would be a linear function of the force exerted by the muscle, increasing as the force diminished. (Hill, 1938)

Written at a time when virtually nothing was known of the biochemistry of the contractile apparatus, and a year before myosin was discovered to have the ability to hydrolyze ATP, Hill's statement explains the energetics of muscular contraction by postulating two states for interactions at hypothetical "active points" within the muscle. To account for the inverse relationship between load and the rate of energy release (Fig. 6.14), Hill postulated that, at any instant, the active points of muscle can exist in either of two states. In one state the active points are attached and are developing tension, much as a man pulling against a rope (Fig. 6.16); in the other, the active points are free to liberate chemical energy and thus are able to move, as when the same man runs freely (Fig. 6.17). To explain the relationship between load and the rate of extra energy release (Fig. 6.14), Hill postulated that the distribution of the active points of muscle between these two states is determined by the load on the muscle.

In an isometric contraction, where the load P is equal to P_o, all active points are in the state in which they develop tension (Fig. 6.18). Under these conditions,

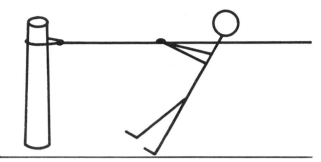

FIG. 6.16. Depiction of one of the active points of muscle in the state in which it develops tension but is not liberating energy.

where the active points are as if they were "locked," force is maximal and the rate of energy liberation is zero. The latter interpretation is tenable because, even though it takes energy to reach the state shown in Fig. 6.18 (the activation energy), according to the Hill equation it costs no energy to *maintain* tension.

When the load on a muscle is zero and the muscle is shortening freely, all of the active points are in the freely running state (Fig. 6.19). As long as there is no resistance to shortening, all of the active points move at their maximal intrinsic rate. Hence the maximal rate of energy turnover during unloaded shortening, which can be looked on as movements of hips, knees, and ankles (Figs. 6.17 and 6.19), is determined by the intrinsic velocity of the interactions between the contractile points (myosin and actin). The rate of energy expenditure therefore is maximal when the load P is zero (Fig. 6.14).

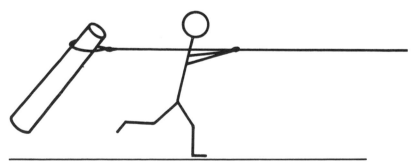

FIG. 6.17. Depiction of one of the active points of muscle in the state in which it is liberating energy but is not developing tension.

$$P = P_o, \quad V = 0$$

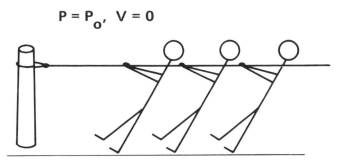

FIG. 6.18. Depiction of the active points of a muscle contracting under isometric conditions $(P = P_o, V = 0)$. All active points are in the state in which they develop tension.

ENERGY WASTAGE AND TENSION-TIME HEAT

The classic Hill equation is, of course, a simplification that assumes that each active point is locked during an isometric contraction, and unable to undergo further chemical change after tension is established. As already pointed out, however, there is a tension-time heat [$f(P,t)$, in Eqs. 6.5 and 6.6] that probably arises from the slow turnover of active points during isometric tension, much like the "little men" in Fig. 6.18 shifting their feet.

The heat liberated by a muscle during an isometric contraction, the term $f(P,t)$, is proportional to myosin ATPase activity because both reflect the intrinsic turnover rate of the cross-bridges. In other words, the energy wastage that occurs when the "little men" shift their feet during an isometric contraction [f(P,t)] is faster in muscles with high myosin ATPase activity. This is because the intrinsic turnover rate of the myosin cross-bridges arises from the same molecular properties of myosin that also determine its ATPase activity *in vitro* (Chapter 8).

$$P = 0, \quad V = V_{max}$$

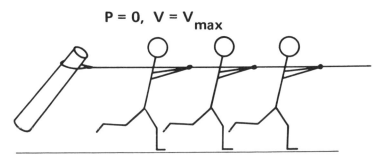

FIG. 6.19. Depiction of the active points of a muscle contracting against zero load $(P = 0, V = V_{max})$. All active points are in the state in which they liberate energy.

"Fast" muscles, which contain a high ATPase myosin (Chapter 3), contract rapidly (as in the rabbit's quick getaway), but are inefficient in generating high levels of tension. Conversely, low myosin ATPase muscles, although slower, are more efficient in developing large forces, probably because of their lower rate of tension-time heat liberation. The importance of these concepts is emphasized in Chapter 25, when we discuss heart failure.

Because a muscle that contains high ATPase myosin contracts more efficiently when lightly loaded than a muscle with a lower myosin ATPase activity, in the context of our analogy of the "little men," it is apparent that when the faster runners lift their feet rapidly from the ground—which is like the rapid cycling of a myosin cross-bridge—they are more efficient. Stated in even simpler terms, we run more slowly and less efficiently if we wear leaded shoes, even though these shoes could help us to sustain tension.

P_o AND V_{max}: THE INTERCEPTS OF THE FORCE-VELOCITY CURVE

On a theoretical basis, and from examination of Fig. 6.19, the shortening velocity of unloaded muscle should be independent of the number of active points in the muscle. Thus, one man capable of a top speed of 10 mph pulls an unloaded rope at the same speed as three (or any number) of such men linked together. For this reason, V_{max} in the force-velocity curve (Fig. 6.15) should reflect only the intrinsic velocity of myosin turnover, and be independent of the number of active points.

The other intercept of the force-velocity curve (P_o) represents the maximal force-generating capacity of the muscle. In terms of the analogy of the "little men" (Figs. 6.16 and 6.19), P_o should depend only on the number of men pulling on the rope, and not on how fast they can run when the load is zero. The experimental finding that the maximal force developed by a muscle bears little or no relationship to its maximal shortening velocity can thus be explained because P_o is theoretically independent of the maximal rate of energy expenditure, but instead reflects the number of active points in the muscle.

It is obvious, of course, that the active points in muscle are interactions between the thick and thin filaments and not little homunculi (Chapter 1). To provide an understanding of the properties of the contractile proteins that make up these filaments, and the biochemical basis for the energetic properties of muscle described in this chapter, the following chapter examines the contractile proteins and their interactions.

REFERENCES

Evans CL, Matsuoka Y. (1914–1915). The effect of the various mechanical conditions on the gaseous metabolism and efficiency of the mammalian heart. *J Physiol (Lond)* 49:378–405.

Fenn WO. (1923). The relation between the work performed and the energy liberated in muscular contraction. *J Physiol (Lond)* 58:373–395.

Fenn WO, Marsh BS. (1935). Muscular force at different speeds of shortening. *J Physiol (Lond)* 85:277–297.

Hill AV. (1938). The heat of shortening and the dynamic constants of muscle. *Proc R Soc Lond [Biol]* 126:136–195.

Mommaerts WFHM. (1969). Energetics of muscular contraction. *Physiol Rev* 49:427–508.

Potter JR, Hsu F-J, Ponwall HJ. (1977). Thermodynamics of Ca^{2+}-binding to troponin-C. *J Biol Chem* 252:2452–2454.

Rall JA. (1982). Sense and nonsense about the Fenn effect. *Am J Physiol* 11:H1–H6.

BIBLIOGRAPHY

Alpert NA, Mulieri LA, Hasenfus G. (1991). Myocardial chemo-mechanical energy transduction. In Fozzard H, Haber E, Katz A, Jennings R, Morgan HE, eds.: (1991). *The heart and cardiovascular system,* 2nd ed. New York: Raven Press.

Curtin NA, Woledge RC. (1978). Energy changes and molecular contraction. *Physiol Rev* 58:690–761.

7

Contractile Proteins

As the focus of our discussion moves from the liberation of heat and work by living muscle to adenosine triphosphate (ATP) hydrolysis and the chemistry of contractile protein interactions, it may seem that we have drastically shifted our subject. Yet energetics and chemistry are but different ways of looking at a single process: the function of muscle as a mechanochemical transducer.

The properties of the contractile proteins that effect this mechanochemical transduction are described in this chapter, which also begins our discussion of the control of their interactions. The latter defines the molecular basis for excitation-contraction coupling, the transitions between rest and activity in muscle, and the regulation of myocardial contractility.

Myocardial contraction and its control are now understood in terms of the interactions between six proteins (Table 7.1). When assembled *in vitro*, these proteins exhibit properties that reflect the three salient features of cardiac contraction: (a) they hydrolyze ATP and thus are able to liberate chemical energy; (b) when they hydrolyze ATP, they undergo physiocochemical changes that are manifestations of tension development and shortening in living muscle; and (c) their interactions are controlled by calcium ions in a manner that reflects the ability of this cation to couple excitation at the cell surface to the initiation of contraction in the living muscle.

In seeking to understand the molecular basis for each of these characteristics— adenosine triphosphatase (ATPase) activity, contraction, and excitation-contraction coupling—we first examine the structural and functional features of each of these proteins.

MYOSIN

Myosin is the major protein of the thick filament of muscle. The rigid "tails" of the elongated myosin molecules are woven in the backbone of this filament, whereas the enzymatically active "heads" project as the cross-bridges. A close functional relationship exists between the enzymatic characteristics of myosin and the

151

TABLE 7.1. *Contractile proteins*

Protein	Location	Approximate molecular weight	Number of components	Salient biochemical properties
Myosin	Thick filament	480,000	Two heavy chains, 200,000 each; four light chains, two 19,000; two 27,000	ATP hydrolysis; interacts with actin
Actin	Thin filament	41,700	One	Activates myosin ATPase; interacts with myosin
Tropomyosin	Thin filament	67,000	Two nonidentical 33,500 chains	Modulates actin-myosin interaction
Troponin C	Thin filament	18,400	One, contains four "E-F hands"	Calcium binding
Troponin I	Thin filament	23,500	One	Inhibits actin-myosin interactions
Troponin T	Thin filament	38,000	One	Binds troponin complex to the thin filament

expression of its biochemical properties in the force-velocity curve of the intact muscle.

Molecular Characteristics

Myosin is a large molecule with a filamentous "tail" that maintains the structural rigidity of the thick filament, and a globular "head" that contains the important biological activities of the protein. The length of cardiac myosin is approximately 1,700 Å, and its molecular weight is ~480,000. The tail of the molecule is organized as a coiled coil, made up of two α-helical peptide chains wound around each other (Fig. 7.1). Each of these α-helices is derived from one of the two ~200,000 dalton heavy chains that make up most of the myosin molecule. The head of the myosin molecule, which has a globular conformation, is also paired, each half being derived from one of the heavy chains. In addition to two heavy chains, cardiac myosin contains two pairs of light chains having molecular weights of approximately 19,000 and 27,000 daltons (Fig. 7.2). The light chains are associated with two "hinge" regions, points of flexibility between the head and the tail.

The myosin heavy chains and the light chains are members of multigene families. Different isoforms of these peptides are found in different muscles, in the same muscle at different stages of development, and even in adjacent cells. Early data suggested that the functional differences between muscle types were determined by the light chains, but it is now clear that the heavy chains are the major determinant of ATPase activity *in vitro,* and shortening velocity in the living muscle.

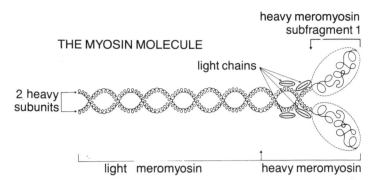

FIG. 7.1. Myosin is an elongated molecule consisting of two heavy chains and four light chains. The "tail" of the molecule (*left*) is a coiled coil (two α-helical chains wound around each other) that extends into the paired globular "head" of the molecule (*right*). Enzymatic cleavage at the point indicated by the *lower arrow* produces heavy and light meromyosins, whereas enzymatic cleavage of heavy meromyosin at the point indicated by the *upper arrow* yields heavy meromyosin subfragment 1.

Myosin Heavy Chains

The atria and ventricles contain their own myosin heavy chains; and both high and low ATPase heavy chain isoforms can be found in each of these structures (Table 7.2). Fetal and neonatal hearts contain additional heavy chain isoforms. Table 7.2 includes the high ATPase, fast ventricular myosin heavy chain—called α or V_1, and the lower ATPase, slower ventricular myosin heavy chain—called β or V_3; small amounts of hybrid myosin containing one α and one β heavy chain (V_2)

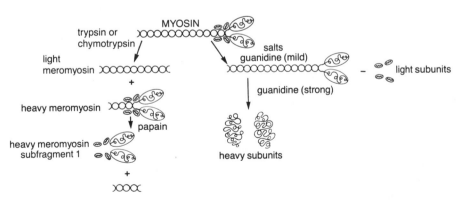

FIG. 7.2. Fragments (*left*) and subunits (*right*) generated from myosin. The fragments are produced by proteolytic digestion, whereas subunits (chains) are released by salts. Mild treatment releases the light chains, whereas stronger denaturing agents are needed to dissociate the two heavy chains.

TABLE 7.2. *Regional diversity of cardiac myosin heavy chains*

Structure	Heavy chain	Myosin characteristics
Atria	A_1 (α)	Very high ATPase
	A_2 (β)	Low ATPase
Ventricles	V_1 (α)	High ATPase
	V_2 (α,β)	Intermediate ATPase
	V_3 (β)	Low ATPase

are also found. Both α and β heavy chains can be found in large amounts in the rodent ventricle; however, the ventricles of larger animals, including man, normally contain little or no α myosin heavy chain. Human atria contain both atrial isoforms. In humans, the genes for both the α and β heavy chains are found on chromosome 14 (Saez et al., 1987).

The ability of the heart to express genes that encode different myosin heavy chain isoforms plays an important role in long-term adaptation of cardiac performance to such conditions as chronic overload, aging and endocrinopathies (Chapter 14). As noted above, different myosin heavy chains are also found in adjacent cells. The significance of this "mosaicism" is not well understood, but may contribute to the homogeneity of function that is essential for cardiac performance (Katz and Katz, 1989).

Myosin Light Chains

Each myosin molecule contains two pairs of light chains that, from an evolutionary standpoint, are closely related to one another, both pairs being members of a family of calcium-binding proteins, of which more is said later in this chapter.

The nomenclature for the myosin light chains is confusing; one pair (MLC-2) is relatively easily removed from the myosin molecule by nondenaturing agents like DTNB, a sulfhydryl reagent, and by the metal chelator EDTA; hence these are often called "DTNB" or "EDTA" light chains. Removal of the other two light chains (MLC-1 and MLC-3) requires exposure of the myosin to high pH; hence the designation "alkali" light chains. The alkali light chains are classified according to size: MLC-1 isoforms have molecular weights of 25,000 to 30,000, MLC-3 are smaller, ranging from 15,000 to 20,000. A fascinating insight into the basis for biological variability is provided by the finding that MLC-1 and MLC-3 are produced from a single gene by alternative splicing (Periasamy et al., 1984).

The MLC-2 molecules in some muscles are substrates for calcium, calmodulin-dependent protein kinases; in other muscles, they can bind calcium (see below). Cardiac MLC-2 can be phosphorylated by calcium, calmodulin-dependent protein kinases (Bárány et al., 1983). As phosphorylation of MLC-2 increases the extent and rate of force development in skeletal muscle (Sweeney and Stull, 1990), it is likely that phosphorylation of cardiac MLC-2 amplifies force development during systole, when cytosolic Ca^{2+} is increased.

In smooth muscle, phosphorylation of a MLC-2 isoform plays a central role in activation. Unlike skeletal and cardiac muscle, where a calcium-binding protein of the thin filament (troponin C, see below) is the calcium-receptor of the contractile machinery, calcium does not bind to any of the smooth muscle contractile proteins. Instead, smooth muscle contraction is initiated when calcium binds to a cytosolic calcium-binding protein called *calmodulin,* which like the myosin light chains and troponin C, is a member of the family of calcium-binding proteins. The calcium-calmodulin complex then activates a *myosin light chain kinase* that phosphorylates smooth muscle MLC-2. This calcium, calmodulin-dependent phosphorylation reaction represents the critical step in smooth muscle activation (Adelstein et al., 1982).

An unusual form of regulation is found in some invertebrates, where a MLC-2 isoform has retained its ability to bind calcium, and so is able to serve as the calcium receptor for the contractile apparatus.

In the human heart three types of light chain having molecular weights of 25,000, 19,000, and 15,000 have been described (Klotz et al., 1982). The atria and ventricles contain different light chains, and a light chain similar to the atrial isoform is normally found in the developing ventricle, in developing skeletal muscle, and in adult slow skeletal muscle. Two ventricular isoforms (VLC-1 and VLC-2) are found in equal amounts in the human ventricle. An atrial light chain (ALC-1) is expressed in the ventricles during fetal life, but by adolescence it is almost entirely replaced with VLC-2. In the pressure-overloaded human atrium, VLC-1 appears to be induced (Kurabayashi et al., 1988). The gene that encodes human ventricular MLC-1 has been localized to chromosome 3 (Fodor et al., 1989).

Architecture

The proteolytic enzymes *trypsin* and *chymotrypsin* split myosin into two fragments (Fig. 7.2). *Light meromyosin,* the smaller of these fragments, is derived from the "tail" of the molecule and exhibits the solubility properties of native myosin. The larger fragment, *heavy meromyosin,* consists of the "head" of the molecule along with a portion of the tail. Further proteolysis of heavy meromyosin with *papain* removes the rest of the tail; the remaining globular protein, called *heavy meromyosin subfragment 1,* includes the head of the molecule (Fig. 7.2) along with the myosin light chains; the important biochemical activities of the molecule reside in this subfragment.

In early studies, light and heavy meromyosins were often referred to as "subunits" of myosin. However, if one accepts the usual definition of a subunit as a discrete polypeptide chain within the parent molecule, this designation is incorrect because the meromyosins are really proteolytic fragments.

The point at which myosin is cleaved into the meromyosins represents a flexible (or "hinge") region of the tail at which susceptibility to proteolysis is increased because the coiled-coil conformation is less rigid in this region. The other point of proteolytic cleavage, which corresponds to a second region of flexibility in the tail, near the base of the head, separates heavy meromyosin subfragment 1 from the

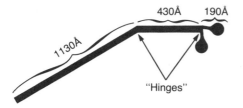

FIG. 7.3. Shape of a myosin molecule showing the paired heads, each approximately 190 Å in length, at the base of which is a point of flexibility, or "hinge." A second hinge divides the tail of the molecule into two unequal lengths as shown in the figure. These hinges represent points of proteolytic cleavage.

remainder of the tail. Morphologic studies have confirmed the presence of two points of flexibility in the myosin molecule: one at the base of the two heads, which are pear-shaped structures approximately 190 Å in length; the other within the tail (de la Torre and Bloomfield, 1980; Elliott and Offer, 1978) (Fig. 7.3). As discussed below, these two hinges allow the myosin head to interact with actin at short sarcomere lengths, where thickening of the muscle separates the thick and thin filaments (Highsmith et al., 1979).

Biological Properties

Purified myosin possesses two important biological properties. The first, discovered in 1939 by Engelhardt and Ljubimova, is its ATPase activity, the ability to hydrolyze the terminal phosphate of ATP thereby releasing the chemical energy of the nucleotide. The ability of myosin to bind actin, the second of the biological properties of myosin, represents an *in vitro* manifestation of the interactions between the thick and thin filaments of the sarcomere that are responsible for muscular contraction. Both of these biological properties are found in heavy meromyosin and heavy meromyosin subfragment 1, and so can be localized to the globular head of the myosin molecule. This location is seen later to be of central importance to the contractile process.

The filamentous tail of the myosin molecule, which lacks enzymatic and actin-binding activities, aggregates under the ionic conditions that exist in the muscle. Its coiled-coil conformation confers rigidity to this portion of the molecule and so strengthens the aggregated myosin tails that make up the backbone of the thick filament of the sarcomere (see below).

Organization in the Sarcomere

Myosin is found as a regular aggregate in the myocardial cell, the *thick filament* (Fig. 7.4), in which the myosin tails are wound together to form a rigid backbone and the myosin heads project as the cross-bridges. The orientation of the elongated myosin molecules becomes reversed at the center of the thick filament so that the myosin cross-bridges in each half of the thick filament project away from the center of the sarcomere (Fig. 7.4).

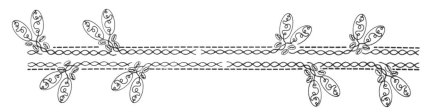

FIG. 7.4. Organization of individual myosin molecules in the thick filament. The "backbone" of the thick filament, delineated by *dashed lines*, is made up of the tails of the individual myosin molecules, which have opposite polarities in the two halves of the sarcomere (*right* and *left*). The bare area in the center of the thick filament is a region devoid of cross-bridges, which can be seen to arise from the "tail-to-tail" organization of myosin molecules unique to the center of the thick filament. The cross-bridges represent the "heads" of the individual myosin molecules, which project from the long axis of the thick filament.

In resting muscle, the cross-bridges are nearly perpendicular to the long axis of the thick filament, whereas in active muscle their tips shift toward the center of the sarcomere (Fig. 7.5). Repeated cycles of this translocation of myosin heads have been postulated to cause a "rowing" motion. Beginning when the thick filaments become attached to the thin filaments, this rowing motion draws the thin filaments toward the center of the sarcomere, causing the sarcomere to shorten. If the ends of the muscle are fixed, the sarcomere cannot shorten and the cross-bridges are prevented from pulling the thin filaments toward the center of the sarcomere; instead, tension is developed.

The shift in orientation of the cross-bridges requires at least one flexible hinge in the myosin molecule. The second hinge explains the finding that the strength of the interactions between thick and thin filaments does not diminish markedly at shorter sarcomere lengths. Because muscle volume remains virtually constant during muscle shortening, the lateral distance between the thick and thin filaments must increase when the sarcomere shortens. Yet the intensity of the interaction between the myosin cross-bridges and the thin filaments appears to be relatively independent of sarcomere length. This finding indicates that the tips of the cross-bridges can extend from the backbone of the thick filament to maintain contact with the thin filaments as the muscle thickens, and the filament lattice widens, during sarcomere shortening. The needed mobility of the cross-bridges is made possible by the two hinges in the myosin molecule (Fig. 7.6).

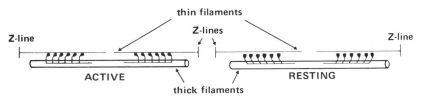

FIG. 7.5. In resting muscle (*right*) the cross-bridges project almost at right angles to the longitudinal axis of the thick filament. In active muscle (*left*) the cross-bridges interact with the thin filaments, which then are "pulled" toward the center of the sarcomere by motion of the myosin heads.

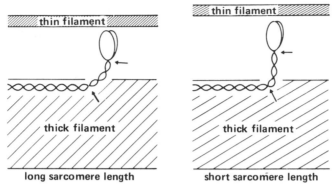

FIG. 7.6. Relationship between cross-bridges and thin filaments in resting muscle at long and short sarcomere lengths. Two flexible hinges in the myosin molecule (*arrows*) allow the relationship between the tip of the cross-bridge and the thin filament to remain the same in spite of changes in separation between the thick and thin filaments.

Functional Implications

It has already been pointed out that myosins purified from muscles that serve different functions exhibit different intrinsic ATPase activities (Chapter 3). In general, shortening is slowest in muscles adapted for sustained activity; e.g., postural muscles, leg muscles of the hare, and pectoral muscles of flying birds. Slow muscles characteristically contain myosins that have a low ATPase activity. In contrast, muscles adapted for brief bursts of rapid acceleration (e.g., leg muscles of the rabbit) generally contract rapidly and contain high ATPase myosins. In this regard, the myocardium is like a slow muscle. The functional significance of these specializations are described in Chapter 3.

Fast and slow myosins contain different light chains, and the light chains of cardiac myosin, which is functionally a slow myosin, are similar to those of slow skeletal muscle. Furthermore, when a fast muscle is innervated surgically with a nerve that originally supplied a slow muscle, muscle shortening velocity and myosin ATPase activity decrease. These changes are accompanied by the replacement of the myosin light chains characteristic of the fast muscle with those whose electrophoretic mobilities are characteristic of the slow muscle; opposite changes being seen in the cross-innervated slow muscle (Streter et al., 1975). These findings were initially interpreted to mean that myosin ATPase and muscle shortening velocity were determined mainly by the light chain composition. It is now apparent, however, that the heavy chains, rather than the light chains, are the major determinants of ATPase activity and shortening velocity.

Data obtained over the past decades have established that differences in the heavy chains contribute to the heart's response to abnormal endocrine states and chronic hemodynamic overloading. Myosin heavy chain isoforms also undergo complex changes during development. These changes provide a long-term "tonic" control of cardiac function, in which the genetic apparatus of myocardial cells is redirected to synthesize altered myosin heavy chains (Chapter 14).

ACTIN

Between 1864, when myosin was first described by Kühne, and the early 1940s, the viscous protein isolated from muscle minces was assumed to consist of a single protein species. As studies of these "myosins" became more searching, however, it became apparent that not all myosin preparations were the same. Most important was that the physicochemical properties of *myosin A,* which were isolated after brief salt extraction of minced muscle, differed from those of *myosin B,* obtained after longer extraction. These differences were explained when Straub, working in the laboratory of Szent-Györgyi, found that the myosin B obtained by prolonged salt extraction contained an additional protein not present in myosin A. This second protein, first purified in 1942, was called *actin* because of its ability to activate myosin ATPase activity.

Molecular Characteristics

Actin is much smaller than myosin, having a molecular weight of 41,700. Unlike the elongated myosin molecule, actin is a globular protein having a slightly ovoid shape with an average diameter of $\sim55\text{Å}$. Actin can be stabilized *in vitro* in either a monomeric form, called G-actin (G = globular), or as a highly asymmetrical polymer, F-actin (F = fibrous). G-actin polymerizes readily when the highly charged actin monomers are allowed to approach each other, e.g., when their negative charges are screened by the addition of salts. Depolymerization of F-actin can be effected most simply by removal of salts.

Actin has a very interesting chemistry that, although not clearly relevant to muscular contraction, probably contributes to its role in the locomotion of single-celled organisms (Stossel, 1989). G-actin contains both a bound nucleotide and a bound divalent cation; the nucleotide that binds to G-actin with greatest stability is ATP, whereas either calcium or magnesium can occupy the cation-binding site. The nucleotide and cation bound to G-actin are both freely exchangeable, although when either is removed, G-actin becomes unstable and rapidly loses its ability to polymerize. F-actin also contains a nucleotide and a cation, but in the polymer both are tightly bound and do not exchange freely with nucleotides and cations in the solution.

During polymerization, actin-bound ATP is hydrolyzed to form adenosine diphosphate (ADP) and inorganic phosphate (P_i); the former remaining bound to F-actin. When F-actin is depolymerized, the bound ADP dissociates and is replaced by free ATP. If actin is sonicated or held at high temperatures, both reactions can alternate rapidly, thereby allowing free ATP to be hydrolyzed. Thus actin can have the properties of an ATPase enzyme. According to the usual definition of the term, however, actin is not an ATPase because under ordinary conditions the protein does not hydrolyze free ATP. Neither actin-bound nucleotide nor cation has been found to have a role in muscular contraction; instead, it is likely that they stabilize the structure of the actin polymer.

Biological Properties

Actin has two biological properties that are directly relevant to muscular contraction: it activates myosin ATPase activity, and it interacts physicochemically with myosin. Together, these properties allow the "two-protein" actomyosin reconstituted from highly purified actin and myosin to liberate chemical energy from ATP and undergo physicochemical changes, two of the three salient features of the contractile process. Except for the ability to respond to calcium (see below), therefore, two-protein actomyosins exhibit the key features of muscle contraction.

Organization in the Sarcomere

Actin is found in the sarcomere as the F-actin polymer, which provides the "backbone" of the thin filament. The basic structure of both F-actin and the thin filament is that of a double-stranded macromolecular helix (Fig. 7.7), each strand being a chain of actin monomers. Thus, the thin filament resembles two strings of beads wound around each other. (This structure differs from the coiled-coil structure of the tail of the myosin molecule, which is made up of chains of amino acids rather than of macromolecules.)

The distance between the nodes of the F-actin filament is ~385 Å, so that each half-turn of the F-actin filament contains seven pairs of 55-Å actin monomers (Fig. 7.7). These quantitative characteristics are important to understanding the functional organization of the thin filament, as will become clear when we examine the interactions between actin and the regulatory proteins tropomyosin and the troponin complex.

Actin, whose structure has been highly conserved during evolution, is found in all eukaryotic cells. The hearts of small mammals contain two isoforms: α-skeletal actin is present during fetal life, and is replaced by α-cardiac actin in the adult. In rat skeletal muscle, the opposite isoform shift occurs, α-cardiac actin is replaced by α-skeletal actin! Human hearts contain mainly α-cardiac actin, along with a smaller amount of α-skeletal actin. The gene that encodes α-cardiac actin is found on chromosome 1, and the gene for α-skeletal actin is on chromosome 15.

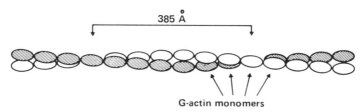

FIG. 7.7. The F-actin polymer is composed of two strands of G-actin monomers (*ovals*) wound around each other. The G-actin monomers in the two strands are identical; one strand is *shaded* here only to illustrate the two-stranded structure of F-actin. The internodal distance is approximately 385 Å.

Actin can combine with a wide variety of proteins. Some, like myosin, are responsible for movement; interactions of actin with myosin-like proteins in nonmotile cells such as the platelet also lead to contraction. Other proteins, like *spectrin* in erythrocytes and *vinculin* in muscle, attach actin to membranes, whereas the combination of *filamen* with actin forms cytoskeletal networks that impart rigidity to the plasma membrane. Some actin-binding proteins play an important role in regulating muscle contraction, for example, *caldesmon* in smooth muscle and the *troponin-tropomyosin complex* in cardiac and skeletal muscle. The latter, discussed below, is a key component of the regulatory proteins of the thin filament, which allow the interactions between the thick and thin filaments to be controlled by calcium.

TROPOMYOSIN

For the first 15 years after its discovery in 1948, tropomyosin was an "orphan." Purified tropomyosin had no biological activity, and neither hydrolyzed ATP nor did it interact with myosin. However, its structure proved to be of considerable interest to physical chemists, for like the tail of the myosin molecule, tropomyosin forms a rigid coiled coil.

Molecular Characteristics

Tropomyosin is a filamentous molecule, ~400 Å in length, made up of two helical peptide chains linked by a single disulfide bridge (Lehrer, 1978) (Fig. 7.8). The molecule can be a homodimer or heterodimer containing either or both of two isoforms, α and β, that have slightly different amino acid compositions. Both isoforms have the same molecular weight, 34,000 daltons, so that the total molecular weight of tropomyosin is 68,000. Different proportions of these two isoforms are found in fast and slow skeletal muscle; cardiac tropomyosin in smaller mammals is made up of α_2-dimers (Lewis and Smillie, 1980), but the hearts of larger mammals contain significant amounts of the β-subunit (Leger et al., 1976). Human atria and ventricles contain similar proportions of the α- and β-isoforms, but β-isoform content increases during development. It is of interest that the content of the β-isoform

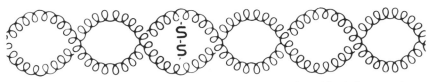

FIG. 7.8. The tropomyosin molecule is made up of two α-helical peptide chains wound around each other in a coiled coil conformation. Unlike the tail of the myosin molecule (Fig. 7.1), the two polypeptide chains are joined by a single disulfide bond (-S-S-).

in a number of species and developmental stages is inversely correlated with heart rate (Humphreys and Cummins, 1984).

> The remarkable pleiomorphism of muscle protein structure is apparent in the case of the α-subunit of tropomyosin, which can exist as at least three isoforms that are tissue specific and developmentally regulated; like the myosin light chains, these are produced by alternate gene splicing (Ruiz-Opazo et al., 1985).

Biological Properties

Tropomyosin is a relatively inflexible elongated molecule that regulates the interactions between actin and myosin (Murray et al., 1982). These effects are complex, and can be either stimulatory or inhibitory, depending on the state of the actin-myosin interaction (Chapter 8). Most important is the ability of tropomyosin, along with troponin, to mediate the signal initiated by an increase in cytosolic Ca^{2+}, which activates the actin-myosin interactions responsible for muscle contraction.

> Tropomyosin can be phosphorylated by a calcium, calmodulin-dependent protein kinase; however, this reaction appears to play a role in the structural organization of the thin filament rather than in the contraction-relaxation cycle (Heeley et al., 1989).

Organization in the Sarcomere

Tropomyosin binds stoichiometrically to F-actin in the thin filament; one molecule of tropomyosin lies in each of the two grooves that run longitudinally between the two strands of actin in the thin filament (Fig. 7.9). In this position, tropomyosin adds structural rigidity to the thin filament. More importantly, through cooperative interactions with the other proteins of the thin filament, tropomyosin participates in the regulation of contraction.

THE TROPONIN COMPLEX

The troponin complex, first described in 1965 by Ebashi, is now known to be made up of three discrete proteins. *Troponin I*, in concert with tropomyosin, regu-

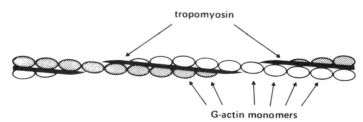

FIG. 7.9. Tropomyosin is found along with actin in the thin filament, where it is located in the "groove" between the two strands of the F-actin polymer.

TABLE 7.3. *Approximate molecular weight of the troponin components*

Component	Fast skeletal muscle	Cardiac muscl
Troponin C	18,000	18,400
Troponin I	21,000	23,500
Troponin T	33,000	38,000

lates the interactions between actin and myosin; as the most important of these regulatory effects is to inhibit the interactions between actin and myosin, this protein was named troponin I. *Troponin T* serves primarily to bind the troponin complex to tropomyosin, whereas *troponin C* contains the calcium-binding sites that regulate muscular contraction. Although the molecular weights of cardiac and fast skeletal muscle troponins T and I differ (Table 7.3), and several isoforms are found for each of the troponin components, all muscles contain the full complement of three troponin components. These three troponin components interact in a cooperative manner with each other, with tropomyosin and actin, and even with myosin (see below).

Molecular and Biological Characteristics

Troponin C

Troponin C is a dumbbell-shaped protein (Fig. 7.10) that contains four similar amino acid sequences (I–IV), each of which is a member of the "family" of calcium-binding proteins that includes calmodulin and the myosin light chains. These amino acid sequences are of two types: some bind only calcium and are designated Ca^{2+}*-specific sites;* others that also bind magnesium are called Ca^{2+}*-Mg^{2+} sites.*

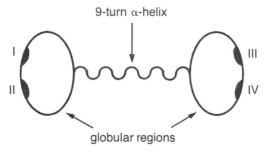

FIG. 7.10. Schematic diagram of troponin C showing the two globular regions separated by a 9-turn α-helix. Each globular region contains two of the four sites that can bind a metal ion. Each of these sites is formed by a polypeptide chain homologous to the primitive calcium-binding protein. In cardiac troponin C, site I has lost its metal ion-binding properties, site II is Ca^{2+} specific, whereas sites III and IV are Ca^{2+}-Mg^{2+} sites.

As the Mg^{2+} concentration in muscle is several orders of magnitude higher than that of Ca^{2+}, the Ca^{2+}-Mg^{2+} sites are normally occupied by magnesium and so do not play a role in excitation-contraction coupling. Instead, binding of magnesium to the Ca^{2+}-Mg^{2+} sites probably stabilizes the interaction of troponin C with the other two components of troponin. Thus, it is the Ca^{2+}-specific sites that serve the critical function of troponin C: recognition of a rise in cytosolic Ca^{2+} concentration as a signal to initiate the interactions between actin and myosin that activate muscular contraction.

The troponin C isoform in fast skeletal muscle contains two Ca^{2+}-Mg^{2+} sites and two Ca^{2+}-specific sites. Mammalian cardiac troponin C also contains four of these amino acid sequences; two (sites III and IV) are Ca^{2+}-Mg^{2+} sites. Site II, one of the Ca^{2+}-specific sites in cardiac troponin C, is the physiological calcium receptor of the heart's contractile proteins. However, replacement of two aspartic acid residues by leucine and alanine in site I, the other Ca^{2+}-specific site of cardiac troponin C, has abolished its high-affinity calcium binding (Holroyde et al., 1980). Recent studies using site-directed mutations, suggest that site I modifies the cooperativity of the response to calcium (Putkey et al., 1989).

Troponin I

Troponin I, which alone is a weak inhibitor of actin-myosin interactions, becomes a powerful regulator when combined with tropomyosin. Cardiac, fast skeletal, and slow skeletal muscle contain different isoforms of troponin I; a fourth troponin I isoform has recently been identified in developing muscle (Sabry and Dhoot, 1989, Saggin et al., 1989).

The cardiac isoform of troponin I contains a serine at position 20 that is not present in fast skeletal troponin I; this serine is a substrate for phosphorylation by protein kinase A. Phosphorylation of cardiac troponin I, through cooperative interactions in the troponin complex, reduces the calcium affinity of troponin C. The resulting desensitization of the response to calcium in the heart under the influence of β-adrenergic agonists favors relaxation (see Chapter 14). Calcium, calmodulin–dependent protein kinases and protein kinase C can phosphorylate other serine residues in cardiac troponin I (Noland et al., 1989), but the functional significance of these phosphorylations is not yet clear.

Troponin T

Troponin T, the largest of the three troponin components, is an asymmetrical molecule that binds the troponin complex to tropomyosin. As is the case for the myosin light chains and tropomyosin, troponin T isoforms are produced by alternate gene splicing; the variable amino acid sequence so produced can give rise to more than 30 isoforms. Although troponin T itself does not bind calcium, the calcium sensitivity of tension development is influenced by this protein; as a result, isoform switches of troponin T alter the response of the heart to calcium. This indirect influence of troponin T on calcium sensitivity provides a clear example of the cooperativity of the interactions between the myofibrillar proteins.

Switching of two isoforms that confer slightly different calcium sensitivities to the contractile proteins probably plays a role in the adaptation of the hypertrophied heart to sustained overload (Chapter 25). This marked variability of troponin T gene expression has made this protein a useful model in the search for mechanisms that control cell growth and differentiation. A short nucleotide sequence CATTCCT, found in the promoter region of the troponin T gene, appears to be among the relatively small number of elements that regulate gene transcription in developing muscle (Mar and Ordahl, 1988).

Organization in the Sarcomere

The three components of troponin are found along with tropomyosin and actin in the thin filament of the sarcomere, where the troponin complex is distributed along the thin filament at approximately 400 Å intervals (Fig. 7.11). The probable cross-sectional organization of the three components of troponin, actin, and tropomyosin in the thin filament is shown schematically in Fig. 7.12 (Warber and Potter, 1986).

The key to calcium regulation of the thin filament lies in the lability of the bond linking troponin I and actin, which allows reversible conformational changes to occur in the thin filament. The strength of this bond is influenced by the binding of calcium to troponin C. In the relaxed heart, when the Ca^{2+}-specific site of cardiac troponin C is not bound to calcium, the affinity of troponin I for actin is high; the resulting interaction between troponin I and actin causes the thin filament to assume a conformation in which the myosin-binding sites of actin are "blocked" by the regulatory proteins. Systole begins when the binding of calcium to troponin C induces an allosteric change that loosens the bond linking troponin I to actin; the

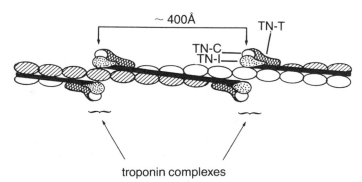

FIG. 7.11. Troponin complexes are distributed along with actin and tropomyosin in the thin filament, appearing at ~400 Å intervals.

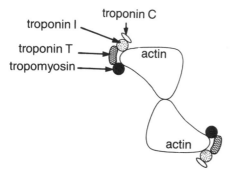

FIG. 7.12. Cross section of the thin filament at the level where the troponin complexes are located shows proposed relationships between actin, tropomyosin, and the three components of the troponin complex. The strength of the bond linking troponin I and actin has been postulated to vary, depending on whether calcium is bound to troponin C.

resulting dissociation of troponin I from actin causes a rearrangement of the proteins of the thin filament that allows interactions between actin and myosin to generate tension (Tao et al., 1990). Stated simply, the variable affinity of troponin I for actin provides a calcium-dependent molecular switch that allows a rise in cytosolic Ca^{2+} to trigger contraction. This mechanism is described more fully in Chapter 8.

Cytosolic Calcium-Binding Proteins

Elucidation of the amino acid sequences of the myosin light chains, troponin C, and several calcium-binding proteins has provided a marvelous insight as to the evolution of cellular regulation by calcium. It is now clear that all are members of a "family" of proteins that share a common ancestor that probably appeared some 600 million years ago, when multicellular animals developed in the primitive Precambrian seas (Goodman et al., 1979). This common ancestor was probably a polypeptide chain of ~30 amino acids that contained two α-helical regions (designated E and F) separated by a nonhelical sequence, or loop (Fig. 7.13). The key to the ability of this protein to bind calcium lies in an arrangement of oxygen-containing amino acids that forms the vertices of an octahedron; this forms a "pocket" in which calcium ions are coordinated with very high affinity. These oxygen-containing amino acids are concentrated in the two helical regions, which can be viewed as the extended index finger and thumb of a right hand in which the other folded fingers and palm correspond to the nonhelical loop (Fig. 7.13). This structure is often referred to as an "E-F hand," and proteins containing this structure as "E-F hand proteins."

The "family" of calcium-binding proteins (Table 7.4) includes a variety of proteins that contain two or four E-F hand regions, presumed to be derived from duplication and modification of the ancestral E-F hand protein. Amino acid substitutions in some of these calcium-binding regions have resulted in the loss of their ability to bind calcium; in others, the specificity for calcium, relative to magnesium, has been lost. As already noted, cardiac troponin C contains four E-F hand regions: site I has

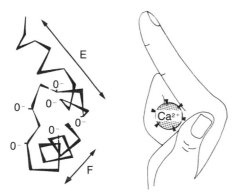

FIG. 7.13. A single calcium-binding site, or the postulated primitive calcium-binding protein (*left*) showing two α-helical regions (E and F) separated by a nonhelical loop. This structure localizes six oxygen atoms (O^-) so that they tightly coordinate a calcium ion (Ca^{2+}). As this structure resembles a right hand (*right*), it is sometimes referred to as an "E-F hand."

lost the ability to bind divalent cations and sites III and IV can bind either calcium or magnesium ions, leaving only site II as calcium specific.

One member of the family of calcium-binding proteins, a myosin light chain, serves as the calcium-receptor of scallop muscle. Even more fascinating is the ability of other members of this family, which have lost the ability to bind calcium, to continue to participate in calcium-dependent regulation. This is the case for the light chains of smooth muscle myosin that, although unable to bind calcium, are substrates for the calcium, calmodulin–dependent protein kinase that participates in the calcium-dependent activation of contraction. These different mechanisms are shown schematically in Fig. 7.14.

Calmodulin

Several calcium, dependent protein kinases have been described in this and earlier chapters; some modify enzymes that regulate the metabolic pathways of energy production (Chapters 4 and 5); others control tension in smooth muscle. Common to most of these protein kinases is a calcium-binding protein called *calmodulin* (Cheung, 1982). First identified as an activator of the enzyme phosphodiesterase, which hydrolyzes cyclic AMP, calmodulin is now recognized as the calcium receptor for a large number of phosphorylation reactions that regulate proteins involved

TABLE 7.4. *Calcium-binding proteins*

Protein	E-F hand regions
Common ancestor (postulated)	1
Parvalbumens	2
Intestinal calcium-binding proteins	2
Troponin C	4
Myosin light chain 1	4
Myosin light chain 2	4
Myosin light chain 3	4
Calmodulin	4

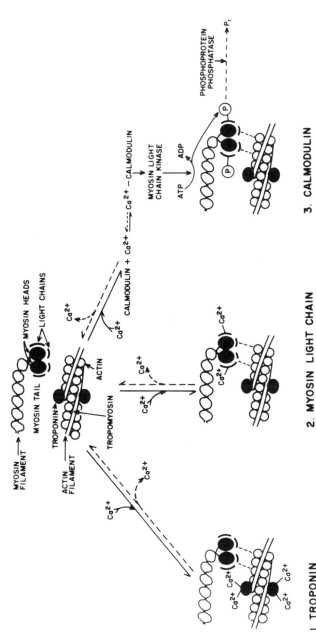

FIG. 7.14. Schematic diagram showing three ways by which calcium-binding proteins mediate excitation-contraction coupling in muscle. In troponin-linked regulation, the calcium-binding protein is incorporated into the thin filament; whereas in myosin-linked regulation, the calcium receptor is a myosin light chain that is part of the thick filament. In smooth muscle, the calcium receptor is the soluble calcium-binding protein calmodulin, although the protein phosphorylated by the calcium, calmodulin–dependent protein kinase is a myosin light chain that, although no longer able to bind calcium, is derived from the family of calcium-binding proteins. (From Katz et al. Cellular actions and pharmacology of the calcium channel blocking drugs. *Am J Med* 1985; 79 (Suppl 4A), pp. 2–10, with permission.)

in such diverse processes as cyclic nucleotide metabolism, intermediary metabolism, muscle contraction, and neurotransmitter release. Calmodulin, which contains four E-F hand regions that are very similar to each other, is a highly conserved protein having little tissue or species specificity.

The ability of calmodulin to respond to a rise in cytosolic Ca^{2+} concentration begins with the formation of a high-affinity calcium-calmodulin complex, which is accompanied by the coalescence of a number of apolar moieties on the surface of the calmodulin molecule. The resulting formation of a large hydrophobic surface allows the calcium-calmodulin complex to interact with hydrophobic domains on the protein or membrane whose function is then altered.

A number of antidepressant drugs, for example tricyclics and phenothiazines, interfere with the functions of the calcium-calmodulin complex, and thus inhibit many of the cellular responses to calcium. This action, sometimes called "calcium antagonism" is quite different from that of calcium channel blocking drugs that inhibit calcium fluxes through membrane calcium channels (Chapter 18). As loose application of this terminology can lead to confusion, the terms used in this text are *calcium-calmodulin inhibitors* and *calcium channel blockers,* which are quite unambiguous.

MINOR PROTEINS OF THE MYOFILAMENTS

A number of additional proteins that have been found in myofibrils are listed in Table 7.5 (Obinata et al., 1981; Pearson and Young, 1989). Many are poorly characterized, and some may be contaminants. Most do not participate in the contractile process, but instead make up the cytoskeleton, which maintains the structure of the sarcomere and provides mechanical linkages that convey the tension developed by the contractile proteins to the surrounding structures and, ultimately, to the ends of the muscle. Glycolytic enzymes associated with the A-band may provide a special source of ATP for the hydrolytic site of myosin ("glycolytic ATP," see Chapter 5).

MODELS OF THE CONTRACTILE PROTEINS

Using only the six proteins described in Table 7.1, it is possible to reconstitute an actomyosin that exhibits properties *in vitro* that are remarkably similar to those of the intact muscle. These properties, noted at the beginning of this chapter, are: (a) ATP hydrolysis, which corresponds to energy liberation in the muscle; (b) physicochemical changes that convert the chemical energy derived from ATP hydrolysis into mechanical work; and (c) regulation by calcium, which corresponds to the response of the contractile proteins to the calcium released into the cytosol during excitation-contraction coupling. The first two properties are seen in the two-protein actomyosins made up only of actin and myosin. The third, control by calcium, requires the four regulatory proteins of the thin filament: tropomyosin and the three proteins of the troponin complex.

TABLE 7.5. *Minor proteins of the sarcomere*[a]

Component	Approx. molecular weight	Probable function
A- and I-bands		
Connectin (titin)	3,000,000	links thick filaments to Z-line; may contribute to passive tension; may be template for myosin assembly
G-(gap) filaments	?	maintains thick filament structure
β-actinin	71,000	controls length of thin filament; may play a role in myogenesis
γ-actinin	35,000	? stabilizes thin filament
Paratropomyosin	34,000	?
M-line		
Myomesin	185,000	links thin filaments to M-line
M-protein	165,000	? thick filament alignment
Thick filaments		
C-protein	150,000	? stabilizes thick filament and/or regulates actin-myosin interactions
X-protein	152,000	? stabilizes thick filament
H-protein	74,000	? organizes thick filament
I-protein	50,000	? regulates actin-myosin interactions
Z-line		
Zeugmatin	500,000	? myofibrillar organization
Filamin	480,000	links actin to Z-line and/or membranes
Synemin	230,000	stabilizes Z-line
a-actinin	200,000	binds thin filaments to Z-line
Vinculin	130,000	? links actin to cell membrane
Vimentin	57,000	stabilizes Z-line
Desmin (skeletin)	55,000	binds thin filaments in Z-line
Eu-actinin	42,000	? links α-actinin to actin
N-line (near Z-line)		
Nebulin	500,000	links thin filaments to Z-line; may be template for myosin assembly

[a]Based on Chapter 5 of Pearson and Young, 1989. A-band associated glycolytic enzymes (creatine kinase, phosphofructokinase [F-protein], glycogen phosphorylase and glycogen debranching enzyme) are not included in this table.

Actin Plus Myosin: The Two-Protein Actomyosin

Actomyosins reconstituted from highly purified actin and myosin are able to utilize energy derived from ATP hydrolysis to generate physicochemical changes analogous to those that lead to tension and shortening in the intact muscle. Many factors govern these interactions *in vitro;* some are of interest only to the biochemist, but others provide insights regarding the contractile process in living muscle.

The ATPase activity of the two-protein actomyosin is stimulated by both calcium and magnesium, whereas the ATPase activity of myosin alone is stimulated by calcium but inhibited by magnesium. The ability of magnesium to stimulate myosin ATPase activity in the presence of actin is accompanied by physicochemical interactions between actin and myosin that represent an *in vitro* manifestation of muscular contraction. Attenuation of this effect may contribute to muscle weakness in patients who are magnesium depleted. High concentrations of alkali metal salts (e.g., NaCl and KCl) inhibit actomyosin ATPase activity and the interactions between actin and myosin.

Dual Effect of ATP

ATP itself has an interesting and important dual effect on actomyosin that reflects two very different roles of this nucleotide. Like the farmer in Aesop's fable who blew hot and cold with the same breath (hot to warm his chilled hands, cold to cool his soup), ATP can either stimulate or inhibit the interactions between actin and myosin (Fig. 7.15). At low concentrations, ATP is a *substrate* for energy-consuming reactions, whereas high concentrations of ATP are inhibitory because of important *regulatory (allosteric)* effects.

Low (micromolar) concentrations of ATP saturate the hydrolytic site on myosin to provide energy needed for the actin-myosin interactions that cause contraction, whereas high ATP concentrations (in the millimolar range) are necessary for the heart to relax. This relaxing effect, induced by the millimolar ATP concentrations found in resting muscle, reflects the ability of the anionic polyphosphate chain of ATP to dissociate actin and myosin. High ATP concentrations, therefore, have a "plasticizing" effect that decreases the interaction between the thick and thin filaments. Loss of this effect explains the ability of a modest reduction in ATP to impair relaxation (Chapter 8). More drastic depletion of ATP in dying muscle is responsible for rigor mortis in skeletal muscle, and ischemic contracture in the heart (Chapter 24).

"Seeing is Believing"

Early investigators in the field of muscle research were often ostracized because, unlike enzyme chemists, they were required to study insoluble proteins. (A soluble muscle would not be of much use.) Although the physical properties of the contractile proteins proved to be an impediment to the study of enzyme kinetics, they did provide striking models of contraction. Most dramatic were the experiments of Szent-Györgyi, who in the early 1940s prepared actomyosin threads oriented so that

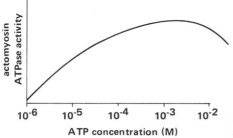

FIG. 7.15. Dependence of actomyosin ATP-ase activity on ATP-ase concentration.

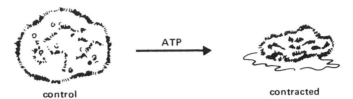

control   contracted

FIG. 7.16. Contraction of a floc of an actomyosin gel *in vitro* (shown here as a sponge), which during syneresis (contraction) squeezes water out of itself to become smaller and denser.

the asymmetrical actin and myosin filaments were parallel to each other. Addition of ATP caused these actomyosin threads to shorten, and if a load was attached, the actomyosin threads could perform work. The mechanical properties of actomyosin threads were similar to those of muscle; in fact, they could even generate hyperbolic force-velocity curves. However, their tensile strength was low, and they broke quite easily.

It is more convenient to study the physicochemical properties of actomyosin gels, where insoluble actomyosin forms flocculent suspensions in which the asymmetrical molecules are randomly oriented. Under these conditions, addition of ATP causes the individual actomyosin flocs to shrink (Fig. 7.16). This process, which resembles a sponge squeezing water out of itself, is called *syneresis* (drawing together of the molecules of the gel). If, after the addition of ATP, gel volume is measured after low-speed centrifugation, the insoluble actomyosin pellet is found to have decreased in volume (Fig. 7.17). Hence the term "superprecipitation" was coined to describe this *in vitro* manifestation of the contractile process.

Another way to study the "contraction" of actomyosin gels is to follow turbidity changes initiated by addition of ATP (Fig. 7.18). Although high ATP concentrations initially dissociate actin and myosin (due to the plasticizing effect; see above), hydrolysis by myosin lowers ATP concentration until its regulatory effect is lost and the substrate effect becomes uncovered, which causes actin and myosin to reassociate, and eventually to superprecipitate. Although largely obsolete, these approaches to the study of actomyosin interactions clearly illustrate the two distinct effects of ATP: a regulatory (allosteric) effect, and a substrate effect. Addition of a high con-

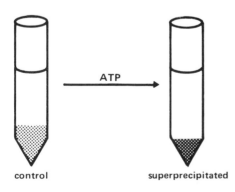

control   superprecipitated

FIG. 7.17. Superprecipitation (contraction) of an actomyosin gel *in vitro*. Shrinkage of the individual flocs of actomyosin (Fig. 7.16) reduces the volume of the pellet that is obtained after centrifugation.

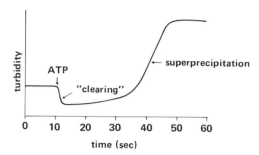

FIG. 7.18. Turbidity changes that follow addition of ATP to an actomyosin gel *in vitro*. Following a brief "clearing" phase, during which actin and myosin are dissociated by high ATP concentration, these proteins become reassociated when ATP levels fall. Under the latter conditions ATP hydrolysis is accelerated and the actomyosin gel contracts (syneresis or superprecipitation) and the suspension becomes more turbid.

centration of ATP initially dissociates actin and myosin, causing an abrupt fall in turbidity, called "clearing" (Fig. 7.18). As ATP concentration falls, due to its hydrolysis by myosin, this plasticizing effect is lost, actin and myosin reassociate, and syneresis increases the turbidity of the actomyosin gels (Fig. 7.18).

Regulation of Actomyosin Interactions

High concentrations of alkali metal salts and ATP, either individually or together, dissociate two-protein actomyosins. These observations led early workers to postulate that the physiological control of the interactions between actin and myosin, and thus the reversible transitions between rest (manifest, for example, as clearing) and activity (manifest as superprecipitation, syneresis, or contraction of actomyosin threads), could be effected by changing intracellular ATP or potassium concentrations. It is now clear, however, that muscular contraction is not normally regulated by changes in these reactants; but instead, by variations in the Ca^{2+} concentration around the myofibrils.

The advantage of control by calcium is apparent if one considers the amounts of ATP, magnesium, or alkali metal salts that would have to be transported to turn muscle on and off. Intracellular concentrations of ATP are in the *millimolar* range, whereas that of K^+ is ~0.1 M; thus, a great deal of energy would be have to be expended to alter the concentration of any of these reactants around the contractile proteins. In the case of Ca^{2+}, on the other hand, cytosolic concentrations are in or below the *micromolar* range, so that much less energy is expended in the calcium fluxes that induce reversible transitions between rest and activity.

At the time that the role of calcium in controlling the activity of the contractile proteins was becoming apparent, it was also recognized that actomyosins made up of highly purified actin and myosin did not respond to calcium. A search for the missing factors responsible for the lost calcium sensitivity was quickly followed by discovery of the role of the regulatory proteins: tropomyosin and the troponin complex.

"Complete" Actomyosin and its Control by Calcium Ion

Each of the major proteins of the sarcomere—myosin, actin, tropomyosin, and the three components of troponin—plays a specific role in the interactions that enable muscle to contract and relax. From the standpoint of the intact muscle, these interactions can be grouped into two types: (a) those responsible for the contractile process itself, and (b) those that permit this process to be controlled. An overview of the way that calcium regulates the contractile process is provided at this point; further details regarding both the regulatory role of calcium and the interactions between actin and myosin that are responsible for contraction are presented in Chapter 8.

Although the ability of calcium to initiate contraction in intact muscle had been known since the 1940s, the mechanism of this stimulatory action became clear only during the early 1960s. At that time, it was recognized that the stimulatory action of calcium arose from a direct effect on the contractile proteins, rather than, as believed earlier, by inactivation of a soluble "relaxing factor." The relaxing factor was actually a sarcoplasmic reticulum contaminant that sequestered calcium in then-unrecognized membrane vesicles (Chapter 11).

Very shortly after the direct stimulatory action of calcium on actomyosin systems came to be understood, it was noted that not all actomyosins responded to this cation. Actomyosins made only of actin and myosin were found to be "calcium insensitive," in that these two-protein actomyosins continued to interact even when Ca^{2+} concentrations were drastically lowered with the then newly discovered calcium chelator EGTA. Realization that calcium removal had no effect on the two-protein actomyosin, whereas complete actomyosins "relaxed" when calcium was removed, was quickly followed by the discovery of the regulatory effects of tropomyosin and troponin.

The role of the regulatory proteins in modulating the interactions between actin and myosin is readily understood by reading downward in column *a* of Table 7.6. When Ca^{2+} concentration is low, actomyosins that do not contain the regulatory proteins are active; ATPase activity is high and they superprecipitate. Inclusion of tropomyosin and the troponin complex inactivates the system as long as Ca^{2+} concentration is low; but when Ca^{2+} concentration is high (column *b*, Table 7.6) the actomyosins remain active, regardless of whether or not the regulatory proteins are included. Table 7.6 thus illustrates two essential aspects of the physiological control of the interactions between actin and myosin: (a) *the regulatory proteins are inhibitory in the absence of calcium,* and (b) *calcium initiates contraction by reversing this inhibitory effect.*

The relationships described in the preceding paragraphs are depicted in Fig. 7.19,

TABLE 7.6. *Actions of calcium on the contractile activity of different actomyosins* in vitro

Actomyosin	(a) Low calcium	(b) High calcium
"Two-protein" (actin + myosin)	Active	Active
"Complete" (actin + myosin + tropomyosin + troponin complex)	Inhibited	Active

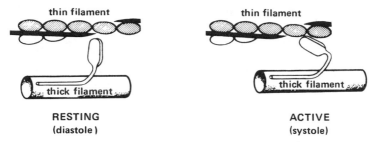

RESTING   ACTIVE
(diastole)   (systole)

FIG. 7.19. Transition from rest (diastole) to activity (systole), showing attachment of the cross-bridges to the thin filament. This interaction can take place only when calcium binds to troponin C and the regulatory proteins (tropomyosin and the troponin complex) undergo a conformational rearrangement that allows actin to interact with the myosin cross-bridge.

which is discussed at length in Chapter 8. On the left are the contractile proteins of the resting heart, in which the myosin cross-bridge projecting from the thick filament (bottom) cannot interact with the actin in the thin filament (top) because of the inhibitory effects of the tropomyosin-troponin complex. This inhibition persists as long as the Ca^{2+}-specific site on troponin C is devoid of calcium. Binding of this cation initiates a series of conformational changes in the regulatory proteins that expose active sites on the actin in the thin filament. Interaction of these active sites with the myosin cross-bridge initiates the processes that effect myocardial contraction (Fig. 7.19, right): transduction of the chemical energy of ATP into mechanical work. Further details of the control exerted by calcium are provided in Chapter 8.

REFERENCES

Adelstein RS, Sellars JR, Conti MA, Pato MD, de Lanerolle P. (1982). Regulation of smooth muscle contractile proteins by calmodulin and cyclic AMP. *Fed Proc* 41:2873–2878.

Bárány K, Bárány M, Hager SR, Sayers ST. (1983). Myosin light chain and membrane protein phosphorylation in various species. *Fed Proc* 42:27–32.

Cheung WY. (1982). Calmodulin: an overview. *Fed Proc* 41:2253–2257.

de la Torre JG, Bloomfield VA. (1980). Conformation of myosin in dilute solution as estimated from hydrodynamic properties. *Biochemistry* 19:5118–5123.

Elliott A, Offer G. (1978). Shape and flexibility of the myosin molecule. *J Mol Biol* 123:505–519.

Fodor WL, Darras B, Seharaseyon J, Falkenthal S, Francke U, Vanin EF. (1989). Human ventricular/slow twitch myosin alkali light chain gene characterization, sequence, and chromosomal location. *J Biol Chem* 264:2143–2149.

Goodman M, Pechere J-F, Haiech J, Demaille J. (1979). Evolutionary diversification of structure and function in the family of intracellular calcium-binding proteins. *J Mol Evol* 13:331–352.

Heeley DH, Watson MH, Mak AS, Dubord P, Smillie LB. (1989). Effect of phosphorylation on the interaction and functional properties of rabbit striated *aa*-tropomyosin. *J Biol Chem* 264:2424–2430.

Highsmith S, Akasake K, Konrad M, Goody R, Holmes K, Wade-Jardetzky N, Jardetzky O. (1979). Internal motions in myosin. *Biochemistry* 18:4238–4244.

Holroyde MJ, Robertson SP, Johnson JD, Solaro RJ, Potter JD. (1980). The calcium and magnesium binding sites on cardiac troponin and their role in the regulation of myofibrillar adenosine triphosphatase. *J Biol Chem* 255:11688–11693.

Humphreys LE, Cummins P. (1984). Regulatory proteins of the myocardium. Atrial and ventricular tropomyosin and troponin-I in the developing and adult bovine and human heart. *J Mol Cell Cardiol* 16:643–657.

Katz AM, Katz PB. (1989). Homogeneity out of heterogeneity. *Circulation* 79:712–717.

Klotz C, Leger JJ, Elzinga M. (1982). Comparative sequence of myosin light chain for normal and hypertrophied human hearts. *Circ Res* 50:201–209.

Kurabayashi M, Komuro I, Tsuchimochi H, Takaku F, Yazaki Y. (1988). Molecular cloning and characterization of human atrial and ventricular myosin alkali light chain cDNA clones. *J Biol Chem* 263:13930–13936.

Leger J, Bouveret P, Schwartz K, Swynghedauw B. (1976). A comparative study of skeletal and cardiac tropomyosins: subunits, thiol group content and biological activities. *Pflugers Arch* 362:271–277.

Lehrer SS. (1978). Effects of an interchain disulfide bond on tropomyosin structure: intrinsic fluorescence and circular dichroism studies. *J Mol Biol* 118:209–226.

Lewis WG, Smillie LB. (1980). The amino acid sequence of rabbit cardiac tropomyosin. *J Biol Chem* 255:6854–6859.

Mar JH, Ordahl CP. (1988). A conserved CATTCCT motif is required for skeletal muscle-specific activity of the cardiac troponin T gene promoter. *Proc Nat Acad Sci USA* 85:6404–6408.

Murray JM, Knox MK, Trueblood CE, Weber A. (1982). Potentiated state of the tropomyosin actin filament and nucleotide-containing myosin subfragment I. *Biochemistry* 21:906–915.

Noland TA Jr, Raynor RL, Kuo JF. (1989). Identification of sites phosphorylated in bovine cardiac troponin I and troponin T by protein kinase C and comparative substrate activity of synthetic peptides containing the phosphorylation sites. *J Biol Chem* 264:20778–20785.

Obinata T, Maruyama K, Sugita H, Kohama K, Ebashi S. (1981). Dynamic aspects of structural protein in vertebrate skeletal muscle. *Muscle Nerve* 4:456–488.

Pearson AM, Young RB. (1989). *Muscle and meat biochemistry.* San Diego: Academic Press.

Periasamy M, Strehler EE, Garfinkel LI, Gubits RM, Ruiz-Opazo N, Nadal-Ginard B. (1984). Fast skeletal muscle myosin light chains 1 and 3 are produced from a single gene by a combined process of differential RNA transcription and splicing. *J Biol Chem* 259:13595–13604.

Putkey JA, Sweeney HL, Campbell ST. (1989). Site-directed mutation of the trigger calcium-binding sites in cardiac troponin C. *J Biol Chem* 264:12370–12378.

Ruiz-Opazo N, Weinberger J, Nadal-Ginard B. (1985). Comparison of α-tropomyosin sequences from smooth and striated muscle. *Nature* 315:67–70.

Sabry MA, Dhoot GK. (1989). Identification and pattern of expression of a developmental isoform of troponin I in chicken and rat cardiac muscle. *J Muscle Res Cell Motil* 10:85–91.

Saez LJ, Gianola KM, McNally EM, Feghali R, Eddy R, Shows TB, Lienwald LA. (1987). Human cardiac myosin heavy chain genes and their linkage in the genome. *Nucleic Acids Res* 15:5443–5459.

Saggin L, Gorza L, Ausoni S, Schiaffino S. (1989). Troponin I switching in the developing heart. *J Biol Chem* 264:16299–16302.

Stossel TP. (1989). From signal to pseudopod. How cells control cytoplasmic actin assembly. *J Biol Chem* 264:18621–18624.

Streter FA, Luff AR, Gergely J. (1975). Effects of cross-reinnervation on physiological parameters and properties of myosin and sarcoplasmic reticulum of fast and slow muscles of the rabbit. *J Gen Physiol* 60:811–821.

Sweeney HL, Stull JT. (1990). Alteration of cross-bridge kinetics by myosin light chain phosphorylation in rabbit skeletal muscle: implications for regulation of actin-myosin interaction. *Proc Nat Acad Sci USA* 87:414–418.

Tao T, Gong B-J, Leavis PC. (1990). Calcium-induced movement of troponin I relative to actin in skeletal muscle thin filaments. *Science* 247:1339–1341.

Warber KD, Potter JD. (1986). Contractile proteins and phosphorylation. In: Fozzard HA, Haber E, Jennings RB, Katz AM, Morgan HE, eds. *The heart and cardiovascular system.* New York: Raven Press; 779–788.

BIBLIOGRAPHY

Bárány M. (1967). ATPase activity of myosin correlated with speed of muscle shortening. *J Gen Physiol* 50(No. 6, Pt. 2):197–216.

Ebashi S. (1979). The Croonian Lecture, 1979. Regulation of muscle contraction. *Proc R Soc Lond [Biol]* 207:259–286.

Katz A. (1970). Contractile proteins of the heart. *Physiol Rev* 50:63–158.

Kretsinger RH (1979). The informational role of calcium in the cytosol. *Adv Cyclic Nucl Res* 11:1–26.

Nadal-Ginard B, Mahdavi V. (1989). Molecular basis of cardiac performance. Plasticity of the myocardium generated through protein isoform switches. *J Clin Invest* 84:1693–1700.

Pollard TD, Cooper JA (1986). Actin and actin-binding proteins. A critical evaluation of mechanisms and functions. *Annu Rev Biochem* 55:987–1035.

Swynghedauw B. (1986). Developmental and functional adaptation of contractile proteins in cardiac and skeletal muscles. *Physiol Rev* 66:710–771.

Swynghedauw B, ed. (1990). *Cardiac hypertrophy and failure*. London. John Libbey.

Weber A, Murray J. (1973). Molecular control mechanisms in muscle contraction. *Physiol Rev* 53:612–673.

8

Mechanism and Control of the Cardiac Contractile Process

The contractile proteins described in Chapter 7 represent the "cast of characters" for the drama to be described in the present chapter: the mechanism and control of muscular contraction in the intact heart. We have already seen that actomyosins reconstituted from highly purified myosin, actin, tropomyosin, and the troponin complex exhibit the three salient properties of muscle. Two are found in the "two-protein" actomyosin mode from actin and myosin, which is able to *hydrolyze adenosine triphosphate (ATP)* and undergo *physicochemical changes* analogous to contraction. The third of these properties, the ability to *respond to calcium*, requires that the regulatory proteins, tropomyosin and the troponin complex, be present in the actomyosin. By assembling contractile systems from individually purified proteins, it has been possible to define functional roles that each of these components play in the theater of contraction in the living heart, where their function is subject to control by a variety of physiologic, pharmacologic and pathophysiologic mechanisms.

In this chapter we first examine the mechanism by which the regulatory proteins recognize a rise in cytosolic Ca^{2+} concentration as a signal that initiates the contractile process. Subsequently, we review our current understanding of the interactions between actin and myosin that give rise to the contractile process itself. Finally these properties are reexamined in terms of the energetics of muscular contraction described in Chapter 6.

CALCIUM AS AN INTRACELLULAR MESSENGER

Calcium ions, by carrying signals generated at the cell surface to a variety of intracellular proteins and organelles, can be viewed as the most important of the intracellular messengers. As already noted, the myocardial cell uses calcium as the essential final step in *excitation-contraction coupling*, the process by which depolarization of the cell surface membrane initiates the interactions between the contractile proteins that lead to tension development and shortening in the walls of the heart. Calcium serves a similar role as activator of motility in single-celled organisms, where this cation initiates cytoplasmic streaming and motion of cilia and flagellae. Calcium also mediates stimulus-secretion coupling in a variety of nonmotile cells. A diverse group of mechanisms, both electrical and chemical, can lead to the appearance of activator calcium within cells, but the final step in stimulation seems always to occur when calcium binds to one or another member of the family of calcium-binding proteins described in Chapter 7.

A series of hypotheses set forth by Kretsinger (1977) may explain why calcium has become an intracellular messenger. These hypotheses start with the fact that cytosolic Ca^{2+} concentration in eukaryotic cells is in the micromolar range; in the resting heart, for example, cytosolic Ca^{2+} concentration is approximately 0.2 μM. In contrast, the Ca^{2+} concentration in the extracellular space, as in sea water, is in the millimolar range. Noting the low solubility of calcium phosphate, Kretsinger suggested that cells originally excluded calcium in order to concentrate phosphate in the cytosol, where this ion served as the chemical energy currency and to "trap" anionic phosphosugars to which the cell membrane is impermeable (Chapter 4). Another reason that primitive cells may have excluded calcium lies in their need to concentrate phosphate for the nucleic acids that transmit genetic information.

Once cells had evolved a "calcium-free" cytosol, calcium leakage by passive diffusion became both a problem and an opportunity. While requiring energy-dependent ion pumps to transport unwanted calcium out of the cell, calcium entry through regulated ion channels in the plasma membrane became a useful means for signaling various processes inside the cell. As calcium ions carry a positive charge, this signal is "two-for-one": electrical as well as chemical. The family of calcium-binding proteins—perhaps initially helping to trap unwanted calcium that leaked into the cytosol—would then have evolved to become intracellular calcium "sensors."

Although obviously speculative, this scenario is useful in understanding the importance of the appearance of measured amounts of calcium in the cytosol, and the ability of this cation, by binding to intracellular calcium-binding proteins, to serve as a ubiquitous cytosolic messenger.

RESPONSE OF THE CONTRACTILE PROTEINS TO CALCIUM IONS

It has already been pointed out that calcium, by binding to troponin C, reverses an inhibitory effect of the regulatory proteins that triggers interactions between actin and myosin. This response of the contractile machinery to calcium begins with a series of cooperative interactions between calcium-bound troponin C and troponin I, troponin T, and tropomyosin. The final step in these allosteric interactions among the regulatory proteins is a shift in the position of tropomyosin in the grooves between the double-standard F-actin polymer in the thin filament (Fig. 8.1). However, the actin-tropomyosin complex, shown in longitudinal view in Fig. 7.9, and in cross section in Fig. 8.1, cannot respond to the calcium released during excitation-con-

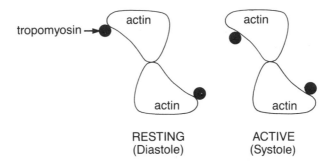

FIG. 8.1. Cross section of a thin filament at a level away from a region containing the troponin complex, showing the location of tropomyosin molecules in the groove between adjacent strands of actin monomers in muscle at rest (*left*) and during activity (*right*).

traction coupling. Instead, the ability of calcium to regulate the contractile process requires that the troponin complex also be present in the thin filament.

The cooperative interactions among the proteins of the thin filament that mediate excitation-contraction coupling begin when calcium binds to troponin C. This initiates a series of allosteric changes that leads to a shift in the position of tropomyosin, which exposes active sites on actin, allowing the latter to interact with myosin. A hypothetical model for this process is provided in Fig. 8.2. According to this model, in resting muscle, where troponin C is not bound to calcium, the tropomyosin fila-

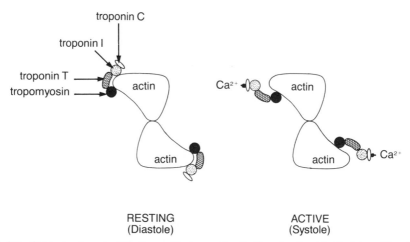

FIG. 8.2. Cross section of a thin filament in the resting (*left*) and active (*right*) states. At rest, the troponin complex holds the tropomyosin molecules toward the periphery of the groove between adjacent actin strands in a manner that prevents actin from interacting with the myosin cross-bridges. In active muscle, calcium binding to troponin C weakens the bond linking troponin I to actin, causing a structural rearrangement of the regulatory proteins that shifts the tropomyosin deeper into the groove between the strands of actin. This rearrangement exposes active sites on actin for interaction with the myosin cross-bridges.

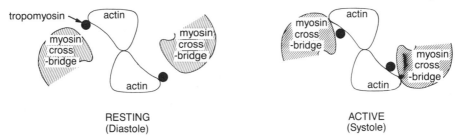

RESTING   ACTIVE
(Diastole)   (Systole)

FIG. 8.3. Cross section of a point of potential interaction between actin and adjacent myosin cross-bridges at rest (*left*) and during activity (*right*). A shift in the position of the tropomyosin molecules toward the center of the groove between adjacent actin strands in the thin filament allows active sites on actin to interact with the myosin cross-bridges.

ments lie toward the outside of the grooves between the two chains of actin where they "block" the development of actin-myosin interactions. When calcium binds to troponin C, the bond connecting troponin I to actin is weakened and these two proteins become dissociated. This cooperative interaction causes the elongated tropomyosin molecules to shift toward the center of the groove between the two strands of actin (Taylor and Amos, 1981) (Figs. 8.1 and 8.2). As this structural rearrangement moves tropomyosin away from its "blocking" position, physical and chemical interactions develop between the myosin cross-bridges and active sites on actin (Fig. 8.3). The muscle returns to its relaxed state when removal of calcium from troponin C causes tropomyosin to return to its original inhibitory position in the thin filament (Fig. 8.3).

Each of the troponin complexes, which are spaced ~400 Å from neighboring troponin complexes along the long axis of the thin filament (Fig. 7.9), influences a tropomyosin molecule that is also ~400 Å long. Thus, calcium binding to each troponin complex exerts an effect along approximately seven pairs of actin monomers, so that these cooperative interactions involve an amplification.

OTHER COOPERATIVE INTERACTIONS

Inhibition of the contractile process by tropomyosin and the troponin complex is only one of many cooperative interactions between these regulatory proteins, actin, and myosin. Although sensitizing the contractile machinery is the most important, the allosteric interactions among these proteins are rich and varied; thus, the regulatory proteins do more than serve as an "on-off" switch that translates the appearance of calcium in the cytosol into a signal that initiates contraction. For example, once the contractile process has begun and actin is interacting with myosin, the regulatory proteins actually stimulate actomyosin. In this way the regulatory proteins can amplify tension development and shortening while the muscle is contracting (Katz, 1964; Weber and Murray, 1973). The development of interactions between actin and myosin also influences the calcium sensitivity of the contractile process (Brandt et al., 1982). Other important allosteric effects include the ability of troponin I phosphorylation to reduce the calcium sensitivity of cardiac troponin C (Chapter 14) and troponin T isoform shifts to alter the response of the hypertrophied heart to calcium. The well-known ability of acidosis to reduce myocardial contractility (Chapter 14) is not due to a direct interaction of protons with the calcium-binding site of troponin C; but instead, arises from an allosteric effect initiated by proton binding to troponin I.

CHEMISTRY OF CARDIAC CONTRACTION

As the actomyosins made up only of actin and myosin can convert the chemical energy derived from ATP hydrolysis into mechanical work (Chapter 7), it is clear that the contractile process can result from interactions involving actin, myosin, and ATP. The following discussion reviews the currently accepted view of the mechanism of muscular contraction, which is based on interactions between the myosin cross-bridge, actin, ATP, and the products of ATP hydrolysis: adenosine diphosphate (ADP) and inorganic phosphate (P_i).

The existence of paired heads in each myosin cross-bridge (Chapter 7) has given rise to a number of complex theories regarding a possible interaction between myosin heads in the contractile process. However, actomyosins containing "one-headed" myosins can exhibit the salient properties of contraction, so that cooperative interactions between the two heavy chains in the normal paired head of myosin seem most likely to play a role in the many allosteric interactions between the contractile proteins.

Motion of the Myosin Cross-Bridge

Changes in cross-bridge orientation relative to the long axis of the thick filament in activated muscle (Figs. 1.20 and 7.5) correspond to the observed flexibility of single myosin molecules and the sites of susceptibility to proteolytic cleavage believed to represent "hinges" in the molecule (Chapter 7). As described below, changing cross-bridge orientation can be related to altered interactions between the myosin cross-bridges and the thin filament. These morphological observations are in accord with the overall mechanism for muscular contraction described below: that cross-bridge movement, linked to changing interactions with the thin filament, arise from a sequence of specific steps in the reaction of myosin with ATP and its hydrolytic products. This mechanism is very complex; for simplicity, this chapter describes only four such states: two of strong binding between actin and myosin ("active" and "rigor" complexes) and two of weak actin-myosin binding ("relaxed" and "relaxed, energized").

Is ATP Essential for Contraction or Relaxation?

It has been apparent since the 1960s that ATP provides the energy for muscular contraction (Chapter 6); thus, a high-energy phosphate bond must be cleaved at some point in the cycle of chemical reactions that underlies muscle's function as a mechanochemical transducer. Early theories of muscular contraction, such as the new elastic body theory (Chapter 6), would require that the energy derived from ATP hydrolysis be used to establish cross-links in the molecular machinery that give rise to the ability to shorten and develop tension according to the general reaction scheme:

$$\text{Actin} + \text{myosin} + \text{ATP} \rightarrow \text{actomyosin} + \text{ADP} + \text{P}_i. \qquad [8.1]$$
$$\text{(relaxed)} \qquad\qquad\qquad \text{(active)}$$

$$\text{Actomyosin} \qquad\qquad \rightarrow \text{actin} + \text{myosin}. \qquad [8.2]$$
$$\text{(active)} \qquad\qquad\qquad \text{(relaxed)}$$

Identification of the plasticizing effect of ATP (Chapter 7), which reflects a requirement for ATP in maintaining the contractile machinery in a relaxed state, suggested the opposite view: that the role of ATP (shown below as related to its binding to myosin) is primarily to cause actomyosin systems to relax:

$$\text{Actomyosin} + \text{ATP} \qquad \rightarrow \text{Actin} + \text{myosin-ATP}. \qquad [8.3]$$
$$\text{(active)} \qquad\qquad\qquad \text{(relaxed)}$$

$$\text{Actin} + \text{myosin-ATP} \qquad \rightarrow \text{actomyosin} + \text{ADP} + \text{P}_i. \qquad [8.4]$$
$$\text{(relaxed)} \qquad\qquad\qquad \text{(active)}$$

As the reader will learn in the following discussion, ATP really is like Aesop's elf (Chapter 7); both models are correct! Detailed analyses of the many steps in the interactions between myosin, actin, ATP, ADP, and P_i, have added new dimensions to this question. The number of known steps in the sequence of chemical reactions responsible for muscular contraction has grown, and it is now apparent that ATP and the products of its hydrolysis, ADP and P_i, interact with the contractile proteins at several steps in this process. Some of these nucleotide effects are related to contraction, others to relaxation. Thus, attempts to answer the simple question posed in the heading to this section have lost much of their relevance. However, in terms of pathophysiology—especially in the energy-starved heart—this remains an important question. For this reason, we return to this question later in the chapter, after details of the reaction mechanism have been presented.

Reaction Mechanisms

The reaction mechanism involved in myosin adenosine triphosphatase (ATPase) activity has assumed considerable functional significance because of the direct relationship between myosin ATPase activity and shortening velocity in unloaded muscle (Chapter 7). This relationship indicates that the same rate-limiting step in the chemical reactions by which actomyosin hydrolyzes ATP (which is also rate limiting for the ATPase activity of myosin alone), is rate limiting for unloaded shortening of the intact muscle.

A number of elaborate schemes for the actomyosin ATPase reaction have been presented. For simplicity, this chapter considers only four steps in the reaction mechanisms that allow the contractile protein to utilize ATP to generate mechanical work. These steps are: (1) binding of ATP to myosin; (2) hydrolysis of myosin-bound ATP in a step where the hydrolytic products (ADP and P_i) remain bound to myosin; (3) formation of an "active" actomyosin complex that begins mechanochemical transduction; and (4) release of hydrolytic products, the actual step where the myosin cross-bridge changes position. The sequence, of course, can be repeated when ATP again binds to myosin.

Before examining the reactions that involve both actin and myosin, it is useful first to examine the simpler ATPase reaction of myosin alone. By comparing the steps in this reaction with those of the two-protein actomyosin, the rate-limiting steps and the role of actin should become clear.

Myosin ATPase Reaction

Like the reactions involving both actin and myosin, the hydrolysis of ATP by myosin alone can be described in several steps. In the following discussion only three steps are described; the fourth, actomyosin formation (step 2 of the actomyosin reaction, see below) is, of course, impossible in the ATPase reaction of myosin alone.

Step 1: Binding of ATP to Myosin

Myosin binds with high affinity to ATP according to the reaction:

$$\text{Myosin} + \text{ATP} \rightarrow \text{myosin-ATP}. \quad [8.5]$$

The affinity of myosin for ATP is very high, so that virtually all of the myosin cross-bridges in resting muscle are bound either to ATP or the products of ATP hydrolysis (see below). As discussed below, when myosin binds to ATP, its ability to interact with actin is inhibited; this means that ATP dissociates actin and myosin, which accounts for its "plasticizing" effect (Chapter 7).

The myosin-ATP complex can exist in two states. In one, the chemical energy of ATP in the complex remains in the terminal phosphate of the nucleotide. In the second state, much of the energy of ATP is transferred to the myosin molecule.

Step 2: Hydrolysis of Myosin-Bound ATP

Hydrolysis of ATP by the enzymatic site of myosin is not followed by the immediate dissociation of the products of ATP hydrolysis (ADP and P_i) from myosin. Instead, a complex is formed in which ADP and P_i remain attached to myosin, which energizes the molecule:

$$\text{Myosin-ATP} \quad \rightarrow \quad \text{myosin} \diagup^{\text{ADP}}_{\diagdown P_i} \quad [8.6]$$

Step 3: Release of ADP and P_i

The hydrolytic products ADP and P_i dissociate very slowly from myosin, which returns to its basal state according to the reaction:

$$\text{Myosin} \overset{\displaystyle ADP}{\underset{\displaystyle P_i}{\big<}} \quad \rightarrow \quad \text{myosin} + \text{ADP} + P_i \qquad . \qquad [8.7]$$

The myosin-product complex is quite stable; so stable, in fact, that dissociation of ADP and P_i are rate limiting for the low ATPase activity of myosin alone. The key role of actin in the living muscle is its ability to accelerate step 3, which because this step is rate limiting, increases the overall rate of ATP hydrolysis.

This simplified three-step myosin ATPase reaction provides a basis for understanding the four-step reaction of actomyosin ATPase described below. Although the latter has also been simplified for presentation in this text, the abbreviated scheme can explain the role of actin, as well as the dual role of ATP: to dissociate actomyosin and so cause relaxation, while at the same time contributing chemical energy for the performance of mechanical work.

Activation of Myosin ATPase by Actin

The well-known ability of actin to increase myosin ATPase activity (Chapter 7) arises from the ability of actin to accelerate the rate-limiting step in this reaction (step 3: release of ADP and P_i, or product dissociation). This critical role begins when actin interacts with myosin still bound to the products of ATP hydrolysis:

$$\text{Myosin} \overset{\displaystyle ADP}{\underset{\displaystyle P_i}{\big<}} \qquad .$$

Actin accelerates product dissociation from this complex, while at the same time converting the low myosin ATPase activity to the much higher activity of actomyosin. Of course, actin does much more than simply accelerate a hydrolytic reaction; the interactions between actin and myosin utilize energy derived from ATP hydrolysis to effect the contractile process.

Actomyosin ATPase Reaction

The essential features of the *cross-bridge cycle* can be summarized in four steps that characterize the interactions between myosin, actin, and ATP. Although the following description is intended to provide insights as to how muscle serves as a mechanochemical transducer, the actual reactions are more complex than the four-step sequence described below (Reaction 8.8 and Fig. 8.4). The reader who wishes to learn more of this subject is referred to a recent review by Taylor (1991).

The simplified four-step reaction depicts two states of myosin and two of the combination of actin and myosin (actomyosin). Both of the former, where myosin is shown in combination with ATP and with ADP + P_i, represent relaxed states of muscle because the cross-bridges are detached from actin. The cross-bridges are attached in the other two states, which therefore involve actomyosin. In one (the active complex), the energy of ATP is still in the myosin cross-bridge; in the other (the rigor complex), mechanochemical energy transduction has taken place, and the energy has been used to shift the position of the cross-bridge.

The steps depicted in Reaction 8.8 should be related to Fig. 8.4, in which four sketches have been positioned to correspond to the "corners" of the reaction scheme.

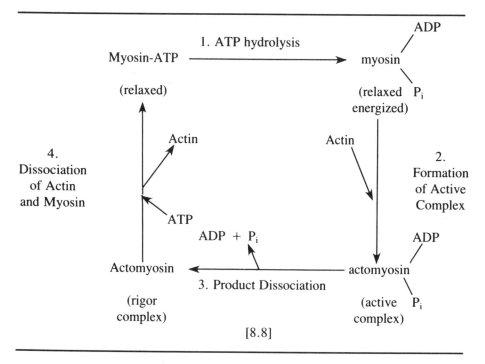

[8.8]

In choosing where to enter this cycle, we follow the cardiac physiologist, who generally views the cardiac cycle as beginning in diastole. Our analysis of the actomyosin cycle begins after the rapid binding of ATP to the cross-bridge in the rigor complex, which forms the myosin-ATP complex, has caused dissociation of actin from myosin. The four steps that follow are (1) hydrolysis of myosin-bound ATP, (2) formation of the active complex with actin, (3) dissociation of the products of ATP hydrolysis, and (4) dissociation of actin and myosin.

As described above, the heart relaxes when the regulatory proteins "block" the interactions between actin and myosin. Although the regulatory proteins are not considered in Reaction 8.8, their ability to maintain the heart in a resting state arises from their inhibition of step 2, formation of the active complex between actin and myosin.

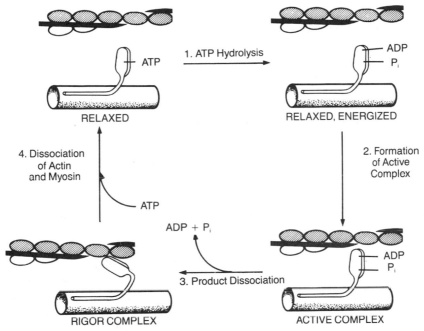

FIG. 8.4. Reaction mechanism for actomyosin ATPase (simplified) showing four steps that should be compared to Reaction 8.8. The sequence begins at the *upper left*, where ATP binding to myosin has dissociated the thick and thin filaments, causing the muscle to relax. Hydrolysis of myosin-bound ATP (step 1) transfers the energy of the nucleotide to the cross-bridge in a relaxed, energized state (*upper right*). Interaction of the cross-bridge with actin in the thin filament (step 2) leads to the formation of the active complex (*lower right*) in which the energy derived from ATP is still associated with the cross-bridge. Dissociation of ADP and P_i, the products of ATP hydrolysis (step 3), leads to the formation of a rigor bond, in which the chemical energy has been expended to perform mechanical work: the motion of the cross-bridge. The cycle ends, and the muscle returns to its resting state, when ATP binding to the rigor complex (step 4) dissociates the cross-bridge from the thin filament.

Step 1. Hydrolysis of Myosin-Bound ATP

As noted above, we enter the scene just after the high concentrations of ATP in the normal heart have dissociated the rigor complexes left over from the preceding cycle, which, of course, has caused the thick and thin filaments to dissociate. This ATP has bound to the catalytic site of myosin, forming the myosin-ATP complex that begins this analysis.

The ATP bound to the dissociated cross-bridge is rapidly hydrolyzed by the catalytic site of myosin. As in the case of ATP hydrolysis by myosin alone, the hydrolytic products, ADP and P_i, remain attached to myosin so that this first step can be described as:

$$\text{Myosin-ATP} \quad \rightarrow \quad \text{myosin} \Big\langle {\,}^{\text{ADP}}_{\text{P}_i} \qquad . \qquad [8.9]$$

(relaxed)   (relaxed
                              energized)

In this step, the energy present in the terminal phosphate bond of ATP is transferred to the myosin cross-bridge. Thus, the complex:

$$\text{myosin} \Big\langle {\,}^{\text{ADP}}_{\text{P}_i}$$

remains "energized"; that is, the chemical energy of the terminal phosphate bond of ATP has not been expended, but has been transferred to the cross-bridge.

Although the reaction depicted in Reaction 8.9 is the same as that shown for myosin alone (Reaction 8.6), the situation in muscle is more complex in that actin and the regulatory proteins can exert subtle allosteric effects that influence the myosin cross-bridge, even after it is "formally" dissociated from the thin filament. In the relaxed muscle, where calcium is not bound to troponin C, the regulatory proteins inhibit the next step: the interaction between myosin and actin that would otherwise allow an interaction with actin to convert the energy in the "energized" cross-bridge to mechanical work.

Step 2. Formation of the Active Complex with Actin

When excitation-contraction coupling provides calcium that binds to troponin C, actin joins the action. The interaction of actin with the myosin cross-bridge initiates the next step in the cross-bridge cycle: the formation of an active complex between actin and myosin:

$$\text{Myosin} \Big\langle {\,}^{\text{ADP}}_{\text{P}_i} \quad + \text{ actin} \rightarrow \quad \text{actomyosin} \Big\langle {\,}^{\text{ADP}}_{\text{P}_i} \qquad . \qquad [8.10]$$

(relaxed   (active
energized)   complex)

In the active complex, the myosin cross-bridge is bound to the thin filament but the mechanical transformation has not taken place; in other words, the cross-bridge has not yet executed the "rowing" motion that pulls the thin filament toward the center of the sarcomere (Fig. 7.19). Because this interaction between actin and myosin neither releases energy nor induces a shift in the orientation of the myosin cross-bridge, the chemical energy available from ATP hydrolysis has not yet been expended; thus, the active complex contains considerable potential energy. It is apparent, therefore, that the active complex is not a stable or long-lived state of the contractile proteins. Transduction of the chemical energy of the active complex to mechanical work, which occurs in the next step, is responsible for the cross-bridge movement that accompanies formation of a much more stable, low energy, rigor complex.

Step 3. Dissociation of the Products of ATP Hydrolysis

It is at this third step in our simplified reaction sequence that the muscle actually behaves like a muscle; that is, it performs mechanical work. At this critical step of mechanochemical transduction, the chemical energy of ATP (now trapped in the active complex) is used to shift the position of the cross-bridge. This occurs when the hydrolytic products, ADP and P_i, are released in the following reaction:

$$\text{Actomyosin} \begin{matrix} {}^{\text{ADP}} \\ {}_{P_i} \end{matrix} \quad \rightarrow \quad \text{actomyosin} + \text{ADP} + P_i \ . \qquad [8.11]$$

(active complex)   (rigor complex)

The new conformation formed between actin and the cross-bridge after the release of ADP and P_i is called the "rigor complex." In this complex, the heads of the myosin molecules have shifted their orientation in a manner that allows the myosin cross-bridges to pull the attached thin filaments toward the center of the sarcomere (Fig. 8.4). This is the slowest of the reactions involved in the cross-bridge cycle in active muscle; it is about 1,000 times slower than the hydrolysis of myosin-bound ATP. Like Reaction 8.7 involving myosin alone, therefore, the release of products $(\text{ADP} + P_i)$ from myosin (Reaction 8.11) is rate limiting.

The rigor complex represents the low-energy state of muscle. It is very different from the active complex, although actin is attached to myosin in both. The main difference is that the active complex is in a high-energy state, whereas the rigor complex is a low-energy complex. This change in state can be readily appreciated because the motion of the cross-bridge during the conversion of the active complex to the rigor complex is accompanied by the expenditure of chemical energy in the performance of mechanical work. Stated simply, the muscle, having expended mechanical energy, has lost chemical energy and is tired.

The rigor complex is so stable that when there is no ATP to dissociate the rigor bond and restart the cycle, it is the final resting place of the contractile machinery. This low-energy state of the contractile proteins accounts for the skeletal muscle rigidity in *rigor mortis*, and *ischemic contracture* in the heart (also called the "stone heart").

Step 4. Dissociation of Actin and Myosin

The cross-bridge cycle returns to its starting point when ATP again binds to myosin. This can be viewed simply (but not correctly) as a competition between ATP and actin for a site on the cross-bridge in the rigor bond. Although the mechanism is more complex, the fact is that ATP does detach the myosin cross-bridge from actin according to the reaction:

$$\text{Actomyosin} + \text{ATP} \qquad \rightarrow \qquad \text{myosin-ATP} + \text{actin} \qquad [8.12]$$

| (rigor | (relaxed) |
| complex) | |

This rapid reaction, which releases the bonds linking myosin to actin (Fig. 8.4), is responsible for the "plasticizing effect of ATP described in Chapter 7; thus, rebinding of ATP to the rigor complex has caused the muscle to relax.

As noted in Chapter 7, high-energy phosphates are not essential to dissociate rigor bonds; inorganic polyphosphates and nonhydrolyzable ATP analogues also dissociate actin and myosin *in vitro*, due possibly to the charge effects of these anionic compounds (Oriel-Audit et al., 1981). In the cells of living muscle, or course, the soluble polyanion available in largest amounts is ATP.

Is ATP Essential for Contraction or Relaxation?

It is appropriate now to return to this question, posed earlier in this chapter. If one reflects on the overall reactions involved in cross-bridge cycling, it is apparent that ATP is essential for *both* contraction and relaxation; one might state that ATP itself is essential for relaxation, whereas its hydrolysis is essential for contraction. These effects represent important manifestations of the dual effect of ATP described in Chapter 7.

It is important to note that the concentrations of ATP needed to dissociate rigor bonds are much higher than those needed to saturate the substrate site of myosin (Chapter 7). This explains why rigor develops in ATP-depleted muscle, where the high-affinity binding of ATP to myosin can maintain the cross-bridge in an energized state that can form rigor bonds with the thin filament even when there is insufficient ATP to dissociate actomyosin. The fact that high, allosteric, ATP concentrations are needed to relax the heart whereas much lower concentrations can lead to the formation of the rigor bonds partly explains the clinical observation that relaxation abnormalities are generally more prominent than depressed contractility in the energy-starved heart (see Chapter 24).

CONTROL OF THE CROSS-BRIDGE CYCLE IN THE INTACT HEART

In the living heart, the cross-bridge cycle can be limited by two mechanisms: the number of troponin C molecules that are bound to calcium, and the properties of the myosin molecule. Both are of importance in cardiac regulation, although each involves a different principle of control.

Rapid changes in the performance of the heart are brought about by variations in the amount of calcium released during excitation-contraction coupling, and by changes in the sensitivity of the contractile proteins to this activation messenger; as noted in Chapter 14, these can be viewed as arising from "phasic" control of the heart. Changes in the expression of the genes that encode the many isoforms of these proteins take place more slowly, and so represent a more "tonic" regulation (see Chapter 14).

Control by Calcium Binding to Troponin C

As discussed at the beginning of this chapter, when troponin C is not bound to calcium the regulatory proteins inhibit the cross-bridge cycle at step 2 in Reaction 8.8, before actin forms the active complex with myosin. Lifting of this inhibitory effect when calcium is delivered to the contractile proteins during excitation-contraction coupling shifts the rate-limiting reaction in the cross-bridge cycle to step 3, where the products of ATP hydrolysis $(ADP + P_i)$ are released and the cross-bridges form rigor bonds. In normal muscle, the cycle continues when ATP dissociates the rigor bonds, ending with myosin in the relaxed, energized state when calcium removal from the cytosol causes the regulatory proteins to return to their "blocking position" (Fig. 8.2).

Control by Myosin

As noted in Chapter 7, both myosin ATPase activity and muscle shortening velocity are determined largely by the myosin heavy chain isoform in the thick filament. When myosin ATPase activity is high, the muscle shortens rapidly, whereas when myosin ATPase activity is low, shortening is slow (Bárány, 1967). Thus, the same property that determines myosin ATPase activity *in vitro* also governs the maximal velocity of shortening in the unloaded muscle.

It is now clear that myosin heavy chain isoform characteristics determine the rate of product dissociation, which determines both the maximum rate of cross-bridge cycling and maximal shortening velocity in the unloaded muscle. This follows because both reflect the same property of myosin: the rate at which ADP and P_i are released.

A calcium, calmodulin-dependent phosphorylation of one of the myosin light chains may have an additional effect to amplify the reactions of the cross-bridge cycle (Chapter 7). Reports that other myofibrillar proteins can be phosphorylated by protein kinase C indicate additional ways that myocardial performance could be regulated. In fact, the cooperativity of the interactions between the myofibrillar proteins is so complex that it is not surprising that a growing number of modifications involving the myofibrillar proteins are being found to influence the cross-bridge cycle.

RELATIONSHIP BETWEEN THE CROSS-BRIDGE CYCLE AND THE ENERGETICS OF CONTRACTION

The ability of the load to determine energy expenditure during contraction (the Fenn effect) was described in Chapter 6, where the rate of energy release was shown to be inversely proportional to load (Fig. 6.14). The remarkably prescient interpretation of this relationship over 50 years ago by A. V. Hill—that the load on an active muscle determines the distribution of "active points" between two different states—is now reexamined in terms of the chemical processes reviewed in this and the preceding chapter.

In attempting to explain the inverse relationship between the rate of energy liberation and load in a contracting muscle, Hill postulated that when the load is great, more of the active points are attached to each other and so are in a state in which chemical energy is not being released. Conversely, virtually all of the active points are free to liberate chemical energy in the freely shortening, unloaded muscle. This interpretation can be tentatively related to the reaction mechanism of the cross-bridge cycle illustrated in Fig. 8.4.

Active Points Maintaining Tension

Slowing of the rate of energy liberation when a muscle lifts a heavy load (Chapter 6) indicates that increasing the tension on an active muscle reduces the rate of ATP hydrolyses. Because the amount of energy liberated per unit time is decreased at higher loads, where actin and myosin are required to interact in a manner that gives rise to more active tension, it is reasonable to postulate that the lifting of a heavy load favors the maintenance of rigor complexes. As increasing tension on the ends of the muscle inhibits the dissociation of actin and myosin, resistance to shortening appears to prevent the breaking of rigor bonds. Using the analogy described in Chapter 6 of "little men" pulling on the rope, holding the men in place by not allowing the rope to move keeps their feet firmly on the ground, and they are unable to liberate energy (Fig. 8.5).

This analysis is also in accord with evidence that maximal shortening velocity is not related to the ability of a muscle to generate tension. In terms of our analogy, the ability of a "little man" to pull on a rope is unrelated to how fast he runs freely if the rope breaks, or the post is pulled out of the ground.

Active Points Liberating Chemical Energy

Hill found that the rate of energy liberation per unit time was maximal in freely shortening muscle, which by definition was contracting against zero load. Furthermore, the maximal shortening velocity (V_{max}) of a given muscle is characteristic of that muscle type, and correlates closely with the intrinsic ATPase activity of its myosin (see above). This means that the maximal speed at which the "little men"

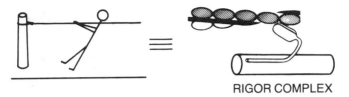

RIGOR COMPLEX

FIG. 8.5. The state of the active points in muscle when they are holding tension is identical to that of the rigor complex.

can run corresponds to the limiting rate of the cross-bridge cycle (Fig. 8.6). As already noted, this rate-limiting step is step 3 in Reaction 8.8, where the hydrolytic products, ADP and P_i, dissociate from the myosin.

Relationship of the Cross-Bridge Cycle to the Force-Velocity Curve

This brief discussion brings us full circle. The reader should recall the Hill equations (Chapter 6), and how measurements of heat liberation and work performance enabled Hill to predict key features of muscle chemistry. According to this analysis, the two intercepts of the force-velocity curve are determined by quite different properties of the muscle. The maximal isometric tension generated by a fully activated muscle, P_0, which is independent of maximal shortening velocity and myosin ATPase activity, reflects the number of active cross-bridges (Fig. 8.7). Thus, P_0 will be determined largely by the amount of calcium available for binding to troponin C and the calcium affinity of the regulatory proteins. Maximal shortening velocity, on the other hand, should be influenced only by the rate of cross-bridge cycling because recruitment of additional runners will not increase this velocity as long as the muscle is fully unloaded. For this reason, variations in the amount of calcium bound to troponin C should not influence V_{max}. Other effects of calcium, such as activation of a calcium, calmodulin-dependent protein kinase that phosphorylates a myosin light chain could, however, alter V_{max}.

These interpretations define two independent mechanisms that can control muscular performance. One depends on the number of active cross-bridges, the other on

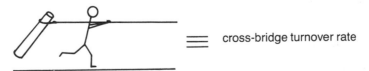

cross-bridge turnover rate

FIG. 8.6. The active points in muscle when the muscle is shortening against zero load are passing repeatedly through the cycle shown in Fig. 8.4 at a rate determined by the intrinsic properties of myosin.

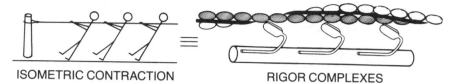

ISOMETRIC CONTRACTION   RIGOR COMPLEXES

FIG. 8.7. During an isometric contraction, where all active points are maintaining tension (*left*), the myosin cross-bridges are linked to the thin filament by rigor bonds.

the characteristics of the myosin heavy chain. We return to this analysis in Chapter 14, where the control of myocardial contractility is discussed in detail.

OTHER MODELS OF THE CONTRACTILE PROCESS

This chapter has relied on the sliding filament model and cross-bridge cycle to explain the contractile process. Although doubts are still expressed regarding the ability of the interactions between actin and myosin described above to explain mechanochemical transduction (Pollack, 1983, 1990), it has been shown that myosin linked to a fluorescent bead can "walk" along an actin filament (Sheetz and Spudich, 1983). Although discussion of alternative theories of muscular contraction is beyond the scope of this book, it seems appropriate to end this chapter with the reminder that, like so many areas of science, the field of muscle contraction is littered with the bones of dead theories. Thus, the reader should be warned that the explanations provided in this chapter might someday have to be revised.

REFERENCES

Bárány M. (1967). ATPase activity of myosin correlated with speed of muscle shortening. *J Gen Physiol* 50(No 6, Pt 2):197–216.

Brandt PW, Cox RN, Kawai M, Robinson T. (1982). Regulation of tension in skinned muscle fibers. Effect of cross-bridge kinetics on apparent Ca^{2+} sensitivity. *J Gen Physiol* 79:997–1016.

Katz AM. (1964). Influence of tropomyosin upon the reactions of actomyosin at low ionic strength. *J Biol Chem* 239:3304–3311.

Kretsinger R. (1977). Evolution of the informational role of calcium in eukaryocytes. In: Wasserman, RH, Corradino, RA, Carafoli E, Kretsinger RH, MacLennan DH, Siegel, FL, eds. *Calcium binding proteins and calcium function*. New York: North Holland, 63–72.

Oriol-Audit C, Lake JA, and Reisler E. (1981). Structural changes in synthetic myosin minifilaments and their dissociation by adenosine triphosphate and pyrophosphate. *Biochemistry* 20:679–686.

Pollack GH. (1983). The cross-bridge theory. *Physiol Rev* 63:1049–1113.

Pollack GH. (1990). *Muscles & molecules. Uncovering the principles of biological motion.* Seattle: Ebner.

Sheetz MP, Spudich JA. (1983). Movement of myosin-coated fluorescent beads on actin cables *in vitro*. *Nature* 305:31–35.

Taylor EW. (1991). Mechanism and energetics of actomyosin ATPase. In: Fozzard H, Haber E, Katz AM, Jennings RB, Morgan HE, eds. *The heart and cardiovascular system*, 2nd ed. New York: Raven Press; In Press.

Taylor KA, Amos LA. (1981). A new model for the geometry of the binding of myosin cross-bridges to muscle thin filaments. *J Mol Biol* 147:297–324.

Weber A, Murray JM. (1973). Molecular control mechanisms in muscle contraction. *Physiol Rev* 53:612–673.

BIBLIOGRAPHY

Brenner B. (1987). Mechanical and structural approaches to correlation of cross-bridge action in muscle with actomyosin ATPase in solution. *Annu Rev Physiol* 49:655–672.

Huxley AF. (1974). Muscular contraction. *J Physiol (Lond)* 243:1–43.

Julian FJ, Moss RL, Sollins MR. (1978). The mechanism for vertebrate striated muscle contraction. *Circ Res* 42:2–14.

Zot AS, Potter JD. (1987). Structural aspects of troponin-tropomyosin regulation of skeletal muscle contraction. *Annu Rev Biophys Biophys Chem* 16:535–559.

Also see bibliography to Chapter 7.

9

Series Elasticity, "Active State," Length–Tension Relationship, and Cardiac Mechanics

In Chapters 6 through 8, we examined the relationship between the chemical inter-actions of the contractile proteins and the energetics of contracting muscle. The frog sartorius muscle was chosen for most of the thermal and mechanical measurements described earlier because of its simple geometry and ability to respond with brief tetani. The latter, especially, simplified the analyses of mechanical performance because the study of tetanized muscle eliminates the complications of time-depen-dent and length-dependent changes in the interactions between the contractile pro-teins. In the heart, however, analyses of muscle energetics are difficult, and proba-bly impossible, for several reasons. In the first place, the complex architecture of the heart (Chapter 1) creates problems in relating the tension on the ends of the muscle to the force generated by its sarcomeres. Internal elasticities cause diffi-culties, even in isolated preparations, because sarcomere length can change during an isometric contraction, where the ends of the muscle are fixed. Another formida-ble obstacle to analysis of cardiac muscle mechanics is the fact that the heart cannot normally be tetanized, which of course would be a disaster in terms of its function as a pump. Because cardiac mechanics must ordinarily be evaluated during the rise and fall of tension that occurs during each cardiac cycle, time-dependent changes in the interactions between the contractile proteins create serious analytical problems. This chapter, therefore, continues our focus on the interplay between energetics and chemistry in amphibian skeletal muscle, where important concepts are clearly dem-onstrated. When we attempt to apply the principles of skeletal muscle energetics to the heart, a most remarkable conclusion emerges: the influence of changing tension and length on actin-myosin interactions in cardiac muscle may be almost as impor-tant as that of the regulatory proteins, tropomyosin and the troponin complex.

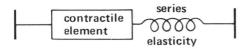

SERIES ELASTICITY

Several features of the time-dependent properties of the mechanical response of a skeletal muscle during a twitch can be explained by postulating an elasticity in series between the contractile element and the ends of the muscle (Fig. 9.1). When the sarcomere shortens, extension of this "series elasticity" absorbs some of the energy generated by the contractile element. As a result, elongation of the series elasticity at the start of contraction delays the transmission of tension developed by the contractile proteins to the ends of the muscle. Thus, the appearance of tension at the ends of the muscle during a twitch (in which activation of the contractile element is very brief) is both attenuated and delayed.

Latent Period

The role of the series elasticity is clearly seen in the latent period, a significant delay between the stimulation of a skeletal muscle and the first appearance of ten- sion. In a muscle that is stimulated under isometric conditions, a slight fall in ten- sion precedes tension development (Fig. 9.2). The brief interval before tension begins to increase is called the *latent period*, and the fall of tension is often called *latency relaxation*.

These phenomena cannot be attributed simply to the time needed for the impulse to reach the contractile elements, because important alterations take place within the muscle during the latent period; for example, optical birefringence changes before

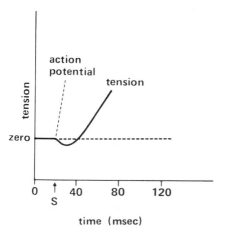

FIG. 9.2. Latency relaxation in a skeletal muscle contracting under isometric condi- tions. The initial decline in tension during the first few milliseconds after stimulation (S) is the latency relaxation. (The time scales in this and other figures in this chapter are adapted from studies of amphibian muscle at 0°C. These events occur much more rapidly in mammalian muscles contracting at 37°C.)

tension develops. Measurements of muscle stiffness indicate that the contractile process begins during the latent period. Even before the muscle develops tension, it becomes less plastic so that a given stretch generates more tension than in the unstimulated muscle. This increased stiffness indicates that actin and myosin have begun their interactions before tension has appeared at the ends of the muscle.

The delay between the onset of actin-myosin interactions and the development of tension during the latent period is due largely to extension of the series elasticity. For this reason, the activity of the contractile elements cannot be measured unless the effects of this elasticity are first eliminated (see below).

Twitch, Summation, and Tentanization

In a skeletal muscle, where the action potential is much briefer than the mechanical response, it is possible to restimulate the muscle before it has relaxed, while tension is still high (Fig. 9.3). The response to a single stimulus (S_1 in Fig. 9.3) is the *twitch*. If a second stimulus is applied before relaxation is complete, a second contraction becomes superimposed on the first; as a result, the tension developed in the second phase of the contraction (S_2 in Fig. 9.3) exceeds that developed during the twitch. Because the tension response to the second stimulus has been added to that of the first, the term *summation* has been introduced to describe this phenomenon.

When a muscle is stimulated so rapidly that each successive stimulus arrives before the muscle can begin to relax, tension continues to rise until it reaches a new steady-state level. Under isometric conditions, the tension developed in this new

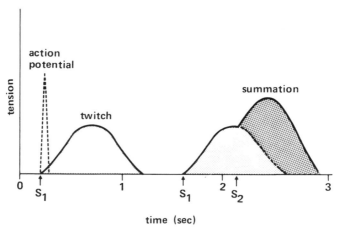

time (sec)

FIG. 9.3. Twitch and summation in a skeletal muscle contracting under isometric conditions. (Left) The symmetrical contraction (solid line) following a single action potential (dashed line) produced by a single stimulus (S_1) is a twitch. (Right) The application of a second stimulus (S_2) during the falling phase of the twitch produces a second action potential (not shown), which causes the renewed development of tension, a phenomenon called summation.

steady state exceeds twitch tension two-or threefold (Fig. 9.4). The stronger sustained contraction is called a *tetanus*, and the new level of tension—*tetanic tension*—corresponds to P_0 of the force-velocity curve discussed in the preceding chapters.

> Confusion can arise regarding the terms *tetanus* and *tetany*. The distinction between the tetanus (or tetanic contraction) shown in Fig. 9.4 and the disease caused by the endotoxin of the bacteria *Clostridium tetani* (a condition sometimes called lockjaw) is obvious. *Tetany*, which is quite different from the tetanus shown in Fig. 9.4, arises from a lowered threshold of the motor end plate to physical and chemical stimuli, rather than the summation of mechanical responses to a train of rapidly applied stimuli. This pathological condition often accompanies systemic alkalosis or hypocalcemia.

The fact that tetanic tension is much higher than that developed in a twitch remained unexplained for many years, but it is now clear that tension is "lost" in a twitch because much of the force developed by the interactions between actin and myosin is absorbed when the series elasticity is stretched.

Figure 9.1 implies that the series elasticity lies outside the contractile element. To some extent this is correct in that the tendinous ends of the muscles contribute an elasticity in experimental muscle preparations. Elasticities in isolated muscles may also arise from damaged regions of the muscle adjacent to the clamps used to hold the muscle to the recording apparatus, and from asynchrony of contraction caused by uneven or incomplete stimulation. Even when all of these artifacts are eliminated or compensated for, a significant elasticity remains in the muscle cell itself. Although some of this elasticity is attributable to the cytoskeleton, significant elasticity also appears to arise from interactions between the cross-bridges and the thin filaments, which persist even in resting muscle (see below).

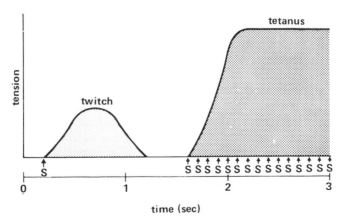

FIG. 9.4. Twitch and tetanic contractions in a skeletal muscle contracting under isometric conditions. (Left) Twitch, as shown in Fig. 9.3. (Right) Application of a train of stimuli (S) causes tension to rise to a higher level than that developed during the twitch. Tension remains at this high level until the train of stimuli is interrupted or the muscle fatigues.

ACTIVE STATE

Because the series elasticity absorbs mechanical energy generated by the contractile proteins, the tension recorded at the ends of a muscle during a twitch does not accurately describe the interactions between the myosin cross-bridges and actin described in Chapter 8; thus, special experimental techniques are needed to analyze the mechanical behavior of the contractile element during a twitch. Suddenly imposed changes in muscle length, by overcoming the effects of the series elasticity, reveal the surprisingly rapid development of actin-myosin interactions after stimulation. The following discussion focuses on the behavior of skeletal muscle, which as already pointed out is relatively simple. As seen later, the results of similar studies in cardiac muscle are quite different from those in skeletal muscle.

Quick-Stretch Experiments

If the tension developed by the contractile elements fails to reach its maximum because energy is absorbed by extension of the series elasticity, one way to compensate for this damping effect would be to eliminate the elasticity early in the contraction. In practical terms this can be achieved if the muscle is suddenly stretched. By "pulling out" the series elasticity, "quick stretches" reveal the full potential for tension development by the contractile element even before tension becomes apparent at the ends of the muscle. Interpretation of quick-strength experiments simply assumes that a steady state is quickly reached between tension at three places in the stretched muscle: the tension at the ends of the muscle, the tension developed by the contractile element, and the tension that has stretched the series elasticity. Since the first of these, muscle tension, is easily determined, the latter two are readily quantified.

When a muscle is stretched immediately after stimulation, the tension that appears at the ends of the muscle depends on the length to which the muscle is stretched. The response to stretching a skeletal muscle to three different lengths is shown in Fig. 9.5. Following a short stretch, in which the tension applied to the series elasticity fails to reach the maximal tension developed by the contractile element, muscle tension keeps rising because of continued shortening by the contractile element (curve 1 in Fig. 9.5). On the other hand, if a quick stretch to a longer length causes muscle tension to exceed the maximum that can be developed by the contractile proteins, the muscle lengthens and tension falls until the latter reaches a level that can be maintained by the contractile element (curve 2 in Fig. 9.5). When an intermediate stretch brings muscle tension to a level equal to that developed by the contractile element, the muscle neither lengthens nor shortens; instead, tension remains at a relatively stable level during the initial period of the contraction (curve 3 in Fig. 9.5). This level of tension, which the muscle can hold without lengthening or shortening, represents the *active state*. Active-state intensity can thus be understood most simply as the tension developed by the undampened

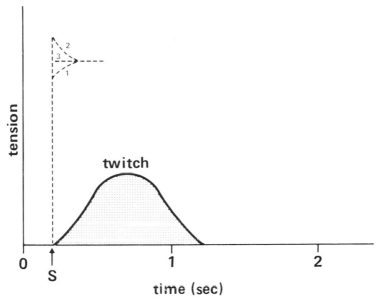

FIG. 9.5. Measurement of the active state by application of quick stretches to a skeletal muscle contracting under isometric conditions. *Solid line*: Twitch, as shown in Fig. 9.3. *Dashed lines*: 1: The muscle is quickly stretched a short distance immediately after stimulation. Tension continues to develop showly after the stretch as the tension at the end of the quick stretch is less than that produced by the contractile element. 2: The muscle is quickly stretched a long distance immediately after stimulation. Tension declines slowly after the stretch as the tension at the end of the quick stretch exceeds that developed by the contractile element. 3: The muscle is quickly stretched immediately after stimulation to a length where the tension maintains a plateau equal to that developed by the contractile element. This tension is the "active-state intensity."

contractile element, measured in experiments that eliminate the absorbtion of energy by the series elasticity. The finding that maximum active-state intensity appears shortly after stimulation is in accord with the finding that "initial" heat is produced mainly in the early stages of the mechanical response (Chapter 6).

The time course of active state development can be estimated by applying a series of quick stretches at different times during tension development (Fig. 9.6). These experiments show that the active state develops very rapidly in a skeletal muscle, reaches a maximum well before the time that twitch tension reaches its peak, and has declined significantly at the time of peak twitch tension.

The concept of active state explains why so much more tension is developed during a tetanus than during a twitch. As the maximum intensity of the active state measured by quick-stretch experiments at the start of a twitch is essentially the same as the tension developed during a tetanus (Fig. 9.7), the high level of tetanic tension reflects the true intensity of the active state. Tetanic stimulation, by preventing the active state from declining, brings the tension on the contractile element, the series elasticity, and the ends of the muscle to equilibrium.

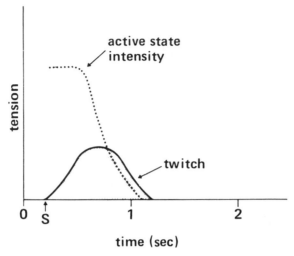

FIG. 9.6. Time course of active-state intensity in a skeletal muscle contracting under isometric conditions. The tension developed by the contractile element (active-state intensity) greatly exceeds that which appears at the ends of the muscle during an isometric twitch because in the twitch a significant amount of energy is absorbed by the series elasticity. This energy is returned as tension during the latter period of the twitch, when twitch tension exceeds the active-state intensity.

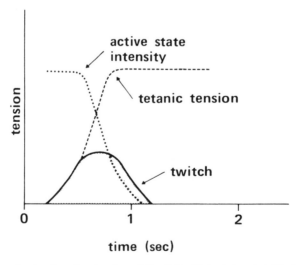

FIG. 9.7. Composite drawing showing the relationship of tetanic tension (*dashed line*; see also Fig. 9.5) and the active-state intensity (*dotted line*; see also Fig. 9.6). By maintaining the contractile element in a constant state of activity, the train of stimuli that produces the tetanic contraction allows the full intensity of the active state to appear at the ends of the muscle.

Quick-Release Experiments

We have already seen that the contractile state of a muscle, the ability of the muscle to lift a load and to shorten, reflects at least two properties of the contractile proteins (Chapter 8). One of these, the number of rigor bonds, is responsible for the ability of a muscle to generate tension. This manifestation of the active state is measured as tension in quick-stretch experiments that eliminate the damping effects of the series elasticity (see above). Quick stretches, however, do not provide information as to the maximal speed at which the contractile element is able to shorten. This second property of the contractile proteins, which is an index of the rate of cross-bridge turnover, can be evaluated in "quick-release" experiments where an isometrically contracting muscle is suddenly presented with a series of new, reduced loads.

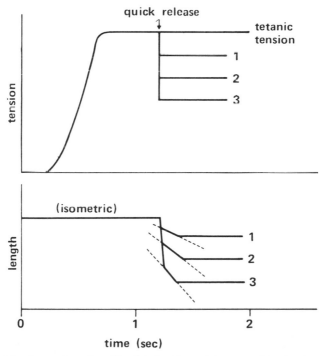

FIG. 9.8. Quick releases to reduced load during the maintenance of tension by a skeletal muscle contracting under isometric conditions. *Top*: The tension developed during a tetanic contraction (Fig. 9.4) abruptly falls when the muscle, during quick releases, is allowed to shorten against a slightly reduced load (1), against a moderately reduced load (2), or against a markedly reduced load (3). *Bottom*: The quick releases allow the muscle to shorten to the new lengths that are inversely proportional to the new load. The initial, rapid length changes are due to shortening of the series elasticity. Subsequently rates of shortening, to which tangents are drawn (*dashed lines*), represent shortening rates of the contractile element at the levels of tension shown in the top diagram. Shortening of the contractile element is more rapid when the quick release is to a shorter length, i.e., when the contractile element shortens at a lower tension.

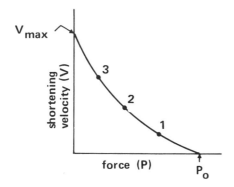

FIG. 9.9. Force-velocity curve constructed from the quick-release experiment shown in Fig. 9.8. The forces at points 1, 2, and 3 are the tensions achieved after the quick releases to different lengths (Fig. 9.8, top). Shortening velocities are the rates of the length change shown by the *dashed lines* in the bottom part of Fig. 9.8. This hyperbolic curve is similar to that shown in Fig. 6.15.

After a quick release, the abrupt fall in tension allows the muscle to shorten. The resulting length changes can be divided into two phases (Fig. 9.8). The first is a very rapid decrease in length that is due to shortening of the series elasticity. This is followed by a slower phase of shortening, the velocity of which is determined by the new load that the muscle encounters after the quick release (dashed lines are drawn tangentially to this second phase of shortening in Fig. 9.8). The second phase of shortening, which provides a measure of the rate of cross-bridge cycle (Chapter 8), becomes more rapid as quick releases are made to progressively lighter loads (1, 2, and 3 in Fig. 9.8, going from heaviest to lightest). When the relationship between this shortening velocity and the load against which the muscle shortens is plotted after a quick release, the familiar hyperbolic force-velocity curve is obtained (Fig. 9.9; see also Fig. 6.15). Thus quick-release experiments in a skeletal muscle provide a means to evaluate both the maximal number of active force-generating sites and the turnover of actin-myosin interactions. As we see later, however, the results of this experiment are very different in cardiac muscle.

LENGTH-TENSION RELATIONSHIP

The dependence of tetanic tension on muscle length, which is referred to as the *length-tension relationship* (Fig. 9.10), has been recognized since the middle of the 19th century. This relationship, shown in Fig. 9.10 for tetanic contractions of skeletal muscle, indicates that the intensity of the active state is maximal at intermediate muscle lengths (l_{max} or l_0), declining at muscle lengths that are both longer and shorter than l_{max}.

The rest length of most skeletal muscles, which is determined by the architecture of the bones and joints, is at or near the peak of their length-tension curves (l_{max}, Fig. 9.10). The heart, however, has no skeletal attachments to determine a rest length; as a result, chamber geometry is the major determinant of resting sarcomere length in its muscular walls. This has important consequences, among which is that the ventricles normally function at sarcomere lengths below l_{max} (see Chapter 16).

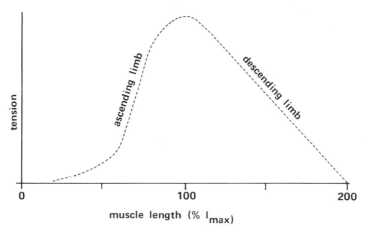

FIG. 9.10. Length-tension curve for a whole muscle, which defines the tension developed when the muscle contracts isometrically during tetanic contractions at different rest lengths. Muscle length is expressed as percent of $_{max}$, which is defined as that rest length at which developed tension is maximal. Curves of this sort are conventionally scanned from left to right; thus the ascending limb is to the *left*, where tension rises with increasing muscle length, and the descending limb is to the *right*, where tension declines with increasing muscle length.

Shortly after the sliding filament hypothesis of muscular contraction (Chapter 1) became widely accepted, attempts were made to explain the length-tension relationship in terms of changing positions of the thick and thin filaments. These explanations, referred to in this text as *ultrastructural mechanisms*, account for the decline of tension when skeletal muscle is stretched at high sarcomere lengths; as length-tension curves are customarily read from left to right, this is referred to as the *descending limb*. The rise in tension that occurs with stretch at shorter sarcomere lengths, the *ascending limb*, is not, however, adequately explained by the ultrastructural mechanism described below.

The classic ultrastructural mechanism of the length-tension curve of skeletal muscle, published in 1966 by Gordon, Huxley, and Julian, is described in the following pages. Although it explains only part of the length-tension curve, this mechanism provides a valuable starting point for understanding the more complex molecular basis of the length-tension curve in cardiac muscle.

Ultrastructural Mechanism

Initial studies of the length-tension relationship in skeletal muscle yielded rather broad curves (Fig. 9.10), due in part to inhomogeneities within the muscle and artifactual elasticities arising from damaged ends of the muscle that were attached to the recording devices. With the development of techniques that permitted the length-tension relationship of a small group of sarcomeres to be recorded, which avoided these problems, it became apparent that this relationship was due in part to length-dependent changes in the positions of the thick and thin filaments.

Length-tension curves for single sarcomeres, or small groups of sarcomeres, are narrower along the length axis than are the curves for the whole muscle (Fig. 9.11). This difference is due largely to inhomogeneities in sarcomere length in the whole muscle. At longer lengths in the whole muscle, not all sarcomeres are equally stretched, so that declining tension caused by lengthening of the longer sarcomeres is partly compensated for by the increased tension developed by the relatively shorter sarcomeres. A similar deviation between the sarcomere length-tension curve and that for the whole muscle is also seen at shorter lengths, where stretch lengthens some sarcomeres more than others.

To understand the ultrastructural mechanism for the sarcomere length-tension curve it is best to begin with the descending limb, at the right of the sarcomere length-tension curve, where developed tension is zero (A in Fig. 9.11). Examination of sarcomere structure at point A in Fig. 9.11, which in the frog semitendinous muscle corresponds to a sarcomere length of about 3.65 μm, shows no overlap between the thick filaments (length = 1.65 μm) and the two thin filaments (length = 2 × 1.0 μm) at this sarcomere length (Fig. 9.12). This absence of overlap does not allow any myosin cross-bridges to interact with actin, so that it is easy to understand why no tension is developed.

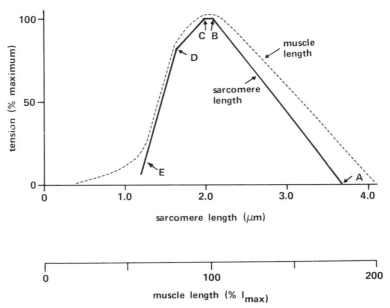

FIG. 9.11. Length-tension curve for a small group of sarcomeres in a frog semitendinous muscle (*solid line*) compared with that for the whole muscle shown in Fig. 9.10 (*dashed line*). Sarcomere length is shown as the upper abscissa. At a sarcomere length of 3.65 μm, no tension is developed (A). Tension becomes maximal as the sarcomere shortens to a length of approximately 2.2 μm (B). As the sarcomere length decreases below approximately 2.0 μm (C), tension begins to decline with further shortening. At lengths below approximately 1.65 μm (D), tension declines more rapidly with extreme sarcomere shortening (E).

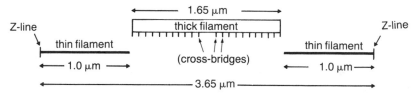

FIG. 9.12. Portion of a single sarcomere at a length of 3.65 μm (A in Fig. 9.11). At this sarcomere length there is no overlap between the thick filament (*above*) and the thin filaments (*below*), so that no interactions are possible between the myosin cross-bridges and actin.

As sarcomere length is reduced (Fig. 9.11, A→B), tension increases, reaching a maximum at a sarcomere length of approximately 2.2μm (B in Fig. 9.11). At this sarcomere length (l_{max}, see above) all of the myosin cross-bridges are adjacent to one of the thin filaments in the two halves of the sarcomere (Fig. 9.13). A small, ~0.20 μm, gap that remains between the ends of the thin filaments, corresponds to a "bare" area in the center of the thick filament that is devoid of cross-bridges (Fig. 7.4).

Reduction in sarcomere length from 2.2 μm to approximately 2.0 μm (Fig. 9.11, B→C) is associated with no change in active tension. This gives rise to a plateau in the sarcomere length-tension curve that is explained by the ultrastructural mechanism because the number of potential interactions between the cross-bridges and the thin filament neither increases nor decreases in this narrow part of the curve. This is because, as the thin filaments enter the bare area in the center of the sarcomere where the thick filament lacks cross-bridges, the peripheral portions of the thin filaments gain the same number of new interactions with cross-bridges at the ends of the thick filament as are lost in the center of the sarcomere (Fig. 9.14). As sarcomere shortening from 2.2 to 2.0 μm causes neither an increase nor a decrease in the number of potential interactions between thick and thin filaments, it does not alter tension.

Although it explains the descending limb and plateau of the length-tension relationship, the ultrastructural mechanism fails to account for the decline in tension that occurs as the sarcomere shortens to lengths below 1.9 to 2.0 μm (C→D in Fig. 9.11). The ascending limb of the length-tension relationship was initially attributed

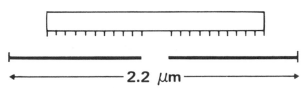

FIG. 9.13. Portion of a sarcomere at a length of 2.2 μm (B in Fig. 9.11). All myosin cross-bridges are adjacent to the thin filaments, so the number of potential interactions between the contractile proteins is maximal.

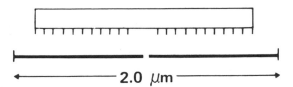

FIG. 9.14. Portion of a sarcomere at a length of 2.0 μm (C in Fig. 9.11). Compared to Fig. 9.13, there has been a loss of cross-bridge interactions with the tips of the thin filaments in the center of the sarcomere, but this has been matched by a corresponding gain at the ends of the thick filaments. Thus, all myosin cross-bridges remain able to interact with the thin filaments.

to "double overlap" of the thin filaments, seen at sarcomere lengths below l_{max}. At these short sarcomere lengths, where the thin filaments from opposite halves of the sarcomers have crossed into the domains of the "wrong" halves of the thick filament (Fig. 9.15), the polarity of the cross-bridges does not allow interactions with the thin filament.

The ultrastructural explanation for the steep decline in tension at very short sarcomere lengths, below ~1.65 μm (D→E in Fig. 9.11), is that the Z-lines collide with the thick filaments (Fig. 9.16). As the length of the thick filament is ~1.65 μm, extremely short sarcomere lengths can be reached only when the thick filament "crumples," causing "contraction bands" (Fig. 9.16). It is now apparent, however, that contraction bands in the heart are abnormal, appearing only after the contractile process has become so intense as to have "gone out of control." This occurs, for example, during reperfusion after prolonged ischemia when large amounts of calcium that enter the cytosol lead to a violent contraction that tears the muscle apart (Chapter 24). The contraction bands seen under these conditions are, in fact, markers of cell death.

A number of ultrastructural explanations have been proposed to explain the decline of developed tension as the sarcomere shortens just below the apex of the ascending limb of its length-tension curve. These include internal resistances caused by flexion of thin filaments where they encounter other thin filaments that had entered the "wrong half" of the sarcomere in the region of double overlap, separa-

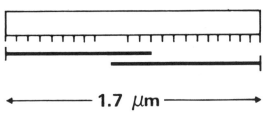

FIG. 9.15. Portion of a sarcomere at a length of 1.7 μm (segment C-D in Fig. 9.11). The central ends of the thin filaments have crossed in the middle of the sarcomere ("double overlap").

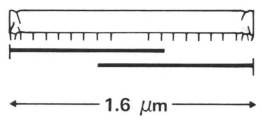

FIG. 9.16. Portion of a sarcomere at a length of 1.6 μm (segment D-E in Fig. 9.11). At this sarcomere length the Z-lines (*vertical lines* at the peripheral ends of the thin filaments) encroach on the ends of thick filaments. This causes the latter to "crumple," giving rise to contraction bands at the periphery of the A-band. These deformations contribute to the precipitous fall of tension as the sarcomere shortens further on this unphysiological portion of the sarcomere length-tension curve.

tion of thick and thin filaments that accompanies sarcomere shortening, and crumpling of the ends of the thick filaments at extremely short sarcomere lengths. However, it is now clear that internal resistances do not adequately explain the fall in tension at short sarcomere lengths. Instead, the ascending limb is due mainly to length-dependent changes in both the calcium sensitivity of the contractile proteins and calcium release from the sarcoplasmic reticulum. This dependence of the intensity of excitation-contraction coupling on sarcomere length is especially important in the heart, which normally functions only on the ascending limb of its length-tension relationship.

Length-Tension Relationship in Cardiac Muscle

As in skeletal muscle, the heart's sarcomeres operate at or near the apex of their length-tension curves. Cardiac contraction begins with the sarcomeres at or near a length where all of the myosin cross-bridges are able to interact with actin in the thin filaments (Fig. 9.17), so that as the myocardial cells shorten, the thin filaments enter the opposite halves of the sarcomere, causing double overlap (see Fig. 9.15). Variability in the lengths of the thin filaments (Robinson and Winegrad, 1979) may help them to pass each other when cardiac sarcomeres reach very short lengths.

Unlike skeletal muscle, the myocardium has a high internal resistance to stretch that accounts for a steep resting length-tension curve (see below). It is, in fact, very difficult, and perhaps impossible, to pull the heart's sarcomeres onto their descending limbs. Because extremely high wall tensions are needed to bring the heart's sarcomeres to their "descending limbs," the diastolic pressures needed to generate such high wall tensions would be encountered only in severe heart failure, and probably only in states of acute decompensation such as pulmonary edema (Chapter 25).

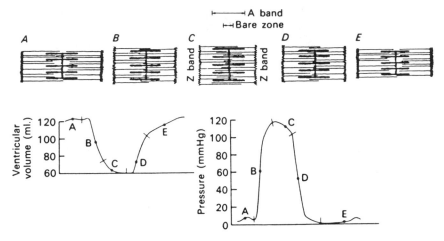

FIG. 9.17. Relationship between sarcomere length (A-E, *upper figures*) and changes in ventricular volume (*lower left*) and pressure (*lower right*) during the cardiac cycle. The positions of the thick and thin filaments shown in A-E are indicated by the corresponding letters on the volume and pressure curves. Shortening of the sarcomere (B, C, D) causes double overlap of the thin filaments that is especially marked in C. Note the variation in thin filament length in the upper figures. (Modified from Robinson and Winegrad, 1979.)

Length-Dependent Variations in Excitation-Contraction Coupling

It is now apparent that length-dependent changes in cardiac ultrastructure cannot explain the ascending limb of the heart's length-tension curve. Instead, this part of the length-tension curve reflects variations in excitation-contraction coupling that could result from length-dependent changes in one or more of three different mechanisms: the action potential that initiates calcium release from the sarcoplasmic reticulum, the opening of calcium-release channels in the sarcoplasmic reticulum, and the calcium sensitivity of the contractile proteins.

Length-Dependent Changes in the Action Potential

Changes in muscle length alter the geometry of the sarcolemma, for example by altering the folding of this membrane. However, in skeletal muscle neither the action potential nor intramembrane charge movement appears to depend on muscle length. Length changes do affect the cardiac action potential, but these effects are seen only when shortening is actually taking place. Rest length itself appears not to influence the cardiac action potential (Hennekes et al. 1981), and no direct influence of sarcomere length on calcium entry during cardiac excitation-contraction coupling has been shown.

Length-Dependent Changes in Calcium Release from the Sarcoplasmic Reticulum

When a "skinned" cardiac muscle fiber (from which the sarcolemma has been removed) is stretched, calcium release from the sarcoplasmic reticulum is increased (Fabiato and Fabiato, 1975). This effect appears to be due to changes in the amount of stored calcium that is released from this intracellular membrane system, rather than to length-dependent changes in its calcium content. Tight ultrastructural coupling between the sarcolemma and sarcoplasmic reticulum (Chapter 1) makes it unlikely that length-dependent changes in the relationship between the plasma membrane, which transmits the action potential, and the sarcoplasmic reticulum play a role in the ascending limb of the length-tension relationship. This response may, in some way, be related to the stretch sensitivity seen in some ion channels (Chapter 25).

Length-Dependent Changes in the Calcium Sensitivity of the Contractile Proteins

The ability of a given Ca^{2+} concentration to activate tension in skinned cardiac fibers is increased when the muscle is stretched (Fig. 9.18), indicating that the calcium sensitivity of the contractile proteins is length dependent (Hibberd and Jewell, 1982). The increased ability of a given amount of calcium released during excitation-contraction coupling to activate the cross-bridge cycle at longer sar-

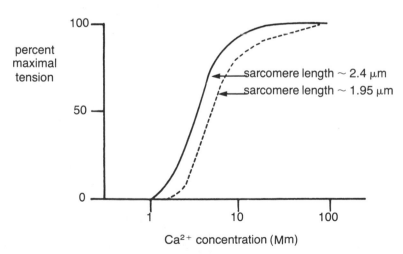

FIG. 9.18. Calcium dependence of tension developed by a cat papillary muscle at two sarcomere lengths. The Ca^{2+} concentration at which tension is half-maximal decreased from 4.90 to 3.02 μm when sarcomere length was increased from ~2.0 to ~2.4 μm. (Data from Hibberd and Jewell, 1982.)

comere lengths provides yet another example of an allosteric interaction among the contractile proteins (Chapter 8). In this case, an allosteric effect of changing sarcomere length ultimately influences the calcium affinity of troponin C. Although details regarding the molecular mechanisms by which changing sarcomere length alters the calcium sensitivity of the contractile proteins are not available, this probably represents the most important explanation for the ascending limbs of the length-tension relationship.

The existence of length-dependent variations in the calcium sensitivity of the contractile proteins has blurred the distinction between two types of regulation, once believed to arise from entirely different mechanisms. These are control by changing initial muscle length, and control by changing myocardial contractility; both can now be explained by variations in excitation-contraction coupling. We return to this subject in Chapter 16, when we examine the regulation of the intact heart.

CARDIAC MECHANICS

The advent of cardiac surgery in the years immediately following World War II, coupled with the recognition that prolonged hemodynamic overloading could irreversibly damage the myocardium (Chapter 25), led to a search for improved means to evaluate and characterize myocardial function. Such techniques, it was hoped, would allow cardiologists to select the optimal time for palliative procedures like valve replacement. It was thought that identification of the time when myocardial function began to deteriorate would allow cardiac surgeons to intervene before the development of irreversible myocardial damage, but not so early as to expose patients prematurely to the many complications caused by prosthetic valves.

It was quickly recognized that simple hemodynamic measurements, like cardiac output and atrial pressure, did not define the state of the myocardium. This was especially true in patients with damaged cardiac valves, where hemodynamic abnormalities were determined more by the valve abnormality than the contractile properties of the heart muscle (Chapter 17). Equally difficult was the challenge of distinguishing between changes in myocardial function caused by abnormalities in the intrinsic contractile properties of the myocardium (myocardial contractility), and those caused simply by changes in muscle length (length-tension relationship). Against this background a new field, *cardiac mechanics*, emerged in the early 1960s.

Cardiac mechanics initially offered promise for the quantification of the "true" length-independent contractile properties of the heart, called *myocardial contractility*, but it quickly became clear that difficulties in measuring the active state in cardiac muscle precluded the routine clinical application of this approach. However, by requiring cardiologists to redefine their view of the contractile behavior of the heart so as to include the biochemical and biophysical properties of the myocardium, cardiac mechanics had a major impact on cardiology (Katz, 1983).

In keeping with the general rule that all aspects of the contractile process are more complex in cardiac than in skeletal muscle, the relatively straightforward time-dependent and length-dependent features of skeletal muscle mechanics described in Chapter 6 are virtually impossible to discern in the heart. In skeletal muscle, it is possible to analyze contractions of muscles where the fibers parallel each other, and where the active state is extremely rapid in onset. More importantly, the ability to tetanize skeletal muscles allows force, velocity, heat, and length to be measured at reasonably constant levels of active state. In the heart, however, the active state is slow in onset and the muscle cannot ordinarily be tetanized. As a result, analyses of cardiac mechanics must chase a moving target, caused by changing time-dependent contractile properties. To make matters worse, the elasticity and spiral arrangement of the muscle fibers of the heart preclude the attainment of true isometric conditions, even when the ends of the muscle are fixed; thus, cardiac mechanics are also complicated by length-dependent changes in contractile conditions.

Quick Stretch in Cardiac Muscle

Fundamental differences between the mechanical properties of cardiac and skeletal muscle are clearly seen when the effects of a quick stretch are compared. Whereas sudden stretching of a skeletal muscle uncovers a steady state of tension that follows the rapid onset of active state in the contractile element (Fig. 9.5), no such plateau is seen after a quick stretch in cardiac muscle (Fig. 9.19). Instead, an

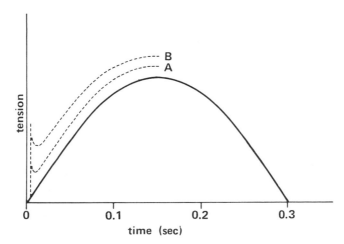

FIG. 9.19. Results of a quick-stretch experiment in cardiac muscle (compare with Fig. 9.5). *Solid line*, normal isometric contraction. *Dashed lines*, tension developed after quick stretches to two different lengths (B is stretched to a longer length than A). Even though the quick stretches cause the muscle initially to reach a length that causes total tension to exceed that developed by the contractile element—as evidenced by a transient fall in tension—total tension resumes its rise and no plateau of tension is seen.

early quick stretch that initially exceeds the ability of cardiac muscle to hold tension (as evidenced by the fall in tension immediately after the stretch) is not followed by a plateau of tension; instead, after a brief fall, tension rises slowly so as to follow a time course similar to the contraction in the unstretched muscle (A in Fig. 9.19). A quick stretch to a longer length is followed by an even greater initial drop in tension before the subsequent slow rise (B in Fig. 9.19). Furthermore, the slow phase of tension development in cardiac muscle after a quick stretch follows a time course that is virtually independent of the time at which stretch is applied, and the tension responses to two stretches to the same length that are applied at different times (A and B in Fig. 9.20) are virtually superimposable.

Even more striking is the finding that when cardiac muscle is stretched to a new length before stimulation (X in Fig. 9.20), the increased tension is the same as that seen after later quick stretches to the same length (A and B in Fig. 9.20). This means that the tension increase following a quick stretch (dotted lines in Figs. 9.19 and 9.20) is due mainly to the length-tension relationship!

These experiments show that unlike skeletal muscle, where quick stretches reveal an active state that develops rapidly and is sustained (Fig. 9.6), active state in cardiac muscle develops slowly. The slow increase in tension following a quick stretch in cardiac muscle (Figs. 9.19 and 9.20) thus reflects continuing development of the active state. The slow onset of the active state explains the finding that heat liberation at the start of contraction in cardiac muscle is slower than in skeletal muscle.

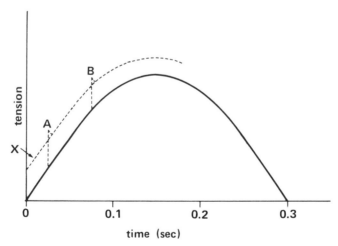

FIG. 9.20. Results of a quick-stretch experiment in cardiac muscle where a quick stretch is applied at two times after stimulation (A and B). Although the tension developed in each stretch initially exceeds that developed by the contractile element—as evidenced by a transient fall in tension—total tension resumes its rise so that both curves become superimposed by the time tension reaches its peak. This increment in tension is the same when the muscle is stretched to the same increased length prior to stimulation (X).

EFFECTS OF CHANGING MUSCLE LENGTH ON ACTIVE STATE

Length changes imposed during contraction have complex effects on the subsequent behavior of the cardiac contractile proteins (Brutsaert and Sys, 1989). As shown in Fig. 9.21, a quick stretch applied early during tension development, in addition to increasing tension (see above), prolongs the active state (Fig. 9.21A). However, when the stretch is applied later, contraction is shortened (Fig. 9.21B). The ability of the late stretch to "destroy" the active state can be explained if the change in muscle length breaks rigor bonds linking actin and myosin at a time, late in the cross-bridge cycle, when new bonds are no longer being formed. The opposite effect of the early stretch to prolong tension implies that rigor bonds are still being formed during the initial phase of the contraction.

Shortening of active heart muscle also modifies subsequent contractile protein interactions. As shown in Fig. 9.21C and D, prevention of subsequent tension development when the muscle is allowed to shorten in an afterloaded contraction abbreviates the active state; and similar effects are caused by quick release. The earlier the myocardium is allowed to shorten, the greater is the abbreviation of systole (compare Fig. 9.21C and D); as a result, an isotonic contraction is much briefer than an isometric contraction.

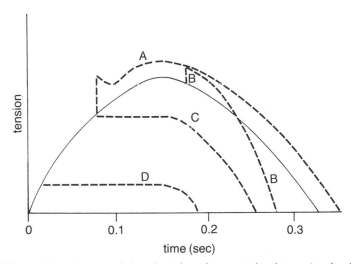

FIG. 9.21. Effects of changing muscle length on the subsequent development and maintenance of tension. When an isometrically contracting muscle (*solid line*) is stretched early during systole, tension is increased and systole is prolonged (A); a similar stretch applied later during systole also increases tension but abbreviates the subsequent maintenance of tension (B). When the muscle is unloaded by allowing it to shorten against loads that are less than maximal isometric tension (C, D; length changes are not shown), the duration of the contraction is abbreviated. Unlike the situation following stretch, the earlier the muscle is allowed to shorten, the greater the abbreviation of systole.

These effects of changing muscle length on the subsequent interactions between the cardiac contractile proteins are, in some ways, reminiscent of the important effects of tension that give rise to the Fenn effect. Both demonstrate that muscle loading influences its chemistry. For this reason, changes in both length and tension can be viewed as additional participants in the cooperative interactions between actin, myosin, tropomyosin, and the troponin complex that control the mechanical behavior of the heart (see Chapter 8). Although the importance of changing sarcomere length in the physiology of the intact heart is not clear, hemodynamic alterations such as a sudden reduction in afterload and even ejection per se may have important effects on contraction, and especially relaxation.

DIASTOLIC PROPERTIES OF THE MYOCARDIUM

The high level of resting tension and low diastolic compliance of cardiac muscle represent additional important features that distinguish the heart from skeletal muscle. Unlike skeletal muscle, in which resting tension is practically zero at muscle lengths below l_{max}, cardiac muscle has a high resting tension at all lengths along its resting length-tension curve (Fig. 9.22). Although the relationships between sar-

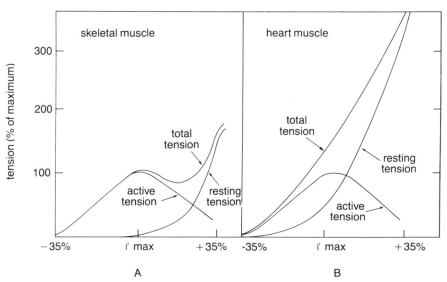

FIG. 9.22. Comparison of total and active length-tension curves in skeletal (A) and cardiac (B) muscle allowed to contract under isometric conditions. Active tension, which is the tension developed during contraction, equals total tension after stimulation minus the tension recorded in the resting muscle prior to stimulation. Although the active length-tension curves are similar for the two muscle types, the resting tension in cardiac muscle is much higher and, unlike skeletal muscle, is significant at lengths below $_{max}$. (Modified from Jewell, *The Physiological Basis of Starling's Law of the Heart*, 1974, Ciba Foundation Syposium, 24, Elsevier, Amsterdam.)

comere length and active tension are similar in cardiac and skeletal muscle, the curve relating muscle length to active tension in the myocardium is superimposed on high levels of resting tension. Stated another way, owing to the fact that it has a much lower resting compliance than skeletal muscle, the heart has a very steep resting length-tension curve.

A number of terms are used to describe the passive properties of the myocardium (Mirsky and Parmley, 1973). These include:

Stress: Force per unit of cross-sectional area, e.g., dynes/cm^2.

Strain: A fractional, or percent, change in dimension caused by the application of stress.

Compliance or *distensibility*: The change in volume that accompanies a change in pressure: dV/dP, or $(dP/dV) - 1$.

Specific compliance: The change in volume per unit of total volume (dV/V) that accompanies a change in pressure: dV/VdP.

Elastic stiffness (or tangent modulus): The slope of a stress-strain curve; that is the amount of stress needed to cause a given strain. In nonphysical terms this can be viewed simply as *stiffness*, the tendency of the myocardium to resist stretching (a strain) in response to an increase in tension (a stress).

Elasticity: The property of a material to return from a stressed state to an original conformation when the stresses are removed.

The exact cause of the high diastolic stiffness of cardiac muscle is still not clearly understood, but probably arises from more than one feature of the myocardium. Some of the high resistance to stretch can be attributed to the extracellular matrix, notably collagen, that lies outside the myocardial cells (Weber, 1989). The cytoskeleton within the cells (Chapter 7) also appears to contribute to the high diastolic stiffness of the myocardium; and as noted in Chapter 7, residual interactions between the thick and thin filaments, even in resting muscle, may contribute to resting tension. A dynamic mechanism for the low compliance of the myocardium is suggested by the finding of spontaneous oscillations in sarcomere length in unstimulated myocardial cells. These oscillations, which can generate significant levels of diastolic tension, are due to cyclical interactions between the thick and thin filaments initiated by cyclic release and reuptake of calcium by the sarcoplasmic reticulum (Lakatta et al., 1985).

The high resting stiffness of the myocardium is of considerable functional significance because the heart determines its own leverage, and because of the energetic disadvantage in a ventricle that ejects from high diastolic volumes (The Law of Laplace, Chapter 15). It is also essential that the heart respond to an increase in filling by improving its ability to eject (Chapter 13), so that the ventricles must function on the ascending limb of their length-tension curves. The low compliance of the myocardium, by making it difficult to pull the normal myocardial cell onto the descending limb of its sarcomere length-tension curve, thus plays an essential role in the physiology of the heart.

REFERENCES

Brutsaert DL, Sys SU. (1989). Relaxation and diastole of the heart. *Physiol Rev* 69:1228–1315.

Fabiato A, Fabiato F. (1975). Dependence of the contractile activation of skinned cardiac cells on the sarcomere length *Nature* 256:54–56.

Gordon AM, Huxley AF, Julian FG. (1966). The variation in isometric tension with sarcomere length in vertebrate muscle fibers. *J Physiol (Lond)* 184:170–192.

Hennekes R, Kaufmann R, Lab M. (1981). The dependence of cardiac membrane excitation and contractile ability on active muscle shortening (cat papillary muscle). *Pflugers Arch* 392:22–28.

Hibberd MG, Jewell BR. (1982). Calcium- and length-dependent force production in rat ventricular muscle. *J Physiol (Lond)* 329:527–540.

Katz AM. (1983). Regulation of myocardial contractility 1958–1983. An odyssey. *J Am Coll Cardiol* 1:42–51.

Lakatta EG, Capogrossi MC, Kort AA, Stern MD. (1985). Spontaneous myocardial Ca oscillations: an overview with emphasis on ryanodine and caffeine. *Fed Proc* 44:2977–2983.

Mirsky I, Parmley WW. (1973). Assessment of passive elastic stiffness for isolated heart muscle and the intact heart. *Circ Res* 33:233–243.

Robinson T, Winegrad S. (1979). The measurement and dynamic implications of thin filament lengths in heart muscle. *J Physiol (Lond)* 286:607–619.

Weber KT. (1989). Cardiac interstitium in health and disease: the fibrillar collagen network. *J Am Coll Cardiol* 13:1637–1652.

BIBLIOGRAPHY

Allen DG, Kentish JC. (1985). The cellular basis for the length-tension relation in cardiac muscle. *J Mol Cell Cardiol* 17:821–840.

Brady AJ. (1965). Time and displacement dependence of cardiac contractility: problems in defining the active state and force velocity relations. *Fed Proc* 24:1410–1420.

Davson H. (1964). *A textbook of general physiology*, Chap. XXI. Boston: Little, Brown.

Katz AM, Smith VE, Weisfeldt ML. (1986). Relaxation and diastolic properties of the heart. In: Fozzard H, Haber E, Katz A, Jennings R, Morgan HE, eds. *The heart and cardiovascular system*. New York: Raven Press; 803–818.

Lakatta EG. (1987). Starling's law of the heart is explained by intimate interaction of muscle length and myofilament calcium activation. *J Am Coll Cardiol* 10:1157–1164.

Sonnenblick EH. (1965). Determinants of active state in heart muscle: force, velocity, instantaneous muscle length, time. *Fed Proc* 24:1396–1409.

Stephenson DG, Wendt IR. (1984). Length dependence of changes in sarcomere calcium concentration and myofibrillar calcium sensitivity in striated muscle fibres. *J Muscle Res Cell Motil* 5:243–272.

10

Excitation–Contraction Coupling

Calcium and Other Ion Fluxes Across the Plasma Membrane

It is quite . . . impossible to explain the rapid development of full activity in a [skeletal muscle] twitch by assuming that it is set up by the arrival at any point of some substance diffusing from the surface [of the muscle]: diffusion is far too slow. Either we must suppose that excitation . . . is produced by excitation (natural or artificial) throughout the interior, not merely at the surface; or we must look for some physical or physicochemical process which is released by excitation at the surface and then propagated inwards. (A. V. Hill, 1949)

The pumping action of the heart, like contraction in skeletal muscle, is initiated by a complex system that rapidly delivers a highly regulated signal to the contractile proteins. The sequence of steps that ends when calcium binds to troponin C is referred to as "excitation-contraction coupling." The complexity of this system was anticipated by Hill (1949), who noted that simple diffusion was not sufficiently rapid to account for the abrupt onset of the active state in frog sartorius muscle (Chapter 9).

By definition, excitation-contraction coupling encompasses the sequence of steps that begins when an action potential depolarizes the plasma membrane, and ends with the binding of calcium to troponin C, the calcium receptor of the cardiac contractile proteins (Chapter 7). In recent years, the concept of excitation-contraction coupling has come to include the processes that cause the heart to relax. Key structures and their function in excitation-contraction coupling are summarized in Table 10.1, and their ultrastructural relationships in the myocardial cell are shown in Figure 10.1.

The complex reactions of excitation-contraction coupling described in this chapter may appear, at first sight, to represent an overly elaborate means for delivering calcium to troponin. This complexity can be especially puzzling when it is remembered that the calcium fluxes that activate the heart involve passive, downhill move-

TABLE 10.1. *Structure-function relationships in excitation-contraction coupling*

Structure	Function in activation	Function in relaxation
Plasma membrane		
Sarcolemma		
Na channel	Propagation of action potential	
Ca channel	Propagation of action potential, calcium entry	
Ca pump		Calcium removal
Na/Ca exchange	Calcium entry	Calcium removal
Na pump		Calcium removal (indirect)
Transverse tubule[a]		
Na channel	Propagation of action potential	
Ca channel	Propagation of action potential, calcium entry	
Sarcoplasmic reticulum		
Subsarcolemmal cisternae		
Ca channel	Calcium release	
Sarcotubular network		
Ca pump		Calcium removal, filling of intracellular calcium stores
Myofilaments		
Troponin C	Calcium receptor	
Other proteins	Allosteric regulation	Allosteric regulation

[a]The t-tubules may also participate in other plasma membrane functions.

ments of this ion through membrane channels. This follows because the level of ionized calcium in the extracellular fluid is about 1 mM, whereas the Ca^{2+} concentration needed to saturate troponin is about 100-fold less ($<10\mu m$), both being considerably higher than the Ca^{2+} concentration in the cytosol of the resting heart, is ~ 0.2 μM.

In view of the large Ca^{2+} concentration gradient across the plasma membrane, it is reasonable to ask why it is necessary to have a complex system for calcium delivery that relies on a specialized intracellular membrane system, the sarcoplasmic reticulum, to store activator calcium within the cell. The answers to these questions lie primarily in the inability of diffusion, the simplest mechanism by which calcium entering the cell would ultimately reach the contractile proteins, to provide for a sufficiently rapid delivery of calcium to troponin C. Although diffusion is a very fast process that can effect rapid movements of solute over short distances, this passive process is of limited value in large structures. As noted by Hill (1949), its limitations are apparent in mammalian skeletal muscle, where the large fiber size and rapidity of active-state development do not allow diffusion of extracellular calcium to explain the rapid onset of contraction.

The abrupt onset of the active state in large, rapidly contracting skeletal muscles (Chapter 9) is now known to depend not on calcium entry from the extracellular space, but on the release of calcium stored within the cell. Utilization of an intracellular store allows activator calcium to reach its binding sites on troponin C by a much shortened diffusion path in skeletal muscle. In the heart, where cells are

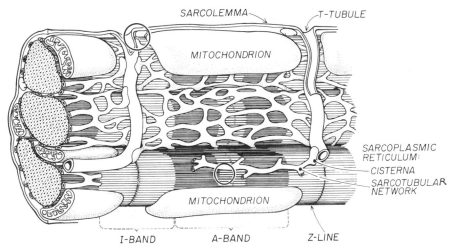

FIG. 10.1. Ultrastructure of the working myocardial cell. Contractile proteins are arranged in a regular array of thick and thin filaments (see in cross section at the *left*). The A-band represents the region of the sarcomere occupied by the thick filaments into which thin filaments extend from either side. The I-band is the region of the sarcomere occupied only by thin filaments; these extend toward the center of the sarcomere from the Z-lines, which bisect each I-band. The sarcoplasmic reticulum, a membrane network that surrounds the contractile proteins, consists of the sarcotubular network at the center of the sarcomere and the cisternae, which abut the t-tubules and the sarcolemma. The transverse tubular system (t-tubule) is lined by a membrane that extends from the sarcolemma and carries the extracellular space into the myocardial cell. Mitochondria are shown in the central sarcomere and in cross section at the *left* side of the figure. (From Katz, *N Engl J Med*, 1975; 293:1184.)

smaller and the onset of contraction slower, the requirement for an internal store of activator calcium is less absolute. Although adult mammalian cardiac muscle cells generally contain an extensive sarcoplasmic reticulum, this membrane system is less well developed than that in skeletal muscles; in the smaller cells of fetal hearts, this internal membrane system is sparse, and may be absent. The slowly contracting cells of the hearts of some amphibians also lack an internal sarcoplasmic reticulum, so that the calcium that enters the myocardium from the extracellular fluid in these hearts participates directly in activating the contractile proteins. In the majority of adult mammalian hearts, including that of humans, most of the activator calcium is derived from internal stores in the sarcoplasmic reticulum.

The complexity of the systems that control excitation-contraction coupling makes possible a remarkably complex control of the heart's contractile performance. The interlocking systems of calcium pumps and calcium channels that control cardiac excitation-contraction coupling allow the heart to adjust its mechanical behavior in response to a variety of physiological and pharmacological stimuli. The resulting "fine-tuning" of cardiac performance, which is detailed in later chapters, is now understood in terms of changes in the many systems that participate in the delivery and subsequent removal of the activator calcium that enters the cytosol for binding to troponin C.

THE PLASMA MEMBRANE

The heart's plasma membrane contains several structurally distinct regions. In this chapter, the term *sarcolemma* refers to unspecialized regions of the plasma membrane that separate the cell interior from the extracellular space. There are, however, at least two specialized regions of the plasma membrane. The first is the *intercalated disc* (Chapter 1), which provides both mechanical linkages between adjacent cells and nonselective channels that allow electrical current and small molecules to flow from one cell to another. The second specialized regions of the plasma membrane, the *t-tubules*, play a special role in excitation-contraction coupling that is described later in this chapter.

EXCITATION-CONTRACTION COUPLING

The processes that signal the heart to contract (excitation-contraction coupling) begin when an action potential depolarizes the plasma membrane surrounding the myocardial cell. This electrical signal is generated by the passage of ions through channels in the plasma membrane that change the electrical potential of the interior of the cardiac cell relative to the extracellular space. These ion fluxes include two major inward currents that depolarize the heart (Chapter 19). (As an inward current, by definition, carries positive charge into the electronegative interior of the resting cell, inward currents reduce the resting potential.) The initial inward current is carried by sodium ions, which enter the cell through sodium-specific channels that open and close very quickly. Membrane depolarization caused by the fast inward sodium current initiates a second inward current; the latter, which is carried by calcium ions, begins later and follows a more prolonged course than the sodium current, and so is called the slow inward current or i_{si}. In addition to carrying positively charged calcium ions into the cytosol, the slow inward current delivers activator calcium to the interior of the cell. Although some of this calcium binds to troponin C in the adult mammalian heart, most is retained in the sarcoplasmic reticulum for release in subsequent contractions. A key function of the small amount of calcium that enters myocardial cells by way of the slow inward current is to "trigger" the release of a much larger amount of calcium from stores in the sarcoplasmic reticulum (Chapter 11).

Ion Currents Responsible for the Cardiac Action Potential

The ion currents that cause the cells of the heart to depolarize and repolarize during each cardiac cycle are described briefly at this point; for additional details, see Chapters 18 and 19. During diastole the plasma membrane is highly permeable to potassium but both sodium and calcium channels are closed. As a result, the normal resting electronegativity of the cell interior is determined largely by the potassium gradient across the plasma membrane. In the working cells of the atria and ventricles, and in the His-Purkinje system, excitation begins when an inward sodium current depolarizes the cell; this sodium current has a rapid onset and brief duration, and so is called the fast inward current. Neutralization of the resting electronegativity of the cell interior by entry of positively charged sodium ions causes the opening of voltage-gated calcium channels and the closing of potassium channels. The action potential ends, and the cell interior returns to its normal resting electronegativity, when the sodium and calcium channels close and the potassium channels reopen, allowing potassium ions to carry positive charge back out of the cell during the repolarization phase of the action potential.

Three general principles govern the ion fluxes that are responsible for the action potential. The first is that all of the ions move downhill; that is, the ion fluxes are "passive" and depend on diffusion. Second, because the ions move through selective channels, they are not accompanied by counter-ions that would neutralize the charge that they carry across the plasma membrane. Finally, when the action potential has ended and the cell has returned to its resting state, small amounts of the ions that have moved across the plasma membrane must be returned to their original locations. These "restorative processes" require that the ions be moved uphill, and are effected by a variety of ion pumps and ion exchangers that, in different ways, require the expenditure of energy.

Calcium Influx Across the Plasma Membrane: The Slow Inward Current

The opening of the calcium channels allows this ion to diffuse rapidly into the cell. The driving force for calcium entry is the large electrochemical gradient across the plasma membrane, which as noted above is created by both the electronegativity of the cell interior in the resting heart, and the large, $\sim 10,000$-fold, Ca^{2+} concentration gradient across the plasma membrane (Chapter 19).

> Even though diffusion is too slow to account for the rapid onset of the active state in large skeletal muscle cells, the reader should not assume that the diffusion of a single ion through a membrane channel is a slow process. Because the membrane bilayer is a very thin structure (Chapter 2), calcium entry is, in a manner of speaking, like the sea rushing through a broken dike. This analogy should help to understand Hill's concern, for even when the seas pour through a breach in a dike on the coast of Holland, it takes some time before Amsterdam is flooded.

The slow inward current serves a number of functions; in fact, the calcium that enters the cells during the action potential plays at least five key roles (Table 10.2). The first is simply to carry positive charge into the cell, which allows calcium entry to contribute to the electrical signal responsible for depolarization. In the working cells of the atria and ventricles, and in the His-Purkinje system, the calcium current turns off slowly, and so maintains a depolarized state that gives rise to the plateau of the cardiac action potential. In the cells of the atrioventricular node, which lack funtioning sodium channels, the calcium current is responsible for impulse propagation and conduction; in the sinoatrial node, where a sodium current is also absent,

TABLE 10.2. *Functions of calcium entry during the cardiac action potential*

Carries positive charge into the cell	Depolarization
Working cells (atria and ventricles)	Action potential plateau
His-Purkinje system	Action potential plateau
Sinoatrial node	Conduction, pacemaker activity
Atrioventricular node	Conduction
Activates potassium channels	Initiates repolarization
Provides calcium for binding to troponin C	Activates contraction
Provides calcium for storage in the sarcoplasmic reticulum	Excitation-contraction coupling
Signals calcium release from the sarcoplasmic reticulum	Calcium-triggered calcium release

calcium entry plays an important role in pacemaker activity (Chapter 19). The calcium that enters the cell by way of the slow inward current also signals the opening of potassium channels which, by allowing the outward movement of positively charged potassium ions, restores the resting electronegativity within the cardiac cell. The slow inward current provides activator calcium for binding to troponin C, but in most cells of the adult mammalian heart, the amount of calcium entering the cytosol in this manner is quite small and makes only a minor contribution to the direct activation of the contractile process (Fabiato, 1983). An important fraction of this calcium is taken up by the sarcoplasmic reticulum, where it contributes to the filling of internal stores for release in subsequent contractions. Finally, but by no means least important, is the role of calcium entry to trigger the release of a much larger amount of calcium from the internal stores in the sarcoplasmic reticulum (Chapter 11).

The structure and regulation of cardiac calcium channels are discussed in more detail in Chapter 18, where we examine the many different members of a growing family of membrane channel proteins.

CALCIUM EFFLUX ACROSS THE PLASMA MEMBRANE

Calcium entry during each cardiac action potential obviously requires that some mechanism exist to transport this calcium back out of the cell during diastole. As noted above, calcium moves into the cell down a steep electrochemical gradient, so that calcium efflux must take place against both a concentration and an electrical gradient; thus, calcium efflux from the myocardium requires the expenditure of energy. The heart actively extrudes calcium by two quite different mechanisms. One of these is an adenosine triphosphate (ATP)-dependent calcium pump that utilizes the energy derived from ATP hydrolysis to perform the chemiosmotic work involved in uphill calcium transport. This adenosine triphosphatase (ATPase) has a low capacity but high affinity for calcium transport. The other mechanism, a sodium/calcium exchanger, uses the energy of the sodium gradient across the plasma membrane to move calcium uphill, out of the cell. This exchanger has a greater capacity than the ATP-dependent calcium pump to move calcium out of the cell, but a somewhat lower affinity for this ion.

ATP-dependent calcium pumps are probably the only mechanism for calcium efflux in nonexcitable cells, such as the erythrocyte, in which an influx of activator calcium does not tax this low capacity, high-affinity transport system. In excitable cells, where large amounts of calcium enter the cell to play a major role in signaling, and especially in the heart where this signal continues without pause, calcium entry could overwhelm the limited capacity for calcium pumping. For this reason, the need for a second, high-capacity calcium efflux system is readily understood. In the heart, as in other excitable mammalian cells, this second system is the sodium/calcium exchange.

ATP-DEPENDENT CATION PUMPS

Three important cation pumps are described in this and the following chapters. These are the calcium pump ATPases of the plasma membrane and sarcoplasmic reticulum, and the sodium pump ATPase, which have similar molecular mechanisms and considerable structural homology. Recent structural information indicates that a variety of cation transporters that play a central role in cardiac regulation arose from a primitive protein that appeared 3 to 4 billion years ago; like the calcium-binding proteins described in Chapter 7, this family of proteins has diverged widely (Table 10.3). We have, in fact, already encountered several members of this family of ion pump ATPase proteins. One is the F_1 ATPase of the mitochondrial inner membrane which, as described in Chapter 5, normally runs in "reverse" so as to use the energy stored in the proton gradient created by oxidative phosphorylation to form high-energy phosphate bonds in ATP. The mitochondrial ATP-ADP exchanger is also a member of this family, and sequences in both actin and phosphofructokinase indicate that these too are derived from the same primitive ancestor. In some cases, primitive proteins appear to have split, giving rise to distinct proteins that can be shown to have been derived from subunits of parental pump proteins. This diversity reflects the processes of gene duplication, gene drift, and fusion and alternate splicing of these genes, which contain many *introns*. We meet several other members of this extended family later in this chapter and in Chapter 11.

TABLE 10.3. *The family of cation pump proteins*

Protein	Function	Appearance or divergence (million years)
Primitive ancestor		4,000–3,000
F_1ATPase	Oxidative phosphorylation	3,000–2,000
Actin	Motion	3,000–2,000
ATP-ADP exchanger	Nucleotide transport	3,000–2,000
Phosphofructokinase	Carbohydrate metabolism	3,000–2,000
Ca pump	Calcium transport	1,000
H,K pump	Acid secretion	500
α-subunit of the Na pump	Sodium and potassium transport	300

Modified from Jørgensen and Andersen (1988). Not listed are potassium and proton pumps found in prokaryocytes, which diverged 2,500 to 4,000 million years ago.

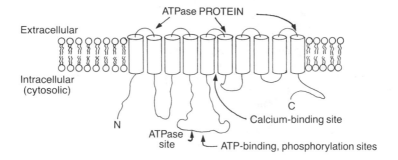

PLASMA MEMBRANE CALCIUM PUMP

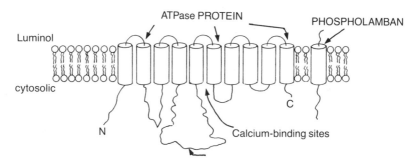

SARCOPLASMIC RETICULUM CALCIUM PUMP

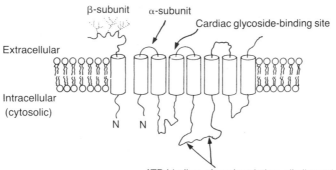

PLASMA MEMBRANE SODIUM PUMP

FIG. 10.2. Models of three membrane cation pump ATPase proteins. Membrane-spanning helical loops are shown as cylinders. Both the plasma membrane and sarcoplasmic reticulum calcium pumps are believed to consist of a single protein containing ten membrane-spanning regions (shown as cylinders). The ATP-binding, calcium-binding, and phosphoenzyme sites all face the cytosolic surface of the membrane. A small portion of the C-terminal region of the peptide chain plays a key regulatory role. In the plasmalemmal calcium pump, this segment is attached to the ATPase protein, whereas in the sarcoplasmic reticulum calcium pump this peptide has split off to become a separate protein called phospholamban. The sodium pump ATPase contains two subunits: a larger α-subunit that contains the ATP-binding, calcium-binding, and phosphoenzyme sites on the cytosolic surface, and a cardiac glycoside-binding site on the extracellular surface. The active pumps are dimers of the structures depicted in this figure, and phospholamban is a pentamer.

The calcium pump ATPases of the plasma membrane and sarcoplasmic reticulum, and the sodium pump ATPase are intrinsic membrane proteins having molecular weights somewhat in excess of 100,000 daltons; each contains several putative transmembrane segments with ATP-binding, phosphorylation, and cation-binding sites with the cytosol (Fig. 10.2). In each case, the functional ion pump appears to be a dimeric structure.

Plasmalemmal Calcium Pump

Calcium efflux from myocardial cells is effected in part by an ATP-dependent calcium pump that is, in many ways, similar to the calcium pump of the sarcoplasmic reticulum described in Chapter 11. However, the plasmalemmal calcium pump is a larger molecule than that of the sarcoplasmic reticulum (Caroni et al., 1983), and is regulated differently. Whereas the calcium pump of the sarcoplasmic reticulum is stimulated by a phosphorylation reaction catalyzed by protein kinase A, the plasmalemmal calcium pump is regulated by the calcium-calmodulin complex, not through a phosphorylation reaction, but instead by the direct binding of the complex to the protein (see below). Because this calcium-dependent regulation allows elevated intracellular Ca^{2+} concentration to increase both the calcium sensitivity and maximal velocity of the pump, it provides a negative feedback by which calcium entry stimulates calcium efflux. In contrast to the sarcoplasmic reticulum, the plasmalemmal calcium pump is not stimulated by cyclic AMP.

The complete amino acid sequence of the plasmalemmal calcium pump, which has been determined in several tissues, indicates that it is a member of the P-class of transport proteins that form an acyl-phosphate intermediate during the transport reaction (see below). Hydropathy plots based on these structural data indicate that the plasmalemmal calcium pump contains ten membrane-spanning domains (Fig. 10.2), with both the N-terminal and C-terminal ends in the cytosol. The latter arrangement is important because the C-terminal region, which contains the site that binds the calcium-calmodulin complex, must lie inside the cell.

The role of the C-terminal calmodulin-binding domain of the plasmalemmal calcium pump offers a fascinating insight into the manner in which nature has conserved structural information for specialized use in different systems. It is now clear that this C-terminal domain interacts with the ATPase and calcium-binding sites of the protein so as to inhibit calcium transport, and that this inhibition is attenuated when this part of the molecule is bound to the calcium-calmodulin complex (Fig. 10.3). What is so fascinating is that the inhibitory domain of the plasmalemmal calcium pump is homologous to *phospholamban*, a regulatory protein that inhibits another calcium pump: that of the sarcoplasmic reticulum (Chapter 11). In phospholamban this inhibitory domain is a separate protein, whereas in the plasmalemmal calcium pump it is an integral part of a larger molecule (Chiesi et al., 1990). Yet both play comparable roles in regulation; the inhibitory effect of phospholamban is reversed when it is phosphorylated by protein kinase A, whereas that of the cal-

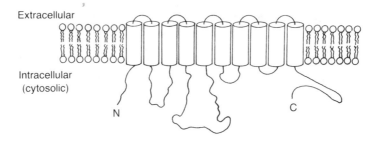

BASAL STATE

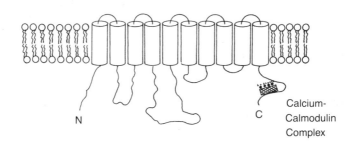

CALCIUM ACTIVATED STATE

FIG. 10.3. Regulation of the plasmalemmal calcium pump by the calcium-calmodulin complex. In the basal state (*top*), the conformation of the C-terminal region slows the pump and reduces its calcium sensitivity. Binding of calcium and calmodulin to this segment of the molecule (*bottom*) attenuates this inhibitory effect and so stimulates calcium efflux.

modulin-binding domain of the plasmalemmal calcium pump is reversed when cytosolic Ca^{2+} concentration rises. It is therefore apparent that the same region of the ancestral calcium pump has been adapted differently to mediate two different signals: in the plasmalemmal protein, this domain remains attached to the ion pump and responds to a calcium signal; in the sarcoplasmic reticulum is has become a separate protein that mediates a signal initiated by cyclic AMP.

Sodium/Calcium Exchange

More than 25 years ago it was observed that the properties expected of an ATP-dependent plasmalemmal calcium pump could not account for several properties of calcium transport out of the myocardial cell. For example, the Q_{10} (i.e., the change in reaction velocity for a 10°C change in temperature) of calcium efflux in the intact cell is only approximately 1.35, a value much lower than that expected from an ATP-dependent ion pump. More surprising, metabolic inhibitors like cyanide and

2,4-dinitrophenol increase, rather than inhibit, calcium efflux from the heart. These properties indicate that systems other than an ATP-dependent calcium pump must play an important role in the uphill movement of calcium out of myocardial cells.

An important role for sodium in regulating the tension developed by the heart has been recognized since the 1920s, when it was found that reducing extracellular Na^+ concentration, like elevation of extracellular Ca^+, increases the force of cardiac contraction. The subsequent finding of a direct relationship between the ratio $[Ca^{2+}]_o/[Na^+]_o$ and myocardial contractility led to the hypothesis that an ion exchanger in the plasma membrane determined intracellular calcium content. This exchanger was postulated to carry either sodium or calcium in both directions across the plasma membrane, the relative amounts of either ion carried being determined by their relative concentrations on either side of the membrane. In other words, sodium and calcium *compete* for a transport site on this exchanger.

> The ability of metabolic inhibitors to increase the rate of calcium efflux is readily explained by sodium/calcium exchange. In metabolically poisoned cells, intracellular calcium rises because the ATP-dependent calcium pump of the sarcoplasmic reticulum is slowed. The resulting increased Ca^{2+} concentration at the inner surface of the plasma membrane makes more of this ion available to leave the poisoned cell in exchange for sodium.

Direct evidence for an exchanger that exchanged intracellular calcium for either extracellular sodium or calcium came with the finding that calcium efflux from the heart, which was slowed by removal of either sodium and calcium, was inhibited to 20% of the control rate when both ions were absent in the extracellular fluid (Reuter and Seitz, 1968). These and other data suggest that about 80% of the calcium efflux from the myocardium occurs via the sodium/calcium exchanger.

The major driving force for calcium efflux via sodium/calcium exchange in the resting cell is the sodium gradient, $[Na^+]_i/[Na^+]_o$. As this gradient is established by the Na-K-ATPase (see below), the ultimate energy source for the uphill transport of calcium out of the cell via the sodium/calcium exchanger is the ATP that is hydrolyzed when the sodium pump establishes this sodium gradient.

Electrogenicity of Sodium/Calcium Exchange

It is now apparent that the sodium/calcium exchange transports three sodium ions in one direction across the membrane in exchange for a single calcium ion that moves in the opposite direction. For this reason, sodium/calcium exchange is electrogenic; that is, each time three sodium ions are exchanged for one calcium ion, there is a net movement of charge across the plasma membrane (Fig. 10.4).

The relationship between the current generated by this exchange and the directions of the ion fluxes can be confusing because, unlike calcium flux through a calcium channel, where calcium and positive charge move in the same direction, the sodium/calcium exchanger moves charge in a direction opposite to that of the calcium flux. This is because the charge movement follows the flux of sodium, rather

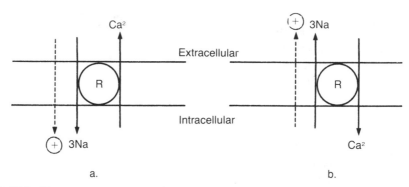

FIG. 10.4. Charge movements associated with sodium/calcium exchange (R) having a stoichiometry of 3 Na$^+$:1 Ca^{2+}. In *a*, the inward movement of sodium would be associated with an inward cationic current that generates a *depolarizing* current. When the efflux of sodium is outward (*b*) the ionic current is also outward, and so would tend to *repolarize*, or *hyperpolarize* the cell.

than of calcium; this is easily understood because of the stoichiometry: three Na$^+$ ions for each Ca^{2+} ion.

The fact that sodium/calcium exchange is associated with a charge movement makes this an extremely complex system. Not only does the exchanger influence membrane potential, but conversely, membrane potential influences the exchange between the two ions. Again, a few simple rules will help the reader to understand how this system operates. A negative intracellular potential, as occurs in the resting cell, represents an electrical gradient that tends to "pull" sodium ions into the cell; thus, *the exchanger favors calcium efflux during diastole.* Reversal of membrane potential during the plateau of the cardiac action potential, when the inside of the cell becomes positively charged, has the opposite effect, so that *the exchanger favors calcium influx during systole.* Stated simply, it is as if, whatever the state of the cell—relaxed or contracting—the direction of the calcium flux favored by the electrogenic sodium/calcium exchanger helps to maintain that state: calcium efflux during diastole, calcium influx during systole!

Not only does membrane potential influence sodium/calcium exchange, but because the exchanger transports three sodium ions in one direction in exchange for one calcium ion moving in the opposite direction, this electrogenic ion exchange mechanism influences membrane potential. Thus, the charge imbalance that occurs when one calcium ion moves in one direction in exchange for three sodium ions generates an ionic current across the plasma membrane; as noted above, current flows in the same direction as the sodium flux, and opposite to the movement of calcium (Fig. 10.4). The currents generated by sodium/calcium exchange are small (Sjodin, 1980), and probably contribute much less than a few millivolts to the membrane potential in the heart.

Mechanism of Sodium/Calcium Exchange

A simple scheme to explain sodium/calcium exchange is shown in Fig. 10.5. A negatively charged carrier (*R*), which can bind either sodium or calcium inside or

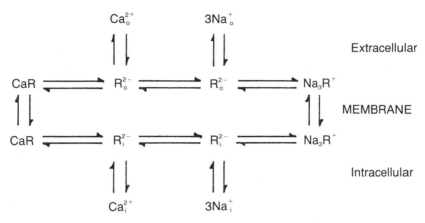

FIG. 10.5. Sodium/calcium exchange by the cardiac plasma membrane occurs through the competitive binding of sodium and calcium at both the inside and outside of the plasma membrane. The amount of each cation moving into the cell in this exchange is determined by the ratio $[Na^+]^3/[Ca^{2+}]$ at the outside of the cell; similarly, the relative amounts of these two cations that leave the cell is determined by the same ratio at the inner surface of the membrane. Abbreviations: o, extracellular; i, intracellular; R, carrier depicted here as having two negative charges.

outside the plasma membrane, is postulated to act as a "shuttle" that can move either ion in either direction across the membrane. If we assume that the carrier carries two negative charges, and that only CaR and Na_3R^+ move freely across the membrane, the driving force for calcium efflux is determined by three variables: the Ca^{2+} and Na^+ concentration gradients across the plasma membrane, and transmembrane potential (*Em*). If the carrier shown in Fig. 10.5 acts as a simple catalyst that establishes a gradient for calcium, and if the affinities of both cations for the carrier are the same on both sides of the membrane, the ratio $[Ca^{2+}]_i/[Ca^{2+}]_o$ will be directly proportional to that of the cube of the sodium gradient and membrane potential (E_m) according to the equation:

$$\frac{[Ca^{2+}]_i}{[Ca^{2+}]_o} = \frac{[Na^+]_i^3}{[Na^+]_o^3} \times \exp\frac{(E_mF)}{(RT)}.$$ [10.1]

Effects of Sodium/Calcium Exchange on Contractility

Increased $[Na^+]_i$, by shifting the equilibrium described in Eq. 10.1, can be seen to increase the ratio $[Ca^{2+}]_i/[Ca^{2+}]_o$. Thus, at constant levels of $[Ca^{2+}]_o$ and membrane potential, Eq. 10.1 states that a rise in $[Na^+]_i$ increases $[Ca^{2+}]_i$. This is readily understood by examining Fig. 10.5, where it can be seen how elevation of $[Na^+]_i$, which provides more sodium ions within the cell to compete with intracellular calcium for binding to the receptor, decreases calcium efflux until a new equilibrium is reached. This effect increases contractility by retaining calcium within the cell. Conversely, a fall in $[Na^+]_i$ favors calcium efflux via this exchanger, and so decreases contractility.

The early finding that cardiac contractility is proportional to the ratio $[Ca^{2+}]_o/[Na^+]_o$ can be readily explained by the model shown in Fig. 10.5 and Eq. 10.1. This proportionality is due simply to competition between $[Ca^{2+}]_o$ and $[Na^+]_o$ for binding to the extracellular sites of the exchanger. If both $[Na^{2+}]_o$ and $[Ca^{2+}]_o$ are changed proportionately, maintaining a constant ratio $[Ca^{2+}]_o/[Na^+]_o^3$, the relative rates of sodium and calcium influx remain constant, and there is no change in contractility. This follows from Eq. 10.1, in which a proportionate change in the denominators of both sides of the equation has no effect on the numerators.

Sodium/calcium exchange also explains why contractility is increased by agents that inhibit the sodium pump or that increase sodium entry into myocardial cells. The ability of the cardiac glycosides to increase contractility is due to their ability to inhibit sodium efflux (see below); this increases $[Na^+]_i$ and the ration $[Na^+]_i/[Na^+]_o$. According to Eq. 10.1, this increases the ratio $[Ca^{2+}]_i/[Ca^{2+}]_o$ so as to maintain the same relationship between Na^+ and Ca^{2+} concentrations on either side of the plasma membrane. Thus, sodium pump inhibition, by causing a net gain in intracellular calcium, increases myocardial contractility (Chapter 14). A similar mechanism explains the ability of drugs that open sodium channels to increase contractility.

Effects of ATP in Sodium/Calcium Exchange

Sodium/calcium exchange is energetically "neutral" because the exchanger simply facilitates a steady state between Na^+ and Ca^{2+} concentrations and electrical potential across the plasma membrane. However, even though no ATP is hydrolyzed during this exchange, ATP does influence the rate of ion transport. Studies of internally perfused squid axons have shown that sodium/calcium exchange is promoted by ATP within the cell, most likely as the result of an increased affinity of the exchanger for binding to intracellular calcium and extracellular sodium (Blaustein, 1977). This effect of ATP, however, does not require that the nucleotide contribute energy to this ion transport system as the exchanger functions, although at a reduced rate, in the absence of this nucleotide; furthermore, it is stimulated by nonhydrolyzable ATP analogues (DiPolo, 1977). Thus, this stimulatory effect is yet another example of an allosteric effect of ATP. As is true for the many regulatory effects of ATP, high nucleotide concentrations are needed to promote sodium/calcium exchange, the Michaelis constant (K_m) for ATP being between 0.1 and 1.0 mM (DiPolo, 1974).

Stimulation of sodium/calcium exchange by ATP reflects a general property of ATP to promote ion fluxes through a variety of ion channels, as well as sodium and calcium pumps (see below). A simple, but not entirely fanciful way to view this action of ATP is to view high concentrations of this nucleotide as a "lubricant" that facilitates many types of ion flux through membrane proteins.

The sodium/calcium exchanger has been reported to be influenced by a calcium, calmodulin–dependent phosphorylation (Caroni and Carafoli, 1983), but the significance of this observation remains unclear.

The recent discovery that the sodium/calcium exchanger can mediate rapid calcium fluxes (Gruver et al., 1990) raises the possibility that this system does more than restore diastolic levels of intracellular calcium. A suggestion that calcium entry via this exchanger can initiate calcium release from the sarcoplasmic reticulum (LeBlanc and Hume, 1990) is, however, still controversial (Lederer et al., 1990).

THE SODIUM PUMP

The sodium pump, which is responsible for the Na-K-ATPase activity of isolated plasma membrane preparations, utilizes the energy derived from ATP hydrolysis to generate a sodium gradient across the plasma membrane. This ion pump represents one of the most important of the transport systems in the cardiac plasma membrane because the potential energy stored in the sodium ion gradient plays a central role in the maintenance of cellular composition and, indirectly, participates in the regulation of myocardial contractility. The sodium gradient is also essential for the electrical activity of the heart as it provides the driving force for the sodium flux that generates the major depolarizing current in the working cells of the atria and ventricles, and the rapidly conducting cells of the His-Purkinje system (Chapter 19).

The direct role of the sodium pump is to clear the cytosol of the small amount of sodium that enters the cell during each action potential. At the same time, the sodium pump returns the small amount of potassium lost from the cytosol during repolarization of the action potential. Although only small amounts of sodium are exchanged for potassium during each cardiac cycle, the fact that both sodium efflux and potassium influx are uphill requires an active transport mechanism to restore cell composition at the end of each systole. Because the sodium pump moves positively charged ions in opposite directions across the membrane, the electrochemical work of this pump is minimized. This sodium/potassium exchange is quite different from the ATP-dependent transport of calcium because transport of a counter-ion, potassium, is an essential part of the ATP-dependent reaction of the sodium pump.

The sodium pump contributes to a number of transport reactions across the plasma membrane because it creates a sodium gradient across the plasma membrane that can be coupled to the uphill fluxes of other substances. We have already examined one such transport reaction, sodium/calcium exchange, which is a "countertransport" or "antiport" that utilizes the downhill movement of sodium into the myocardial cell to "lift" calcium out of the cell against a large electrochemical gradient. The sodium gradient thus provides a reserve of osmotic energy that can be "tapped" by coupling downhill sodium entry to the uphill transport of other substances across the plasma membrane.

The sodium gradient is essential for the uptake of glucose and amino acids by the intestinal brush border, which utilizes the sodium gradient to provide energy for the active transport of these substances. Like the sodium/calcium exchanger, these transport mechanisms couple the energy provided when sodium moves down its electrochemical gradient to the active transport of substrates into the cytosol. Because the sodium and these substrates cross the membrane in the same direction, these are called "cotransport" or "symport" mechanisms.

Electrogenicity of the Sodium Pump

Although the sodium pump catalyzes the exchange of sodium and potassium in opposite directions across the membrane, the amounts of these ions moved during each turnover of the pump are not the same. Instead, three sodium ions are transported out of the cell in exchange for only two potassium ions that are brought into the cell according to the scheme shown in Fig. 10.6.

Because different amounts of sodium and potassium are moved in opposite directions across the plasma membrane, the sodium pump generates an electric current; in other words, the sodium pump is electrogenic. Like the sodium/calcium exchanger (Fig. 10.4), the net flux of positive charge is in the same direction as the net flux of sodium (Fig. 10.6). As a result, the sodium pump generates a current in which positive charge moves out of the cell; according to electrophysiological convention, this represents an outward (repolarizing) current. The electrogenicity of the sodium pump tends to increase the negativity of the cell interior, and so helps to maintain the normal resting potential of the myocardial cells, and when the heart is depolarized, the outward ionic current generated by the sodium pump favors repolarization.

> The potential generated by the sodium pump is small, probably less than 10 mV. However, under some circumstances this outward current can be of considerable functional significance. For example, in injured cells, where resting potential is low and the normally small sodium "leak" into the cell is increased, the outward current generated by the sodium pump may make a significant contribution to maintaining resting potential. In this setting, sodium pump inhibition, by reducing this outward current, would tend to depolarize the cell. However, a more important depolarizing effect of sodium pump inhibition arises from the increase in $[K^+]_i$, the main determinant of resting potential in the heart (Chapter 19).

Cation-Binding Sites on the Sodium Pump

The sodium contains two different types of alkali metal ion-binding site. As would be predicted from the ability of this ion pump to exchange intracellular sodium for extracellular potassium, sodium binds to a site that faces the intracellular

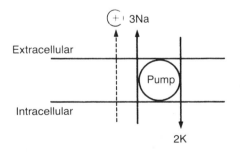

FIG. 10.6. Charge movements caused by the sodium pump reflect its stoichiometry of 3 Na⁺ : 2 K⁺. Thus, the outward movement of sodium is associated with an outward cationic current that tends to *repolarize*, or *hyperpolarize*, the cell.

side of the membrane and potassium binds to an extracellular site. It is not known whether there are, in fact, two discrete sites on the pump, or whether a single cation-binding site loses its affinity for sodium and increases its affinity for potassium after sodium is transported from the cytosol to the extracellular space.

Reaction Mechanism of the Sodium Pump[1]

The sodium pump couples the energy derived from the hydrolysis of ATP to the movements of sodium and potassium in a Na-K-ATPase reaction that involves the formation of a series of intermediates between the sodium pump protein and its substrates. This reaction mechanism can be depicted as a series of steps that describe sequential transitions in the interactions of the sodium pump enzyme with its various substrates. In the overall reaction, depicted in Eq. 10.2, the enzyme is designated as E; E_1 and E_2, and E_1P and E_2P represent different forms of the enzyme in its nonphosphorylated and phosphorylated forms, respectively. These designations are used later, Chapter 11, in our discussion of the calcium pump of the sarcoplasmic reticulum.

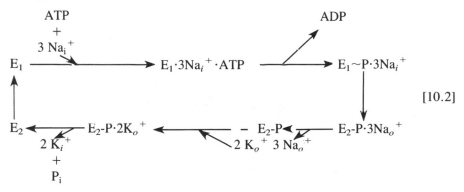

$$[10.2]$$

In the nonphosphorylated enzyme, E_1 and E_2 represent states of the enzyme having different reactivities to ATP and cations. The distinction between E_1P and E_2P is of fundamental importance because these phosphorylated intermediates are quite different in terms of their bond energies.

The entire reaction sequence shown in Eq. 10.2, like that of the calcium pump of the sarcoplasmic reticulum (Chapter 11), can be made to run in reverse. These reverse reactions, which use the ion gradients to synthesize ATP from ADP and inorganic phosphate (P_i), are not seen under physiological conditions because the reverse reactions are strongly inhibited by ATP.

The phosphorylated reaction intermediates formed by the sodium pump are analogous to those formed by the myosin cross-bridge (Chapter 8). Unlike myosin, where the physiological expression of the liberation of chemical energy from ATP is motion, the

---

[1]This section is modified from a review by the author (Katz, 1985). Magnesium ion, which is essential for this reaction, has been omitted for simplicity.

sodium pump uses the chemical energy of ATP to perform osmotic work. Thus, the sequence of steps in the Na-K-ATPase reaction reflect the formation and translocation of complexes between the enzyme and the cations it transports. Overall, however, these steps resemble the complexes formed between myosin and actin during the cross-bridge cycle; as discussed in Chapter 11, they are also quite similar to the reaction intermediates formed by the sarcoplasmic reticulum calcium pump.

High- and Low-Energy Phosphoenzyme Intermediates

At this point, a small digression is in order; this is useful in explaining the mechanism by which chemical energy is transduced to perform different types of work. We have already seen one such transduction in the cross-bridge cycle, where the active complex becomes a rigor bond (Chapter 8). In the case of the sodium pump, the phosphorylated intermediate E_1P is in a high-energy state, where the energy of the terminal phosphate of ATP is retained in a high-energy bond linking the enzyme-bound phosphate to the protein. This high-energy bond, like that in the "active complex" between myosin and actin, is an acyl phosphate, in which the phosphate is linked to the carboxyl group of an acidic amino acid like aspartate:

$$
\begin{array}{ccc}
\text{O} & & \text{OH} \\
\parallel & & | \\
\text{R} - \text{C} & \sim \text{O} - \text{P} - \text{O}^- & \qquad (E_1{\sim}P, \text{ or } E_1P) \\
& \parallel & \\
& \text{O} &
\end{array}
$$

The intermediate E_2P, like E_1P, is an acyl phosphate except that the high-energy bond ($\sim$) is replaced by a low-energy bond ($-$). E_2P, which is like the rigor complex formed between myosin and actin, can be depicted as:

$$
\begin{array}{ccc}
\text{O} & & \text{OH} \\
\parallel & & | \\
\text{R} - \text{C} - \text{O} - \text{P} - \text{O}^- & & \qquad (E_2\text{-}P, \text{ or } E_2P) \\
& \parallel & \\
& \text{O} &
\end{array}
$$

Experimentally, E_1P and E_2P are readily distinguished in terms of their ability to transfer inorganic phosphate (P_i) to ADP to form ATP. Because the high-energy phosphate bond of E_1P is readily transferred to ADP, P_i release from E_1P is accelerated in the presence of ADP and leads to the formation of ATP. For this reason, E_1P is often referred to as "ADP-sensitive." On the other hand, E_2P is a low-energy compound that cannot transfer P_i to ADP; hence, E_2P is an "ADP-insensitive" intermediate whose breakdown is not accelerated by ADP because the phosphate moiety bound to E_2P cannot be transferred to ADP to form ATP.

The Steps of the Sodium Pump Reaction Mechanism

The reaction scheme shown in Eq. 10.2 begins with the formation of $E_1 \cdot 3Na^+{}_i \cdot$ ATP, in which the enzyme forms a complex with ATP and three sodium ions, the latter being bound to sites at the intracellular surface of the enzyme:

$$E_1 + 3Na^+{}_i + ATP \rightarrow E_1 \cdot 3Na^+{}_i \cdot ATP. \qquad [10.3]$$

The enzyme-bound sodium in Eq 10.3 is designated $Na_i{}^+$ because this ion is at its low (intracellular) activity.

Immediately after the formation of $E_1 \cdot 3Na_i{}^+ \cdot ATP$, this complex is converted to another intermediate, $E_1 {\sim} P \cdot 3Na_i{}^+$. In this intermediate, the energy of ATP has been transferred to the enzyme to form $E_1 {\sim} P$, and ADP is liberated according to the reaction:

$$E_1 \cdot 3Na^+{}_i \cdot ATP \rightarrow E_1 {\sim} P \cdot 3Na^+{}_i + ADP. \qquad [10.4]$$

As already pointed out, the $E {\sim} E_1 \cdot 3Na^+{}_i$ intermediate, or $E_1 P$, represents a phosphoenzyme intermediate in which the energy of the terminal phosphate of ATP has been retained in the bond linking the phosphate moiety to the enzyme. As the energy of ATP remains in a high-energy phosphate bond, the enzyme-bound sodium remains at its low, extracellular activity.

The next step in this reaction sequence transfers the phosphate-bond energy of $E_1 P$ to the three sodium ions that are bound to the enzyme. In this way, the enzyme-bound sodium is "raised" to the higher Na^+ activity of the extracellular fluid, thereby making it possible for these ions to be transported out of the cell; thus, this step allows the Na-K-ATPase to pump sodium. Because phosphate bond energy has been transferred to the enzyme-bound sodium, the bond linking the phosphate group to the enzyme becomes a low-energy bond according to the reaction:

$$E_1 {\sim} P \cdot 3Na^+{}_i \rightarrow E_2 \text{-} P \cdot 3Na^+{}_o. \qquad [10.5]$$

The $E_2 \text{-} P \cdot 3Na^+{}_o$ intermediate rapidly releases its bound sodium into the extracellular fluid:

$$E_2 \text{-} P \cdot 3Na^+{}_o \rightarrow E_2 \text{-} P + 3 Na^+{}_o. \qquad [10.6]$$

This leaves a new intermediate, $E_2 \text{-} P$, which binds potassium with high affinity. Thus, immediately after sodium ions are released into the extracellular fluid, potassium ions bind to the extracellar surface of the enzyme, possibly to sites that had previously been bound to sodium, according to the reaction:

$$E_2 \text{-} P + 2 K^+{}_o \rightarrow E_2 \text{-} P \cdot 2K^+{}_o. \qquad [10.7]$$

Phosphate is then released at the same time that the enzyme-bound potassium is translocated and released into the cytosol:

$$E_2 \text{-} P \cdot 2 K^+{}_o \rightarrow E_2 + 2 K^+{}_i + P_i. \qquad [10.8]$$

The cycle is completed when E_2 is reconverted to E_1:

$$E_2 \rightarrow E_1. \qquad [10.9]$$

The overall reaction, which encompasses the steps shown in Eqs. 10.3 through 10.9, is therefore:

$$\overset{E}{3 Na^+{}_i + 2 K^+{}_o + ATP \rightarrow 3 Na^+{}_o + 2 K^+{}_i + ADP + P_i.} \qquad [10.10]$$

Energy Transduction by the Sodium Pump

The step in the reaction scheme shown in Eq. 10.2 in which E_1P is converted to E_2P is believed to represent the step in which active ion transport actually takes place; that is, where sodium ions are "lifted" across the sarcolemmal membrane from the region of low activity inside the cell to that of higher activity in the extracellular space. In other words, this is the step that utilizes the energy obtained from ATP hydrolysis to move sodium across the membrane against its electrochemical gradient.

Effects of ATP on the Sodium Pump

In accord with a now familiar pattern, ATP has two quite different effects on the sodium pump, and as described in Chapter 11, also on the calcium pump of the sarcoplasmic reticulum. These effects arise from two fundamentally different interactions between the nucleotide and these ion pumps. One of these, of course, occurs when ATP binds to the "substrate site" that utilizes the energy of ATP for active cation transport; occupancy of this substrate site occurs in the reaction described in Eq. 10.3. Like other substrate sites, that of E_1 has an extremely high affinity for ATP, being half-saturated at ATP concentrations <1 μM.

The second ATP-binding site represents a "regulatory site" in that the binding of ATP to this site does not provide energy for transport, but instead accelerates the turnover of the ion pumps. In this regard, the allosteric effects of ATP can be viewed as "lubricating effects." The regulatory site, which is described in detail for the sarcoplasmic reticulum calcium pump (Chapter 11), has a much lower affinity for ATP than the substrate site, being half-saturated at approximately 200 μM ATP. It is for this reason that, as noted for other systems, a fall in ATP affects the regulatory site long before substrate binding is reduced by depletion of this nucleotide.

Structure of the Sodium Pump

Each functional unit of the sodium pump is a tetramer made up of two pairs of subunits, designated α and β (Fig. 10.2). The larger α-subunit, which contains the major sites for ATP binding, phosphorylation, alkali metal ion binding, and binding to the cardiac glycosides, has a molecular weight of 112,000 and contains seven hydrophobic, membrane-spanning domains. The cardiac glycosides, which inhibit the sodium pump (see below), bind to the extracellular portions of the peptide chain, whereas phosphorylation and binding of ATP and sodium probably take place at separate sites within the cytosol (Karlish et al., 1990). The potassium-binding sites, which at some point in the reaction sequence must face the extracellular surface of the membrane, may be the same as those which had previously been bound to sodium. There are at least three isoforms of the human α-subunit (Shull and Lingrel, 1987). The β-subunit is a much smaller glycoprotein, having a molecular weight of ~40,000 daltons that includes a single putative membrane-spanning domain.

The α-subunit, which contains the sites for ATP binding, phosphorylation, and sodium and potassium binding, is the catalytic subunit that is responsible for ATP hydrolysis and sodium and potassium transport. The function of the smaller β-subunit, which contains a number of carbohydrate residues that project from the extracellular surface of the plasma membrane, is not clear; this subunit may be involved in the regulation of sodium pump assembly in the plasma membrane (McDonough et al., 1990).

Drug Effects on the Sodium Pump

The sodium pump is inhibited by a fascinating class of drugs called the cardiac glycosides. The prototype of this group of drugs is digitalis, first identified by Withering more than 200 years ago as the active ingredient in an herb tea used to treat dropsy (Chapter 25). Cardiac glycosides, by inhibiting the sodium pump, increase intracellular Na^+ concentration. This effect, by increasing calcium influx and decreasing calcium efflux via the sodium/calcium exchanger (see above), is responsible for the positive inotropic effect of these drugs (Chapter 14). Inhibition of the sodium pump by cardiac glycosides is associated with a decreased rate of the step at which the phosphorylated intermediate $E_2\text{-}P\cdot2K^+_o$ is broken down (Eq. 10.8). The inhibitory actions of these drugs can be partially reversed by increasing extracellular K^+ concentration, which displaces the drug from its extracellular binding site. This effect of extracellular potassium effect explains the clinically significant ability of high serum potassium levels to attenuate the toxic effects of the cardiac glycosides, and conversely, the potentiation of digitalis toxicity by hypokalemia.

Over the past decades occasional reports have described a slight, inconsistent stimulatory effect of very low concentrations of cardiac glycosides on Na-K-ATPase activity in isolated membrane preparations. The author found this effect in the late 1960s, but it was never reproducible. Stimulation of sodium pump activity has also been noted in intact cardiac tissues, but this is best explained by a "side effect" of the cardiac glycosides to release β-adrenergic agonists (Hougen et al., 1981), which themselves increase Na-K-ATPase activity (see below). Although it is now generally agreed that this stimulatory effect is not significant, history warns us not to be too confident in dismissing these observations. Nature may have been playing tricks, and it is not impossible that important actions of this very old drug are still concealed from us. Indeed, as noted in Chapter 25, there is now reason to believe that at least some of the beneficial effects of the cardiac glycosides in the treatment of heart failure may be due to inhibition of the sodium pump in the chemoreceptor trigger zone of the brain, rather than their ability to increase myocardial contractility.

The biochemical mechanism responsible for stimulation of the sodium pump by the sympathetic nervous system (Swann, 1984) and cyclic AMP (Morad, 1982) remains unclear.

SODIUM/HYDROGEN EXCHANGE

The heart, like most vertebrate cells, contains a plasma membrane sodium/hydrogen exchanger that extrudes protons by a countertransport (antiport). Like the sodium/calcium exchanger, this system uses the energy of the sodium gradient for the active transport of protons out of the cell. Sodium/hydrogen exchange can play a role in regulating both intracellular Na^+ concentration and intracellular pH (Lazdunski et al., 1985). Under conditions such as ischemia, where intracellular pH falls (see Chapter 24), the sodium/hydrogen exchanger may help to rid the cell of excess hydrogen ions. The role of this system in mediating sodium entry is not clear; because intracellular H^+ concentration is much less than 1 μM, whereas $[Na^+]_i$ is in the millimolar range, the amounts of sodium that enter the cell in exchange for hydrogen ions by this mechanism are probably very small.

TRANSVERSE TUBULAR SYSTEM

The transverse tubular system of the mammalian myocardium, as described in Chapter 1, is in direct continuity with the extracellular space, so that the "t-system" can be viewed as an extension of the plasma membrane.

As the lumina of the t-tubules open freely into the extracellular space, the composition of the fluid within the transverse tubules is like the extracellular fluid; both contain a solution that is high in calcium and sodium, and low in potassium. This composition of the t-tubular fluid allows these structures to participate in the generation of the action potential.

Transmission of the action potential into the cell interior via the t-tubules allows these sarcolemmal extensions to facilitate the rapid activation of structures deep within the muscle cell. Indeed, the t-tubules provide the best answer to the question posed by Hill that introduced this chapter. Because conduction of the action potential is much more rapid than the diffusion of an activator substance, transmission of the action potential down the t-tubules accelerates activation of the cell interior.

The t-tubules of the heart differ from those of most mammalian skeletal muscles in several important respects. Unlike the corresponding structures in skeletal muscle, which penetrate the sarcomere at the level of the edges of the A-band (the junctions between A- and I-bands), the transverse tubular system of the mammalian myocardium runs alongside the Z-bands. In addition, these tubules can run longitudinally from one sarcomere to the next in the myocardium. A further difference between these muscle types lies in the larger diameter of the cardiac transverse tubular system.

In one of the classic experiments in muscle physiology, A. F. Huxley and R. Taylor demonstrated that localized (nonpropagated) depolarization of a skeletal muscle fiber by a microelectrode placed at an opening of the transverse tubular system caused contraction only of the two half sarcomeres adjacent to the point of stimulation. This finding indicated that the t-tubules transmit the signal of excitation-contraction coupling into the cell interior. Attempts to demonstrate similar localized responses to stimulation of cardiac muscle at the point of opening of the transverse tubular system have failed, however, most likely because the longitudinal extensions of the transverse tubular system in the heart allow activation to spread into adjacent sarcomeres.

> Excitation-contraction coupling is impaired when the connections between the t-tubules and the plasma membrane at the surface of a skeletal muscle cell are disrupted, for example by increasing and then decreasing osmolarity (Eisenberg and Eisenberg, 1968). This loss of excitability, which is accompanied by changes in membrane capacitance caused by the disconnection of the transverse tubular system from the cell surface, indicates that the action potential is transmitted to the cell interior along the t-tubules (Vaughan et al., 1979).

At this point we have reached a critical step in our review of excitation-contraction coupling. This step encompasses the mechanism by which the action potential propagated along the cell surface generates a signal that is transmitted to the cell interior so as to cause the release of activator calcium in the cytosol. In the next chapter, therefore, our focus shifts from the external membranes of the heart to the intracellular membranes of the sarcoplasmic reticulum.

REFERENCES

Blaustein MP. (1977). Effects of internal and external cations and of ATP on sodium-calcium and calcium-calcium exchange in squid axons. *Biophys J* 20:79–111.

Caroni P, Carafoli E. (1983). The regulation of the Na^+-Ca^{2+} exchanger of heart sarcolemma. *Eur J Biochem* 132:451–460.

Caroni P, Zurini M, Clark A, Carafoli E. (1983). Further characterization and reconstitution of the purified Ca^{2+}-pumping ATPase of heart sarcolemma. *J Biol Chem* 258:7305–7310.

Chiesi M, Voherr T, Schwaller R, Carafoli E. (1990). Cardiac phospholamban is related to the inhibitory domain of the plasma membrane Ca-pump. *Circulation* 82(Suppl III):III-349.

DePolo R. (1974). Effect of ATP on the calcium efflux in dialyzed squid giant axons. *J Gen Physiol* 64:503–517.

DiPolo R. (1977). Characterization of the ATP-dependent calcium efflux in dialyzed squid giant axons. *J Gen Physiol* 69:795–813.

Eisenberg B, Eisenberg RS. (1968). Transverse tubular system in glycerol-treated skeletal muscle. *Science* 160:1243–1244.

Fabiato A. (1983). Calcium-induced calcium release from the cardiac sarcoplasmic reticulum. *Am J Physiol* 245:C1–C14.

Gruver C, Katz AM, Messineo FC. (1990). Canine cardiac sarcolemmal vesicles demonstrate rapid initial Na^+-Ca^{++} exchange activity. *Circ Res* 66:1171–1177.

Hill AV. (1949). The abrupt transition from rest to activity in muscle. *Proc R Soc Land [Biol]* 136:399–420.

Hougen TJ, Spicer N, Smith TW. (1981). Stimulation of monovalent cation active transport by low concentrations of cardiac glycosides. Role of catecholamines. *J Clin Invest* 68:1207–1214.

Jørgensen PL, Andersen JP. (1988). Structural basis for E_1-E_2 conformational transitions in Na,K-pump and Ca-pump proteins. *J Membr Biol* 103:95–120.

Karlish SJD, Goldshleger R, Stein WD. (1990). A 19kDa C-terminal tryptic fragment of the α chain of Na/K-ATPase is essential for occlusion and transport of cations. *Proc Natl Acad Sci USA* 87:4566–4570.

Katz AM. (1985). Effect of digitalis on cell biochemistry: sodium pump inhibition. *J Am Cell Cardiol* 5:16A–21A.

Lazdunski M, Frelin C, Vigne P. (1985). The sodium/hydrogen exchange system in cardiac cells: its biochemical and pharmacological properties and its role in regulating internal concentrations of sodium and internal pH. *J Mol Cell Cardiol* 17:1029–1042.

LeBlanc N, Hume TR. (1990). Sodium current-induced release of calcium from cardiac sarcoplasmic reticulum. *Science* 248:372–376.

Lederer WJ, Niggli E, Hadley RW. (1990). Sodium-calcium exchange in excitable cells: fuzzy space. *Science* 248:283.

McDonough AA, Geering K, Farley RA. (1990). The sodium pump needs its beta subunit. *FASEB J* 4:1598–1605.

Morad M. (1982). Ionic mechanisms mediating the inotropic and relaxant effects of adrenaline on the heart muscle. In: Oliver MF, Riemersma RA, eds. *Catecholamines in the non-ischaemic and ischaemic myocardium*. New York: Elsevier; 113–135.

Reuter H, Seitz N. (1968). The dependence of calcium efflux from cardiac muscle on temperature and external ion composition. *J Physiol (Lond)* 195:451–470.

Shull MM, Lingrel JB. (1987). Multiple genes encode the human Na^+, K^+-ATPase catalytic subunit. *Proc Natl Acad Sci USA* 84:4039–4043.

Sjodin RA. (1980). Contribution of Na/Ca transport to the resting membrane potential. *J Gen Physiol* 76:99–108.

Swann AC. (1984). (Na^+,K^+)-adenosine triphosphatase regulation by the sympathetic nervous sytem: effects of noradrenergic stimulation and lesions in vivo. *J Pharmacol Exp Ther* 228:304–311.

Vaughan PC, Howell JN, Eisenberg RS. (1979). The capacitance of skeletal muscle fibers in solutions of low ionic strength. *J Gen Physiol* 59:347–359.

BIBLIOGRAPHY

Carafoli E. (1990). Sarcolemmal calcium pump. In: Langer GA, ed. *Calcium and the heart*. New York: Raven Press; 109–126.

Huxley AF (1959). Local activation of muscle. *Ann NY Acad Sci* 81:446–452.

Philipson KD. (1990). The cardiac Na^+-Ca^{2+} exchanger. In: Langer GA, ed. *Calcium and the heart*. New York: Raven Press; 85–108.

Reeves JP. (1985). The sarcolemmal sodium-calcium exchange system. *Curr Top Membr Trans* 25:77–127.

Reuter H. (1974). Exchange of calcium ions in the mammalian myocardium: mechanisms and physiological significance. *Circ Res* 34:599–605.

Robinson JD, Flashner MS. (1979). The $(Na^+ + K^+)$-activated ATPase, enzymatic and transport properties. *Biochim Biophys Acta* 549:145–176.

Schwartz A, Lindenmayer GE, Allen JC. (1975). The sodium-potassium adenosine triphosphatase: pharmacological, physiological and biochemical aspects. *Pharmacol Rev* 27:3–134.

11

Excitation–Contraction Coupling

Calcium Fluxes Across the Sarcoplasmic Reticulum and Mitochondria

Our description of the signaling mechanisms that initiate muscle contraction has, up to this point, focused on the plasma membrane and its extension into the myocardial cell, the t-tubule. We have seen that this membrane, which separates the cytosol from the extracellular fluid, contains a complex system of ion transport mechanisms that together orchestrate the flow of messenger calcium into and out of the cytosol. However, the amount of calcium that enters the cell from the extracellular fluid is not sufficient to activate the adult mammalian myocardium. Instead, most of the calcium that binds to troponin in the heart is derived from the sarcoplasmic reticulum, an intracellular membrane system that plays a central role in the release and reuptake of activator calcium within these cells.

FUNCTION OF THE SARCOPLASMIC RETICULUM

The sarcoplasmic reticulum, whose main function is regulation of cytosolic Ca^{2+} concentration, is the most important of the systems that deliver activator calcium for binding to troponin C in striated muscle. This membrane system also takes up and stores calcium, and so plays a key role in muscle relaxation. In mammalian fast skeletal muscle, where contraction of individual muscle cells is essentially an all-or-none process (see Chapter 13), the large amount of calcium released by this membrane system saturates the calcium-binding sites of troponin. As regulation in these muscles is effected largely by the recruitment of varying numbers of active motor units by the central nervous system (Chapter 13), calcium fluxes across the sarcoplasmic reticulum membrane are not extensively regulated. In contrast, important changes in the intensity of myocardial contraction are caused by variations in the amount of calcium made available for binding to cardiac troponin C. Thus, it is easy to understand why calcium release from the cardiac sarcoplasmic reticulum is regulated more extensively than in the corresponding system in skeletal muscle.

> Active sarcoplasmic reticulum vesicles that are readily prepared from the microsomal fraction of rabbit white skeletal muscle have come to represent the "gold standard" for work in this field, much like the frog sartorius in muscle mechanics and the squid axon in electrophysiology. The following discussion therefore refers frequently to rabbit skeletal muscle sarcoplasmic reticulum, to which the special properties of cardiac sarcoplasmic reticulum are compared.

ENERGETIC IMPLICATIONS OF CALCIUM FLUXES ACROSS THE SARCOPLASMIC RETICULUM

The Ca^{2+} concentration within the sarcoplasmic reticulum, although not precisely known, is much higher than in the cytosol. For this reason, calcium release during excitation is a passive, downhill, process, whereas calcium uptake requires the expenditure of energy. The calcium fluxes across the sarcoplasmic reticulum are analogous to those across the plasma membrane, where calcium entry into the cytosol is downhill, and energy must be expanded to move calcium back into the extracellular space.

> A significant portion of the calcium contained within the sarcoplasmic reticulum is probably bound to calcium-binding proteins within this membrane structure, and possibly also to the phospholipid head groups of the sarcoplasmic reticulum membrane (see below). A number of anions, notably phosphate and palmitic acid, also form insoluble complexes with calcium and so, under abnormal conditions, may trap this ion within the sarcoplasmic reticulum. As discussed later in this chapter, non-physiological calcium-precipitating anions—notably oxalate—are useful in studying calcium uptake *in vitro*.

STRUCTURE OF THE SARCOPLASMIC RETICULUM

The sarcoplasmic reticulum membrane, like other biological membranes (Chapter 2), consists of a phospholipid bilayer containing a number of intrinsic membrane proteins. From both a structural and a functional standpoint this membrane can be divided into two regions: the *subsarcolemmal cisternae*, which contain the calcium channels through which calcium flows to initiate systole, and the much more extensive *sarcotubular network* that contains a densely packed array of calcium pump adenosine triphosphatase (ATPase) proteins (see Fig. 10.1). In the heart, subsarcolemmal cisternae are found both beneath the plasma membrane and alongside the transverse tubular system, whereas the sarcotubular network surrounds the contractile proteins in the center of the sarcomere.

The Subsarcolemmal Cisternae

The cardiac sarcoplasmic reticulum forms specialized, functionally important junctions where this membrane approaches and parallels the membranes of the sar-

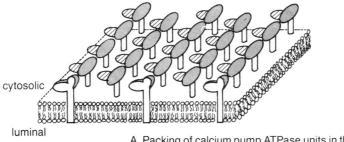

cytosolic

luminal

A. Packing of calcium pump ATPase units in the
sarcotubular network of the sarcoplasmic reticulum.

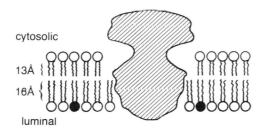

cytosolic

13Å

16Å

luminal

B. Profile of a single calcium pump ATPase unit

FIG. 11.1. Structure of the sarcoplasmic reticulum membrane. A: Three-dimensional depiction of the sarcoplasmic reticulum. The cytosolic surface of the membrane is above the membrane and the lumen into which calcium is pumped is below. The calcium pump ATPase molecules are packed in the bilayer, probably as dimers, in which a large portion of the mass projects from the cytosolic surface of the membrane. (Modified from Stokes and Green, 1990.) B: Cross section through the bilayer showing the cylindrically averaged mass of a single calcium pump ATPase unit; as in A, the cytosolic surface of the membrane is at the *top*. The average length of the fatty acyl chains is slightly longer in the cytosolic leaflet of the bilayer than in the luminal leaflet, and there are more phospholipid molecules in the latter (depicted as phospholipid having black head groups). (Modified from Herbette et al., 1985.)

colemma and the t-tubules; the latter, as described in Chapter 1, represent extensions of the plasma membrane (Fig. 1.22). The sarcoplasmic reticulum assumes a flattened saccular shape at the unctions formed by elements of each of these two membrane systems, called dyads. The *subsarcolemmal cisternae* of cardiac muscle, which are similar to the terminal cisternae of skeletal muscle, are dilated extensions of the sarcoplasmic reticulum. The subsarcolemmal cisternae contain electron-dense proteins that bind calcium and so maintain a store of calcium within this region of the sarcoplasmic reticulum.

Because the calcium-binding proteins that are concentrated within the subsarcolemmal cisternae are much denser than the membrane phospholipids, membrane vesicles derived from this region of skeletal sarcoplasmic reticulum are purified in a *heavy vesicle fraction* that is readily separated from the less dense sarcotubular network, which appears in a *light vesicle fraction*.

Calcium Channels and Calcium Release Channels

The architecture of the subsarcolemmal cisternae (Fig. 1.23) defines a critical relationship between two important proteins in each of the membranes that make up the dyad. The first protein is the *calcium channel* of the plasma membrane and t-tubules, often referred to as the *dihydropyridine receptor* because of its high affinity binding to this class of calcium channel blocking drugs. The second of these proteins is the "foot" protein, which projects from the subsarcolemmal cisternae into the space within the dyad. This protein, often called the *ryanodine receptor* because of its binding to this plant alkaloid, is now known to be the channel through which calcium flows from within the sarcoplasmic reticulum to activate the contractile proteins; thus, the foot protein, or ryanodine receptor, is referred to as the *calcium release channel* of the sarcoplasmic reticulum.

It is now clear that the junctions between the sarcoplasmic reticulum and the t-tubular extensions of the plasma membrane provide a vital functional link between these two membranes. It is at this junction that electrical depolarization of the plasma membrane initiates calcium release from the sarcoplasmic reticulum. As described below, this step in excitation-contraction coupling is effected by different mechanisms in cardiac and skeletal muscle.

The Sarcotubular Network

As noted at the beginning of this chapter, the sarcoplasmic reticulum has two functions. The first, to release activator calcium, is associated with the subsarcolemmal cisternae. The second function, the reuptake of calcium that allows the muscle to relax, is effected by a densely packed array of calcium pump ATPase proteins embedded in the membranes of the sarcotubular network (Fig. 11.1A). These proteins, which actively transport calcium from the cytosol into the sarcoplasmic reticulum, span the membrane and so contact the aqueous spaces on either side of the bilayer.

> The outlines of the calcium pump ATPase protein molecules within the sarcoplasmic reticulum membrane have been defined by a combination of electron microscopy, and x-ray and neutron diffraction (Fig. 11.1B). The calcium pump proteins are arranged, possibly as dimers, such that approximately half of the mass of the protein extends from the cytosolic surface of the phospholipid bilayer into the aqueous space of the cytosol. The portion of the calcium pump ATPase protein that projects into the cytosol contains the phosphorylation and ATP-binding sites that participate in energy transfer during calcium transport; the high-affinity calcium-binding sites are probably associated with the intramembranous region of the molecule (see below). The fact that the calcium pump ATPase spans the membrane allows this protein to function as a pump that moves calcium between the aqueous spaces on the two sides of the membrane.

The calcium pump ATPase molecules in cardiac sarcoplasmic reticulum are less densely packed than those in skeletal muscle; biochemical studies indicate that the density of calcium pump molecules in the cardiac membrane is about a third that in the standard skeletal muscle preparations. Of greater interest is the finding that this density is variable; for example there are fewer calcium pump molecules in the sarcoplasmic reticulum of the failing heart (Chapter 25).

Cardiac, but not fast skeletal, sarcoplasmic reticulum contains a regulatory protein, *phospholamban*, that plays a key role in regulating the cardiac response to β-adrenergic agonists (see below).

The Fluid Within The Sarcoplasmic Reticulum

The composition of the fluid in the lumen of the sarcoplasmic reticulum differs from both the cytosol and extracellular space (Somlyo et al., 1981). By far the most important of these differences is the high Ca^{2+} concentration within this membrane system. From the standpoint of energetics, this means that the calcium fluxes responsible for muscle activation are downhill, and so do not require the expenditure of energy, whereas calcium uptake during relaxation is an active process which, as described later in this chapter, requires the "army" of calcium pump ATPase proteins shown in Fig. 11.1.

CALCIUM RELEASE FROM THE SARCOPLASMIC RETICULUM

Three quite different mechanisms have been postulated to explain how the signal generated by the action potential initiates calcium release from the sarcoplasmic reticulum (Fig. 11.2). The first is an electrical coupling in which a depolarization-

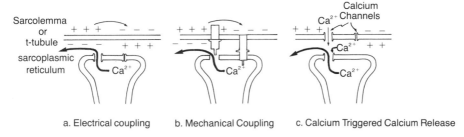

FIG. 11.2. Three possible mechanisms by which depolarization of the plasmalemmal or t-tubular membrane could induce calcium release from the sarcoplasmic reticulum. An action potential is shown to proceed from left to right across the membrane of the t-tubule, the depolarized region of this membrane being shaded. a: *Electrical coupling*. Calcium release is initiated when the sarcoplasmic reticulum membrane is depolarized by charge movements related to passage of the action potential across the adjacent plasma membrane. b: *Mechanical coupling*. Passage of the action potential across the plasma membrane causes a shift in an intrinsic membrane protein that "unplugs" a channel, allowing calcium to flow out of the sarcoplasmic reticulum. c: *Calcium-triggered calcium release*. The small amount of calcium that enters the cell through voltage-dependent plasmalemmal calcium channels, which open in response to the action potential, causes a much larger amount of calcium to be released from within the sarcoplasmic reticulum.

induced alteration in charge distribution across the t-tubule opens a voltage-sensitive calcium channel in the sarcoplasmic reticulum, and is mentioned mainly for historical reasons. Alternatively, a structural rearrangement of a protein or proteins within the t-tubule may allow calcium to leave the sarcoplasmic reticulum by removing a "plug" that occludes the resting channel; this mechanism is sometimes referred to irreverently as the "plumber's helper model," because the plug, as originally drawn, resembled the device used to open a blocked drain (Chandler et al., 1976). According to the third mechanism, a small amount of calcium that enters the cytosol from the extracellular space through a calcium channel in the t-tubule membrane, by increasing Ca^{2+} concentration outside the subsarcolemmal cisternae, triggers the opening of a calcium channel in the sarcoplasmic reticulum. Generally called "calcium-induced calcium release," this mechanism is analogous to the firing of an old flintlock musket as the small calcium entry during the action potential is like the primer charge which, when exploded by the flint striking the primer pan, ignites the much larger amount of powder within the barrel of the musket (analogous to the larger quantity of calcium released from the sarcoplasmic reticulum).

The First Mechanism: Electrical Coupling

The concept of an electrical signal that passes from the plasma membrane to cause calcium release from the sarcoplasmic reticulum follows logically from the well-known role of changing transmembrane potential to open voltage-dependent ion channels in the plasma membrane. Evidence for such an electrical triggering in the sarcoplasmic reticulum comes from the finding that permeant anions, such as chloride, which readily cross the sarcoplasmic reticulum membrane, can cause calcium release when added to calcium-filled sarcoplasmic reticulum vesicles equilibrated in solutions containing an impermeant anion like propionate (Endo, 1977). These effects of anion exchange have been attributed to transient depolarization of the sarcoplasmic reticulum caused by the rapid entry of negatively charged chloride ions; the resulting neutralization of a positive charge within the sarcoplasmic reticulum has been postulated to open calcium channels in this membrane (Figure 11.2A). At this time, however, these anion effects are better explained as being due to their role as counter ions. Thus electrical signaling is not likely to be important for this step in excitation-contraction coupling.

The Second Mechanism: Mechanical Coupling

The second mechanism proposed to explain the coupling between the cardiac action potential and calcium release from the sarcoplasmic reticulum involves a physical interaction between proteins in the membranes of the plasma membrane and t-system, and in the sarcoplasmic reticulum. According to this model, depolarization of the former shifts the position of a "voltage sensor" in the plasma membrane or t-tubule, immediately adjacent to the subsarcolemmal cisternae (Fig. 11.2B).

This mechanism is much less fanciful than once thought as movements of charged regions of voltage-gated ion channels are now known to initiate channel openings in the plasma membrane (Chapter 18). In fact, fast skeletal muscle t-tubules are a rich source of plasmalemmal calcium channels (dihydropyridine receptors), a finding that was initially puzzling because virtually no calcium currents are detected in these muscles. This conundrum has been resolved with the recognition that the role of the dihydropyridine receptors in skeletal muscle is not to mediate a voltage-dependent calcium flux into the cell; instead, the ability of these proteins to serve as voltage-sensors in response to a change in membrane potential (Chapter 18) probably opens the calcium release channel in the foot protein by a mechanism not unlike that depicted in Fig. 11.2B.

The Third Mechanism: Calcium-Triggered Calcium Release

The third possible trigger for calcium release from the sarcoplasmic reticulum is calcium itself. This mechanism postulates that the entry of a small amount of calcium across the plasma membrane, by binding to a calcium receptor at the cytosolic surface of the sarcoplasmic reticulum, induces the release of the much larger amount of activator calcium from the sarcoplasmic reticulum.

> Evidence for this important amplification of the calcium signal has come largely through the meticulous efforts of Fabiato (1983), who studied "skinned" muscle fibers (single cells from which the plasma membrane had been removed without damaging either the sarcoplasmic reticulum or contactile proteins). When a skinned fiber is presoaked in calcium and then placed briefly in a calcium-free solution, the sarcoplasmic reticulum remains filled with calcium. Subsequent addition of a minute amount of calcium, which by itself is too small to evoke a mechanical response, to the solution bathing the fiber, induces a brief contraction. The latter can be shown to have been initiated by the transient release of a larger quantity of the calcium from within the sarcoplasmic reticulum. In this manner, the effect of the small amount of added calcium is amplified to induce the much larger calcium release from the sarcoplasmic reticulum.

There is little doubt that calcium-triggered calcium release provides the most important mechanism that opens calcium release channels in the adult mammalian heart. This difference from the mechanical coupling that opens calcium channels in skeletal muscle provides another example of the ability of our cells to use the same, or similar, structures for different purposes. In skeletal muscle, a voltage-dependent shift in the S4 membrane-spanning of the plasma membrane calcium channel protein opens the channel; this shift, which is described in detail in Chapter 18, is mechanically coupled to the opening of the calcium release channel (Fig. 11.2B). In cardiac muscle, a similar voltage-dependent shift allows calcium to flow through the open plasma membrane calcium channel, thereby generating a chemical signal that opens the calcium release channels in the subsarcolemmal cisternae (Fig. 11.2C). Thus, as we have seen in other systems, different mechanisms are used in these two muscle types to couple the signal initiated by changing transmembrane potential to the opening of calcium release channels in the sarcoplasmic reticulum.

Calcium Release Channels

The past few years have witnessed a rapid growth in our knowledge of the proteins that mediate the release of the activator calcium that initiates and controls myocardial contractility. Supplementing traditional biochemical techniques, the modern tools of molecular biology are providing complete amino acid sequences of these proteins, and electrophysiological studies of single-channel molecules reconstituted into membrane bilayers have led to remarkably detailed functional characterizations of these channels.

Structure of Calcium Release Channels

As noted above, and in Chapter 1, the morphologically described foot protein, the ryanodine receptor, and the calcium release channel of the sarcoplasmic reticulum are all one and the same membrane protein. The calcium release channel is a tetrameric structure, each subunit of which includes a large cytosolic domain and an intramembranous domain that traverses the membrane of the subsarcolemmal cisternae (Block et al., 1988; Saito et al., 1988). The four subunits within the membrane bilayer of the subsarcolemmal cisternae surround a central channel that appears to connect with radial channels within each of the four projections of this molecule into the cytosol (Fig. 11.3). These structures have been proposed to represent the channels through which activator calcium is released to initiate muscle contraction.

The cytoplasmic portions of the calcium release channel, which project as the "feet" within the cytosolic space of the dyad between the subsarcolemmal cisternae and the t-tubule (Fig. 1.22), are closely related to the dihydropyridine receptor proteins (calcium channels) (Fig. 11.4). These plasmalemmal calcium channels, which are described in detail in Chapter 18, are also tetrameric structures. However, there appear to be only half as many calcium channels as foot protein molecules so that only alternate foot proteins are related to the structures that initiate calcium-triggered calcium release.

Elucidation of the complete amino acid sequence of the foot protein has shown that each subunit of this tetrameric protein has a molecular weight of 565,000, and contains four membrane-spanning domains and a huge cytosolic domain (Fig. 11.5). The former represents the stem and the latter the cap of each of the "mushrooms" depicted in Fig. 11.3. A calcium-binding site, probably located in the cytosolic domain of the foot protein, opens the calcium release channel after it interacts with calcium that enters the cytosol through the dihydropyridine receptor (the plasmalemmal calcium channel). The calcium release channel in cardiac muscle is slightly smaller than that of skeletal muscle and has the same topology as shown in Fig. 11.5; however, there is only about 66% identity of the amino acid sequences of these isoforms. The cardiac gene is located on chromosome 1, whereas the skeletal calcium release channel is encoded by a gene on chromosome 19 (Otsu et al., 1990).

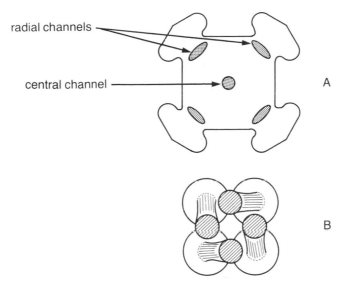

FIG. 11.3. Schematic representation of the calcium release channel (foot protein or ryanodine receptor) of the subsarcolemmal cisternae. A: Image based on negative staining data showing fourfold symmetry. The central channel, which is surrounded by four membrane-spanning sequences within the phospholipid bilayer, has been suggested to connect to four putative radial channels that lie in the "foot" (Fig. 1.22) seen on the cytoplasmic surface of this membrane; these channels are believed to deliver calcium for binding to troponin C. (Based on data of Saito et al., 1988.) B: Reconstruction of the foot protein shown in A, viewed from within the lumen of the subsarcolemmal cisternae, showing four subunits that resemble mushrooms. The putative central channel lies between the "stems" of the mushroom shaped structures, and four radial channels may empty through each of the "caps." (Based on data of Block et al., 1988.)

Recordings from Single Calcium Release Channels

The ability to reconstitute single ion channels into artificial phospholipid bilayers has added an entirely new dimension to the study of channel function. This approach, which provides detailed analyses of the opening and closing of single-channel molecules, is described in our discussion of the voltage-dependent ion channels of the plasma membrane (Chapter 18). In the case of the calcium release channels of the sarcoplasmic reticulum, this method has identified calcium-selective channels that are activated by adenosine triphosphate (ATP), calcium, and caffeine (the latter is a useful drug that opens sarcoplasmic reticulum calcium channels) (Rousseau et al., 1986).

Several types of calcium release channels have been found in the canine heart (Borgatta, 1991); these include "small" channels (defined as having a low slope conductance) that are opened by inositol triphosphate, a second messenger that is described in Chapter 12, rather than by caffeine. More fascinating is the finding that the caffeine-gated calcium release channels of the septum are smaller than those of the free wall, and that the septal channels open more slowly but remain open for a longer time. Thus, like so many other proteins, the calcium release channels are a family of isoforms.

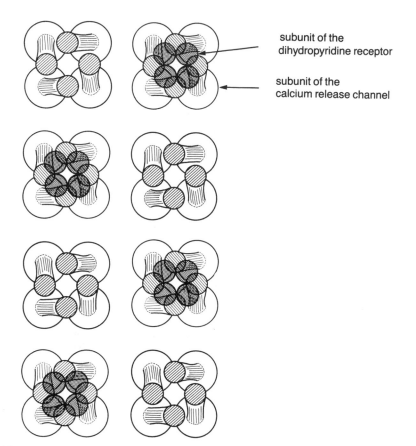

subunit of the
dihydropyridine receptor

subunit of the
calcium release channel

FIG. 11.4. Relationship between the calcium release channels of the subsarcolemmal cisternae (see Fig. 11.3) and the tetrameric calcium channels in the t-tubular membranes. Only half of the former are related to the plasmalemmal calcium channels. (Based on data of Block et al., 1988.)

FIG. 11.5. Structure of each subunit of the tetrameric calcium release channels (foot protein) in the membrane of the subsarcolemmal cisterna (*below*), showing four membrane-spanning regions and the large asymmetrical cytoplasmic domain. Shown is one of the foot proteins that relates to a dihydropyridine receptor (calcium channel) in the t-tubular membrane (*above*). Each of the mushroom-shaped subunits of the calcium release channel depicted in Fig. 11.3B corresponds to the structure shown in this figure, so that the tetrameric calcium release channel of the subsarcolemmal cisternae shown in Fig. 11.3A is made up of four of the subunits depicted in this figure. The dihydropyridine receptor within the t-tubular membrane also consists of four subunits, each of which contains six membrane-spanning helices; one of these membrane-spanning helices, (S4), which is rich in positively charged amino acids, is believed to be the voltage sensor that initiates a conformational change in the plasmalemmal calcium channel when this membrane is depolarized. (Redrawn from Takeshima et al., 1989.)

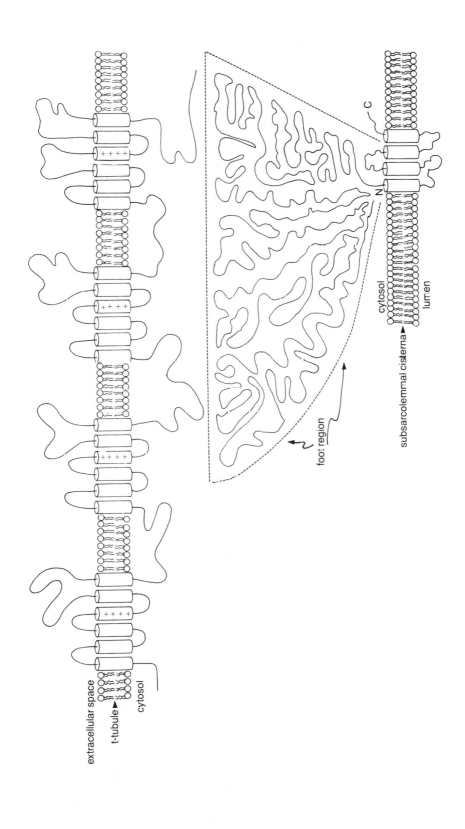

extracellular space

t-tubule

cytosol

+ + + +

foot region

cytosol

lumen

subsarcolemmal cisterna

N

C

Regulation of the Calcium Release Channel

Calcium release from skeletal muscle sarcoplasmic reticulum is inhibited by calcium, calmodulin-dependent phosphorylation, but neither calcium, calmodulin- nor cyclic AMP-dependent phosphorylation appears to influence the calcium release channel of cardiac muscle (Kim et al., 1987). However, the calcium-calmodulin complex itself markedly inhibits the cardiac calcium release channels; this inhibition is due to reduction of the mean open time of the channels, and not a change in channel conductance (Smith et al., 1989). This response provides a mechanism by which an excessive increase in cytosolic calcium can, in effect, shut down further calcium release from the sarcoplasmic reticulum. A different "safety mechanism" was described in Chapter 10, where the calcium-calmodulin complex was noted to stimulate the ATP-dependent calcium pump of the plasma membrane that removes calcium from the cytosol.

CALCIUM UPTAKE INTO THE SARCOPLASMIC RETICULUM

In contrast to excitation, which is mediated by the passive flux of calcium into the cytosol through highly regulated calcium release channels in the sarcoplasmic reticulum membrane, relaxation requires the active transport of this cation back into the sarcoplasmic reticulum. It is now apparent that this uphill process is effected by an ATP-dependent calcium pump that, like the plasmalemmal calcium pump described in Chapter 10, utilizes energy liberated by the hydrolysis of the high-energy phosphate bonds of ATP to perform the osmotic work in transporting calcium against its concentration gradient back into the sarcoplasmic reticulum.

The ability of the sarcoplasmic reticulum to transport calcium *in vitro* was discovered independently during the early 1960s by Hasselbach and Makinose, and by Ebashi and Lipmann, who described the ATP-dependent transport of calcium into microsomal vesicles prepared from cardiac and skeletal muscle. This discovery has an interesting history, for supernatants obtained after high-speed centrifugation of muscle minces had, for the previous decade, been recognized to have a relaxing effect on actomyosin that could be reversed by calcium. It was initially believed that these supernatants contained a "soluble" relaxing factor that was inactivated by calcium. However, it was soon found that these supernatant fractions contained tiny membrane vesicles, or microsomes, which took up calcium in the presence of ATP. The concurrent discovery by A. Weber that actin-myosin interactions were activated by micromolar concentrations of calcium led to the realization that calcium uptake into these membrane vesicles was, in fact, responsible for muscle relaxation. It is now known that this microsomal calcium transport system is derived from the sarcotubular network of the sarcoplasmic reticulum.

The calcium pump of the sarcoplasmic reticulum has a sufficiently high affinity for calcium to reduce cytosolic Ca^{2+} concentrations to levels low enough to dissociate this cation from its high-affinity binding sites on troponin C. In the resting heart, this is ~0.2 to 0.3 μM Ca^{2+}. The rate of calcium uptake is rapid enough to account for the observed rate of relaxation in the intact myocardium, and these membranes can retain sufficient calcium to activate the troponin in cardiac muscle. Furthermore, the calcium pump of cardiac sarcoplasmic reticulum vesicles is regulated in a manner that can explain important changes in the contractile properties of the heart that accompany the response to a variety of physiological, pharmacological, and pathological influences.

Structure of the Sarcoplasmic Reticulum Calcium Pump

The calcium pump of the sarcoplasmic reticulum, like that of the plasma membrane (Chapter 10) is a member of a family of P-type ion pumps that couples the hydrolysis of the terminal phosphate of ATP to active ion transport (Fig. 10.3). The sarcoplasmic reticulum calcium pump is smaller than that of the plasma membrane, having a molecular weight of $\sim$110,000. At the present time, three genes are known to encode at least five isoforms of this important protein (Table 11.1). The gene for the fast-twitch protein can encode two alternatively spliced isoforms, one is found in adult skeletal muscle, the other in neonatal muscle. A second gene encodes two additional isoforms, also by alternate splicing; one is found in cardiac and slow-twitch muscle, the other in the endoplasmic reticulum of smooth muscle and non-muscle tissues (Zarain-Herzberg et al., 1990). The third gene encodes calcium pump ATPase proteins in a diverse range of tissues, including heart, skeletal muscle, uterus, brain, lung, liver, kidney, intestine, pancreas, and testis.

Recent structural information regarding the calcium pump ATPase of the sarcoplasmic reticulum is summarized in Fig. 11.6; this depiction differs from that of the plasmalemmal calcium pump (Fig. 10.3) in that the cytoplasmic surface is shown as above the bilayer and more detail is provided as to the interactions between the cytoplasmic loops and the sites for ATP binding and phosphoenzyme formation. The calcium-binding site itself appears to involve charged amino acid residues within the transmembrane domain of the protein, possibly in the three intramembranous segments M4, M5, and M7 (Clarke et al., 1990).

Although there is a great deal of physical evidence to suggest that the calcium pump ATPase functions as a dimer, most of the pump reactions—including occlusion of calcium—have been seen in detergent solubilized monomers of this pump (Andersen, 1989). Furthermore, no channel openings analogous to that shown for

TABLE 11.1. Genes encoding isoforms of the sarcoplasmic and endoplasmic reticulum calcium pumps

SERCA1[a]	Fast-twitch isoforms
SERCA1a	Adult skeletal
SERCA1b	Neonatal skeletal
SERCA2	Slow-twitch/cardiac isoforms
SERCA2a	Cardiac and slow skeletal isoforms
SERCA2b	Smooth muscle and nonmuscle isoforms
SERCA3	Muscle and nonmuscle isoforms

[a]SERCA: Sarco(endo)plasmic reticulum Ca^{2+}-ATPase

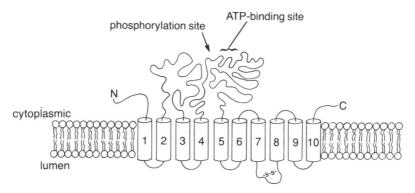

FIG. 11.6. Depiction of the calcium pump ATPase showing ten membrane-spanning segments (M1–M10) and two large cytoplasmic loops. The latter forms the large projections of the protein shown in Fig. 11.1. The phosphorylation site and the site for ATP binding are both found on the large cytoplasmic loop between M4 and M5. The extracellular loop between M7 and M8 contains a disulfide bridge. Polar amino acids in the membrane-spanning loops M4, M5, M6, and M8 may participate in calcium binding and transfer across the bilayer.

the calcium release channel (Fig. 11.3A) have been found, suggesting that calcium is translocated while bound to the pump, as has also been postulated for the sodium pump (Chapter 10). A fundamental difference between ATP-dependent transloca-tion of calcium bound to the pump protein and calcium flux through a preformed channel is consistent with the much slower rate of calcium pumping than calcium flux through a channel (see below).

Reaction Mechanism of the Sarcoplasmic Reticulum Calcium Pump

The coupling of ATP hydrolysis to active ion transport by the sarcoplasmic retic-ulum calcium pump is quite similar to that of the sodium pump described in Chap-ter 10, which also utilizes the energy of the terminal high-energy phosphate bond of ATP to perform osmotic work. In many ways, the interactions of calcium with the sarcoplasmic reticulum calcium pump are analogous to those of sodium with the plasmalemmal sodium pump except that the former does not transport a counter-ion analogous to potassium.

The flux of positively charged calcium ions across the sarcoplasmic reticulum membrane would be expected to generate an electrical current. However, because the sarcoplasmic reticulum is permeable to a variety of anions, concurrent move-ments of chloride and phosphate anions prevent the development of a transmem-brane potential.

The anion permeability of the sarcoplasmic reticulum is useful in studies of calcium transport by vesicles derived from these membranes. Inclusion of calcium-precipitat-ing anions like oxalate and phosphate during calcium pump reactions *in vitro* greatly increases the amount of calcium taken up by the isolated vesicles. This is due simply to the ability of these anions to form precipitates with the calcium transported into the vesicles, thereby preventing intravesicular Ca^{2+} concentration from rising to high levels that inhibit the pump.

The reaction sequence of the calcium pump shown in Eq. 11.1 is quite similar to that of the sodium pump in Eq. 10.2.

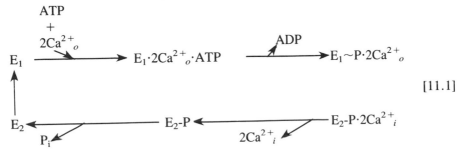

$$[11.1]$$

The subscripts o and i refer to the cytosol, outside the sarcoplasmic reticulum, and the internal lumen of the intracellular membrane system respectively. The designations E_1, E_2, E_1P, and E_2P refer to reaction intermediates analogous to those of the sodium pump: E_1 and E_1P are high-energy intermediates, whereas in E_2 and E_2P energy has been utilized for the uphill movement of calcium. Magnesium is essential for this reaction, but its involvement has been omitted for clarity and simplicity.

A sketch that attempts to provide physical meaning to Eq. 11.1 is presented in Fig. 11.7. In this model, E_1 is labeled E, and E_2 is *E. The functional unit, shown in Fig. 11.7 as a dimer, is likely to be a monomer (see below). Binding of calcium to a site within the membrane bilayer is, however, in accord with current evidence.

The Steps of the Calcium Pump Reaction Mechanism

The initial step in the calcium pump ATPase reaction sequence, like that for the Na-K-ATPase (Eq. 10.3), begins when calcium and ATP bind to the enzyme according to the reaction:

$$E_1 + 2\,Ca^{2+}_o + ATP \rightarrow E \cdot 2Ca^{2+}_o \cdot ATP. \qquad [11.2]$$

It is important to keep in mind that cytosolic Ca^{2+} concentration is very low, so that this step requires that calcium bind to high-affinity sites on the calcium pump.

The initial step of calcium and ATP binding is followed by release of adenosine diphosphate (ADP) and the transfer of the terminal high-energy phosphate of ATP, along with its chemical energy, to the calcium pump ATPase protein through formation of the high-energy acyl phosphoprotein E_1P:

$$E \cdot 2Ca^{2+}_o \cdot ATP \rightarrow E_1 {\sim} P \cdot 2Ca^{2+}_o + ADP. \qquad [11.3]$$

At this step the calcium bound to the enzyme can no longer exchange with free cytosolic Ca^{2+}, and so is referred to as "occluded" calcium. Although nonex-

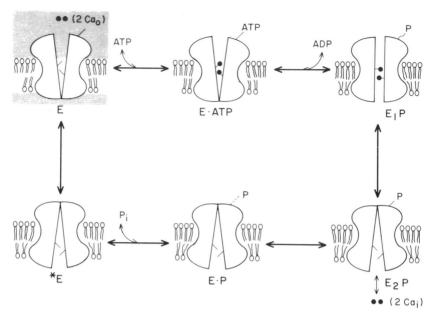

FIG. 11.7. Schematic representation of the calcium pump ATPase reaction showing the movement of two calcium ions (o) between the aqueous spaces on the two sides of the sarcoplasmic reticulum membrane (*shaded, upper left*). The cytosolic side of the membrane is *above* and the interior of the sarcoplasmic reticulum is *below* the bilayer. This figure corresponds to Eq. 11.1 except that E_1 is labeled E, and E_2 is *E. The functional unit of the calcium pump, depicted here as a dimer, is likely to be a monomer.

changeable, the occluded calcium probably remains at the low activity of the cytosolic calcium. Because Eq. 11.3 is reversible (like all of these reaction steps, see below), the high-energy phosphorylated intermediate, $E_1{\sim}P{\cdot}2Ca^{2+}{}_o$, is able to transfer its energy to ADP; as the breakdown of this intermediate is accelerated by ADP, E_iP is referred to as an ADP-sensitive phosphoenzyme.

The next step, in which the enzyme-bound calcium is "lifted" to the higher activity within the sarcoplasmic reticulum, takes place in a reaction where the enzyme-bound phosphate in $E_1{\sim}P$ loses its energy in forming the low-energy intermediate, E_2-P. The energy made available in this step is transferred to the bound calcium, which has thus been "pumped" into the region of high Ca^{2+} concentration in the lumen of the sarcoplasmic reticulum.

$$E_1{\sim}P{\cdot}2Ca^{2+}{}_o \rightarrow E_2\text{-}P{\cdot}2Ca^{2+}{}_i. \qquad [11.4]$$

As E_2-P can no longer react with ADP, this is an "ADP-insensitive" phosphoenzyme.

The mechanisms responsible for the energy transduction that occurs at this critical step in active transport remains unclear. Energy transduction may involve interactions with magnesium that play a role in calcium transport analogous to that of potassium in sodium transport (Suko et al., 1981; Takisawa and Tonomura, 1979). A large entropy change may also be of importance in this transport process (deMeis et al., 1982).

The energy transduction that takes place in the reaction described in Eq. 11.4 is followed by the release of calcium, now at the higher activity within the sarcoplasmic reticulum, according to the reaction:

$$E_2\text{-}P\cdot2Ca^{2+}{}_i \rightarrow E_2\text{-}P + 2Ca^{2+}{}_i. \qquad [11.5]$$

The breakdown of the E_2P complex then proceeds with the release of bound phosphate and the appearance of nonphosphorylated E_2:

$$E_2\text{-}P \rightarrow E_2 + P_i. \qquad [11.6]$$

As was true for the sodium pump reaction, the E_2 intermediate differs from that of E_1, the nonphosphorylated enzyme at the start of the reaction. Thus completion of the calcium pump cycle requires the conversion of E_2 to E_1:

$$E_2 \rightarrow E_1. \qquad [11.7]$$

The overall reaction of the calcium pump ATPase can therefore be written:

$$2Ca^{2+}{}_o + ATP \xrightarrow{E} 2Ca^{2+}{}_i + ADP + P_i. \qquad [11.8]$$

The rate-limiting step in calcium pump turnover *in vitro* is generally agreed to occur at one of the steps of EP degradation, possibly the transition from $E_1\text{-}P\cdot2Ca^{2+}{}_o$ to $E_2\text{-}P + 2Ca^{2+}{}_i$ (Eqs. 11.4 and 11.5). In the intact heart, however, $[Ca^{2+}]_o$ is rate limiting during diastole, whereas during systole calcium transport rate is probably determined by the $E_1P \rightarrow E_2P$ transition.

Reversal of the Calcium Pump Reaction

All of the steps in the calcium pump ATPase reaction, like those of the Na-K-ATPase, are reversible. Thus, when the calcium pump is made to run backward, the energy of the calcium gradient across the sarcoplasmic reticulum is coupled to the synthesis of ATP from ADP and P_i in a manner that is analogous to the chemiosmotic synthesis of ATP during oxidative phosphorylation (Chapter 5). However, special conditions are needed to run the calcium pump in reverse: *all* of the following must be met: high $Ca^{2+}{}_i$, ADP, and P_i; low $Ca^{2+}{}_o$ and ATP. Although these conditions allow downhill calcium efflux from the sarcoplasmic reticulum to be coupled to the synthesis of high-energy phosphate bonds, they are highly artificial and not found in normal muscle; for this reason, "pump reversal" is an interesting *in vitro* phenomenon that probably has no role in muscle physiology.

Differences Between Cardiac and Skeletal Sarcoplasmic Reticulum

The overall reaction mechanism for calcium transport by fast skeletal sarcoplasmic reticulum is the same as that of cardiac muscle except that the calcium sensitivity of the cardiac pump is less than that of skeletal sarcoplasmic reticulum

(Shigekawa et al., 1976). This difference, however, is due to the effects of phospholamban, a regulatory protein that is present in cardiac, but not fast skeletal muscle, sarcoplasmic reticulum (see below). The content of the calcium pump ATPase protein in the cardiac sarcoplasmic reticulum, which as noted above (Table 11.1) is a different gene product than the fast skeletal muscle calcium pump, is also less than in the skeletal muscle membrane.

Regulatory Effects of ATP

As already described for many other systems, ATP has a dual effect on calcium transport by cardiac and skeletal sarcoplasmic reticulum. Low concentrations of ATP represent the substrate for calcium transport, whereas at higher concentrations this nucleotide stimulates the calcium pump (Shigekawa et al., 1978). These effects reflect the presence of two types of ATP-binding sites in these membranes (Nakamura and Tonomura, 1982): a *high-affinity catalytic site*, which is half-saturated at micromolar ATP concentrations, and a *low-affinity regulatory site*, which is half-saturated at ATP concentrations of about 100 μM. The regulatory sites, which appear to stimulate calcium transport by accelerating the conversion of E_1P to E_2P (Scofano et al., 1979), may play a role in slowing relaxation when ATP levels fall in an energy-starved heart (see Chapters 24 and 25).

Retention of Calcium Within the Sarcoplasmic Reticulum

Although much of the calcium taken up by the sarcoplasmic reticulum is stored in the free, ionized form, some is associated with several calcium-binding proteins within these membranes. Most important is *calsequestrin*, a 45,000 dalton that traps calcium within this membrane system. Cardiac muscle calsequestrin is slightly smaller than the skeletal muscle isoform (Scott et al., 1988), neither contains the high-affinity (E-F hand) calcium-binding domain that is characteristic of the family of calcium-binding proteins described in Chapter 7. Other calcium-binding proteins found in smaller amounts include the 44,000 dalton protein *calreticulin* and a 170,000 dalton, *histidine-rich calcium-binding protein* that may also help to retain calcium within the sarcoplasmic reticulum; a 26,000 dalton protein appears to play an as-yet-undefined role in the interactions between calcium and calsequestrin in the terminal cisternae (Mitchell et al., 1988). All of the calcium-binding proteins are concentrated in the terminal cisternae of skeletal muscle sarcoplasmic reticulum, where they maintain a calcium store that is readily released through the calcium release channels during excitation-contraction coupling. Some of the calcium within this membrane system may be bound to the anionic head groups of phospholipids; however, these components of the bilayer have a low affinity for calcium.

Two glycoproteins having molecular weights of 53,000 and 160,000 (*sarcalumenin*), which are derived by alternate splicing from the same gene, have been found in skeletal sarcoplasmic reticulum; these proteins may be involved in the transfer of calcium from the sarcotubular network back to the subsarcolemmal cisternae (Leberer et al., 1990). Enzymes that catalyze the reactions of glycogenolysis and glycolysis co-purify with sarcoplasmic reticulum membrane preparations *in vitro*. The significance of these proteins remains poorly understood; they could be contaminants, but their association with these calcium transporting membranes might be related to an apparent special role for "glycolytic" ATP (see Chapter 5).

"Calcium Uptake" and "Calcium Binding"

Understanding of the reactions of isolated sarcoplasmic reticulum vesicles *in vitro* has been confounded by two terms: calcium uptake and calcium binding. Although seemingly appropriate when introduced over 20 years ago, they are now known to be misleading.

Calcium binding: Because high Ca^{2+} concentrations within the sarcoplasmic reticulum markedly inhibit ATP-supported calcium transport, only small amounts of calcium are taken up by vesicles prepared from the sarcotubular network, which do not contain calcium-binding proteins. This very limited calcium transport was initially called *calcium binding*; however, this term is a misnomer as most of the calcium associated with the vesicles under these conditions is free. In fact, the amount of calcium retained by isolated sarcoplasmic reticulum vesicles under these conditions is determined largely by the relative rates of calcium influx and efflux in the rapid exchange reaction catalyzed by the reaction shown in Eq. 11.4 (Takenaka et al., 1982). *Calcium uptake*: Calcium transport by sarcoplasmic reticulum vesicles *in vitro* is greatly increased in the presence of a calcium-precipitating anion such as oxalate or phosphate. This enhanced calcium transport (often called *calcium uptake*) reflects the ability of these anions to precipitate the calcium taken up by sarcoplasmic reticulum vesicles, and thus to maintain a low internal Ca^{2+} concentration. By preventing high Ca^{2+} concentrations within the sarcoplasmic reticulum from inhibiting the calcium pump, calcium-precipitating anions greatly increase the amount of this cation that can be taken up by this membrane system.

Energetic Implications of the Active and Passive Calcium Fluxes Involved in the Regulation of Contraction

The fact that the delivery of activator calcium to the contractile proteins is a passive, downhill process, whereas relaxation requires that calcium be actively transported against a concentration gradient, has important consequences, especially when the ability of the myocardium to generate energy becomes impaired. These consequences of energy starvation reflect the fact that activation is a passive process in which calcium diffuses through membrane channels from the extracellular space and sarcoplasmic reticulum, where Ca^{2+} concentration is in the millimolar range; into the cytosol, where Ca^{2+} concentration is ~ 0.2 μM. These downhill fluxes of activator calcium are extremely rapid; for example, calcium entry via a single plasmalemmal calcium channel has been estimated to be $\sim 3,000,000$ ions per second (Tsien, 1983). In contrast, the ATP-dependent calcium pumps that are largely responsible for relaxation are much slower; for example, the maximal flux of calcium through a single calcium pump site of the sarcoplasmic reticulum at 37° is ~30 ions per second (Katz, 1986), or 1/100,000 the rate of calcium entry through a calcium channel.

Estimates of the relative rates of the calcium fluxes that effect relaxation and those that activate the heart (Table 11.2), although only crude estimates, reveal a precarious situation that may help to explain why the energy-starved heart is susceptible to calcium overload. This is because the maximal rate at which calcium can be removed from the cytosol to relax the heart is about an order of magnitude slower than that of the calcium fluxes during activation. The reason for this disparity is simply that diffusion is so much faster than active transport that even the densely packed calcium pump proteins in the sarcoplasmic reticulum membrane (Figure 11.1), which resemble the army of terra-cotta soldiers in the underground tombs of Xian, cannot overcome the ~100,000-fold greater rate of diffusion through the limited number of channels that allow calcium to enter the cytosol.

Probably the most accurate representation of the balance between the calcium fluxes during activation and relaxation is presented in line K of Table 11.2. As calcium efflux via the calcium pump is highly dependent on cytosolic Ca^{2+} concen-

TABLE 11.2. *Balances between calcium fluxes during activation and relaxation in the myocardium*

Activation	
A. Plasmalemmal dihydropyridine receptors/cell[a]	90,000
B. Functional plasmalemmal calcium channels/cell[b]	2,500
C. Sarcoplasmic reticulum calcium release channels/cell[c]	11,500
D. Total calcium channels/cell (B + C)	14,000
E. Rate of calcium flux through a calcium channel[d]	3×10^6 ions/sec
F. Maximal calcium entry/cell during systole (D × E)	4×10^{10} ions/sec
Relaxation	
G. Sarcoplasmic reticulum calcium pump sites/cell[a]	166,000,000
H. Rate of calcium transport during relaxation[e]	30 ions/sec
I. Maximal calcium removal/cell during diastole (G × H)[f]	5×10^9 ions/sec
J. Ratio *Maximal rate of calcium entry during systole* / *Maximal rate of calcium removal during diastole*	~8 (~6)[g]
K. Ratio *Maximal rate of calcium entry during systole* / *Average rate of calcium removal during diastole*[h]	~16 (~13)[g]

[a]From Swynghedauw (1990).

[b]Assumes 3% of dihydropyridine receptors are functional calcium channels (Schwartz et al., 1985).

[c]Assumes one (tetrameric) calcium release channel/8 dihydropyridine receptors.

[d]From Tsien (1983).

[e]Estimated by Katz (1986) from data of Shigekawa et al. (1976).

[f]This estimate ignores plasmalemmal calcium pumps and sodium/calcium exchange. Assuming that calcium efflux via the latter equals calcium influx across the plasma membrane, which contains ~20% of the total calcium channels (B/B + C), would add only ~20% to the maximal rate of calcium efflux from the cytosol.

[g]Corrected for plasma membrane calcium efflux (see footnote f).

[h]Assumes that, because $[Ca^{2+}]_i$ decreases during diastole, the *average* rate of calcium efflux is 50% of the *maximal* rate of the calcium pump.

tration, this line assumes that this pump operates at half-maximal velocity during relaxation of the heart. This seems reasonable as the calcium pump operates near 50% of its maximal velocity at Ca^{2+} concentrations in the range of $1\mu M$, where tension developed by the cardiac contractile proteins remains high.

> Table 11.2 assumes that Ca^{2+} concentration outside the cytosol does not change during the cardiac cycle, and that calcium flux through the heart's calcium channels is independent of changes in cytosolic Ca^{2+} concentration because the ~10,000-fold calcium gradient is like a waterfall. This table also does not take into account the fact that activation is much briefer than relaxation, which is, of course, the reason that the heart is able to remain at a steady state in which the normal oscillations in cytosolic calcium content do not led to a net gain in this cytotoxic cation.

Regulation of Calcium Transport by the Cardiac Sarcoplasmic Reticulum

Variations in the rate and extent of calcium transport by the sarcoplasmic reticulum play an important role in cardiac regulation. The most important regulator of this calcium pump is calcium itself. Calcium transport is quite sensitive to changing cystolic Ca^{2+} concentration due largely to the role of calcium as a substrate for the reaction shown in Eq. 11.2, which is probably rate limiting in the resting heart. Calcium has a second action to stimulate this calcium pump that is mediated by a calcium, calmodulin-dependent protein kinase (see below). Slowing of this ion pump by a small deficit in myocardial ATP supply, due to attenuation of the allosteric stimulation by ATP, may play a role in abnormal states where the heart is in an energy-starved state (Chapters 24 and 25).

Phospholamban

The response of the heart to the sympathetic nervous system, which from a physiological standpoint is one of the most important components of the cardiovascular adjustment to exercise, includes an important change in the calcium pump of the sarcoplasmic reticulum. This response is mediated by cyclic AMP, the intracellular second messenger that appears in cells when they are stimulated by a variety of agents, including the β-adrenergic agonists and glucagon, that activate adenylyl cyclase. Phosphodiesterase inhibitors, which inhibit cyclic AMP breakdown (Chapter 12), also stimulate the calcium pump. The signal initiated by increased cytosolic levels of cyclic AMP is mediated by a protein called *phospholamban*, which serves as a substrate for several protein kinases, including that stimulated by the calcium-calmodulin complex (Tada and Katz, 1982).

Phospholamban, like the C-terminal portion of the plasmalemmal calcium pump ATPase discussed in Chapter 10, inhibits the basal rate of calcium transport by cardiac sarcoplasmic reticulum. In the heart, this inhibition is reversed when phospholamban is phosphorylated by either cyclic AMP– or calcium, calmodulin-dependent protein kinase. The inhibitory effect reappears when phospholamban is dephosphorylated by one of a number of phosphoprotein phosphatases.

Like so many forms of regulation, the effects of cyclic AMP are indirect, involving a protein that is not directly involved in the function that is modified. In another response to β-adrenergic agonists, protein kinase A alters the calcium sensitivity of the cardiac contractile proteins by phosphorylating troponin I, rather than troponin C, the actual calcium receptor (Chapter 7). This principle is clearly seen in the cardiac sarcoplasmic reticulum, where the substrate for protein kinase A is not the calcium pump ATPase protein, but a separate protein: phospholamban. Evidence that phospholamban represents a part of the primitive calcium pump ATPase that has split off from the parent protein, to be encoded by a different gene (Chapter 10) provides a fascinating clue as to how some of these regulatory systems may have evolved.

Structure of Phospholamban

Phospholamban is found in cardiac, slow skeletal, and smooth muscle, but is absent in fast skeletal muscle where regulation is organized in the central nervous system rather than by changes in the biochemistry of the muscle (Chapter 13). Phospholamban is a pentamer made up of five identical subunits having molecular weights of 6,000 (Fujii et al., 1987), slow skeletal muscle phospholamban is identical to that of the heart, but smooth muscle phospholamban appears to be slightly different (Watras, 1988).

The C-terminal domain of phospholamban is hydrophobic and lies within the sarcoplasmic reticulum membrane bilayer, whereas the N-terminal region contains two sites that, when phosphorylated, stimulate calcium transport. The substrate for cyclic AMP–dependent phosphorylation is serine at position 16, whereas threonine at position 17 is phosphorylated by calcium, calmodulin-dependent protein kinase (Fujii et al., 1989). The bond formed in these phosphorylation reactions is a phosphoester which, as described in Chapter 8, differs from the acyl phosphate intermediates of the calcium pump described earlier in this chapter.

Regulation of the Calcium Pump of the Cardiac Sarcoplasmic Reticulum by Cyclic AMP–Dependent Phosphorylation of Phospholamban

Phosphorylation of phospholamban by cyclic AMP–dependent protein kinase increases the rate of calcium transport by effects on several steps in the reaction mechanism shown in Eq. 11.1; these include both an increase in the calcium sensitivity of the cardiac calcium pump and acceleration of the rate of the overall calcium pump cycle (Hicks et al., 1979). Increased turnover of the cardiac sarcoplasmic reticulum calcium pump when phospholamban is phosphorylated is associated with acceleration of both the formation of E_1 from E_2 (Eq. 11.5) and the $E_1P{\rightarrow}E_2P$ transition (Eq. 11.3) (Tada et al., 1983). The effect of phospholamban phosphorylation to increase the calcium sensitivity of the calcium pump is accompanied by the loss of a positive cooperativity for the binding of the two $Ca^{2+}{}_o$ to the enzyme (Eq. 11.2) seen when phospholamban is in its dephospho- form. Together, accelerated turnover and increased calcium sensitivity of the calcium pump facilitate relaxation when the heart comes under the influence of β-adrenergic agonists.

Phosphorylation of phospholamban causes the calcium sensitivity of calcium uptake to resemble that of skeletal sarcoplasmic reticulum, which lacks phospholamban (Hicks et al., 1979); recent direct evidence that the dephospho- form of phospholamban inhibits the calcium pump (Inui et al., 1986; James et al., 1990) provides further support for the model of the interaction between phospholamban and the calcium pump shown in Fig. 11.8. Dephospho-phospholamban is probably an inhibitor of the calcium pump of cardiac sarcoplasmic reticulum, whereas phosphorylation of this regulatory protein reverses this inhibitory effect.

Phosphorylation of phospholamban probably increases the calcium content of the heart's sarcoplasmic reticulum by favoring calcium retention in intracellular stores at the expense of calcium efflux via the plasma membrane calcium pump and sodium/calcium exchange. This would allow cyclic AMP not only to promote relaxation by accelerating calcium transport into the sarcoplasmic reticulum (7A in Fig. 11.9), but also to increase myocardial contractility by retaining calcium within the myocardial cell (7B in Fig. 11.9).

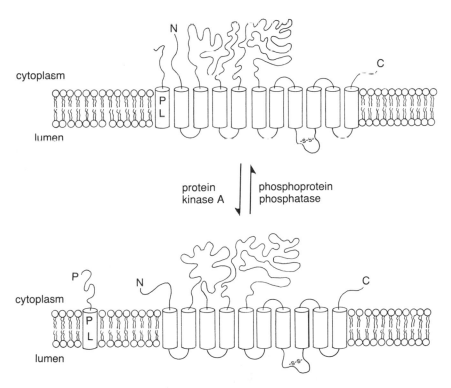

FIG. 11.8. Schematic representation of the effects of phospholamban (PL) on the calcium pump of the cardiac sarcoplasmic reticulum. *Top*: Phospholamban in the dephosphorylated form interacts with the calcium pump so as to decrease the calcium sensitivity of calcium transport and slow its turnover. *Bottom*: Phosphorylation of phospholamban, probably by dissociating this regulatory protein from the calcium pump, accelerates calcium transport by abolishing these effects.

Effects of Catecholamines on the Cardiac Sarcoplasmic Reticulum

1. Catecholamine Binding to the Sarcolemmal β-Receptor
   ↓
2. Activation of Adenylyl Cyclase
   ↓
3. Increased Intracellular Cyclic AMP
   ↓
4. Activation of Cyclic AMP-Dependent Protein Kinase
   ↓
5. Phosphorylation of Phospholamban
   ↓
6. Increased Ca^{2+} - Sensitivity and Acceleration of the Calcium Pump
   ⋀
7A: Accelerated Calcium Transport   7B: Increased Calcium Stores

FIG. 11.9. Cascade of reactions by which β-adrenergic agonists modify calcium transport by the sarcoplasmic reticulum so as to regulate the mechanical properties of the heart.

The physiological importance of the cascade initiated by the binding of the β-adrenergic agonists to their plasma membrane receptors (Fig. 11.9) reflects a powerful effect of sympathetic stimulation to increase heart rate and myocardial contractility. This physiological response not only increases the amount of calcium released during excitation-contraction coupling (see Chapter 14), but also shortens diastole, during which calcium is pumped back into the sarcoplasmic reticulum. Mechanisms that increase heart rate abbreviate each cardiac cycle, which shortens diastole more than systole, thereby tending to impair the ability of the ventricle to fill. Because the reserve of the calcium fluxes that effect relaxation is more "precarious" than that of the systolic calcium fluxes (Table 11.2), it is not surprising that the heart has evolved a number of mechanisms that accelerate relaxation when the heart is driven by sympathetic stimulation. The increased rate of calcium transport and increased calcium sensitivity of calcium transport into the cardiac sarcoplasmic reticulum help the heart to fill during β-adrenergic stimulation. These responses are essential in maintaining a high cardiac output during intense sympathetic activity, such as normally occurs during exercise.

Regulation of the Calcium Pump of the Cardiac Sarcoplasmic Reticulum by Calcium, Calmodulin-Dependent Phosphorylation of Phospholamban

Phospholamban is also phosphorylated by a protein kinase whose activity is stimulated by the calcium-calmodulin complex. This phosphorylation reaction, like that catalyzed by protein kinase A, stimulates calcium uptake by cardiac sarcoplasmic reticulum vesicles *in vitro*. Although the physiological significance of this stimulation of calcium transport is not clear, it appears that calcium, calmodulin-dependent phosphorylation occurs in the intact heart when cyclic AMP levels are high (Wegener et al., 1989). A cooperative interaction with cyclic AMP thus appears to accelerate the removal of activator calcium in the intact heart, and so facilitate calcium removal from the cytosol of the heart when calcium entry is increased during sympathetic stimulation.

Regulation of the Calcium Pump of the Cardiac Sarcoplasmic Reticulum by
Protein Kinase C–Dependent Phosphorylation of Phospholamban

Phospholamban can also be phosphorylated *in vitro* by a phospholipid-dependent protein kinase (Movsesian et al., 1984). This enzyme, called *protein kinase C*, is activated when calcium is present along with diacylglycerol, one of the products of phosphatidylinositol hydrolysis (Chapter 12). A role for this reaction in regulation of cardiac function has not yet been defined, however.

Phosphoprotein Phosphatases

In order for the phosphorylation of phospholamban to play a physiological role in the regulation of myocardial function, a mechanism must exist to "turn off" the signal initiated by this phosphorylation reaction; in other words, a system is also needed to dephosphorylate this protein. This requirement is filled by another class of enzymes, the *phosphoprotein phosphatases*, which hydrolyze the phosphoester bonds formed by the protein kinases according to the general reaction:

$$\text{Protein} + \text{ATP} \xrightarrow{\substack{\text{Protein} \\ \text{kinase}}} \text{Protein-P} \xrightarrow{\substack{\text{Phosphoprotein} \\ \text{phosphatase}}} \text{Protein} + P_i.$$

The phosphoprotein phosphatases are a diverse and complex group of highly regulated enzymes. As their ability to dephosphorylate the many phosphoesters in the cell can modify a wide range of activities, intricate control systems have evolved for the inhibitory regulation of the phosphoprotein phosphatases. It has been suggested that these systems, whose complexity and diversity are beyond the scope of this text, protect the cell from the accidental activation of "a hydrolytic enzyme that would create havoc within the cell if allowed to operate unchecked" (Villa-Moruzzi et al., 1984).

A number of phosphoprotein phosphatases can dephosphorylate phospholamban. One such enzyme, which has been purified from cardiac cytosol, is a heterotrimer made up of three subunits having molecular weights of 63,000, 55,000, and 38,000; this enzyme has been designated as a phospholamban phosphatase (Kranias et al., 1988).

MITOCHONDRIA

The well-known ability of mitochondria to take up large amounts of calcium led to the hypothesis that mitochondrial calcium transport and release might play a role in cardiac excitation-contraction coupling and the regulation of myocardial contractility. However, the calcium affinity of the mitochondrial calcium pump is low, and the rate of calcium transport is slow at physiological cytosolic Ca^{2+} concentrations

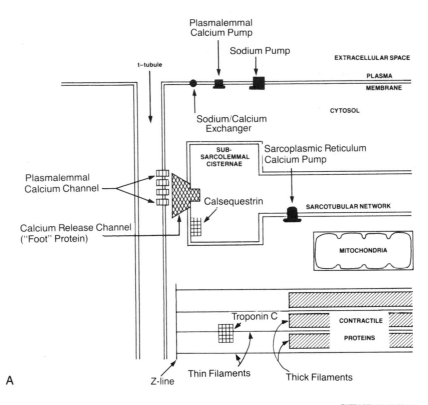

A

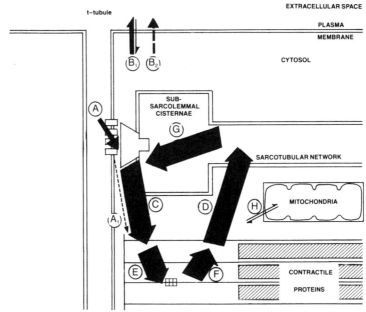

B

(Ebashi et al., 1978); for these reasons, it is unlikely that these structures normally play a role in the calcium fluxes involved in excitation-contraction coupling. As the uptake and release of calcium by the mitochondria are in dynamic equilibrium with cytosolic calcium (Williamson et al., 1983), the mitochondria can "buffer" cytosolic calcium and so protect the myocardium from the detrimental effects of calcium overload when abnormally large amounts of this ion gain access to the cytosol. Mitochondrial calcium uptake and storage may blunt the calcium overloading that occurs in pathological states such as myocardial ischemia. It must be remembered, however, that calcium loading of mitochondria inhibits their capacity to participate in oxidative phosphorylation (see Chapter 5).

CALCIUM FLUXES DURING EXCITATION-CONTRACTION COUPLING

The data reviewed in this and the previous chapters allow the calcium fluxes involved in excitation-contraction coupling to be understood in terms of the movement of this ion between five pools, or compartments, within the heart. These are the *extracellular space*, the *sarcoplasmic reticulum*, the *cytosol*, *troponin*, and the *mitochondria* (Figure 11.10). Movements of calcium between these pools are responsible for the initiation and termination of the contractile event; in addition, these calcium fluxes play a major role in regulating the intensity of tension development and shortening in the heart.

The diagram in Figure 11.10 illustrates both transsarcolemmal and "internal" circulations of calcium. As shown by the thicknesses of the arrows in this figure, the amount of calcium that moves within the cell is much greater than that which enters and leaves the cell with each cardiac cycle. Thus, in the mammalian heart, the amount of calcium that enters the cytosol via the slow (calcium) channels in the

---

FIG. 11.10. Schematic diagram showing **(A)** key structures and **(B)** major calcium fluxes involved in cardiac excitation-contraction coupling. The thickness of the *arrows* indicates the magnitude of the calcium fluxes, and their directions describe the "energetics" of the calcium fluxes: *downward arrows* describe passive calcium fluxes and *upward arrows* describe energy-dependent calcium transport. Calcium enters the cell from the extracellular fluid via plasmalemmal calcium channels (A); although most of this calcium triggers calcium release from the sarcoplasmic reticulum, a small portion directly activates the contractile proteins (A_1). Calcium transport back into the extracellular fluid involves two plasma membrane systems: sodium/calcium exchange (B_1), and the plasmalemmal calcium pump (B_2). The sarcoplasmic reticulum membrane regulates two calcium fluxes: calcium release from the subsarcolemmal cisternae (C), and active calcium uptake by the calcium pump of the sarcotubular network (D). Calcium diffuses within the sarcoplasmic reticulum in a third calcium flux (G), returning to the subsarcolemmal cisternae where it is stored in complex with calsequestrin and other calcium-binding proteins. Binding (E) and dissociation (F) of calcium with the high-affinity calcium-binding sites of troponin C define its affinity for calcium, which is the ratio E:F. Movements of calcium into and out of mitochondria (H) buffer cytosolic Ca^{2+} concentration.

plasma membrane is only a fraction of the total amount of calcium liberated into the cytosol during excitation-contraction coupling (Table 11.2).

> The functional significance of the circulation of calcium within the myocardial cell is seen in the quotation that heads Chapter 10. This is simply to shorten the distances this ion must move to provide for the rapid onset of both systole and diastole essential in the hearts of warm-blooded animals.

The calcium fluxes depicted in Figure 11.10 serve as the basis for our subsequent discussion of the regulation of myocardial contractility (Chapter 14). There are three calcium fluxes across the plasma membrane. One (A) allows calcium influx into the cytosol, whereas the other two (B_1 and B_2) are responsible for the return of this calcium to the extracellular space. The major mechanism for calcium entry, the slow inward current (A), initiates calcium-triggered calcium release from the sarcoplasmic reticulum; a smaller amount of this calcium contributes to the calcium delivered to the contractile proteins (dotted arrow A_1). Although calcium can enter the cytosol via sodium/calcium exchange (B_1), as pointed out in Chapter 10 this countertransport serves mainly to move calcium out of the cytosol. The plasma membrane calcium pump, shown as arrow B_2, also participates in calcium efflux, but appears to be less important quantitatively.

The more important internal circulation of calcium during excitation-contraction coupling and relaxation is described by arrows C, D, E, F, and G. Arrows C and D represent calcium fluxes across the sarcoplasmic reticulum membrane, while G describes the movement of calcium taken up by the sarcotubular network back to the subsarcolemmal cisternae. Arrows E and F represent the binding and dissociation of calcium from troponin C. The buffering role of the mitochondria is shown by the double arrow H, which represents calcium fluxes between the cytosol and the interior of the mitochondria.

A rough depiction of the energetics of the calcium fluxes involved in excitation-contraction is also given in Figure 11.10. The downward arrows A, C, and E represent passive calcium fluxes "powered" either by diffusion (A, C) or, in the case of calcium binding to the contractile proteins, by association with high-affinity Ca^{2+}-binding sites. The corresponding uphill calcium fluxes are shown by arrows B_1, B_2, D, and F. Calcium returns from the sarcotubular network to the subsarcolemmal cisternae by diffusion; as the Ca^{2+} concentration gradient within this membrane structure is small, arrow G is nearly horizontal. The two components of arrow H are also drawn nearly horizontal because Ca^{2+} concentration within the mitochondria is normally low (Chapter 5).

We return to this figure in Chapter 14, when we discuss the regulation of myocardial contractility in terms of changes in these calcium fluxes, and the systems by which they are controlled.

REFERENCES

Andersen JP. (1989). Monomer-oligomer equilibrium of sarcoplasmic reticulum Ca^{2+}-ATPase and the role of subunit interactions in the Ca^{2+} pump mechanism. *Biochim Biophys Acta* 988:47–72.

Block BA, Imagawa T, Campbell KP, Franzini-Armstrong C. (1988). Structural evidence for direct interaction between the molecular components of the transverse tubule/sarcoplasmic reticulum junction in skeletal muscle. *J Cell Biol* 107:2587–2600.

Borgatta L, Watras J, Katz AM, Ehrlich BE. (1991). Regional differences in calcium release channels from heart. *Proc Natl Acad Sci USA* 88:2486–2487.

Chandler WL, Rakowski RF, Schneider MF. (1976). Effects of glycerol treatment and maintained depolarization on charge movement in skeletal muscle. *J Physiol* 254:285–316.

Clarke DM, Loo TW, MacLennan DH. (1990). Functional consequences of alterations to polar amino acids located in the transmembrane domain of the Ca^{2+}-ATPase of sarcoplasmic reticulum. *J Biol Chem* 264:6262–6267.

deMeis L, deSouza Otero A, Martins OB, Alves EW, Inesi G, Nakamoto R. (1982). Phosphorylation of sarcoplasmic reticulum ATPase by orthophosphate in the absence of Ca^{2+} gradient: contribution of water activity to the enthalpy and the entropy changes. *J Biol Chem* 257:4993–4998.

Ebashi S, Kitazawa T, Kodama K, Van Eerd P-C. (1978). Calcium ion in cardiac contractility. In: Kobayashi T, Sano T, Dhalla NS, eds. *Recent advances in studies on cardiac structure and metabolism, vol 11: Heart function and metabolism.* Baltimore: University Park Press; 93–101.

Endo M. (1977). Calcium release from the sarcoplasmic reticulum. *Physiol Rev* 57:71–108.

Fabiato A. (1983). Calcium-induced release of calcium from the cardiac sarcoplasmic reticulum. *Am J Physiol* 245:C1–C14.

Fujii J, Maruyama K, Tada M, MacLennan DH. (1989). Expression and site-specific mutagenesis of phospholamban. Studies of residues involved in phosphorylation and pentamer formation. *J Biol Chem* 264:12950–12955.

Fujii J, Ueno A, Kitano K, Tanaka S, Kadoma M, Tada M. (1987). Complete complementary DNA-derived amino acid sequence of canine cardiac phospholamban. *J Clin Invest* 79:301–304.

Herbette LG, DeFoor P, Fleischer S, Pascolini D, Scarpa A, Blasie JK. (1985). The separate profile structures of the functional calcium pump protein and the phospholipid bilayer within insolated sarcoplasmic reticulum membranes determined by x-ray and neutron diffraction. *Biochim Biophys Acta* 817:103–122.

Hicks M, Shigekawa M, Katz AM. (1979). Mechanism by which cyclic adenosine 3′:5′-monophosphate–dependent protein kinase stimulates calcium transport in cardiac sarcoplasmic reticulum. *Circ Res* 44:384–391.

Inui M, Chamberlain BK, Saito A, Fleischer S. (1986). The nature of the modulation of Ca^{2+} transport as studied by reconstitution of cardiac sarcoplasmic reticulum. *J Biol Chem* 261:1794–1800.

James P, Inui M, Tada M, Ciesi M, Carafoli E. (1990). Nature and site of phospholamban regulation of the Ca^{2+} pump of sarcoplasmic reticulum. *Nature* 342:90–92.

Katz AM. (1986). Potential deleterious effects of inotropic agents in the therapy of heart failure. *Circulation* 73 (Suppl 3):184–190.

Kim HW, Kim DH, Ikemoto N, Kranias EG. (1987). Lack of effects of calcium-calmodulin–dependent phosphorylation on Ca^{2+} release from cardiac sarcoplasmic reticulum. *Biochim Biophys Acta* 903:333–340.

Kranias EG, Steenaart NAE, Di Salvo J. (1988). Purification and characterization of phospholamban phosphatase from cardiac muscle. *J Biol Chem* 263:15681–15687.

Leberer E, Timms BG, Campbell KP, MacLennan DH. (1990). Purification, calcium binding properties, and ultrastructural localization of the 53,000- and 160,000 (sarcalumenin)-dalton glycoproteins of the sarcoplasmic reticulum. *J Biol Chem* 265:10118–10124.

Mitchell RD, Simmerman HKB, Jones LR. (1988). Ca^{2+}-binding effects on protein conformation and protein interactions of canine cardiac calsequestrin. *J Biol Chem* 263:1376–1381.

Movsesian MA, Nishikawa M, Adelstein RS. (1984). Phosphorylation of phospholamban by calcium-activated, phospholipid-dependent protein kinase. Stimulation of cardiac sarcoplasmic reticulum calcium uptake. *J Biol Chem* 259:8029–8032.

Nakamura Y, Tonomura Y. (1982). The binding of ATP to the catalytic and the regulatory site of Ca^{2+}, Mg^{2+}-dependent ATPase of the sarcoplasmic reticulum. *J Bioenerg Biomemb* 14:307–318.

Otsu K, Willard HF, Khanna VK, Zorzato F, Green NM, MacLennan DH. (1990). Molecular cloning of cDNA encoding the Ca^{2+} release channel (ryanodine receptor) rabbit cardiac muscle sarcoplasmic reticulum. *J Biol Chem* 265:13472–13483.

Rousseau E, Smith JS, Henderson JS, Meissner G. (1986). Single channel and $^{45}Ca^{2+}$ flux measurements of the cardiac sarcoplasmic reticulum calcium channel. *Biophys J* 50:1009–1014.

Saito A, Inui M, Radermacher M, Frank J, Fleischer S. (1988). Ultrastructure of the calcium release channel of sarcoplasmic reticulum. *J Cell Biol* 107:211–219.
Schwartz IM, McCleskey EW, Almers W. (1985). Dihydropyridine receptors in muscle are voltage-dependent but most are functional calcium channels. *Nature* 314:747–751.
Scofano HM, Vieyra A, deMeis L. (1979). Substrate regulation of the sarcoplasmic reticulum ATPase. Transient kinetic studies. *J Biol Chem* 254:10227–10231.
Scott BT, Simmermann HKB, Collins JH, Nadal-Ginard B, Jones LR. (1988). Complete amino acid sequence of canine cardiac calsequestrin deduced by cDNA cloning. *J Biol Chem* 263:8958–8964.
Shigekawa M, Dougherty JP, Katz AM. (1978). Reaction mechanism of Ca^{2+}-dependent ATP hydrolysis of skeletal muscle sarcoplasmic reticulum in the absence of added alkali metal salts. I. Characterization of steady state ATP hydrolysis and comparison with that in the presence of KCl. *J Biol Chem* 253:1442–1450.
Shigekawa M, Finegan J-AM, Katz AM. (1976). Calcium transport ATPase of canine cardiac sarcoplasmic reticulum. A comparison with that of rabbit fast skeletal muscle sarcoplasmic reticulum. *J Biol Chem* 251:6894–6900.
Smith JS, Rousseau E, Meissner G. (1989). Calmodulin modulation of single sarcoplasmic reticulum Ca^{2+}-release channels from cardiac and skeletal muscle. *Circ Res* 64:352–359.
Somlyo AV, Gonzales-Serratos H, Shuman H, McClellan G, Somlyo AP. (1981). Calcium release and ionic changes in the sarcoplasmic reticulum of tetanized muscle: an electron probe study. *J Cell Biol* 90:577–594.
Stokes DL, Green NM. (1990). Three dimensional crystals of Ca-ATPase from sarcoplasmic reticulum. Symmetry and packing. *Biophys J* 57:1–14.
Suko J, Plank B, Preis P, Kolassa N, Hellmann G, Conca W. (1981). Formation of magnesium-phosphoenzyme and magnesium-calcium-phosphoenzyme in the phosphorylation of adenosine triphosphatase of orthophosphate in sarcoplasmic reticulum: Model of a reaction sequence. *Eur J Biochem* 119:225–226.
Swann AC. (1984). (Na^+,K^+)-adenosine triphosphatase regulation by the sympathetic nervous system: effects of noradrenergic stimulation and lesions in vivo. *J Pharmacol Expo Ther* 228:304–311.
Swynghedauw B. (1990). Changes in membrane proteins in chronic mechanical overload of the heart. *Am J Cardiol* 65:30G–33G.
Tada M, Inui M, Yamada M, Kadoma M, Kuzuya T, Abe H, Kakiuchi S. (1983). Effects of phospholamban phosphorylation catalyzed by adenosine 3′:5′-monophosphate- and calmodulin-dependent protein kinases on calcium transport ATPase of cardiac sarcoplasmic reticulum. *J Mol Cell Cardiol* 15:335–346.
Tada M, Katz AM. (1982). Phosphorylation of the sarcoplasmic reticulum and sarcolemma. *Annu Rev Physiol* 44:401–423.
Takenaka H, Adler PN, Katz AM. (1982). Calcium fluxes across the membrane of sarcoplasmic reticulum vesicles. *J Biol Chem* 257:12649–12656.
Takeshima H, Nishimura S, Matsumoto T, Ishida H, Kangawa K, Minamino N, Matsuo H, Ueda M, Hanaoka M, Hirose T, Numa S. (1989). Primary structure and expression from complementary DNA of skeletal muscle ryanodine receptor. *Nature* 339:439–445.
Takisawa H, Tonomura Y. (1979). ADP-sensitive and -insensitive phosphorylated intermediates of solubilized Ca^{2+}, Mg^{2+}-dependent ATPase of the sarcoplasmic reticulum from skeletal muscle. *J Biochem* 86:425–441.
Tsien RW. (1983). Calcium channels in excitable cell membranes. *Annu Rev Physiol* 45:341–358.
Villa-Moruzzi E, Ballou LM, Fischer EH. (1984). Phosphorylase phosphatase. Interconversion of active and inactive forms. *J Biol Chem* 259:5857–5863.
Watras J. (1988). Regulation of calcium uptake in bovine aortic sarcoplasmic reticulum by cyclic AMP–dependent protein kinase. *J Mol Cell Cardiol* 20:711–723.
Wegener AD, Simmerman HKB, Lindemann JP, Jones LR. (1989). Phospholamban phosphorylation in intact ventricles. Phosphorylation of serine 16 and threonine 17 in response to β-adrenergic stimulation. *J Biol Chem* 264:11468–11474.
Williamson JR, Williams RJ, Coll KE, Thomas AP. (1983). Cytosolic free Ca^{2+} concentration and intracellular calcium distribution of Ca^{2+}-tolerant isolated heart cells. *J Biol Chem* 258:13411–13414.
Zerain-Herzberg A, MacLennan DH, Periasamy M. (1990). Characterization of rabbit cardiac sarco-(endo)plasmic reticulum Ca^{2+}-ATPase gene. *J Biol Chem* 265:4670–4677.

BIBLIOGRAPHY

Feher JJ, Fabiato A. (1990). Cardiac sarcoplasmic reticulum: calcium uptake and release. In: Langer GA, ed. *Calcium and the heart*. New York: Raven Press; 199–268.

Glass DB, Krebs EG. (1980). Protein phosphorylation catalyzed by cyclic AMP–dependent and cyclic GMP–dependent protein kinases. *Annu Rev Pharmacol Toxicol* 20:363–388.

Katz AM. (1979). Role of the contractile proteins and sarcoplasmic reticulum in the response of the heart to catecholamines: an historical review. *Adv Cyclic Nucl Res* 11:303–343.

Katz AM. (1983). Cyclic adenosine monophosphate effects on the myocardium: a man who blows hot and cold with one breath. *J Am Coll Cardiol* 2:143–149.

Lytton J, MacLennan DH. (1991). Sarcoplasmic reticulum. In: Fozzard H, Haber E, Katz A, Jennings R, Morgan HE, eds. *The heart and circulation*, 2nd ed. New York: Raven Press. In Press.

Mathias RT, Levis RA, Eisenberg RS. (1980). Electrical models of excitation-contraction coupling and charge movement in skeletal muscle. *J Gen Physiol* 76:1–31.

Tada M, Yamamoto T, Tonomura Y. (1978). Molecular mechanisms of active calcium transport by sarcoplasmic reticulum. *Physiol Rev* 58:1–79.

12

Receptors, Coupling Proteins, and Second Messengers

The electrical and mechanical performance of the heart is regulated by a dazzling fabric of systems that adjust the cardiac pump to the continually changing needs of the body. These interlocking systems avoid the consequences of "Murphy's law": "If anything can go wrong, it will, and at the worst possible time." The way that we are able to survive a failure in one or another component of our hearts is through this network of overlapping, and often redundant, controls. It is as if Murphy's law is met by a law of the heart that states: "If something is worth doing, it will be done in a number of different ways." This is, after all the design of a modern airplane, where, as with the heart, total failure in a critical system can lead to a fatal crash.

Key to understanding the regulation of the cardiac performance, the major subject of most of the remainder of this text, is the following general mechanism by which a signal reaching the heart elicits a response:

$$
\text{Signal} \rightarrow \text{Receptor} \rightarrow \text{Coupling protein} \underset{\searrow}{\overset{\nearrow}{}} \begin{array}{l} \text{Response} \\ \text{Second messenger} \rightarrow \text{Response} \end{array}
$$

The present chapter focuses on the initial steps in this sequence: the manner by which various signals alter the response of effector proteins, either directly or through the production of intracellular second messengers.

Regulation of cardiac performance begins when a signal, generally a small molecule, arrives at the outer surface of a myocardial cell. These *extracellular (first) messengers* bind to specific plasma membrane proteins called *receptors*; because they generally form tight bonds with the receptors, these small molecules are referred to as *ligands*.

The formation of a ligand-receptor complex in the plasma membrane does not, itself, usually modify cardiac function. Instead, other systems "translate" the binding of the ligand to its specific receptor to generate a signal that modifies cell function, often by the production of additional messengers. These processes of signal transduction generally involve *coupling proteins* that, when activated by the ligand-receptor complex, can modify directly the function of other membrane proteins. More often, however, activated coupling proteins interact with membrane-bound enzymes that produce *intracellular second messengers* that transmit the signal elsewhere within the cell.

Intracellular (second) messengers, which are quite different from the extracellular (first) messengers, are synthesized within the cytosol by membrane-bound enzymes. Some of these enzymes use membrane lipids as precursors for the second messenger; for example, the response to α-adrenergic receptor agonists is generally mediated by two intracellular second messengers, diacylglycerol and inositol 1,4,5-trisphosphate, which are derived from phosphatidylinositol 4,5-bisphosphate, one of the membrane phospholipids discussed in Chapter 2. The second messenger produced in response to β-adrenergic receptor neurotransmitters, adenosine 3',5'-cyclic monophosphate (cyclic AMP), is produced from adenosine triphosphate (ATP). In contrast acetylcholine, the parasympathetic neurotransmitter, does not have a second messenger; instead acetylcholine binds to a special class of cholinergic receptors in the heart that, through a group of inhibitory coupling proteins discussed later, reduce cyclic AMP production and influence several effector systems.

SYMPATHETIC AND PARASYMPATHETIC INFLUENCES ON THE HEART

Autonomic regulation of the heart is effected mainly by two systems: the sympathetic and parasympathetic nervous systems (Chapter 1). In the resting heart, the major influence is parasympathetic, whereas during exercise the situation is reversed and sympathetic stimulation becomes predominant.

The sympathetic and parasympathetic subdivisions of the autonomic nervous system can be viewed, in general terms, as opposing each other. For example, sympathetic stimulation increases heart rate, blood pressure, and myocardial contractility, whereas parasympathetic stimulation slows the heart, decreases blood pressure, and causes a marked negative inotropic effect on the atria. Until recently, it was generally taught that the ventricles were insensitive to both parasympathetic stimulation and acetylcholine; however, it is now apparent that cholinergic nerves supply the ventricles and conducting tissues of the His-Purkinje system (Loffenholz and Pappano, 1985). The inhibitory effects of cholinergic stimulation on the ventricles and His-Purkinje system are much more prominent following β-adrenergic receptor stimulation, so that parasympathetic stimulation blunts the response to sympathetic stimulation.

Discovery of the Neurotransmitters

A role for chemical mediators in cardiac regulation was discovered in 1894, when Oliver and Shäfer found that adrenal extracts increased heart rate in cats. A decade later, Elliott suggested that sympathetic nerve stimulation, which had effects quite similar to those of adrenal extracts, might also involve chemical mediators. However, it was not until 1921 that Otto Loewi performed a remarkably simple experiment that proved conclusively that a chemical mediator was indeed involved in neural regulation—in this case by the vagus nerve.

> Loewi's experiment illustrates how a clever, yet simple experiment solved a difficult problem. Earlier efforts to isolate a chemical substance from hearts after vagal stimulation had proved fruitless; as we now know, this was because acetylcholine—the parasympathetic neurotransmitter—is so labile that it could not have remained active during early attempts to collect and transfer the hypothetical chemical mediator. Loewi simply placed two frog hearts a short distance apart in a slowly moving stream of Ringer's solution, and then stimulated the vagus nerve supplying the "upstream" heart. He not only observed the expected slowing of the upstream heart, but in the unstimulated "downstream" heart as well; of course, stimulation of the vagus supplying the downstream heart did not slow the upstream heart. This simple experiment proved that cardiac slowing caused by vagal stimulation was mediated by a chemical, which Loewi called "vagusstoff."

Loewi's demonstration that vagal stimulation could liberate a chemical mediator was followed in a few years by his demonstration that vagusstoff was *acetylcholine*.

In the 1930s, Cannon and Rosenblueth showed that sympathetic stimulation also released a mediator that was subsequently shown to be a *catecholamine* with properties similar to *epinephrine* (adrenaline), the cardioaccelerator substance found in adrenal extracts. Shortly after World War II, von Euler found that the major sympathetic neurotransmitter was *norepinephrine*. Since that time, the number of known neurotransmitters and other extracellular messengers has grown rapidly to include small molecules like *dopamine, histamine, serotonin, glucagon, glutamate*, and *gamma-aminobutyrate*, as well as peptides such as *angiotensin II, bradykinin*, and *vasopressin*. In order for these and other neurotransmitters to modify cardiac function, however, they must first bind to specific receptor molecules in the heart's plasma membrane.

RECEPTORS

Loewi's seminal discovery that nerve stimulation could lead to the release of chemical transmitters also set the stage for the identification of cellular mechanisms that recognize the arrival of a neurotransmitter as a signal to modify cell function. Long before the receptor molecules were purified, it had become apparent that signal-recognition by a cell was, itself, a very complex process. A number of puzzling differences in the responses of various tissues to epinephrine and norepinephrine indicated that factors other than the neurotransmitter determined specific cellular responses; for example, norepinephrine caused some smooth muscles to contract, whereas other muscles responded with relaxation. These and other confusing observations were explained by Ahlquist's postulate that specific responses to chemical signals were determined not only by the structure of the neurotransmitters, but also by the nature of a "receptor" that recognized these specific structures.

Ahlquist thus explained the ability of norepinephrine to cause contraction in some smooth muscles, and relaxation in others, by postulating the existence of two types of receptor that bound this catecholamine. One, which he called the α-receptor, mediated the constrictor action; the other, named the β-receptor, mediated the relaxing response.

The correctness of this hypothesis has now been proved by the recent elucidation of the structures of these and many other receptor molecules. The heart contains mainly β-adrenergic receptors although α-adrenergic receptors are also present; blood vessels, on the other hand, contain more vasoconstrictor α- than vasodilator β-adrenergic receptors.

Receptor Subtypes

It is now clear that receptors are members of a large and diverse group of closely related membrane proteins, and that different receptor subtypes often bind to a given neurotransmitter. Receptor subtypes were initially postulated because different responses could be produced by a single neurotransmitter. The recent elucidation of the amino acid sequences of a large number of receptor molecules has provided conclusive proof that functionally different receptor subtypes are, in fact structurally different members of a single class of proteins.

The β-adrenergic receptors are classified as β_1-, β_2-, and β_3-subtypes; most cardiac β-adrenergic receptors are of the β_1-subtype, β_2-receptors predominate in bronchial and vascular smooth muscle, and β_3-receptors are found in adipose tissue. Many tissues, including the heart, contain more than one β-adrenergic receptor subtype.

There are two important types of parasympathetic (cholinergic) receptors: the *nicotinic* receptors, which are found mainly in skeletal muscle and ganglial cells, and the *muscarinic* receptors that mediate parasympathetic influences on the heart. The nicotinic receptors, whose structures are quite different from those of the muscarinic receptors, are not considered further in this text. Muscarinic receptors, like β-adrenergic receptors, are encoded by a number of different genes; most important are the M_1-subtype, found mainly in autonomic ganglia and the central nervous system, the M_2-subtype found in the heart, and the M_3-subtype in smooth muscle and secretory cells; all are blocked by *atropine*. Further discussion of the pharmacology of these and other receptor subtypes, which is beyond the scope of this text, can be found in standard pharmacology texts.

Structure of Receptors

Almost a half-century elapsed between the postulation that specific receptor molecules mediated neurotransmitter effects and the actual elucidation of their structures. Rapid advances in molecular biology have now proved that most cardiac receptors are members of an extensive family of membrane proteins containing

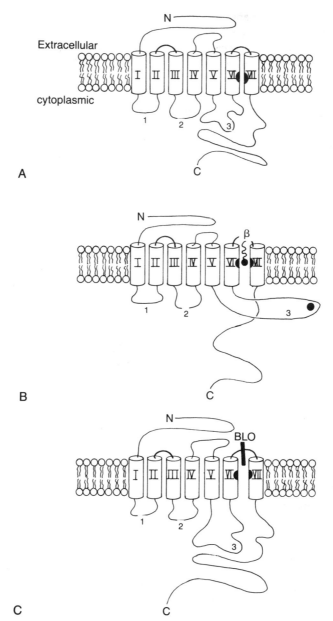

FIG. 12.1. A: Structure of the β-adrenergic receptor protein showing seven membrane-span-ning helices (I–VII) three intracellular loops (1–3), the cytosolic C-terminal peptide chain, and the extracellular N-terminal region. B: Binding of the agonist (β), which probably involves three membrane-spanning domains (IV, VI, VII) alters the structure of the large intracellular peptide chain (3), allowing the latter to interact with the G proteins as indicated by the *solid circle* in cytoplasmic loop 3. C: Binding of a blocker (BLO) to the same site as the one that binds the agonist prevents agonist molecules from gaining access to this site, but does not induce the conformational changes that allow the ligand-receptor complex to activate the G proteins.

seven hydrophobic membrane-spanning regions (Fig. 12.1A). This family includes all known subtypes of the α- and β-adrenergic receptors, the muscarinic cholinergic receptors, receptors for a number of peptide hormones, and even rhodopsin, which responds not to chemical transmitters, but to photons.

> The genes that encode the many members of this family of receptor proteins are found on a number of chromosomes. Although this might seem surprising (as it was, initially, to the author), migration of these genes actually illuminates the processes of evolution. Analysis of sequence homologies among the various receptors indicates that both gene and chromosomal duplication, as well as chromosomal rearrangements, account for the divergences within this widely distributed class of regulatory proteins (Yang-Feng et al., 1990).

Homologies among the different members of the family of receptor proteins provide clues regarding structure-function relationships in their amino acid sequences. Homology is especially close in the seven membrane-spanning regions and in the two shorter intracellular loops, whereas the longest of the cytoplasmic loops and both the C- and N-terminal peptide chains show extensive variability. Binding of the β-adrenergic neurotransmitters appears to be determined largely by the amino acids in the hydrophobic membrane-spanning helices IV, VI, and VII (Fig. 12.1B), whereas coupling with the G proteins (see below) involves the third intracellular loop. Binding of the muscarinic receptor to acetylcholine also appears to involve transmembrane helices; in this case, with helices II, III, VI, and VII (Fig. 12.2). As is the case for the β-receptor, cytoplasmic loop 3 appears to be critical for the functional interactions between the muscarinic ligand-receptor complex and the G proteins. Although many details of these structure-function relationships are still tentative, it appears that binding of extracellular messengers occurs within a "pocket" formed by some of the hydrophobic, membrane-spanning regions within the membrane bilayer. This leads to a conformational change within the cytoplasmic peptide chains that effects the next step in signal transduction: interaction of the ligand-receptor complex with the G proteins (see below).

The Ligand-Receptor Complex

As already discussed, regulation of cardiac function begins when a ligand reaches the heart by way of the extracellular fluid, either via the circulation, or by release

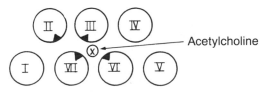

FIG. 12.2. Cross section through a muscarinic receptor showing seven transmembrane helices and the putative acteylcholine-binding sites on helices II, III, VI, and VII (*solid wedges*). (Based on Hulme et al., 1988.)

from adjacent nerve endings. The ability of very small amounts of these ligands to be recognized by the plasma membrane receptors depends on the formation of high-affinity ligand-receptor complexes. The extent to which a ligand modifies cardiac function depends on its concentration, increasing when more ligand is present. This concentration-dependence of the response to a ligand is due simply to the fact that increasing the number of ligand molecules makes it more likely that a ligand molecule will locate and bind to a receptor. This probability is increased when there are more ligand molecules in the medium surrounding the receptor.

Specific and Nonspecific Ligand-Receptor Interactions with Membranes

The binding of various ligands to membranes differs widely, indicating that the mechanisms for ligand-membrane interactions are not all the same. *Nonspecific binding* generally refers to interactions between a ligand and membrane lipids; this is the "anesthetic effect" described in Chapter 2. *Specific binding* implies that the ligand has interacted with a binding protein or receptor. The affinities of receptors for different ligands vary considerably; some toxins, for example, bind tightly to membrane proteins at concentrations below 10^{-12} M, whereas most organic drug molecules bind at concentrations between 10^{-6} and 10^{-8} M. Compounds, like ethanol, whose actions are nonspecific bind to membranes at concentrations around 10^{-3} M (Table 12.1).

As might be expected, ligands with high binding affinities have fewer side effects than those that only bind at high concentrations. This is readily understood because a high binding affinity implies a high degree of "recognition" between ligand and receptor, which minimizes interactions with other components of the membrane.

Except for side effects that are due to allergic, or sensitivity reactions (which often depend little on the dose of a drug), most toxic effects are seen at higher drug concentrations than those that produce desired therapeutic effects. The "toxic/therapeutic ratio" is the ratio of ligand concentrations at which these effects are seen; the greater this ratio, the less likely is the drug to cause toxicity at doses that yield desirable therapeutic effects.

TABLE 12.1. *Range of binding affinities of several ligands to the cardiac plasma membrane*

Ligand	Receptor	Approximate K_d
Tetrodotoxin	Sodium channel	10^{-12} M
Nitrendipine	Calcium channel	10^{-10} M
Epinephrine	β-adrenergic receptor	10^{-8} M
Ouabain	Sodium pump	10^{-6} M
Ethanol	Nonspecific	10^{-3} M

Receptor Agonists and Antagonists

The concept that specific receptor molecules mediate the responses to neurotransmitters led to the development of drugs to inhibit the effects of physiological stimulation. Thus, compounds with structures similar to the neurotransmitters were developed to inhibit their effects. Because the inhibitory effects of these molecules exhibit competitive kinetics, and can be reversed by high concentration of the physiologic neurotransmitters, the inhibitors are known as *antagonists*, or simply as *blockers*, whereas the neurotransmitters are called *agonists*.

Kinetics of Ligand-Receptor Interactions

Direct measurements of the binding of a variety of agonists and antagonists to receptors in cells and isolated plasma membranes show that structurally related compounds bind to a limited number of high-affinity binding sites, which are, of course, the receptors. The ligand concentration at which 50% of receptors are bound to a ligand molecule is the *dissociation constant* (k_d), which defines the "affinity" of the receptor for the ligand; thus, k_d is analogous to K_m, the Michaelis constant in enzyme kinetics. The lower the k_d, the higher is the affinity of the receptor for its ligand. Ligand-receptor binding can also be expressed as an *association*, or *binding, constant* (k_b), which is simply the reciprocal of the dissociation constant.

Values for k_b are proportional to the ratio of the rate of binding of the ligand of the receptor (the "on-rate") to the rate of ligand dissociation (the "off-rate").

While k_d and k_b define the "tightness" to which the ligand binds to the receptor, another term, B_{max}, provides a measure of the number of receptors. Values for B_{max}, determined as the maximal amount of ligand that can bind to specific membrane receptors, can be estimated by extrapolating curves of the concentration-dependence of ligand binding to infinite ligand concentration. B_{max} is generally expressed as pmoles or μmoles ligand bound per mg membrane protein.

The kinetics of ligand-receptor interactions can be extremely complex because the binding affinity of most receptors to their natural neurotransmitters is not constant, but instead changes when the receptors interact with the G proteins (see below). For simplicity, the terms k_d and B_{max} are used in this text in their simplest forms: to describe ligand binding that follows classical first-order kinetics.

Pathways by Which a Ligand Gains Access to its Receptor

The "pathway" by which a ligand reaches its plasma membrane receptor can involve simple diffusion through the aqueous medium outside of the cell, or a more elaborate diffusion pathway in which the ligand dissolves in the much greater surface of membrane bilayer lipids before reaching the receptor. Although the aqueous pathway would seem intuitively to be the most likely, there is growing reason to believe that many membrane-active drugs utilize the lipid pathway (Herbette et al., 1989; also see Chapter 2). This hypothesis finds strong support in the evidence, cited above, that the ligand-binding sites of many members of the receptor proteins depicted in Figs. 12.1 and 12.2 involve membrane-spanning domains located within the hydrophobic core of the bilayer.

Most cardiac drugs have extremely high partition coefficients, which means that a vast majority of the drug molecules in an aqueous solution are located within the membrane bilayer. For example, when a cell is exposed to 10,001 molecules of a drug having a partition coefficient of 10,000, then 10,000 molecules will dissolve in the membrane bilayer leaving only 1 in the aqueous medium outside the cell. This characteristic is in accord with the view that the pharmacokinetics of a drug may be influenced by its interaction with the membrane bilayer (Herbette et al., 1988).

Coupling Proteins

At this point in our description of signaling mechanisms in the heart, the reader should recall the general pathways of signaling described at the beginning of this chapter:

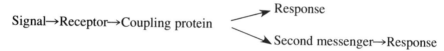

The process described above, in which a ligand is recognized by its receptor and forms a ligand-receptor complex, is generally only the first step in the mechanism that ultimately modifies cell function. The next step, *coupling* or *transduction*, occurs when the ligand-receptor complex interacts with another class of membrane proteins called *coupling proteins*.

The coupling proteins should be viewed as providing a vital step in a series of "translations" that begins when a ligand arrives at the cell surface and binds to its specific receptor. The role of the coupling proteins is to translate the formation of the ligand-receptor complex into a "language" that can be recognized by intracellular effector systems whose function is modified; in other words, it is the coupling proteins, rather than the receptor, that "inform" effector systems within the cell that a ligand has reached the cell and has been recognized by binding to a surface receptor.

Coupling proteins can mediate the signal generated by the formation of a ligand receptor complex in several ways. In some cases, the coupling proteins interact with a membrane-bound enzyme that synthesizes a second messenger within the cell, whereas other coupling proteins modify directly a membrane protein such as an ion channel. In some cases, a single coupling protein can do both.

The G Proteins: A Family of Signal Transducers

By far the most important of the coupling proteins are the *G proteins*, another widely distributed group of related proteins that serves diverse roles in signal transduction. Once called "N proteins," this family of membrane proteins is now referred to as *G proteins* because guanine nucleotides play a vital role in their actions. As noted above, in most signaling systems it is the G proteins, not the ligand-receptor complex, that interact physically with the effectors whose function is modified when extracellular messengers bind to their receptors.

The G proteins interact with a number of effector systems that control the performance of the heart; some of these are listed in Table 12.2. It is noteworthy that different G proteins mediate the excitatory effects of sympathetic stimulation and the inhibitory effects of the parasympathetic nervous system.

> G proteins not only play a central role in the regulation of cell function as this family also includes proto-oncogenes that regulate cell growth and protein synthesis. One of these proteins, the *ras* oncogene product, probably promotes tumors because it cannot hydrolyze guanosine triphosphate (GTP), which is essential to shut off the signal generated by most G proteins (see below).

Structure of the G Proteins

The G proteins are heterotrimers made up of three subunits called G_α, G_β, and G_γ. Each of these subunits is a member of an extended family of proteins that is encoded by several genes, many of whose products are modified by alternative splicing. The G_α subunits range in molecular weight from 40,000 to 46,000; the G_β and G_γ subunits are smaller having molecular weights of 37,400 and 8,000 to 10,000, respectively. While the G_α subunits are most variable in structure [a recent review lists 12 isoforms derived from nine genes (Birnbaumer, 1990b)], the other subunits are by no means constant in structure (the same review describes four cloned G_β subunits and three cloned G_γ subunits). The reader may not be surprised to learn that there is strong evidence of many more to come. Current terminology for the many different G proteins, as well as for the isoforms of the G_α subunits, is confusing; for simplicity this text considers only G_s and G_i, the stimulatory and inhibitory G protein complexes, respectively.

The larger G_α subunits are the major participants in the coupling function of the G proteins; they are also largely responsible for the specificity of the G protein. These subunits possess the more interesting of the biochemical features of the G proteins,

TABLE 12.2. *Some G protein-mediated signal transduction systems in the heart*

Ligand	Receptor	Effector	Effect[a]	Secondary messenger
β-agonists	β-adrenergic	Adenylyl cyclase	+	Cyclic AMP
		Ca channel	+	Inward Ca current
α-agonists	α-adrenergic	Phospholipase C	+	Diacylglycerol, InsP$_3$[b]
Acetylcholine	Muscarinic	K channel	+	Outward K current
	Muscarinic	Adenylyl cyclase	−	Cyclic AMP
Adenosine	P$_1$-purinergic	K channel	+	Outward K current
		Adenylyl cyclase	+	Cyclic AMP
Angiotensin II	Angiotensin	Phospholipase C	+	Diacylglycerol, InsP$_3$

[a] +, activates; −, inhibits.
[b] Inositol 1,4,5-trisphosphate

including the ability to bind and hydrolyze GTP, and to serve as substrates for adenosine diphosphate (ADP)-ribosylation reactions that are useful in the identification and study of the G proteins.

> Nicotinamide-adenine dinucleotide (NAD)-dependent ribosylation, in which the ADP-ribose complex derived from NAD is transferred to G_α, can be catalyzed by both cholera and pertussis toxins. The ability of cholera toxin to produce severe, and sometimes fatal, diarrhea occurs when ADP-ribosylation of a stimulatory G protein in the intestine leads to the persistent activation of intestinal secretion and motility. Pertussis toxin catalyzes an ADP-ribosylation that blocks inhibitory G proteins; however, the pathogenic role of pertussis toxin in causing the symptoms of whooping cough is not clearly understood.

Function of the G Protein Subunits

In coupling the signal generated by the binding of a ligand to its receptor, the G proteins act as two "units": G_α and the $G_{\beta\gamma}$ complex. By far the most important function is that of G_α which, when stimulated to bind GTP by its specific ligand-receptor complex, forms an activated $G_\alpha{}^*GTP$ complex that modifies various effector systems. *It is this action of $G_\alpha{}^*GTP$ that accounts for the vital role of the G proteins in signal transduction.*

Together, G_β and G_γ function as a regulatory $G_{\beta\gamma}$ complex. The effects of this complex on the interactions between the ligand, its receptor, G_α, and the effector whose function is ultimately regulated, are less clear but it may participate in binding G_α to the plasma membrane. As described below, the $G_{\beta\gamma}$ complex is needed for G_α to interact with the receptor; this complex also inhibits the overall cycling of the interactions between the ligand-receptor complex and the G proteins.

Interactions Between a Ligand, its Receptor, and the G Proteins

The interactions between the G proteins and the ligand-receptor complex that lead to effector stimulation involve a series of reactions that are simplified in the seven-step sequence depicted schematically in Fig. 12.3.

Step 1: Binding of the Ligand (L) to its Receptor (R). In the basal states of most cells, where receptors are not bound to their ligands, the free receptors are bound to the nucleotide-free G protein ($G_{\alpha\beta\gamma}$). This interaction between the receptor and the G protein increases the affinity of the receptor (depicted as R^*) for its ligand (L), thus favoring ligand-receptor binding, the first step in the activation sequence.

$$R^*\text{-}G_{\alpha\beta\gamma} + L \rightarrow R^*\text{-}L\text{-}G_{\alpha\beta\gamma}. \qquad [12.1]$$

Step 2: Activation of G_α. When complexed with the ligand-receptor complex formed in step 1, G_α is activated and binds to GTP, thereby forming $G_\alpha{}^*GTP$. At this step, the activated $G_\alpha{}^*GTP$ complex remains bound to $G_{\alpha\beta\gamma}$.

$$R^*\text{-}L\text{-}G_{\alpha\beta\gamma} + GTP \rightarrow R^*\text{-}L\text{-}G_\alpha{}^*GTP\text{-}G_{\beta\gamma}. \qquad [12.2]$$

Step 3: Dissociation of $G_{\beta\gamma}$. Activated G_α^*GTP dissociates from its complex with $G_{\beta\gamma}$, but remains bound to the ligand-receptor complex.

$$R^*\text{-}L\text{-}G_\alpha^*GTP\text{-}G_{\beta\gamma} \rightarrow R^*\text{-}L\text{-}G_\alpha^*GTP + G_{\beta\gamma}. \qquad [12.3]$$

Step 4: Dissociation of R^*-L from G_α^*GTP. After $R^*\text{-}L\text{-}G_\alpha^*GTP$ becomes disso-ciated from $G_{\beta\gamma}$, the ligand-receptor complex also separates from G_α^*GTP. Disso-ciation of the receptor from the G proteins reduces its affinity for binding to the ligand ($R^* \rightarrow R$).

$$R^*\text{-}L\text{-}G_\alpha^*GTP \rightarrow R + L + G_\alpha^*GTP. \qquad [12.4]$$

Step 5: Interaction of activated G_α^* with the effector (E). The activated G_α^*GTP complex, now separated from the ligand-receptor complex, carries out its critical role in signal transduction. This occurs when G_α^*GTP interacts with the effector (E) so as to modify effector function (E^*).

$$G_\alpha^*GTP + E \rightarrow G_\alpha^*GTP\text{-}E^*. \qquad [12.5]$$

Step 6: Dephosphorylation of bound GTP. When the G_α^*GTP complex is disso-ciated from the receptor, it becomes a guanosine triphosphatase (GTPase); as a result, the GTP bound in G_α^*GTP is dephosphorylated. The resulting $G_\alpha GDP$ com-plex returns to its basal state, which causes $G_\alpha GDP$ to dissociate from the activated effector and E^* to return to its resting state. The $G_\alpha GDP$ regenerated in this step then rebinds to $G_{\beta\gamma}$.

$$G_\alpha^*GTP\text{-}E^* + G_{\beta\gamma} \rightarrow G_\alpha GDP\text{-}G_{\beta\gamma} + P_i + E. \qquad [12.6]$$

Step 7: Dissociation of $G_{\alpha\beta\gamma}$ and GDP. When $G_\alpha GDP$ reforms its complex with $G_{\beta\gamma}$, GDP becomes dissociated. The $G_{\alpha\beta\gamma}$ formed in this step then rebinds to the receptor, increasing its affinity for the ligand.

$$R + G_\alpha GDP\text{-}G_{\beta\gamma} \rightarrow R^*\text{-}G_{\alpha\beta\gamma} + GDP. \qquad [12.7]$$

Regulatory Effects of the Guanine Nucleotides

In the reaction sequence described above and depicted in Fig. 12.3, the guanine nucleotides have two important effects: they modify both the affinity of the receptor for its ligand and the affinity of the G proteins for the effector.

Effects of Guanine Nucleotides on Ligand-Receptor Binding. The affinity of the receptor for its ligand is increased when the receptor is complexed with the nucle-otide-free G proteins ($G_{\alpha\beta\gamma}$); this, of course favors ligand binding to the receptor. However, after ligand binding to the receptor releases G_α, the latter binds GTP; this in turn separates the ligand-receptor complex from the G proteins, which reduces the ligand-binding affinity of the receptor (step 4). The latter is restored when the free receptor again binds to the nucleotide-free G protein (step 7). In this way, the guanine nucleotides modify the affinity of the receptor for its ligand.

Effects of Guanine Nucleotides on the Interaction of G_α with the Effector. The

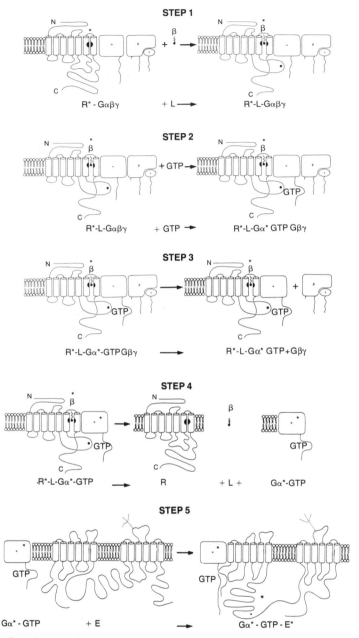

FIG. 12.3. Seven steps by which the three subunits of the G protein (G_α, G_β, G_γ) couple the binding of a β-adrenergic agonist (β) to the activation of adenylyl cyclase (E). Step 1: Binding of the ligand to the activated receptor in its complex with the nucleotide-free G protein. Step 2: Binding of GTP and activation of G_α. Step 3: Dissociation of $G_{\beta\gamma}$ complex from activated, receptor-bound, G_α*-GTP. Step 4: Dissociation of activated G_α*-GTP and the ligand from the receptor. Step 5: Interaction between G_α*-GTP and the cyclase, which activates the latter. Step 6: Dephosphorylation of GTP bound to activated G_α*-GTP returns E to its basal state and allows the $G_{\beta\gamma}$ complex to rebind G_α. Step 7: Dissociation of GDP from $G_{\alpha\beta\gamma}$ allows the nucleotide-free G protein to rebind the receptor, which increases its affinity for the ligand.

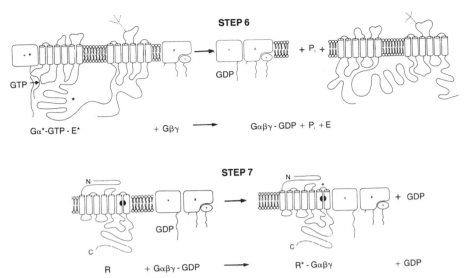

FIG. 12.3. Continued. When activated, G_α and E are indicated with asterisks. As in Fig. 12.1, the ability of the receptor to interact with the G protein is indicated by a *solid circle* in cytoplasmic loop 3. The depiction of adenylyl cyclase (E), which shows a polysaccharide attached to one extracellular loop of the protein (*dashed lines*), is modifed from Krupinski et al. (1989).

binding of G_α to GTP is vital to the ability of the G proteins to activate the effector (step 5). However, because $G_\alpha{}^*$GTP hydrolyzes GTP to form the inactive G_αGDP complex (step 6), activation by the G proteins is short-lived. Thus, interactions of G_α with the guanine nucleotides first initiate (with GTP), and then terminate (with GDP), its ability to activate the effector.

Ending the Signal

It is apparent that, like the "play within the play" in *Hamlet*, guanine nucleotide-induced changes in ligand-receptor affinity and G_α-effector interactions operate within the overall reaction to bring the major actions of the G proteins in signal transduction to an appropriate ending. Changes in the affinity of the receptor for the ligand after the G proteins have been activated help to "turn off" receptor-mediated stimuli by dissociating the ligand from the receptor. Similarly, loss of the ability of G_α to activate the effector after activated $G_\alpha{}^*$GTP has hydrolyzed its bound guanine nucleotide also "turns off" the G proteins. Both of these actions limit the effects of ligand binding. As noted above, the tumor-promoting action of the *ras* oncogene product appears to be related to the fact that it cannot hydrolyze GTP, and so generates a signal that is not turned off.

Other mechanisms also help to prevent "runaway signaling." In addition to dissociation of the ligand-receptor complex at step 4, and hydrolysis and subsequent dissociation of the guanine nucleotide at steps 6 and 7, which tend to shut off this system, enzymatic degradation and reuptake of neurotransmitters, along with diffusion of ligands away from their receptors, play an important role in terminating the effects of neurotransmitters and other extracellular messengers. Prolonged activation is also avoided by desensitization of receptors (see below).

Overview of the Role of the G Proteins

Lest the forest be lost in the trees, it should be reemphasized that the best way to appreciate the interplay between the ligand, the receptor, and the G proteins is to view the latter as the ultimate mediator of the ligand-receptor interaction. Thus, to appreciate the role of the G proteins in signal transduction, one must realize that *it is the G_α^*GTP complex, rather than either the neurotransmitter or the ligand-receptor complex, that modifies the heart's performance in response to autonomic and other stimuli.*

RECEPTORS AND THEIR INTERACTIONS WITH LIGANDS

Having reviewed the effects of the G proteins on the affinity of ligand-receptor binding, we can understand important differences between receptor interactions with agonists and antagonists. Because of their importance in the heart, our focus is on the β-adrenergic receptor and its agonists and antagonists.

Receptor Interactions With Agonists and Antagonists

Although β-adrenergic agonists (physiological hormones and neurotransmitters such as epinephrine and norepinephrine) and β-blockers bind to the same site, the latter do not activate the effector (adenylyl cyclase), but instead block the effects of the agonists. In isolated membranes, β-blockers displace β-adrenergic agonists from their binding sites, whereas in living cells the blockers competitively inhibit both the physiological effects and binding of the agonists. The fundamental difference between a β-adrenergic agonist and a β-blocker therefore does not arise from where they bind, but what they do after binding has occurred. Although agonists, through the interactions with the G protein described above, ultimately activate the effector, blockers (like Aesop's dog in the manger, who selfishly kept the farmer's cattle from eating the hay that the dog himself was unable to eat) occupy the receptor without changing its interaction with the G proteins. The clinical value of a drug like a β-blocker is simply that when the blocker is bound to the receptor, the subsequent binding, and thus the functional effects, of the β-adrenergic agonists are prevented.

The molecules that interact with β-adrenergic receptors do not all fall into the two simple classes of agonists and blockers. Instead some compounds that bind to the β-adrenergic receptor weakly activate adenylyl cyclase. Such drugs are called "partial agonists," and the minor stimulatory effect that accompanies their β-blocking activity is referred to as "intrinsic sympathomimetic activity" (ISA). Partial agonists may be useful clinically as, by blocking the more potent activation of adenylyl cyclase by the physiological neurotransmitter, they cause enough β-blockade to inhibit surges of agonist activity, yet provide some stimulatory support in the basal state.

Because the β-blockers do not alter the interactions of the β-adrenergic receptor with the G proteins, the G proteins do not modify the affinity of the receptor for these ligands. Thus, the affinity of the receptor for the β-blockers is generally constant, and follows simple first-order kinetics. This is in contrast to the complex interactions of the receptor with physiological signaling molecules, which reflect changes in receptor affinity caused by the dissociation and reassociation of the G proteins.

Desensitization

Up to this point, our discussion of the regulation of cardiac performance by extracellular messengers has focused on interactions between the ligands, their receptors, and the G proteins. There is, however, an additional, and entirely different, type of regulation, in which the receptors themselves are modified in response to a persistent signal. In the case of sympathetic stimulation, for example, the β-adrenergic receptors lose their ability to generate a response when a neurotransmitter like norepinephrine is continually delivered to the heart. This can occur when the sympathetic system becomes chronically overactive, for example in patients with chronic heart failure (Chapter 25).

The opposite of desensitization (called "resensitization" in this text) explains the "rebound" seen when chronically administered β-blockers are stopped suddenly; this causes the heart to become exquisitely, and sometimes dangerously, sensitive to β-adrenergic agonists. Both desensitization and resensitization generally occur when changes in the β-adrenergic receptor alter its ability to interact with the ligand, but desensitization can also arise from changes elsewhere in the processes of signal recognition, coupling, and response.

> Anyone who has used a β-adrenergic agonist-containing nasal spray is aware that the spray loses its efficacy after excessive use, and that there can be a "rebound" rhinorrhea when the spray is no longer administered. These effects reflect desensitization and resensitization of the nasal β-adrenergic receptors, as described below. Another example of desensitization is adaptation to light, which occurs by mechanisms quite similar to the attenuation of β-adrenergic receptor responsiveness. This is not surprising as rhodopsin, which is one of the family of the receptor proteins shown in Fig. 12.1, responds to protons by generating a signal that is mediated by members of the family of G proteins.

The ability of an agonist both to turn on (activate) and turn off (desensitize) a receptor may seem paradoxical, or even inimical, in the orderly regulation of cellular function. However, this dual response is actually a general property of biological regulation. In the case of voltage-regulated ion channels, for example, the same depolarizing signal that opens an ion channel also leads to channel inactivation (Chapter 18). These seemingly self-defeating responses, in fact, reflect the very important regulatory principle that when a messenger turns on a signal, it should also see to it that the signal is turned off to protect against a "runaway" response. To use a simple analogy, when a signal to turn on a water tap is coupled to one that subsequently shuts it off, the possibility of a flood caused by an absentminded bather is avoided.

The importance of β-adrenergic receptor desensitization is apparent in situations where this process is overridden, as occurs when very high concentrations of β-adrenergic agonists are infused chronically, or in patients with a pheochromocytoma (a β-adrenergic agonist secreting tumor). In these conditions, excessive and prolonged sympathetic stimulation leads to a cardiomyopathy caused by catecholamine-induced myocardial cell death.

Mechanisms for Desensitization

The attenuation of the response to chronic administration of a β-adrenergic agonist, once called "tachyphylaxis" or "refractoriness," is now known to be caused by several quite different mechanisms. These are referred to collectively as *desensitization*, but unfortunately the terminology in this field can be difficult. Two frequently used terms are *homologous desensitization*, which refers to a receptor-specific loss of sensitivity to a single class of ligand, such as the β-adrenergic agonists, and *heterologous desensitization*, where prolonged exposure to one agonist attenuates the response to agonists that interact with other, different, receptor types.

The term *down regulation*, which commonly refers to a reduction in the number of functional receptors, has been restricted by some authorities to those mechanisms in which the receptors are either destroyed or partially degraded by proteolytic digestion.

The ability of a receptor to bind to its physiological agonist can be attenuated by three quite different mechanisms: uncoupling, internalization, and digestion, which appear to occur in the sequence shown in Fig. 12.4. These are described below mainly in terms of changes in the β-adrenergic receptor, for which our understanding is most complete. There is, however, growing evidence for desensitization of other receptors, including the α-adrenergic, muscarinic, and some peptide receptors.

Uncoupling

Uncoupling of β-adrenergic receptors, the first step in the process of desensitization shown in Fig. 12.4, is due largely to cyclic AMP–stimulated phosphorylation of the receptor. This reaction is catalyzed by a cyclic AMP–dependent protein kinase having a high degree of specificity for the β-adrenergic receptor. This β-adrenergic receptor protein kinase (abbreviated "βARK") thus provides a negative feedback in which the signaling sequence initiated by binding of the β-adrenergic agonist to its receptor uses cyclic AMP, the product of the agonist-induced stimulation, to inactivate the receptor that had initiated the sequence. Inactivation of the receptor when it is phosphorylated by β-adrenergic receptor kinase involves a cofactor called *arrestin*, which blocks the interaction between the phosphorylated receptor and the G protein (Fig. 12.4).

Internalization

A second step in desensitization, which occurs after phosphorylation uncouples the receptors from the cyclase, is disappearance of the receptor molecules from the plasma membrane (Fig. 12.4). As the full complement of receptors can be recovered when cells are homogenized, these receptors are transferred to another membrane system, presumably within the cell; for this reason, this process is called "internalization." Initially, the internalized receptors remain structurally intact, even though they have lost their ability to interact with their agonists, the G protein, and/or the cyclase.

Phosphorylated receptors probably remain internalized until they are either destroyed (see below), or dephosphorylated by a phosphoprotein phosphatase which, as noted in Chapter 11, is one of a class of enzymes that generally turn off signals. Once the receptor is dephosphorylated, arrestin becomes dissociated and the receptor can return to the plasma membrane. Thus, when sympathetic stimulation of the heart ceases and the phosphoprotein phosphatases begin their task of "undoing" the effects of the many cyclic AMP–induced phosphorylations, the β-adrenergic receptors are resensitized.

Loss of Receptors

If exposure of the cell to the agonist is prolonged, the return of active receptors to the cell surface becomes impaired. This is because the internalized receptors begin to disappear, due most likely to their proteolysis by lysosomal enzymes within the cell. Unlike uncoupling and internalization, this mechanism is irreversible, so that full return of function after prolonged exposure to high concentrations of an agonist requires that new receptors by synthesized.

The preceding discussion has focused on desensitization of the β-adrenergic receptors, but there is also evidence for α_1-receptor desensitization; in this case the mediator appears to be protein kinase C, which is activated by α_1-receptor agonists. Similarly, muscarinic receptors are desensitized after prolonged exposure to muscarinic agonists; although probably involving receptor phosphorylation, the mechanism for muscarinic desensitization is less well understood.

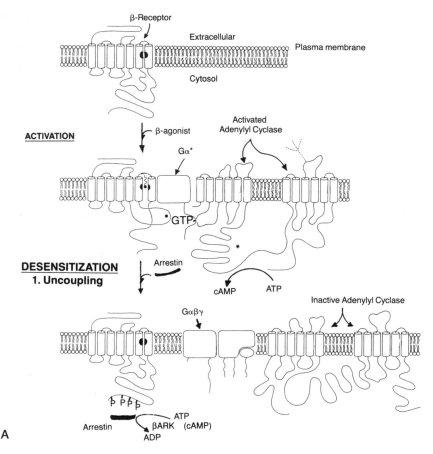

FIG. 12.4. Mechanisms that can desensitize the β-adrenergic receptor. *Activation*: Binding of the β-adrenergic agonist to its receptor stimulates adenylyl cyclase to produce cyclic AMP (see Fig. 12.2). *Desensitization* then procedes through three sequential steps: *1. Uncoupling*, which begins when cyclic AMP produced by the activated adenylyl cyclase stimulates a cyclic AMP–dependent protein kinase (β-adrenergic receptor kinase, or βARK), to phosphorylate the β-receptor. The phosphorylated receptor then binds arrestin, an inhibitor protein that prevents further interaction of the receptor with the G proteins. *2. Internalization*, which occurs when the phosphorylated receptor-arrestin complex is detached from the plasma membrane and moves into the cytosol. *3. Loss of receptors*, which is irreversible, occurs when the internalized receptors are digested by proteolytic enzymes. *Resensitization* occurs when the internalized receptors are dephosphorylated by a phosphoprotein phosphatase, which causes arrestin to dissociate and the receptor to return to the plasma membrane.

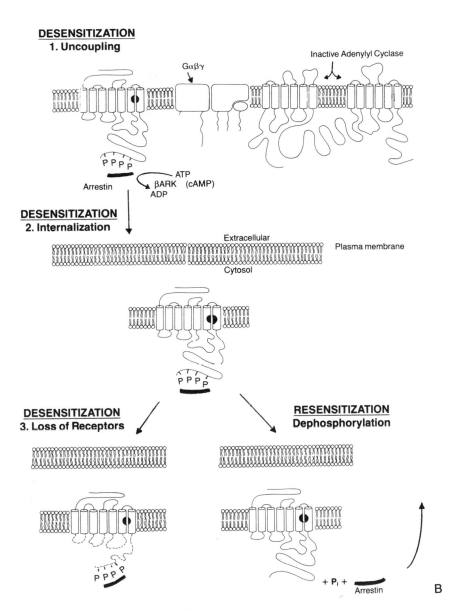

FIG. 12.4. Continued

Changes in Coupling Proteins and Effectors

Desensitization can also be caused by changes in the G proteins and such effectors as adenylyl cyclase. These are, of course, examples of heterologous desensitization, as they would impair the responses to all ligands that act through the desensitized component of the cell's signaling system. These mechanisms have not been as clearly described as the receptor alterations described above.

Enhanced β-Adrenergic Sensitivity

As noted earlier, effects opposite to desensitization are also seen. Thus, the sensitivity of the heart to β-adrenergic agonists is increased following prolonged administration of β-blockers or after the heart is denervated (sometimes called "denervation sensitivity"). This heightened sensitivity to β-adrenergic agonists appears to result from the ability of β-blockade to increase β-adrenergic receptor number, due possibly to externalization of receptors that, under normal conditions, are held in reserve within the cell. For this reason it is dangerous to discontinue suddenly the administration of a β-blocker in patients who have received long-term β-blocker therapy.

A number of other mechanisms, besides chronic administration of β-adrenergic agonists, can modify the number of β-receptors in the heart. For example, β-receptors are desensitized in patients with hypothyroidism, whereas sensitivity of the receptors is enhanced in hyperthyroid patients (see also Chapter 23).

Spare Receptors

The concept of "spare receptors" is mentioned at this point mainly to distinguish a spare receptor from a desensitized receptor. In contrast to the latter, which represent receptors that have lost the ability to activate their effectors, spare receptors are excess receptors at the cell surface that, although able to bind to their agonists and initiate normal signaling, are present in excess and so are not needed for full activation of their effectors.

> The concept of spare receptors is readily understood by considering a membrane containing 100 β-adrenergic receptors that surrounds a cell where full activation of adenylyl cyclase by β-adrenergic agonists occurs when only 60 receptors are bound to their ligand. The remaining 40 are considered to represent spare receptors. Unlike a desensitized receptor, which is unable to elicit a response, a spare receptor is a functional receptor that when bound to its agonist does not modify cell function because agonist-binding to other receptors has already produced a maximal response.

Functional Effects of Ligand-Receptor Interactions

The following discussion provides a brief introduction to the effects of ligand binding to different classes of receptor. Emphasis at this point is on the general effects of the various classes of agonists. More complete descriptions are found in later chapters, where many of the key effector systems in the heart are described.

Functional Effects of β-Adrenergic Receptors

The interactions between β-adrenergic receptors and G_s stimulate adenylyl cyclase to synthesize cyclic AMP, the major intracellular messenger that mediates the stimulatory effects of the sympathetic nervous system. There are, however, additional mechanisms by which activation of G_s by β-adrenergic stimulation can modify cardiac function; these involve direct interactions between the activated G protein and specific effector systems. Most important is probably the ability of the G_s that is activated by β-adrenergic agonists to interact directly with plasma membrane calcium channels (Table 12.2).

Functional Effects of α-Adrenergic Receptors

The effects of α-adrenergic agonists on the heart are not as dramatic as those of the β-adrenergic agonists. The most important cardiovascular effects of α-adrenergic agonists are on vascular smooth muscle, where they induce vasoconstriction. Binding of α-adrenergic agonists to cardiac $α_1$-receptors has a weak positive inotropic action that, although mediated by a G protein, generates a different second messenger. The G protein that is activated by α-adrenergic agonist binding to its receptor increases the catalytic activity of phospholipase C, a lipolytic enzyme that hydrolyzes phosphatidylinositol 4,5-bisphosphate (PIP_2), one of the membrane lipids described in Chapter 2. This, in turn, leads to the production of two intracellular messengers: inositol 1,4,5-trisphosphate ($InsP_3$) and diacylglycerol (DAG) (see below).

Functional Effects of Muscarinic Receptors

Binding of acetylcholine to muscarinic-receptors has at least two important effects (Table 12.2). Both oppose the effects of the sympathetic nervous system, although by different mechanisms. The first, which is much more prominent in the atria than the ventricles, is to open potassium channels. Because the potassium currents carried by these channels promote repolarization, this response turns off the electrical signal caused by plasma membrane depolarization and so shortens systole and reduces contractility. This interaction between the muscarinic receptor and the potassium channel is mediated by a G protein that, when activated by agonist binding to the receptor, interacts directly with the channel.

Of greater interest in the context of the present chapter is the other effect of agonist binding to the muscarinic receptor, inhibition of adenylyl cyclase. This effect, which is opposite to that produced by agonist binding to the β-adrenergic receptor, is mediated by the inhibitory G_i mentioned earlier in this chapter. Inhibition of calcium channel opening, which is due at least in part to this effect to reduce cyclic AMP levels, has effects on impulse generation and conduction in the sino-atrial and atrioventricular nodes that are important in the management of certain arrhythmias (see Chapter 23).

The differences between G_s and G_i highlight the role of the G proteins in signal transduction. Their opposing effects on cyclic AMP production, which are due mainly to differences in the G_α subunit, clearly document the pivotal role of the coupling proteins in cell regulation.

Functional Effects of Other Ligand-Receptor Interactions

Two other members of the family of receptor proteins listed in Table 12.2, the adenosine and angiotensin receptors, are described briefly at this point. Although quite different in their actions, both play important roles in the regulation of cardiac performance.

Adenosine and its Receptors

Adenosine binds to a subclass of purinergic receptor, called A or P_1 (the other class, P_2, includes ATP-binding receptors in smooth muscle and endothelial cells.) The adenosine receptors are heterogeneous; those in the heart (A_1) are inhibitory and exert effects that are quite similar to those of acetylcholine; namely, inhibition of adenylyl cyclase and activation of potassium channels that carry outward, re-polarizing, ionic currents. In other tissues, it should be noted, another adenosine receptor subtype, A_2, activates adenylyl cyclase. The response of the heart to aden-osine, which is mediated by G proteins, includes an important effect on conduction that is similar to that of the muscarinic agonists. Most likely by inhibiting the in-ward current through calcium channels (Cerbai et al., 1988), adenosine slows con-duction in the atrioventricular node; because its effects are very brief, adenosine is proving to be almost ideal for the treatment of arrhythmias that involve abnormal atrioventricular conduction (see Chapter 23).

Adenosine has an extremely important vasodilatory action that arises from its interac-tion with inhibitory receptors on the blood vessels. This effect appears to play a major role in adjusting coronary flow to the metabolic needs of the heart, notably during ischemia. The ability of adenosine to cause smooth muscle relaxation may also play a role in *autoregulation*, the process whereby an increase in perfusion pressure induces vasoconstriction so as to maintain a constant rate of blood flow through a vascular bed.

Angiotensin II and its Receptors

Angiotensin II, which plays a number of key roles in the regulation of cardio-vascular function, is a powerful vasopressor formed by *renin*, a protease produced by the kidney. Renin hydrolyzes angiotensinogen, an α_2-globulin, to liberate the decapeptide, angiotensin I; the latter, which like angiotensinogen is pharmacologically inactive, is a substrate for another class of proteolytic enzymes, the *angiotensin converting enzymes*, which release the active octapeptide angiotensin II. Although its most prominent effects are on smooth muscle, angiotensin II also has a weak positive inotropic effect on the heart.

The angiotensin II receptor, like other members of its family, acts through a G protein that allows the ligand-bound angiotensin II receptor to increase the catalytic activity of a phospholipase C to produce InsP$_3$ and DAG; thus, the response to these peptide hormones is quite similar to those of the α-adrenergic agonists described above.

A novel view of the angiotensin II receptor emerged a few years ago when the *mas* oncogene, which causes tumors in nude mice, was found to encode one of the family of membrane proteins depicted in Fig. 12.1. Although this *mas* oncogene product is a functional angiotensin receptor, it now appears unlikely that the *mas* oncogene product is the cardiac angiotensin II receptor. There is growing evidence that angiotensin II plays an important role in regulating protein synthesis and gene expression in both the heart and blood vessels (Katz, 1990).

The Eicosanoids

Several important extracellular messengers, called eicosanoids, are produced from the 20-carbon fatty acid arachidonic acid, which is released from the plasma membrane by another lipolytic enzyme, phospholipase A$_2$. The eicosanoids, which include prostaglandins, thromboxane, and leukotrienes, are rapidly degraded, and so probably act locally. Little is known of the structures of the receptors for the many compounds in this class; their second messengers appear to include cyclic AMP, InsP$_3$, and DAG. The prostaglandins play an important role in vascular regulation, and may have a weak inotropic effect.

Second Messengers

In this and previous chapters, we have encountered a number of intracellular messengers that mediate a variety of regulatory processes. Although all share the ability to transmit signals within the cell, these messengers are quite dissimilar from each other, as well as from the extracellular messengers like epinephrine, acetylcholine, and angiotensin II. Several of the second messengers are listed in Table 12.3; this table is not complete, nor are all of these intracellular second messengers of equal importance in regulating the performance of the heart. It is apparent, however, that the second messengers listed in Table 12.3 have diverse origins: *calcium*, which enters the cytosol from the extracellular space and sarcoplasmic reticulum; *cyclic AMP*, which is made from ATP; and *InsP$_3$* and *DAG*, which are cleaved from phospholipids in the plasma membrane.

TABLE 12.3. *Intracellular messengers*

Second messenger	Initiation of signal	Termination of signal
Calcium	Diffuses into the cytosol from a region of high concentration	Pumped out of the cytosol
Cyclic AMP	Synthesized from ATP by adenylyl cyclase	Degraded by AMP by phosphodiesterase
$InsP_3$	Synthesized from PIP_2 by a phospholipase C	Dephosphorylated by a phosphatase
DAG	Synthesized from PIP_2 by a phospholipase C	Phosphorylated to form phosphatide or hydrolyzed to form monoglyceride

Abbreviations: PIP_2, phosphatidylinositol 4,5-bisphosphate; $InsP_3$, inositol 1,4,5-trisphosphate; DAG, diacylglycerol.

Cyclic AMP

Aside from calcium, the most important second messenger in the regulation of the heart's performance is cyclic AMP. Several actions of cyclic AMP increase calcium entry into the cytosol; in addition to these effects, which increase contractility, cyclic AMP has effects that promote relaxation (Chapter 14). Elevation of cyclic AMP levels also has important arrhythmogenic effects on the heart.

Cytosolic levels of cyclic AMP are regulated not only by the production of this second messenger, but also by its breakdown. Thus, the signal generated by cyclic AMP is controlled both by *adenylyl cyclase*, which synthesizes cyclic AMP, and by the *phosphodiesterases*, which degrade cyclic AMP by hydrolyzing one of the two ester bonds linking phosphate to ribose in the cyclic nucleotide.

Intracellular Ca^{2+} levels have important effects to regulate cyclic AMP levels in the heart (Fig. 12.5). As cardiac phosphodiesterases are stimulated by the calcium-calmodulin complex, elevation of cytosolic Ca^{2+} concentration, central to the cardiac response to cyclic AMP, promotes cyclic AMP degradation (Tada et al., 1976). Calcium can also reduce cyclic AMP levels by inhibiting adenylyl cyclase. These interactions provide further examples of the intricate and interlocking mechanisms that, as described earlier in this chapter, help to prevent runaway activation.

Adenylyl Cyclase

The recently published amino acid sequence of adenylyl cyclase (see Fig. 12.3) has several features in common with ion channel proteins (Krupinski et al., 1989). The significance of these similarities is not yet clear, but suggests that this enzyme is related to the family of ion channel and transporter proteins that are oligomers (usually four) of peptides having six membrane-spanning domains (Chapter 18).

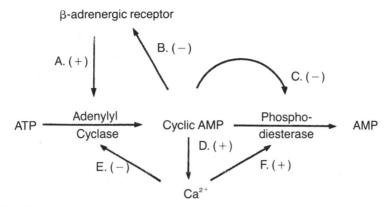

β-adrenergic receptor

FIG. 12.5. Feedback loops involved in the regulation of cyclic AMP levels in the heart. A: β-adrenergic agonists activate adenylyl cyclase, thereby increasing cellular levels of cyclic AMP. B: Cyclic AMP, by promoting the phosphorylation of β-receptors by the cyclic AMP–dependent protein kinase βARK, desensitizes the β-receptors after prolonged exposure to β-adrenergic agonists. C: Cyclic AMP also accelerates its own destruction by activating phosphodiesterase. D: Cyclic AMP leads to an increase in cytosolic calcium that reduces cyclic AMP levels both by inhibiting adenylyl cyclase (E) and activating phosphodiesterase activity (F). Steps that increase cyclic AMP levels are indicated by ($+$); those that decrease cyclic AMP by ($-$).

Protein Kinases

As has already been pointed out in earlier chapters, notably in the description of the control of glycogen synthesis and breakdown (Chapter 4), cyclic AMP itself, while a "second messenger," is not the "final messenger" as its signal often involves an additional step of protein phosphorylation. This is also often true for calcium, and almost always true for diacylglycerol. Thus, second messengers represent additional intermediaries in the complex mechanisms that modify effector systems. Different second messengers activate different classes of *protein kinase* (Table 12.4).

Protein kinases, as already described in this text, are enzymes that catalyze the transfer of the terminal phosphate of ATP to serine and threonine hydroxyl groups in proteins according to the reaction:

$$\text{Protein} + \text{ATP} \xrightarrow{\text{Protein kinase}} \text{Protein phosphoester.}$$

The signal generated by the formation of these protein phosphoesters, as noted in Chapter 11, is "turned off" when the phosphoesters are broken down by phosphoprotein phosphatases according to the general reaction:

$$\text{Protein phosphoester} \xrightarrow{\text{Phosphoprotein phosphatase}} \text{Protein} + P_i.$$

Most of these enzymes contain a number of different subunits. The cyclic AMP–

TABLE 12.4. *Protein kinases*

Second messenger	Protein kinase
Calcium	Calcium, calmodulin–dependent protein kinase
Cyclic AMP	Cyclic AMP–dependent protein kinase (protein kinase A)
Diacylglycerol	Phospholipid–dependent protein kinase (protein kinase C)

dependent protein kinases are tetramers made up of two *catalytic subunits*, responsible for the transfer of the terminal phosphate of ATP to the effector protein, and two *regulatory subunits*. Each of the latter contains two cyclic AMP–binding sites (R) that control the activity of the catalytic subunits (C). Under basal conditions, the regulatory subunits bind to and inhibit protein kinase activity. In response to sympathetic stimulation, or other mechanisms that increase cyclic AMP levels, protein kinase A activity is increased when binding of the second messenger to the regulatory subunits causes the latter to dissociate from the catalytic subunits. Thus, cyclic AMP (cAMP) stimulates protein kinase A activity according to the general reaction:

$$R_2C_2 + 4 \ cAMP \rightarrow cAMP_4R_2C_2 \rightarrow cAMP_4R_2 + 2 \ C^*$$

where C is the catalytic subunit in inactive (C) and active (C^*) states. Activation of protein kinase A ends when a fall in cytosolic cyclic AMP levels causes the nucleotide to dissociate from the regulatory subunits, thereby restoring the inactive R_2C_2 complex.

Inositol 1,4,5-Trisphosphate and Diacylglycerol

Diacylglycerol (DAG) and inositol 1,4,5-trisphosphate (InsP$_3$), the second messengers produced as a result of the binding of α-adrenergic agonists and angiotensin II to their receptors can be viewed as an "unmatched pair" of intracellular messengers (Fig. 12.6). Both are produced in a single lipolytic reaction, the hydrolysis of phosphatidylinositol 4,5-bisphosphate (PIP$_2$) by a phospholipase C:

$$PIP_2 \xrightarrow{\text{Phospholipase C}} InsP_3 + DAG.$$

However, InsP$_3$ and DAG are entirely different in both structure and mechanism of action. Each of these two second messengers controls a separate intracellular signal transduction pathway. In general, InsP$_3$ releases calcium from intracellular stores, whereas DAG activates protein kinase C; this latter effect can be promoted by calcium.

> The effects of DAG are mimicked by the phorbol esters, a group of plant lipids known to cause tumors in animals. This oncogenic effect is related to a role of protein kinase C activation in mediating stimuli that promote hypertrophy in the heart and vascular smooth muscle (Dzau, 1988).

Perhaps reflecting their common origin from PIP$_2$, the regulatory cascades initiated by DAG and InsP$_3$ often interact (Fig. 12.6); for example, activation of protein

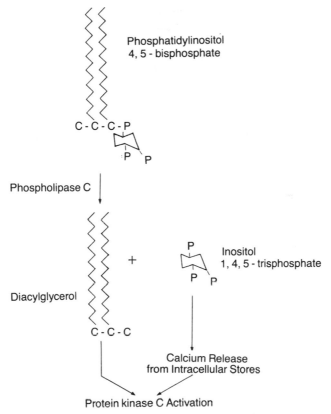

FIG. 12.6. Two second messengers are liberated from phosphatidylinositol 4,5-bisphosphate by a phospholipase; these are diacylglycerol and inositol 1,4,5-trisphosphate, each of which has a separate signaling pathway. These signaling pathways interact because calcium can participate in the activation of protein kinase C by diacylglycerol, and activated protein kinase C can increase intracellular calcium. These reactions are simplified in that phosphorylations of phosphatidylinositol are involved in regulating these signals, and additional phosphoinositols may serve as second messengers.

kinase C often depends on, or is increased by the calcium released in the response to InsP$_3$. Conversely, protein kinase C can influence cellular calcium levels by promoting the opening of calcium channels in the cardiac plasma membrane (Dösemeci et al., 1988).

CONCLUSIONS

The complex and interacting systems described up to this point in our text provide a basis for the remainder of this test, in which we examine the regulation of the performance of the heart. The importance of these systems in determining the mechanical performance of the heart is the subject of Chapters 13 to 17, and Chapters 17 to 23 review the operation of these same mechanisms in controlling both the normal and abnormal electrical behavior of the heart. The final two chapters turn to the two most important pathophysiological abnormalities of cardiac function: ischemia and heart failure. In all of these discussions, the important regulatory principles discussed in these initial chapters are seen to be seminal in understanding not only pathophysiology, but also therapy.

REFERENCES

Brückner R, Mügge A, Scholz H. (1985). Existence and functional role of alpha$_1$-adrenoceptors in the mammalian heart. *J Mol Cell Cardiol* 17:639–645.
Cerbai E, Klockner U, Isenberg G. (1988). Ca-antagonistic effects of adenosine in guinea pig atrial cells. *Am J Physiol* 255:H872–H878.
Döşemeci A, Dhallen RS, Cohen NM, Lederer WJ, Rogers TB. (1988). Phorbol ester increases calcium current and stimulates the effects of angiotensin II on cultured neonatal rat heart myocytes. *Circ Res* 62:347–357.
Dzau VJ. (1988). Cardiac renin-angiotensin system. Molecular and functional aspects. *Am J Med* 84(Suppl 3A):22–27.
Herbette LG, Trumbore M, Chester DW, Katz AM. (1988). Possible molecular basis for the pharmacodynamics of three membrane active drugs: propranolol, nimodipine, amiodarone. *J Mol Cell Cardiol* 20:373–378.
Herbette LG, Vant Erve YMH, Rhodes DG. (1989). Interaction of 1,4 dihydropyridine calcium channel antagonists with biological membranes: lipid bilayer partitioning could occur before drug binding to receptors. *J Mol Cell Cardiol* 21:187–201.
Katz AM. (1990). Angiotensin II: hemodynamic regulator or growth factor? *J Mol Cell Cardiol* 22:739–747.
Krupinski J, Coussen F, Bakalyar HA, Tang W-J, Feinstein PG, Orth K, Slaughter C, Reed RR, Gilman AG. (1989). Adenylyl cyclase amino acid sequence: possible channel or transporter-like structure. *Science* 244:1558–1564.
Loffenholz K, Pappano AJ. (1985). The parasympathetic neuroeffector junction of the heart. *Pharmacol Rev* 37:1–24.
Tada M, Kirchberger MA, Iorio J-AM, Katz AM. (1976). Control of cardiac sarcolemmal adenylate cyclase and sodium, potassium activated adenosine triphosphatase activities. *Circ Res* 36:8–17.
Taylor SS, Buechler JA, Yonemoto W. (1990). cAMP-dependent protein kinase: framework for a diverse family of regulatory enzymes. *Annu Rev Biochem* 59:971–1005.
Yang-Feng TL, Xue F, Zhong W, Cotecchia, S, Frielle T, Caron MG, Lefkowitz RJ, Francke U. (1990). Chromosomal organization of adrenergic receptor genes. *Proc Natl Acad Sci USA* 87:1516–1520.

BIBLIOGRAPHY

Benovic JL, Bouvier M, Caron MG, Lefkowitz RJ. (1988). Regulation of adenylyl cyclase-coupled β-adrenergic receptors. *Annu Rev Cell Biol* 4:405–428.
Berridge MJ. (1989). Inositol triphosphate, calcium, lithium, and cell signalling. *JAMA* 262:1834–1841.
Birnbaumer L. (1990a). G proteins in signal transduction. *Annu Rev Pharmacol Toxicol* 30:675–705.
Birnbaumer L. (1990b). Transduction of receptor signal into modulation of effector activity by G proteins: the first 20 years or so. . . *FASEB J* 4:3068–3078.
Frielle T, Caron M, Lefkowitz RJ. (1989). Properties of the β$_1$- and β$_2$-adrenergic receptor subtypes revealed by molecular cloning. *Clin Chem* 35:721–725.
Gilman AG. (1989). G proteins and regulation of adenylyl cyclase. *JAMA* 262:1819–1825.
Halushka PV, Mais DE, Mayeux PR, Morinelli TA. (1990). Thromboxane, prostaglandin and leukotriene receptors. *Annu Rev Pharmacol Toxicol* 10:213–239.
Hulme EC, Birdsall NJM, Buckley NJ. (1988). Muscarinic receptor subtypes. *Annu Rev Pharmacol Toxicol* 30:633–673.
Nishizuka Y. (1989). The family of protein kinase C for signal transduction. *JAMA* 262:1826–1833.
Shearman MS, Sekiguchi K, Nishizuka Y. (1989). Modulation of ion channel activity: a key function of the protein kinase C enzyme family. *Pharmacol Rev* 41:211–237.

13

Myocardial Contractility

Force, Velocity, Length, and Time

Changing myocardial contractility is one of the most important elements of the response to altered circulatory demands. However, the significance of changes in the intrinsic contractile properties of the heart was largely overlooked until the mid-1950s, owing to earlier emphasis on length-dependent changes in myocardial performance (the Frank-Starling relationship; Chapter 16). A number of early observations had suggested that the intrinsic contractile properties of cardiac muscle could change in response to interventions such as neurohumoral stimulation, but the importance of these early observations did not become apparent until 1955, when Sarnoff introduced the concept of a "family of Starling curves." This concept, presented in full in Chapter 16, clearly distinguished changes in cardiac function due to altered contractility from the length-dependent regulation of contractile performance described more than a half-century earlier.

Realization that the intrinsic contractile properties of the heart could vary, and that these changes were of considerable functional importance, led cardiovascular physiologists to reexamine the mechanical properties of cardiac muscle in light of new discoveries regarding the biophysics and biochemistry of muscle contraction (Chapters 7 and 8) and excitation-contraction coupling (Chapters 10 and 11). As discussed in the following chapter, recognition of the importance of changing myocardial contractility marked the first of two paradigmatic shifts in our understanding of the regulation of cardiac performance. The result was a major expansion of our understanding of the heart's response to a variety of physiological, pharmacological, and pathological factors.

The relevance of muscle energetics and mechanics (Chapters 6 and 8) to the regulation of cardiac performance reflects the fact that the pumping action of the heart is controlled by mechanisms intrinsic to the myocardial cell. This intrinsic control of myocardial contractility is highlighted in Table 13.1, which compares four mechanisms that are potentially available for the regulation of cardiac and

TABLE 13.1. *Mechanisms regulating muscular performance*

Mechanism	Functional role in skeletal muscle	Functional role in cardiac muscle
Ability to summate individual contractile events (partial and complete tetanus)	Minor	None
Ability to vary number of active motor units	Major	None
Ability to undergo length-dependent changes in contractile properties (length-tension or Frank-Starling relationship)	Usually minor	Major in beat-to-beat regulation; minor in sustained circulatory changes
Ability to change intrinsic contractile properties (contractility)	Minor	Major in sustained circulatory changes; minor in beat-to-beat regulation

skeletal muscle performance. It is apparent that the two types of muscle use these control mechanisms in quite different ways.

SUMMATION OF CONTRACTIONS

The tension developed by a skeletal muscle can be augmented when high stimulation frequencies cause summation (Fig. 9.3) or a tetanic contraction (Fig. 9.4). Although these properties of skeletal muscle allow tension to be regulated by variations in the frequency at which the motor neuron supplying the muscle is discharged, most skeletal muscle contractions are actually brief tetani or summated contractions. Some of the movements of the extraocular muscles may be twitches, but these brief contractile responses generally represent functionally useless contractions; consider, for example, the knee jerk. For this reason, variations in the extent of summation of individual contractile events probably play no more than a minor role in the regulation of skeletal muscle performance.

The cardiac action potential unlike that of skeletal muscle lasts until the end of the active state. Because the heart's plasma membrane does not regain its ability to respond to electrical stimuli until the mechanical response has ended, summation and tetanization are not possible. For this reason, these regulatory mechanisms are not of importance in the heart.

VARIATIONS IN THE NUMBER OF ACTIVE MOTOR UNITS

Each skeletal muscle is composed of a number of motor units, which are groups of muscle cells innervated by a single motor neuron. Because individual motor neurons in the nerve supplying a skeletal muscle can function independently of other motor neurons, the tension generated by the muscle can be modulated by the recruitment of a greater or lesser number of motor units. This control is integrated within the central nervous system, whose output determines the number of active motor units. Thus, when we lift a light load, only a few percent of the motor units are activated, whereas if we use the same muscles to lift a heavy load, a much greater proportion of the motor units in the muscles involved are activated via their motor neurons. On the other hand, the intensity of the contractile event in a skeletal muscle cell tends to be stereotyped, generally as a maximal contractile response. For this reason, skeletal tension is determined by the recruitment of a greater or lesser number of motor neurons by the central nervous system, rather than changes intrinsic to the individual muscle fibers.

Control by variations in the number of active motor units is not possible in the heart, which is a functional syncytium because the intercalated discs contain specialized, highly permeable cell-cell junctions (the nexus or gap junctions described in Chapter 1). As these represent pathways of low electrical resistance, an electrical impulse entering any region of the myocardium is normally conducted throughout the heart; thus, fractional activation of the heart does not normally occur.

CHANGES IN SARCOMERE LENGTH

The dependence of muscle tension on rest-length, which is considered in some detail in Chapter 9, provides a mechanism by which preload can influence the tension output of a muscle. In most skeletal muscles, however, control of muscle performance by varying initial length is of little importance in regulating performance for the simple reason that muscle length is determined by the angles at the joints, rather than by the functional demands on the muscle. When we choose our position during the performance of muscular work, especially when it is isometric, considerations of leverage, rather than sarcomere length, are the main determinants. Thus, skeletal muscle sarcomere length is determined more by the need to achieve optimal leverage than by attempts to set the sarcomeres to the apices of their length-tension curves.

In the heart, which is a hollow viscus whose leverage is determined by the radius of curvature of its muscular walls (Chapter 15), the sarcomere length-tension relationship plays a much more important role in regulating force generation by the walls of the atria and ventricles. Sarcomere length in the heart is determined largely by preload, which in turn is influenced by the volume of blood returning during diastole and that remaining in the ventricle after the preceding systole. This allows the length-tension relationship to play an important role in adjusting the heart's ability to empty to compensate for changes in venous return and residual volume.

The length-tension relationship plays a major role in cardiac regulation by providing a means by which beat-to-beat changes in ejection match the heart's output to changing hemodynamics, and equalize the outputs of the two ventricles. Operation of the length-tension relationship in the heart, which is responsible for Starling's law of the heart discussed in Chapter 16, can therefore be viewed as a passive mechanism by which the heart responds to hemodynamic changes that alter diastolic volume. These are readily understood by considering the following dynamic situations, which illustrate how the length-tension relationship allows the heart to adjust rapidly to changing circulatory hemodynamics.

Responses to Changing Circulatory Hemodynamics

Changes in Venous Return

Raising the legs causes the forces of gravity to increase systemic venous return, which is defined simply as the volume of blood returning to the right atrium. The resulting elevation in right atrial pressure is transmitted to the right ventricle where it increases end-diastolic volume (dilatation) and thus adds to the preload. Operation of the length-tension relationship allows dilatation of the right ventricle to increase the ability of this chamber to eject blood; this will be true as long as the ventricle remains on the ascending limb of its length-tension curve (Fig. 9.10). The ability of the heart to increase its output in response to an increase in venous return establishes a positive feedback in which an increase in the flow of blood returning to the heart leads to a corresponding increase in the flow of blood leaving the heart.

Changes in Impedance to Ejection

A similar positive feedback by the length-tension relationship occurs when impedance to the ejection of blood from the heart is increased.

The terms *resistance* and *impedance* are sometimes used interchangeably, but there is a difference. *Resistance* refers to the forces opposing the movement of blood away from the aortic valve throughout the cardiac cycle, whereas *impedance* describes the forces opposing the movement of blood away from the aortic valve during ejection. This distinction is readily understood by considering two patients in whom cardiac output is the same, but blood pressures are 120/80 and 200/40 mm Hg. As mean aortic pressures are ~93 mm Hg (mean aortic pressure can be estimated as diastolic pressure $+ \frac{1}{3}$ pulse pressure), resistances should be the same; yet the impedance to ejection is obviously much greater in the patient with systolic hypertension.

An abrupt increase in aortic impedance reduces the ejection of blood from the left ventricle, which in turn causes a larger volume of blood to be retained in the ventricle at the end of the systole. This increased end-systolic (or residual) volume is then added to the venous return during the next diastole, thereby increasing end-diastolic volume. Although the accompanying rise in end-diastolic pressure would be expected to diminish venous return, the major effect in the normal heart is to increase sarcomere length beyond that seen before aortic pressure was elevated. The resulting dilatation of the ventricle, according to the length-tension relationship, causes more force to be developed and so allows the ventricle to eject a normal volume of blood even in the face of the increased aortic impedance.

In order for the length-tension relationship to mediate the cardiac response to changing hemodynamics, the heart must be operating on the ascending limb of the sarcomere length-tension curve. As noted in Chapter 9, it is unlikely that the heart normally can function on the descending limb.

Matching the Outputs of the Right and Left Sides of the Heart

The other regulatory function that is served by the length-tension relationship is the matching of the outputs of the two sides of the heart. Without such a control system, the output of the right ventricle might exceed that of the left ventricle, a situation that would prove lethal by literally drowning the individual as blood accumulates in the lungs.

The positive feedback that normally results from the operation of the ventricles on the ascending limbs of their length-tension relationships plays a vital role in equalizing the outputs of the ventricles. For example, if right ventricular output is increased (e.g., by leg raising; see above), the increased flow of blood through the lungs would, by dilating the left ventricle, allow the operation of the length-tension relationship to increase left ventricular ejection. Conversely, reduced ejection by the right ventricle would decrease left ventricular filling, and so reduce left ventricular output.

Although the length-tension relationship plays a major role in adjusting cardiac performance to hemodynamic factors as described above, changes in developed tension due to altered muscle fiber length appear not to be critical to most long-term circulatory changes. During exercise, for example, where cardiac work is increased greatly, the heart often becomes smaller; whereas in heart failure, where cardiac work decreases, the heart becomes enlarged. For this reason other regulatory systems must operate to allow the heart to adjust its performance to major long-term changes in circulatory dynamics, where important neurohumoral mechanisms come into play.

CHANGES IN CONTRACTILITY

Summation and tetanization, along with recruitment of a greater or lesser number of motor units, allow skeletal muscle performance to be regulated by the central nervous system. In the heart, where these mechanisms do not normally operate, performance is regulated by a much more powerful mechanism: altered myocardial contractility.

The distinction between length-dependent changes in cardiac performance and those that arise from changes in contractility have been blurred because the cellular mechanisms responsible for the length-tension relationship (Chapter 9) are now known to resemble those involved in changing contractility. Although the first represents a response to changing sarcomere length, and the second to neurotransmitters, drugs, and other chemical stimuli, both are mediated by alterations in the processes of excitation-contraction coupling. One should therefore view length-dependent regulation of muscle function as a passive adjustment to changing hemodynamics, whereas changing contractility arises from dynamic changes in the signal-response systems that impinge on the cells of the heart (Chapter 12). As the signals that modify contractility are quite different from those that simply cause a change in sarcomere length, this distinction is important.

Changes in the intrinsic contractile properties of most skeletal muscle cells are of little functional significance. Although slight changes in skeletal muscle contractile performance can be shown to occur in the intact animal under special circumstances, the role of these changes in altering the functional capacity of the muscle is much less important than the extrinsic control systems already discussed. For practical purposes, therefore, one can look on skeletal muscle contraction as a maximal response, as if the contractile proteins of a skeletal muscle deliver their "all" in response to any form of physiological stimulation.

The situation in the heart is quite different from that just described for a skeletal muscle. Under basal conditions the normal heart makes available only approximately two-thirds of its maximal contractility to pump blood. Although myocardial contractility can be adjusted in response to a large number of influences, this variability does not mean that the heart does not obey the "all-or-none law," which states that the intensity of a response is not determined by the intensity of the signal. Instead, the amount of the "all" can be changed in response to chemical regulators, as described in Chapter 14.

The term *inotropic* is commonly used in discussing changes in myocardial contractility. A *positive inotropic intervention* is one that causes contractility to increase, whereas a *negative inotropic intervention* reduces contractility. Inotropic changes probably mediate most important changes in the physiological function of the heart and are involved in the response of the heart to a number of drugs and disease states.

What is Myocardial Contractility?

Myocardial contractility is extremely difficult to define because contractility is the manifestation of *all* of the many factors that influence the interactions between the contractile proteins. The simplest definition of contractility is the "*potential to do work,*" which is, in turn, the expression of the actin-myosin interactions during the cross-bridge cycle (Chapter 8). The fact that the cross-bridge cycle in the heart is influenced directly and indirectly by a myriad of factors, however, makes it impossible to provide a crisp definition of this important term. The reader should neither despair nor close this book at this point, however, because *a change in myocardial contractility* is easy to define; this is simply *any change in work performed during the cardiac cycle not caused by a change in initial fiber length.* Any such change, by definition, can be considered to be the result of a change in contractility. For example, in an isolated strip of cardiac muscle contracting at a fixed muscle length, when a drug increases the ability of the muscle to shorten, develop tension, or both, contractility has been increased (Fig. 13.1). Conversely, a drug that reduces the ability of the muscle to do work during each beat at constant rest length can be said

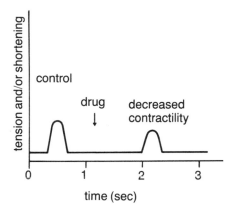

FIG. 13.1. Increased myocardial contractility enhances the amount of tension developed, the rate of shortening, or both, without an increase in rest length.

to have decreased contractility (Fig. 13.2). In the intact heart, a change in contractility can be identified by measuring an increase or decrease in the work performed per beat at a constant end-diastolic volume.

If we accept the definition of a change in myocardial contractility set forth in the preceding paragraph, we are still left with the difficult but important challenge of defining what it is that has in fact been changed. It is at this point that virtually all definitions of contractility fall short of their goal (Chapter 17) because, as already pointed out, myocardial contractility is the aggregate effect of all mechanisms that control the activity of the contractile proteins, and so determine the muscle's "*potential to do work*." Thus, any attempt to characterize myocardial contractility in a patient must take into account the ability of the muscle to develop tension and to shorten, which can vary independently of each other, as well as the rate of onset, overall duration, and decay of both of these variables. To make matters more complex, the characteristics of the contracting myocardium are not the only determinants of the ability of the heart to do work; contractile performance is also influ-

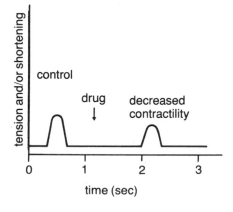

FIG. 13.2. Decreased myocardial contractility reduces the amount of tension developed, the rate of shortening, or both, without a decrease in rest length.

enced by elasticities and heterogeneities in the contraction of the heart as an organ. Finally, even if the heart's contraction were to occur with a fixed set of muscular characteristics, the manifestations of the contraction in terms of pressure and flow within the circulatory system are highly dependent on loading conditions (Chapter 16).

> Because loading conditions influence the extent to which sarcomere length decreases during systole, there being more sarcomere shortening when aortic impedance is low, the distinction between changes due to altered contractility, as opposed to those arising from the length-tension relationship, become blurred. For this reason, the distinctions commonly made between length-dependent and contractility-dependent determinants of cardiac function are, in fact, somewhat artificial.

Although the problems set forth in the preceding paragraphs have created insurmountable impediments to clinical determinations of the "true" level of myocardial contractility, there is no question that, as a concept, contractility is important, and must be understood in order to evaluate the cardiac patient. The many clinical indices of myocardial contractility (Chapter 17), although often only rough approximations, can be of considerable value in following the changing clinical course of patients with conditions such as valvular heart disease and heart failure. It does not follow, however, that the more complex the index, the more useful it is; in fact, as pointed out in Chapter 17, *ejection fraction*, a relatively simple index, is of proven value in assessing these patients.

Two approaches to the understanding of myocardial contractility are provided in this chapter. One is based on extrapolations from the analyses of skeletal muscle mechanics described in Chapter 6, and the other on our knowledge of the interactions between the contractile proteins, set forth in Chapter 8. The reader who can relate these two different ways of looking at the variable contractile response of the heart will have achieved a good working understanding of the meaning of myocardial contractility.

Contractility Defined in Terms of Muscle Mechanics

One of the major challenges in defining the intrinsic properties of a contracting muscle arises from the influence of loading conditions; this is simply because tension and shortening of a muscle are altered by changing load, even when contractility is constant. The concepts of muscle mechanics provide one way to get around these confounding effects of load.

It was pointed out in Chapter 6 that, many years before the discovery of the role of actin-myosin interactions in muscular contraction, Hill postulated two states in the "active points" of muscle. In the first, all of the active points are holding tension, whereas in the second state they are participating in chemical reactions. Hill also postulated that the distribution of active points between these two states is determined by the load on the muscle. This situation in contracting muscle can, therefore, be viewed as a "potential to do work" that can be "tapped" in different ways. When the muscle is presented with a heavy load, this potential to do work appears as tension, so that large loads are moved slowly short distances. At lower loads the muscle performs work in a different manner as the lighter load allows the potential to do work to appear as velocity, so that light loads are moved rapidly over greater distances. Thus, when load is varied, both the total work performed (Fig. 6.3) and the velocity of muscle shortening (Fig. 6.15) also vary. It is important to remember that these load-dependent changes do not represent variations in the potential to do work, but are different ways in which this property of the contracting muscle can be expressed. The perceptive reader should, by this point, realize that the term "potential to do work" is a simple way of stating the elusive concept of contractility.

We now turn to the concepts of muscle mechanics to quantify this term, examining the force-velocity relationship, which defines the mechanical manifestations of muscular contraction at different loads. According to Hill's postulate of two states in active muscle, it is theoretically possible for each state to vary independently of the other. For example, the number of active points in muscle could increase without there being any change in their rate of turnover. This is analogous to an increase in the number of "little men" pulling on the rope shown in Fig. 6.18. Similarly, the maximum rate of energy liberation by these active points could increase, so that the "little men" in Fig. 6.19 move more quickly without there being a change in their number. As discussed in Chapter 8, therefore, it is possible to vary contractility by one or both of two independent mechanisms. Variations in the number of active points would, in theory, alter P_o, the intercept of the force-velocity curve where force is maximal. Variations in the rate of turnover of active points, on the other hand, would shift V_{max}, the intercept of the force-velocity curve at zero load, where velocity is maximal. Either would move the force-velocity curve upward and to the right, which represents an increase in the potential to do work because the muscle is able to develop more tension or to shorten more rapidly. Thus, an increase in contractility that causes an upward and rightward shift in the force-velocity curve can arise from increased V_{max}, P_o, or both (Fig. 13.3).

Figure 13.3 demonstrates that *any mechanism that, at constant muscle length, shifts the force-velocity curve upward and to the right, has increased contractility.* This is readily understood because, regardless of whether P_o or V_{max} has increased, the ability to do work at intermediate loads has been increased. Conversely, a shift in this curve downward and to the left represents a decrease in contractility. The restriction that initial muscle length must remain constant maintains the distinction between length-dependent changes in muscle performance and changes due to altered contractility. The three mechanisms that shift the force-velocity curves in Fig. 13.3 are quite different, and can be differentiated only when the two intercepts of the force-velocity curve are measured and compared. As is apparent from Fig. 13.3, no distinction between these mechanisms is possible if measurements are made only at intermediate loads.

At this point it should be apparent that contractility is determined by at least two theoretically independent properties of the contractile proteins: maximal force-gen-

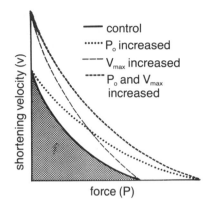

shortening velocity (v)

— control
...... P$_o$ increased
– – – V$_{max}$ increased
---- P$_o$ and V$_{max}$
     increased

force (P)

FIG. 13.3. An increase in myocardial contractility causes an upward shift in the force-velocity curve that can be brought about by increased V$_{max}$, increased P$_o$, or both. Measurements at intermediate forces cannot distinguish between these inotropic mechanisms. The control force-velocity relationship is *shaded*.

erating capacity and maximal shortening velocity. In a tetanized skeletal muscle, it is relatively simple to generate the force-velocity curves needed to quantify each of these parameters. The heart, however, cannot be tetanized; furthermore, the active state is slow in onset and is altered by changes in muscle length and load (Chapter 9). The fact that the interactions between the contractile proteins change during the slow evolution of cardiac systole makes it impossible to obtain data such as shown in Fig. 13.3. Because the performance of the heart is also determined by time-dependent changes in both P_o and V_{max}, measurements of tension and shortening velocity at intermediate loads tell us little about either the number of active points or their rate of interaction in the heart.

Because the active state is both slow in onset and of finite duration in the normal cardiac contraction (Chapter 9), at least three time-dependent properties must be added to the list of variables that determine myocardial contractility. The first is the *rate of onset* of the capacity to generate tension and to shorten, the second is the *duration*, and the third is the *rate of decay*. Viewed in terms of the force-velocity curve, therefore, it is possible to imagine that this relationship undergoes a series of changes that evolve throughout each contraction. We return to these time-dependent properties later in the chapter, after first reexamining the concepts of force and velocity in terms of our current understanding of their relationship to the known interaction between the contractile proteins.

Contractility Defined in Terms of the Interactions Between the Contractile Proteins

The relationship between the molecular interactions of the contractile proteins and the energetics of muscular contraction was discussed at the end of Chapter 8. Here it was postulated that Hill's first state of the active points in muscle, which generates tension, occurs when the actin-myosin interactions are present as the rigor complex, where tension is generated but no energy is being liberated. The second

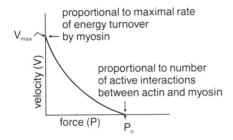

FIG. 13.4. The two intercepts of the force-velocity curve can be related to specific aspects of the interactions between the contractile proteins. V_{max} is determined largely by the rate of energy turnover by myosin, whereas P_o is proportional to the number of active interactions between actin and myosin.

state, in which the active points liberate chemical energy at their maximal intrinsic rate, corresponds to the rapid cycling of actin-myosin-ATP interactions that cause muscle shortening when no tension is being generated. According to this formulation, the intercepts of the force-velocity curve, and thus the determinants of contractility, arise from two quite different aspects of the chemistry of the contractile proteins: P_o is proportional to the number of active cross-bridges, and V_{max} to their turnover rate (Fig. 13.4).

According to the definition set forth in the preceding paragraph, myocardial contractility can be increased when the number of tension-generating rigor complexes is increased, the maximal rate of energy liberation during the cross-bridge cycle is increased, or both. Of course, even this analysis is not simple; the reader need only recall the many cooperative interactions among the contractile proteins that are influenced by such chemical factors as ATP levels, phosphoesters formed by various protein kinases, and even effects of changing muscle length (Chapters 8 and 9). In addition, a growing number of protein isoform shifts are being identified that can modify these variables (Chapter 7). In spite of these complexities, it is useful to view contractility as depending on two major variables: the number of rigor complexes formed during excitation-contraction coupling, and the rate of the cross-bridge cycle. These, of course, correspond to the two intercepts of the force-velocity curve.

Regulation by an Altered Number of Rigor Complexes

By far the most important mechanisms that regulate myocardial contractility are changes in the number of rigor complexes. These are readily explained as the result of variations in the amount of calcium delivered to the contractile proteins at the onset of systole. Because each of the troponin complexes probably determines the ability of seven actin monomers to participate in the contractile process (Chapter 7), variations in the amount of calcium released during excitation-contraction coupling are amplified approximately sevenfold in regulating the number of potential rigor complexes. As the number of rigor complexes is the major determinant of force under isometric conditions, where force is maximal and shortening velocity is zero, changes in P_o can be most easily explained as being due to variations in the availability of calcium for binding to troponin C during systole.

> Although the tension-generating capacity of the rigor complex may be variable, mechanisms that lead to such changes in the heart have not yet been clarified. Such well-documented phenomena as phosphorylation of the myosin light chains are reasonable candidates for such an effect.

Regulation by Altered Cross-Bridge Cycling

Variations in the rate of cross-bridge cycling represent the other major parameter that determines myocardial contractility. This property, which determines both ATP hydrolysis *in vitro* and maximal shortening velocity in a muscle at zero load *in vivo*, also determines V_{max}, the other intercept of the force-velocity curve. Changes in this determinant of muscle shortening velocity arise from alterations in the myosin heavy chains, which in turn, reflect the synthesis of the various isoforms of this protein. As discussed in Chapter 8, posttranslational modification of the contractile proteins, notably protein kinase–catalyzed phosphorylation, may also influence this rate.

Influence of Time-Dependent Properties on Contractility

In addition to the changes in the number and rates of actin-myosin interactions, which determine the two intercepts of the force-velocity curve, alterations in the rates of activation and inactivation of the contractile process can influence myocardial contractility. Each contraction of the heart, like each twitch of a skeletal muscle, has a characteristic rate of onset and termination that is determined both by the rate of development of the active state and by the damping effect of the series elasticity; in the heart, the gradual onset of tension results primarily from the slow rate of activation, rather than damping by the series elasticity. Thus, changes in the time course of delivery and removal of activator calcium can modify the ability of cardiac muscle to do work, and so change myocardial contractility (Fig. 13.5).

> The relationship between cytosolic Ca^{2+} concentration and tension shown in Fig. 13.5 has a number of interesting features. Most important is that Ca^{2+} concentration begins to rise before significant tension has been developed, and that Ca^{2+} levels begin to fall well before tension has reached its maximum. In some preparations, two components in the calcium signal have been seen. Although these findings were initially interpreted as defining a small initial rise in cytosolic Ca^{2+} concentration due to calcium entry across the plasma membrane, followed by a larger component due to calcium release from the sarcoplasmic reticulum, it now appears that both are due to the latter. Studies of regional changes in cytosolic Ca^{2+} concentration in isolated cardiac myocytes have demonstrated spatial heterogeneities even within single cells (Weir et al., 1987).

Both the time course and extent of tension development by the heart can vary with changing rates of calcium release and reuptake by the sarcoplasmic reticulum.

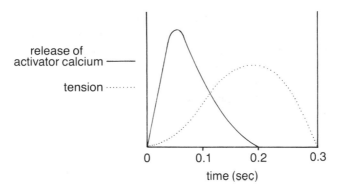

FIG. 13.5. The release of activator calcium (*solid line*) precedes the development of tension in cardiac muscle.

Three hypothetical changes in this time course are depicted in Fig. 13.6, each of which could increase the capacity of the heart to do work, even if the maximum number of active points (P_o) and the intrinsic rate of turnover of the active points (V_{max}) remained constant. These are (a) an increased rate of delivery of activator calcium, (b) a prolonged duration of maximal activator calcium release, and (c) a reduced rate of activator calcium removal. Conversely, a decline in myocardial contractility would occur if the rate of activator calcium delivery was decreased, the duration of its maximal release shortened, or the rate of its removal increased.

Importance of Relaxation

This is an appropriate point at which to reemphasize the importance of relaxation. As noted in Chapter 11, the reserve for the ATP-dependent ion pumps that remove

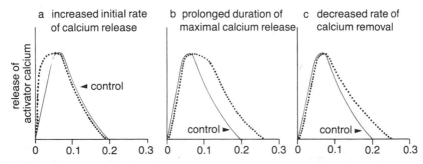

FIG. 13.6. Three ways by which time-dependent changes in the release of activator calcium can increase contractility without a change in the maximal amount of activator calcium released. In each example the *solid line* represents the time course of calcium release in the control state (tension is not shown). More work can be performed in a contraction if (a) the rate of activator calcium release is increased, (b) the duration of maximal activator calcium release is prolonged, or (c) the rate of activator calcium removal is reduced.

calcium from the cytosol to relax the heart is much less than for the downhill calcium fluxes that initiate systole. For this reason, any intervention that increases the amount of calcium delivered to the contractile proteins must tax the systems responsible for relaxation. Although these considerations are of minimal importance for the normal heart, efforts to increase contractility in the ischemic or failing heart may provoke important relaxation abnormalities.

Force-Velocity-Time Relationships

In the preceding discussion we have seen how three independent variables determine myocardial contractility: the number of active cross-bridges (P_o), the rate of the cross-bridge cycle (V_{max}), and the time courses of the onset and offset of cross-bridge interactions. The interplay between these three variables, and thus myocardial contractility, can be visualized as a three-dimensional graph in which each makes up one coordinate (Fig. 13.7). Figure 13.7 has been constructed with a constant V_{max} in view of theoretical evidence that the velocity of shortening becomes maximal as soon as activator calcium reaches the contractile proteins (Chapter 9). Myocardial contractility represents the surface of the solid figure in Fig. 13.7, which defines the time course of the force-velocity curve during each cardiac cycle. This surface, which should be "read" from bottom left to top right, defines the rise and fall of the force-velocity curve, that is, the "potential to do work" described earlier in this chapter.

The depiction of myocardial contractility in Fig. 13.7 is oversimplified because it omits at least two important factors. The first is the length dependence of the active state. Because sarcomere shortening reduces activation by decreasing both calcium release from the sarcoplasmic reticulum and the calcium sensitivity of the contractile proteins (Chapter 9), P_o progressively falls during the cardiac cycle. This process of "deactivation" occurs even when muscle length is held constant as the elasticity of the cardiac muscle allows for some sarcomere shortening as the elastic elements are stretched. Because the heart normally functions at the apex or on the "ascending limb" of its sarcomere length-tension curve (Chapter 9), these length-dependent phenomena cause P_o to decrease. The second complication to the

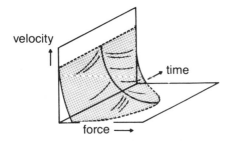

FIG. 13.7. Three-dimensional graph showing the dependence on time (axis moving to the right, away from the reader) of a series of force-velocity curves in which V_{max} is constant (*dashed line* on *vertical axis*), whereas P_o (*dashed line* on *horizontal axis*) first rises and then falls in response to the release and reuptake of activator calcium.

analysis of myocardial contractility presented in Fig. 13.7 arises from internal resistances to shortening, which are especially marked in the heart. These internal resistances would reduce the apparent shortening velocity, especially when the amount of activator released, and thus the number of active cross-bridge interactions, is small. Taking the length dependence of active-state and internal resistances into consideration, a more accurate representation of myocardial contractility is that shown in Fig. 13.8, in which maximal velocity, as well as maximal force, is shown to vary with time.

The determinants of the mechanical performance of the heart are summarized in Table 13.2, which states that cardiac performance is determined both by factors intrinsic to the myocardium, and by external load. The former include at least four variables. One, initial sarcomere length, is generally distinguished from the other three: the number of active cross-bridges (P_o), the rate of cross-bridge cycling (V_{max}), and the time courses of activation and inactivation. The latter three, as described above, contribute to myocardial contractility. As noted earlier, distinctions between the effects of changing initial sarcomere length and those of myocardial contractility fail to take into account the load-dependent changes in sarcomere length that occur when the heart ejects. The influence of load on cardiac performance in considered further in Chapter 16.

Although the complexity of the definition of myocardial contractility makes it difficult to apply this concept to intact cardiac muscle, the simplicity of defining a *change in contractility* must not be forgotten. As long as initial fiber length remains constant, any change in the ability of the heart to do work, by definition, reflects a change in myocardial contractility. Beyond this simple statement, however, our ability to distinguish among the determinants of a change in contractility in cardiac muscle is limited, especially in the clinical setting where the geometry of the heart must also be considered. Yet, estimates of myocardial contractility are part of the clinical evaluation of cardiac performance. We return to this subject in Chapter 17 after first reviewing our current understanding of the regulation of myocardial contractility (Chapter 14) and the manifestations of these changes in simple cardiac muscle preparations (Chapter 15).

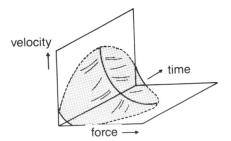

FIG. 13.8. Three-dimensional graph, constructed as in Fig. 13.7, showing time-dependent changes in V_{max} caused by the internal resistances to shortening that are especially marked in the heart. A progressive fall in P_o caused by variable, load-dependent, sarcomere shortening should be superimposed on the rise and fall in P_o that are determined largely by the release and reuptake of activator calcium.

TABLE 13.2. *Determinants of the mechanical performance of the heart*

I. Factors intrinsic to the myocardium
  1. Number of active cross-bridges (P_0)
  2. Rate of cross-bridge cycling (V_{max})
  3. Time courses of activation and inactivation
  4. Initial sarcomere length
II. External factors, most important of which is load

Myocardial contractility, as generally defined, includes I.1 and I.2, and sometimes I.3.

REFERENCES

Sarnoff SJ. (1955). Myocardial contractility as described by ventricular function curves: observations on Starling's Law of the Heart. *Physiol Rev* 35:107–122.
Weir WG, Cannell MB, Berlin JR, Marban E, Lederer WJ. (1987). Cellular and subcellular heterogeneity of $[Ca^{2+}]_i$ in single heart cells revealed by Fura-2. *Science* 245:325–328.

BIBLIOGRAPHY

Abbott BC, Mommaerts WFHM. (1959). A study of inotropic mechanisms in the papillary muscle preparation. *J Gen Physiol* 42:533–541.
Blinks JR. (1986). Intracellular $[Ca^{2+}]$ measurements. In: Fozzard H, Haber E, Katz A, Jennings R, Morgan HE, eds. *The heart and cardiovascular system*. New York: Raven Press; 671–701.
Brady AJ. (1974). Mechanics of the myocardium. In: Langer GA, Brady AJ, eds. *The mammalian myocardium*. New York: Wiley; 163–192.
Julian FJ, Moss RL. (1976). The concept of active state in striated muscle. *Circ Res* 38:53–59.
Katz AM. (1988). Molecular biology in cardiology, a paradigmatic shift. *J Mol Cell Cardiol* 20:355–366.
Katz LN, (chairman). (1955). Symposium on the regulation of the performance of the heart. *Physiol Rev* 35:89–168.
Pollack GH, Krueger JW. (1976). Sarcomere dynamics in intact cardiac muscle. *Eur J Cardiol* 4(Suppl):53–65.
Sonnenblick EH. (1962). Implications of muscle mechanics in the heart. *Fed Proc* 21:975–990.

14

Regulation of
Myocardial Contractility

Our growing knowledge of the regulation of the heart's performance has been accompanied by a shifting emphasis among three quite different types of control: *organ physiology, cell biochemistry and biophysics,* and *gene expression* (Table 14.1) (Katz, 1988). Each can be viewed as a different paradigm, or school of science, that has aided our efforts to understand how the work of the heart is controlled. Furthermore, these three types of control are likely to have appeared sequentially during evolution (Fig. 14.1). Regulation at the *organ* level, the most recent to have evolved, could only operate after the heart had become organized as a tissue. Regulation by changing *cell* biochemistry and biophysics would have appeared earlier, when single-celled organisms had developed to a point where, surrounded by a semipermeable membrane, they gained the ability to control their internal environment. Regulation by synthesis of altered *gene* products, which is almost certainly the oldest, probably aided early life forms, not yet able to control the milieu containing their genes, in adapting to environmental changes. As the most primitive mechanism by which living organisms adapted to a changing environment, regulation by altered gene expression would have had the longest time to evolve. It is not surprising, therefore, that this mechanism is turning out to be the most complex of the three paradigms listed in Table 14.1.

The manifestation of the first paradigm, as it applies to cardiac regulation, is Starling's law of the heart; this is the control at the *organ* level, discussed in Chapters 15 and 16. Changing myocardial contractility, which as defined in Chapter 13 is determined largely by the properties of the *cell*, reflects the second of the paradigms listed in Table 14.1. Myocardial contractility, although regulated mainly by changes in the calcium fluxes involved in excitation-contraction coupling and relaxation (Fig. 14.2), is also influenced by the third paradigm, altered *gene* expression, which adjusts cardiac function to such chronic conditions as aortic stenosis, endocrinopathies, and aging.

TABLE 14.1. *Three paradigms in the development of our knowledge of cardiac performance*

Organ (physiology)	Changing end-diastolic fiber length (the Frank-Starling relationship)
Cell (biochemistry and biophysics)	Changing myocardial contractility, calcium fluxes
Gene (molecular biology)	Altered synthesis of myocardial proteins

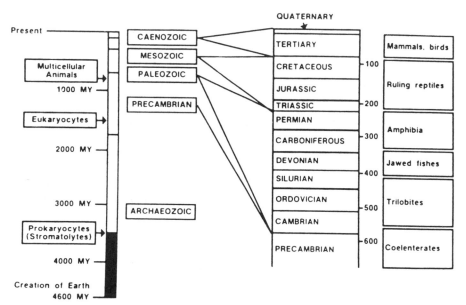

FIG. 14.1. Possible evolutionary basis for the three paradigms that describe the regulation of the performance of the heart. Life on earth probably appeared ~3,500,000,000 years ago with the emergence of *prokaryocytes* that, early in their evolution, lacked highly developed plasma membranes; thus, these early life forms probably adapted to environmental changes mainly by producing altered gene products. With the appearance of *eukaryocytes* ~1,800,000,000 years ago, cell membranes made it possible for living organisms to regulate cytosolic composition, which allowed changes in cell biochemistry and biophysics to regulate function on the adaptation to changing external environment. Only after the appearance of multicellular animals ~800,000,000 years ago, could regulation by changing organ function have come to play a role in the adaptation of life forms to a changing environment. Scales are in millions of years (MY). The time line shown to the *left* is enlarged at the *right* (from Katz, 1990).

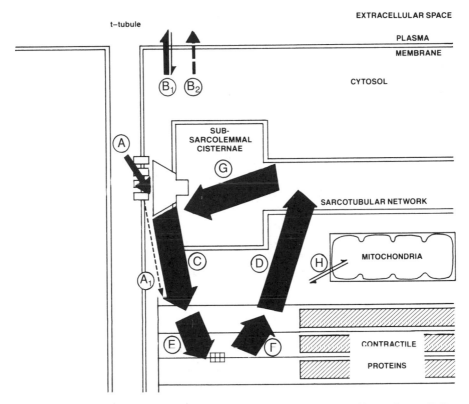

FIG. 14.2. Schematic diagram showing the major calcium fluxes involved in cardiac excitation-contraction coupling. The thickness of the *arrows* indicates the magnitude of the calcium fluxes, and their directions describe the "energetics" of the calcium fluxes: *downward arrows* describe passive calcium fluxes and *upward arrows* describe energy-dependent calcium transport. Calcium enters the cell from the extracellular fluid via plasmalemmal calcium channels, *A*; although most of this calcium triggers calcium release from the sarcoplasmic reticulum, a small portion directly activates the contractile proteins, A_1. Calcium transport back into the extracellular fluid involves two plasma membrane systems: sodium/calcium exchange, B_1, and the plasmalemmal calcium pump, B_2. The sarcoplasmic reticulum membrane regulates two calcium fluxes: calcium release from the subsarcolemmal cisternae, *C*, and active calcium uptake by the calcium pump of the sarcotubular network, *D*. Calcium diffuses within the sarcoplasmic reticulum in a third calcium flux, *G*, returning to the subsarcolemmal cisternae where it is stored in complex with calsequestrin and other calcium-binding proteins. Binding, *E*, and dissociation, *F*, of calcium with the high-affinity calcium-binding sites of troponin C define the affinity for calcium: the ratio *E/F*. Movements of calcium into and out of mitochondria, *H*, buffer cytosolic Ca^{2+} concentration.

MECHANISMS INVOLVED IN THE REGULATION OF MYOCARDIAL CONTRACTILITY

Tonic and Phasic Control

Adaptive responses mediated by the three paradigms listed in Table 14.1 have very different time courses. Regulation of *organ* function by changing rest length is the fastest as it involves beat-to-beat changes in cardiac function (Chapter 13). Less rapid is regulation by changing *cell* biochemistry and biophysics, which is generally brought about by changing interactions between calcium and various cellular components; the responses to the neurotransmitters and drugs that modify myocardial contractility by this second paradigm evolve over several seconds or minutes and have been referred to as "phasic" regulation (Katz, 1976). On the other hand, changes in myocardial contractility that arise from alterations in *gene* expression evolve much more slowly, generally over periods of days, weeks, or even months. For this reason, these have been called "tonic" changes. Although tonic and phasic control seemed to be a useful classification when I introduced these terms in 1976, it now seems more appropriate to classify the fundamentally different mechanisms that regulate myocardial contractility in terms of the three paradigms listed in Table 14.1.

Changes in the amount of calcium that binds to the cardiac contractile proteins play a central role in the regulation of myocardial contractility. These generally involve altered calcium fluxes and calcium-protein interactions at the *cell* level; most are phasic changes that modulate excitation-contraction coupling and relaxation. Alterations in *gene* expression, however, can also play an important role in determining the interactions of calcium with several systems within the myocardial cell; as noted above, these represent long-term, or tonic, adjustments.

Changes in the number of cardiac troponin molecules that bind calcium during excitation-contraction coupling modify the number of interactions between actin and myosin (Chapter 13). The resulting variations in the number of active force-generating sites alter maximum isometric tension so that, on theoretical grounds, these mechanisms should shift P_o of the force-velocity curve. There is growing evidence that isoform shifts involving the myofibrillar proteins can also regulate the number of troponin molecules that bind calcium, due to altered calcium sensitivity of the heart's contractile proteins. Thus, tonic mechanisms can also modify P_o. Quite different mechanisms modify the rate of the cross-bridge cycle, and so would be expected to alter V_{max}. Most known examples of this type of regulation are tonic mechanisms that involve the synthesis of altered myosin heavy-chain isoforms, but calcium-dependent phosphorylations, a phasic mechanism, may also regulate the rate of actin-myosin interactions.

The following discussion reviews several important mechanisms by which altered calcium-troponin interactions regulate myocardial contractility. These lead to changes in the number of active actin-myosin interactions as the result of changes in three systems: the plasma membrane, sarcoplasmic reticulum, and troponin complex.

Regulation of Myocardial Contractility by Changing Calcium Fluxes Across the Plasma Membrane

The discovery that calcium is essential for the heart to contract was accidental. In the 1880s, Ringer found that when distilled water was used to make up the salt solutions with which he perfused isolated hearts, the hearts failed to contract. However, when the same salt solutions were prepared from tap water, the hearts contracted forcefully. This led to the search for a factor in the tap water needed for the heart to develop tension. In a now-classic study, Ringer analyzed the mineral content of the tap water obtained from the New River Water Company and found that, of the many substances present in trace amounts, it was the contaminating calcium salts that were essential for the heart to contract. This requirement for extracellular calcium is now known to arise mainly from its participation in the "calcium-trigger" that opens calcium release channels in the cardiac sarcoplasmic reticulum (Chapter 11). In addition to its critical role in excitation-contraction coupling, extracellular calcium contributes to the filling of calcium stores in the sarcoplasmic reticulum and, in some invertebrate and fetal hearts, to the calcium that binds to the contractile proteins.

> The contractile response of skeletal muscle does not require extracellular calcium because opening of the calcium release channels in the sarcoplasmic reticulum appears to involve a mechanical coupling, rather than a calcium signal, between the t-tubule and the calcium release channel (Chapter 11).

Effects Mediated by Calcium Channels

Most of the calcium that enters the heart crosses the plasma membrane through voltage-dependent, calcium-selective ion channels that are called *calcium channels* in the remainder of this text. The properties of several different types of plasmalemmal calcium channel are discussed in Chapter 18; at this point, we focus on the functional effects of the calcium that they allow to enter the cell. Myocardial contractility can be regulated both by changes in the behavior of these channels, and by changes in the channels themselves. Most known examples of the latter involve posttranslational changes, notably phosphorylations. There is evidence, still incomplete, that the expression of abnormal calcium channel isoforms plays a role in the adaptation of the heart to such tonic influences as chronic hemodynamic overloading.

The Positive Staircase

The positive staircase, which is a manifestation of rate-dependent variations in contractility that are known collectively as the force-frequency relationship, is named after Bowditch, who at the end of the 19th century described rate-dependent variations in the intensity of the contractile response of cardiac muscle.

> It is fitting that Bowditch also described the "all-or-none law," which states that the intensity of a response does not depend on the intensity of the stimulus. Even though

the rate-dependent changes in myocardial contractility noted by Bowditch represent variations in the mechanical response of the myocardium, they do not violate this fundamental property of excitable tissue because it is the *frequency* of stimulation, not the *intensity*, that is responsible for the positive staircase. Thus, changes in myocardial contractility do not violate the "all-or-none law," but instead, reflect variations in the amount of the "all."

Bowditch found that at any given frequency of stimulation, the heart develops a characteristic tension (Fig. 14.3). An increase in frequency at moderate to low heart rates leads to a rise in tension in which each succeeding beat becomes stronger until a new plateau of tension is reached; tension builds up by a series of small steps (Fig. 14.3), hence the designation "staircase," or its German translation *treppe*. Conversely, a decrease in the frequency of stimulation causes developed tension to decrease.

For many years the positive staircase was believed to be causally related to net efflux of potassium observed at higher rates of stimulation. It is now clear, however, that even though increasing the frequency of contraction causes a slight loss of potassium, due to the greater number of action potentials per unit of time, the correlation between loss of cellular potassium and the increase in contractility is indirect, and does not reflect a causal relationship.

It is now clear that the positive staircase is the result of increased calcium entry through plasma membrane calcium channels. This is due simply to the fact that at the higher rates, these channels open more often and so allow more calcium to enter the cell (Fig. 14.4).

Post-extrasystolic Potentiation

The positive inotropic response of the beat following a premature systole (often, but necessarily, occurring as an "extrasystole"), is among the most intense seen in cardiac muscle (Fig. 14.5). This powerful inotropic response, called *post-extra-systolic potentiation*, represents a special manifestation of the positive staircase.

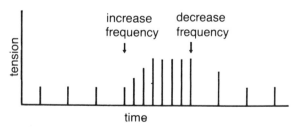

FIG. 14.3. The positive (Bowditch) staircase. The tension developed by a strip of cardiac muscle during a series of isometric contractions (represented as *vertical lines*) increases in a stepwise manner after the frequency of stimulation is increased, and decreases when stimulation frequency is reduced.

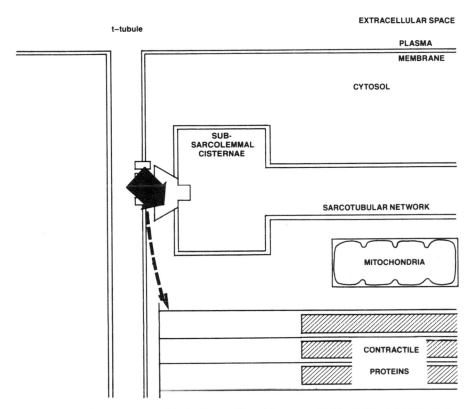

FIG. 14.4. Mechanism responsible for the positive staircase and post-extrasystolic potentiation. In the former, accelerated stimulation frequency causes more calcium channel openings per unit time, which increases calcium influx across the plasma membrane. Post-extrasystolic potentiation, which is also due to increased calcium entry, occurs when premature depolarization of the plasma membrane increases the amount of calcium that enters the cell via this channel. In this and other figures based on Fig. 14.2, only the *initial* changes initiated by different interventions are depicted as changes in the thickness of arrows depicted in Fig. 14.2.

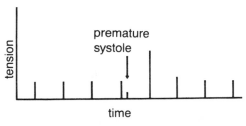

FIG. 14.5. Post-extrasystolic potentiation. The tension developed during the first contraction after a premature systole (the "extrasystole") is markedly potentiated. The positive inotropic state left behind by premature systole decays slowly, and so potentiates tension slightly in the second contraction after its occurrence. (As in Fig. 14.3, each contraction is represented as a *vertical line*.)

The extent to which the post-extrasystolic contraction is potentiated does not depend on the tension developed by the premature systole; in fact, the positive inotropic effect is greater when the early beat is so premature that little or no tension is developed. Post-extrasystolic potentiation can even occur when the premature beat comes so early as merely to delay relaxation of the preceding normal beat.

The mechanism responsible for post-extrasystolic potentiation was clarified in a classical study of Wood, Hepner, and Weidmann (1969), who using intracellular electrodes, induced small currents across the plasma membrane during systole (Fig. 14.6). These currents caused either slight depolarization or hyperpolarization during the absolute refractory period (Chapter 19), when the heart could not respond with a regenerative action potential. Depolarizing currents applied at this time caused membrane potential to become more positive, but did not affect the tension during the systole when the currents were applied; however, the systole that followed the beat during which the depolarizing current was applied was markedly potentiated (1 in Fig. 14.6). Conversely, a hyperpolarizing current that tended to return membrane potential toward its resting level markedly reduced tension developed by the subsequent beat, but again had no effect on the contraction during which this current was applied (2 in Fig. 14.6).

These findings can be explained by voltage-dependent changes in the open state of the calcium channels caused by the small applied currents. Depolarization during or shortly after the end of the plateau of the cardiac action potential increases cal-

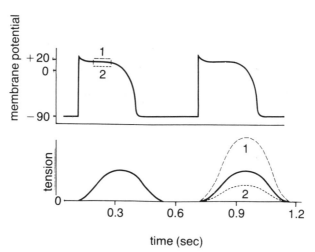

FIG. 14.6. Effects of altered membrane potential (*top*) on mechanical performance (*bottom*). A depolarizing (1) or hyperpolarizing (2) electrical current, which alters membrane potential only during the plateau of the cardiac action potential, has no effect on tension developed during the contraction in which the current was applied. Tension developed in the subsequent contraction is, however, markedly increased following the depolarizing current (1), and markedly decreased following the hyperpolarizing current (2).

cium channel opening, whereas reducing membrane potential during this phase of the action potential accelerates their closing. As noted in Chapter 11, little of this calcium is delivered directly to the contractile proteins; instead, most is added to the stores in the sarcoplasmic reticulum where its effect is seen during subsequent contractions. This experiment, therefore, demonstrates that the calcium that enters the cell during the plateau of the action potential has little influence on the tension developed in the contraction during which the channels are open. Instead, the calcium that crosses the plasma membrane during systole is added to the pool of calcium within the sarcoplasmic reticulum that becomes available for binding to troponin only during the subsequent contractions.

Effects of Cyclic AMP

β-adrenergic agonists and other agents that increase adenosine 3', 5'-cyclic monophosphate (cyclic AMP) levels in the heart also increase calcium entry via plasma

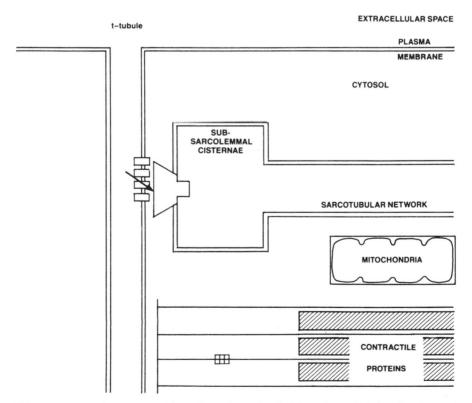

FIG. 14.7. Drugs that inhibit calcium channel opening (calcium channel blockers) reduce calcium entry across the plasma membrane.

membrane channels. The mechanism responsible for this effect, which is due to phosphorylation of the calcium channels by protein kinase A, is discussed in Chapter 18, and integrated with the other effects of cyclic AMP at the conclusion of this chapter.

Effects of Calcium Channel Blocking Drugs

Drugs that block cardiac plasma membrane calcium channels are sometimes called "calcium antagonists," but this is an unfortunate term since the drugs antagonize neither calcium nor its effects on the cell. Instead, by modifying the kinetics of the channels (that is, their opening, closing, inactivation, and reactivation [Chapter 18]), these drugs reduce the amount of calcium that enters the cells of the heart (Fig. 14.7).

Effects Mediated by the Sodium/Calcium Exchanger

As discussed in Chapter 10, a plasma membrane countertransport system exchanges sodium and calcium in both directions across the plasma membrane. Changes in the calcium fluxes mediated by this sodium/calcium exchanger have several important effects on myocardial contractility.

Effects of Extracellular Calcium and Sodium

The opposing actions of extracellular Na^+ and Ca^{2+} concentrations on myocardial contractility can, as discussed in Chapter 10, be expressed by the following relationship:

$$\text{Contractility} \sim [Ca^{2+}]_o/[Na^+]_o{}^3. \qquad [14.1]$$

In other words, myocardial contractility is determined by the ratio between these two cations. The effect of an increase in extracellular calcium, a decrease in extracellular sodium, or both, is shown in Fig. 14.8, where the sodium/calcium exchanger mediates an increased calcium entry (arrow B_1) and so increases contractility. The opposite changes in extracellular calcium and sodium would, of course, have a negative inotropic effect.

Effects of the Cardiac Glycosides

The primary effect of the cardiac glycosides (e.g., digitalis) is to inhibit sodium efflux via the sodium pump (Chapter 10); the resulting increase in the concentration of sodium within the cell (Lee et al., 1985) has indirect, but important, effects on the sodium/calcium exchanger that increase myocardial contractility.

The ability of sodium pump inhibition to increase myocardial contractility in-

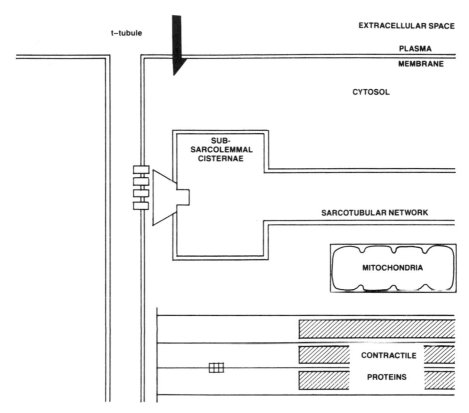

FIG. 14.8. Increasing extracellular Ca^{2+} concentrations and decreasing extracellular Na^+ both augment calcium entry via the sodium/calcium exchanger.

volves two changes in calcium movements across the plasma membrane, both of which are mediated by the sodium/calcium exchanger. The first is competition between the increased intracellular sodium and calcium for transport out of the cell by the sodium/calcium exchanger, which by reducing calcium efflux (Fig. 14.9), retains calcium within the cell. The second effect of the increased cytosolic sodium caused by sodium pump inhibition is related to increased sodium efflux via the exchanger. As some of the sodium that would normally have been transported out of the cell by the sodium pump in exchange for potassium must, instead, be exchanged for calcium, a greater amount of calcium enters via the exchanger (Fig. 14.9).

Inhibitors of Sodium/Calcium Exchange

Progress in studying the molecular properties of the sodium/calcium exchanger has been slow due to the lack of specific inhibitors and drugs that bind covalently to the membrane system(s) that mediate this important countertransport. Several

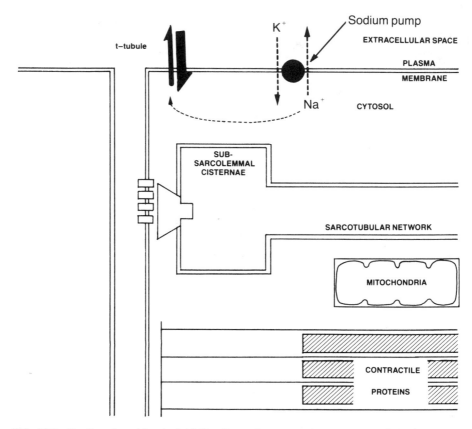

FIG. 14.9. Cardiac glycosides, by inhibiting the sodium pump, increase cytosolic Na$^+$ concentration. This, in turn, increases intracellular Ca^{2+} concentration by reducing calcium efflux via the sodium/calcium exchanger. Because of increased sodium efflux via the exchanger, calcium influx is also increased.

drugs, for example the diuretic amiloride, inhibit the exchanger (Kim and Smith, 1986), but these effects are not highly specific.

Effects of Altered Membrane Potential

The fact that sodium/calcium exchange is electrogenic was emphasized in Chapter 10, where it was noted that because three Na$^+$ ions exchange for one Ca^{2+}, a net positive charge follows the sodium that is exchanged for calcium. It was also pointed out that membrane potential modifies the ion exchange, tending to "pull" sodium into, and calcium out of, the fluid in contact with the negatively charged side of the membrane. This charge effect helps to move calcium out of the resting cell, in which the cell interior has a negative potential. Conversely, the reversal of membrane potential in the depolarized cell favors sodium transport out of, and

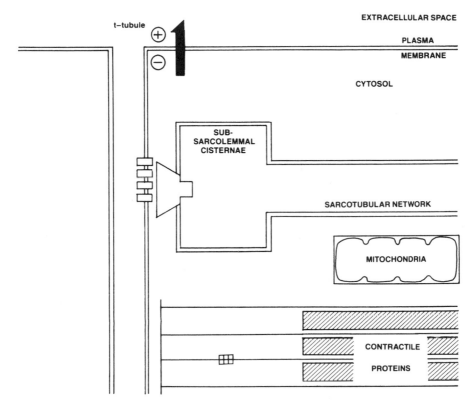

FIG. 14.10. The normal resting potential across the plasma membrane (positive outside, negative inside) favors calcium efflux via the sodium/calcium exchanger. This is due to the electrogenicity of the exchange, which favors a net flux of sodium ions toward, and calcium ions away from, the negative side of the membrane.

calcium transport into, the electropositive cell interior. The most important of these effects is probably that which favors calcium efflux during diastole; this is depicted in Fig. 14.10.

Effects Mediated by the Plasma Membrane Calcium Pump

The plasma membrane calcium pump, which along with the sodium/calcium exchanger, participates in the efflux of activator calcium from the myocardial cell, is stimulated by a calcium,calmodulin-dependent protein kinase (Chapter 10). This effect, which stimulates calcium efflux in the calcium-overloaded cell (Fig. 14.11), is another of the many mechanisms that help to prevent "runaway signaling" associated with an excessive rise in cytosolic Ca^{2+} concentration.

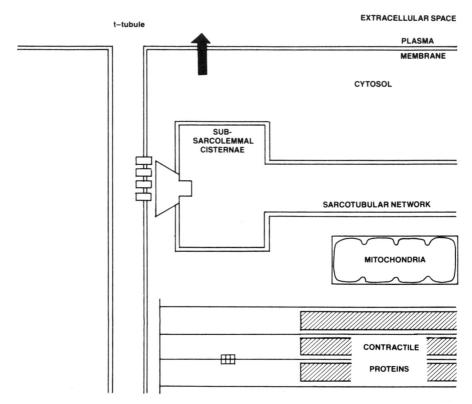

FIG. 14.11. Acceleration of the plasmalemmal calcium pump by calcium-calmodulin–dependent protein kinase increases calcium efflux via this active transport mechanism.

Regulation of Myocardial Contractility by Changing Calcium Fluxes Across the Sarcoplasmic Reticulum

A number of important mechanisms regulate myocardial contractility by modifying calcium release and uptake by these internal membranes. Both fluxes are modified by allosteric effects of adenosine triphosphate (ATP), which have already been noted to act like a "lubricant" to increase ion fluxes across membranes. Calcium itself has direct and indirect effects on both calcium release and reuptake by the sarcoplasmic reticulum, and the calcium pump of the cardiac sarcoplasmic reticulum is regulated by cyclic AMP. Changes in sarcoplasmic reticulum function can also arise from alterations in gene expression; one clearly defined example of this tonic mechanism is not an isoform shift, but an alteration in membrane architecture in which the density of calcium pump molecules is reduced in the chronically overloaded heart (see below). The diffusion of calcium from the sarcotubular network to the subsarcolemmal cisternae may become rate-limiting at rapid heart rates, where a second (negative) staircase can appear.

Effects Mediated by Sarcoplasmic Reticulum Calcium Release Channels

Effects of Calcium

The most important physiologic regulator of calcium release from the heart's sarcoplasmic reticulum is the intensity of the signal that opens the calcium channels in this intracellular membrane. This is, of course, the calcium-triggered calcium release discussed in Chapters 10 and 11. The effect of a reduction in this signal is shown in Fig. 14.7. An increase in the calcium entry that initiates the opening of calcium channels in the "foot proteins" of the subsarcolemmal cisternae would have the opposite effect; this is illustrated later when we consider the integrated response of the heart to cyclic AMP (see Fig. 14.22).

Calcium also has an indirect effect on the cardic calcium release channels (Chapter 11). This effect, to decrease calcium release by reducing the mean open time of the channels, provides yet another means to avoid a "runaway" calcium signal.

Effects of ATP

As the opening of the calcium release channel is stimulated by high concentrations of ATP (Chapter 11), a fall in the concentration of this nucleotide in an energy-starved heart would have a negative inotropic effect, as depicted in Fig. 14.12.

Effects Mediated by the Cardiac Sarcoplasmic Reticulum Calcium Pump

Effects of Calcium

As discussed in Chapter 11, cytosolic Ca^{2+} concentration is a major determinant of the rate of calcium transport by the calcium pump of the sarcoplasmic reticulum. The progressive slowing of calcium removal as cytosolic Ca^{2+} concentration falls during the normal cardiac cycle (Fig. 13.5) is readily explained by attenuation of the ability of calcium to activate the calcium pump as this cation is removed from the cytosol by transport into this internal membrane system.

Effects of Cyclic AMP–Dependent and Other Protein Kinases

Cyclic AMP has an important effect of stimulating calcium transport into the cardiac sarcoplasmic reticulum. This effect, which is the result of phosphorylation of *phospholamban* by protein kinase A, (Chapter 11), is due both to increased calcium sensitivity of the pump, which accelerates calcium removal at low Ca^{2+} concentrations, and more rapid pump turnover. Both effects accelerate relaxation (Fig. 14.13); the increased calcium sensitivity of the calcium pump may also increase the extent of relaxation by reducing cytosolic Ca^{2+} concentration in the fully

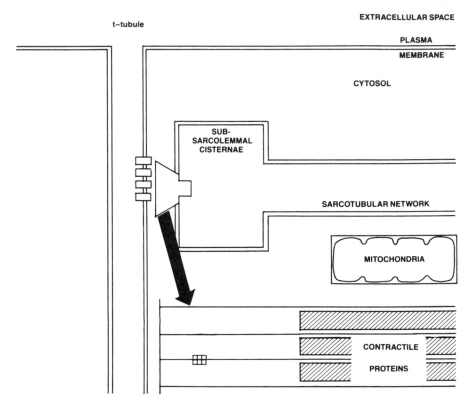

FIG. 14.12. A number of interventions decrease calcium efflux from the sarcoplasmic reticulum; these include reduction in calcium-triggered calcium release and ATP depletion.

relaxed heart. These effects are discussed later in this chapter, when the effects of sympathetic stimulation on the heart are integrated.

> The effects of protein kinase C on the calcium pump of the cardiac sarcoplasmic reticulum are still controversial (Chapter 11). A recent report (Rogers et al., 1990) suggests that activation of this system by diacylglycerol has an inhibitory effect that, by slowing calcium transport into this intracellular membrane system, might contribute to the negative inotropic effects of acetylcholine and adenosine.

Effects of ATP

Calcium uptake by the sarcoplasmic reticulum, like calcium release, is stimulated by the familiar allosteric effects of high concentrations of ATP. Attenuation of this effect, by slowing calcium removal from the cytosol, probably contributes to the marked impairment of relaxation commonly seen in the energy-starved heart (Fig. 14.14).

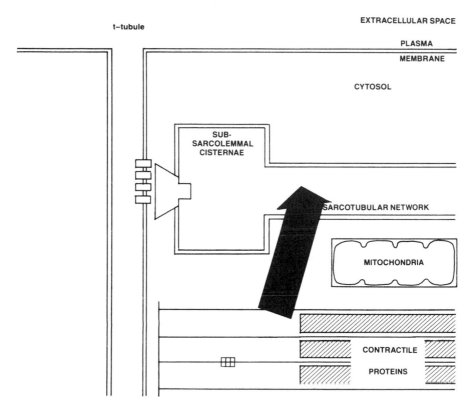

FIG. 14.13. Accelerated calcium uptake into the sarcoplasmic reticulum caused by phosphorylation of phospholamban favors relaxation by increasing the rate and extent of calcium removal from the cytosol.

Changes in Calcium Pump Density

Calcium transport into the cardiac sarcoplasmic reticulum can be modulated by changes involving the calcium pump ATPase itself. At least one such change, an example of the third paradigm of altered *gene* expression discussed at the beginning of this chapter, does not involve an isoform shift even though there are several calcium pump isoforms in the human heart, and isoform shifts occur during development (Chapter 11). Instead, calcium uptake by the sarcoplasmic reticulum is slowed by a quite different mechanism in the chronically overloaded heart (De la Bastie et al., 1990) and in aged animals (Maciel et al., 1990). Here, the abnormality is a change in membrane architecture that reduces the concentration of calcium pump molecules that are normally packed into this intracellular membrane (Chapter 11).

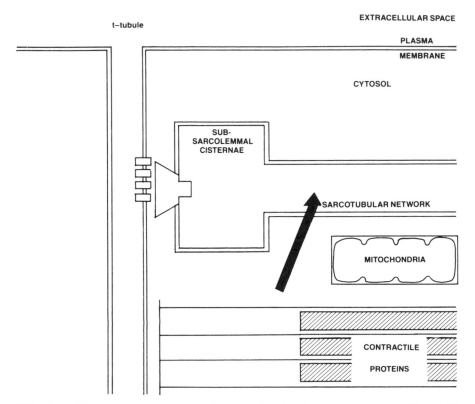

FIG. 14.14. Slowed calcium uptake into the sarcoplasmic reticulum can be caused by a fall in ATP or reduction in the number of calcium pump molecules in this intracellular membrane system. These interventions impair relaxation by slowing calcium removal from the cytosol.

Calcium Transfer Within the Sarcoplasmic Reticulum

Little is known of the regulation of calcium transfer from the sarcotubular network, where calcium is taken up by the calcium pump adenosine triphosphatase (ATPase), to the subsarcolemmal cisternae, from which this ion is released through calcium release channels. Calcium transfer within the sarcoplasmic reticulum, which is almost certainly mediated by passive diffusion, may become rate limiting in the calcium cycle at rapid heart rates. This can be explained by the relatively long distance over which calcium must be moved, compared to the small area within these membranes across which calcium can diffuse.

According to the Fick equation for diffusion, the rate at which a substance diffuses from one region to another (ds/dt) is directly proportional to the area (A) through which diffusion can take place:

$$ds/dt = -DA(dc/dx) \qquad [14.2]$$

where $-D$ is the diffusion coefficient for the substance, and dc/dx is the concentration gradient, or "driving force." Thus, diffusion through a long, narrow tubule is a relatively slow means to transport large quantities of a substance.

The negative staircase, a puzzling feature of the force-frequency relationship seen at rapid heart rates, may occur when slow diffusion of calcium within the sarcoplasmic reticulum becomes rate limiting.

The Negative Staircase

In 1902, shortly after Bowditch described the positive staircase, Woodworth observed a second staircase phenomenon in which tension decreased as rate increased (Fig. 14.15). This aspect of the force-frequency relationship, which is the opposite of the Bowditch staircase, is called the *negative* or *Woodworth staircase*. The negative staircase, which is generally more prominent at higher stimulation frequencies, also causes a transient increase in tension when stimulation frequency is decreased, and heightened tension in the first beat after a pause in stimulation; the latter is sometimes called *the recuperative effect of a pause*.

Both the negative (Woodworth) and positive (Bowditch) staircases can be seen in a single response to a change in stimulation frequency (Fig. 14.16). The negative staircase, however, evolves more rapidly than the positive staircase, so that the former is responsible for the initial fall in tension at an increased stimulation frequency and a transient rise in tension after the rate is decreased. Thus, the decline in tension during the first two beats after the increase in stimulation frequency (1 in Fig. 14.16), which is due to the negative staircase, is subsequently overcome in the following contractions by the more slowly developing positive staircase (2 in Fig. 14.16). Conversely, when rate is decreased, the negative staircase is responsible for the increased tension developed by the first beat following the long diastole (3 in Fig. 14.16); this is "the recuperative effect of a pause" described above. Subsequently, the more slowly evolving positive staircase becomes predominant, over-

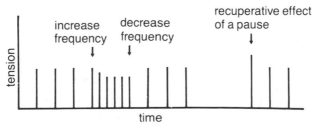

FIG. 14.15. The negative (Woodworth) staircase. The tension developed by a strip of cardiac muscle during a series of contractions decreases during the first few beats after the rate of stimulation is increased, and is augmented when stimulation frequency is slowed. Another manifestation of the negative staircase is the recuperative effect of a pause (*right*), where tension is increased in the first beat that follows an interruption of stimulation.

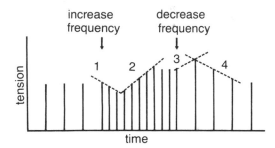

FIG. 14.16. Simultaneous evolution of the positive and negative staircases. The initial response to an increase in stimulation frequency is a transient fall in tension (1, the negative staircase), which is then overcome by a rise in tension caused by the more slowly evolving positve staircase (2). Similarly, the initial response to a decrease in stimulation frequency is a transient rise in tension (3, the negative staircase), followed by a fall in tension as the positive inotropic effect of the positive staircase wears off (4).

coming the transient positive inotropic effect of the negative staircase so as to reduce tension (4 in Fig. 14.16).

As already discussed, the positive staircase is explained by changes in calcium entry through plasma membrane calcium channels that modulate the total content of cellular calcium. The more rapid changes in contractility associated with the negative staircase, in contrast, probably arise from changes in the distribution of calcium within the cell. According to one hypothesis, the rapidly developing effects of the negative staircase are explained by retention of calcium within the sarcotubular network, from where it must first diffuse to the subsarcolemmal cisternae before it can be released to bind to troponin. If this hypothesis is correct, diffusion of calcium within the sarcoplasmic reticulum becomes rate limiting at very high heart rates. By failing to replenish calcium stores in the subsarcolemmal cisternae, this effect reduces the amount of calcium available for release to the contractile proteins (Fig. 14.17). Conversely, a reduction in stimulation frequency or a pause in beating allows calcium that has accumulated in the sarcotubular network to diffuse in increased amounts to the subsarcolemmal cisternae so as to augment the tension developed in subsequent contractions (Fig. 14.18).

> It should be emphasized that the explanation for the negative staircase in the preceding paragraph is speculative. Another plausible mechanism is that slow reactivation of the calcium release channels in the subsarcolemmal cisternae causes these channels to become refractory at high stimulation frequencies, which reduces the flux of activator calcium through these channels at rapid heart rates.

The fact that the negative staircase is eventually overwhelmed by opposing rate-dependent changes in calcium fluxes across the plasma membrane (the positive staircase) can be explained by the paramount importance of the total content of calcium in the sarcoplasmic reticulum. This follows because diffusion of calcium within the sarcoplasmic reticulum, which as noted in Eq. 14.2 is proportional to dc/dx, is increased when additional calcium that enters the cell during the positive

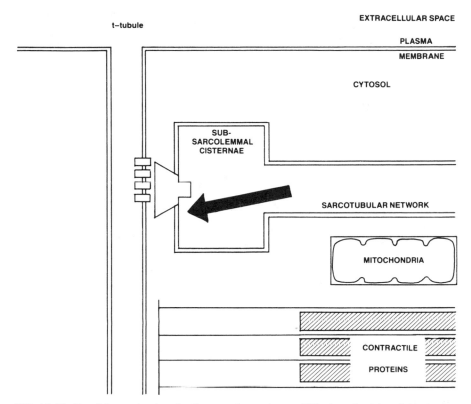

FIG. 14.17. Possible mechanism for the negative staircase. Diffusion of calcium from the sarcotubular network to the calcium release site in the subsarcolemmal cisternae may, at very rapid heart rates, be too slow to allow all of the calcium to move from the former to the latter. Another explanation for the negative staircase (not shown) is the development of a refractory state of the calcium release channels of the sarcoplasmic reticulum.

staircase overcomes the negative staircase. Conversely, when stimulation frequency is reduced, or after the recuperative effects of a pause, any inotropic effect caused by increased calcium release from the subsarcolemmal cisternae will be transient because the excess calcium that is released leaves the cell.

Regulation of Myocardial Contractility by Changing Calcium Binding to the Troponin Complex

Alterations in the calcium-binding affinity of troponin provide yet another mechanism by which the contractile response of the heart is regulated (Fig. 14.19). It is apparent that any change in this property will have opposite effects on contraction and relaxation; that is, an increase in calcium affinity that increases tension developed during systole will make it harder for the heart to relax, and vice versa. It is

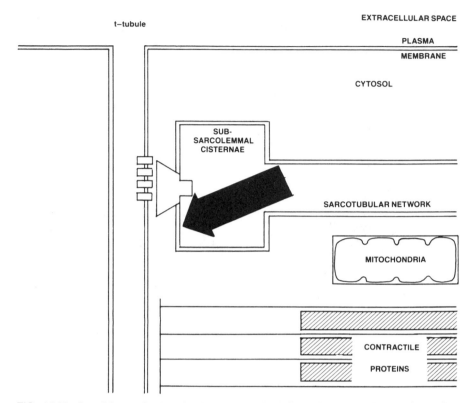

FIG. 14.18. Possible mechanism for the recuperative effect of a pause. In situations where calcium has accumulated in the sarcotubular network, a pause would allow increased amounts of calcium to move as a bolus to the calcium release site in the subsarcolemmal cisternae.

now apparent that such changes participate in a number of physiological responses of the heart. Most important are the effects of α- and β-adrenergic stimulation, which are opposite to each other.

Effects of α-Adrenergic Stimulation

Studies of the relationship between cytosolic Ca^{2+} concentration and contractility have demonstrated that the positive inotropic effects of agents that generate $InsP_3$ and diacylglycerol, the two intracellular messengers produced by hydrolysis of phosphatidylinositol 4,5-bisphosphate (Chapter 12), are due in part to an increase in the calcium affinity of the calcium receptor of the contractile apparatus (Fig. 14.18). A similar effect can be produced by phorbol esters (Gwathmey and Hajjar, 1990), indicating that protein kinase C phosphorylation plays a key role in this response; however, the substrate for this putative phosphorylation has not yet been defined.

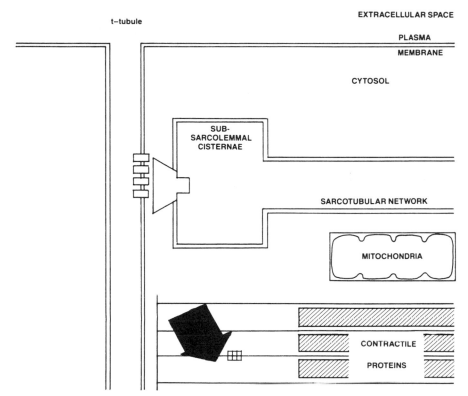

FIG. 14.19. An increase in the calcium affinity of the troponin complex would increase contractility by promoting the binding of activator calcium.

It has recently been noted that muscarinic, but not purinergic, agonists also increase the calcium sensitivity of the cardiac contractile proteins through a mechanism, similar to that described above, that appears to involve a protein kinase C-mediated phosphorylation (Puceat et al., 1990). A number of inotropic drugs, including several phosphodiesterase inhibitors, also increase contractility by this mechanism.

Effects of β-Adrenergic Stimulation

Phosphorylation of the cardiac troponin complex by protein kinase A decreases the calcium affinity of the cardiac troponin complex. This effect, like others we have already examined, involves allosteric interactions among the proteins of the thin filament because troponin I is phosphorylated, rather than the troponin C which actually binds the activator calcium.

Because agents that increase cyclic AMP levels have powerful positive inotropic effects, the ability of cyclic AMP to decrease the calcium sensitivity of the contractile proteins was initially unexpected. However, the physiological significance of this mechanism, which reduces the ability of the calcium released during excitation-contraction coupling to activate the heart's contractile proteins, is readily understood in light of the heart's limited ability to transport calcium out of the cell (Chapter 11). The fact that β-adrenergic agonists increase calcium entry (see above), as well as increase heart rate (see Chapter 22), means that more activator calcium must be removed from the cytosol in a shorter time. This is accomplished in part when calcium uptake into the sarcoplasmic reticulum is accelerated by phosphorylation of phospholamban (see above). At the same time, phosphorylation of troponin I decreases the calcium affinity of the contractile proteins, and so facilitates the ability of the calcium pump to relax the heart by removing calcium from troponin C (Fig. 14.20.).

β-adrenergic stimulation also increases the rate of cross-bridge cycling; the mechanism responsible for this effect, which appears to be mediated by cyclic AMP, is not yet clear (Hoh et al., 1988).

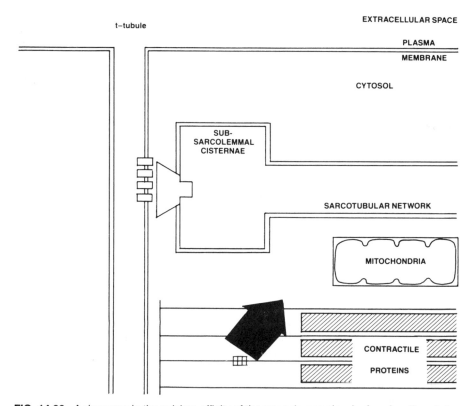

FIG. 14.20. A decrease in the calcium affinity of the troponin complex, by favoring dissociation of this ion from its binding site on the contractile proteins, would accelerate relaxation, albeit at the expense of a decrease in contractility.

Isoform Shifts

Isoform shifts involving the proteins of the thin filaments, which as noted in Chapter 7 are members of multigene families, can alter the calcium sensitivity of the heart's contractile proteins. At this time, the best documented of the isoform shifts that regulate calcium binding to cardiac troponin involve troponin T (McAulliffe et al., 1990). Once again, the protein that is modified is not troponin C, which contains the actual calcium-binding site, so that this tonic mechanism also illustrates the importance of cooperative interactions among the regulatory proteins of the thin filament.

Effects of Altered Intracellular Environment

Potassium Ion

The well-known ability of elevated extracellular K^+ concentration to depress myocardial contractility led, many years ago, to the view that changes in intracellular potassium played a major role in regulating myocardial contractility. It is now apparent, however, that this negative inotropic effect does not arise from a direct action of potassium on the contractile process; but instead is due to depolarization and shortening of the action potential (Chapter 19). Although changing concentrations of potassium both inside and outside the cell have little direct effect on either cardiac contraction or relaxation, indirect effects can be of considerable importance under certain pathological conditions, notably ischemia (Chapter 24).

Hydrogen Ion

Acidosis has been known to have a negative inotropic effect since the work of Gaskell in 1880. Studies of the effects of pH on the calcium sensitivity of actomyosin carried out during the late 1960s indicated that the curve defining the calcium dependence of both actomyosin ATPase and the tension generated by actomyosin preparations *in vitro* was shifted to higher Ca^{2+} concentrations in the acidotic heart. These and other data indicate that protons, by competing with calcium for binding to troponin, reduce tension development in the heart. It should come as no surprise to the reader that this effect is not due to a direct effect on calcium binding to troponin C, but is, instead, mediated by an effect on another protein, in this case troponin I, that by a cooperative interaction reduces the calcium affinity of the troponin complex. As noted in Chapter 24, the negative inotropic effect of acidosis may play a role in the early pump failure of the ischemic heart.

Intracellular acidosis may also reduce the force generated by attached cross-bridges; this effect has been suggested to contribute to muscle fatigue (Edman and Lou, 1990).

Effects of ATP

Recognition that ATP plays a key role in providing chemical energy for the contractile process suggested to early workers that lack of ATP might directly impair the performance of the overloaded heart. In view of the many mechanisms that maintain ATP levels in the normal heart, however, it seems unlikely that changing ATP levels participate in the physiological regulation of myocardial contractility. Furthermore, as noted in Chapter 8, mild ATP depletion impairs relaxation more than contraction by attenuating the "plasticizing" effect that dissociates the contractile proteins. Thus, ATP deficiency is most likely to play an important role in the pathogenesis of relaxation abnormalities in the ischemic heart, where energy demands exceed the ability to regenerate ATP, and in the dying heart, where severe ATP deficiency causes contracture because rigor bonds linking actin and myosin (Chapter 8) cannot be dissociated.

REGULATION OF MYOCARDIAL CONTRACTILITY BY β-ADRENERGIC STIMULATION: AN INTEGRATED RESPONSE

Cyclic AMP has a number of effects on the heart, many of which have been described in the preceding discussion (Table 14.2). Some of these—notably the increased calcium entry through plasmalemmal calcium channels and accelerated

TABLE 14.2. *Effects of β-adrenergic stimulation of the heart*

1. Energy production	
Accelerated glycogenolysis	Increases ATP availability
2. Plasma membrane	
Phosphorylation of Ca channels	
Increased Ca entry	
Atria and ventricles	Increases contractility (+ INO)
Sinoatrial node	Increases heart rate
Atrioventricular node	Accelerates AV conduction
Phosphorylation of the Na pump	
Increased Na efflux	Increases Ca efflux via Na/Ca exchange (LUSI)
3. Sarcoplasmic reticulum	
Phosphorylation of phospholamban	
Increased Ca pump turnover	Increases Ca uptake (LUSI)
Increased Ca sensitivity of the Ca pump	Increases Ca uptake (LUSI)
Increased Ca stores	Increases Ca release (+ INO)
4. Contractile proteins	
Troponin	
Phosphorylation of troponin I	
Decreased Ca sensitivity of the troponin complex	Decreases Ca binding (− INO and LUSI)
Actomyosin	
Increased cross-bridge cycling	Increases shortening velocity (INO)

Abbreviations: + and − INO, positive and negative inotropic effects; LUSI, lusitropic (relaxation-promoting) effects.

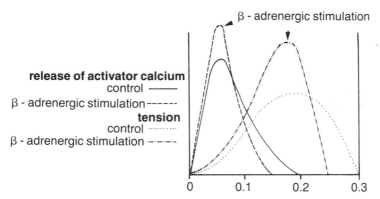

β - adrenergic stimulation

release of activator calcium
control ———
β - adrenergic stimulation ------
tension
control ·········
β - adrenergic stimulation ·—·—·

0   0.1   0.2   0.3

FIG. 14.21. Interventions that increase cellular levels of cyclic AMP, notably β-adrenergic stimulation, increase the rate at which calcium enters and is pumped out of the cytosol, as well as the maximum amount of calcium release. This gives rise to a contraction in which tension, although markedly enhanced, is abbreviated.

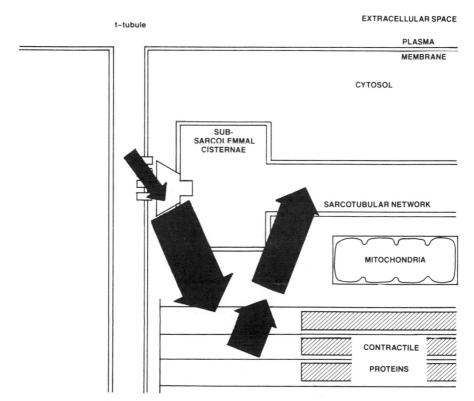

FIG. 14.22. Summary of the major effects of β-adrenergic stimulation. Two effects increase contractility: increased calcium entry across the plasma membrane and increased calcium release from the sarcoplasmic reticulum. Two effects accelerate relaxation: decreased calcium affinity of the troponin complex and increased calcium uptake into the sarcoplasmic reticulum.

cross-bridge cycling—favor contraction, whereas others—decreased calcium affinity of troponin and increased calcium uptake by the sarcoplasmic reticulum following phosphorylation of phospholamban—favor relaxation. Together, these effects provide an integrated response to β-adrenergic stimulation that increases myocardial contractility, while at the same time permitting the heart to relax in the face of the increased binding of activator calcium to the contractile proteins and a shorter time in which to remove enough calcium from the cytosol to allow the ventricles to relax. These responses are shown in Fig. 14.21, where both cytosolic calcium and tension development are seen to be increased, yet both follow abbreviated time courses. The key factors causing these responses are depicted in Fig. 14.22, which shows the increased calcium entry that is largely responsible for the positive inotropic effect, and the facilitated dissociation of calcium from troponin and increased calcium uptake by the sarcoplasmic reticulum that accelerate relaxation.

REGULATION OF MYOCARDIAL CONTRACTILITY BY ALTERED EXPRESSION OF MYOSIN HEAVY-CHAIN ISOFORMS

The tonic changes in myocardial contractility that arise from alterations in *gene* expression, as noted at the beginning of this chapter, develop much more slowly than the phasic changes in calcium fluxes described above. Several isoform shifts that influence calcium fluxes in the heart have already been described, as has the change in the architecture of the sarcoplasmic reticulum membrane that slows relaxation in the hypertrophied heart. Unlike these mechanisms, which ultimately modify the *number* of actin-myosin interactions, a quite different type of regulation is brought about by changes in the expression of the genes that encode the myosin heavy chains. As described in Chapter 7, the latter play a key role in determining two *rates*: myosin ATPase activity and V_{max}, the maximal velocity of shortening of unloaded muscle.

Functional Significance of Altered Expression of Myosin Isoforms

Preferential expression of the gene that encodes the slow β-heavy-chain isoform, by reducing the maximal velocity of contraction, has a negative inotropic effect. Conversely, increased expression of the gene that encodes the fast α-isoform increases myocardial contractility. These isoform switches also have important effects on muscle economy as muscles containing the slow β-myosin heavy chains generate tension more efficiently than muscles with the faster α-isoform (Table 14.3). For this reason, replacement of fast myosin heavy chains with the slow isoform not only reduces myocardial contractility, due to slowing of the cross-bridge cycle, but at the same time improves efficiency by increasing the amount of work that can be done when a given amount of ATP is consumed.

The relationship between the enzymatic properties of myosin and the behavior of the contractile proteins in the intact muscle was discussed in Chapter 8, where it was

TABLE 14.3. *Effects of myosin heavy-chain isoform switching on cross-bridge mechanics*

α/β ratio	Cycling frequency	Tension-time integral	Economy of force development
Increased	Increased	Decreased	Decreased
Decreased	Decreased	Increased	Increased

α/β ratio: ratio of fast to slow myosin heavy-chain isoforms.
Cycling frequency: turnover of the cross-bridge cycle.
Tension-time integral: tension integral during a single contraction.
Economy of force development: an index of "efficiency" is equal to the tension-time integral divided by the tension-dependent initial heat.

pointed out that the same rate-limiting step determines ATP hydrolysis *in vitro* and cross-bridge cycling *in vivo*. The energy-sparing effect of slowing this rate-limiting step is due to a reduced rate at which the cross-bridge hydrolyzes ATP during the maintenance of tension.

> This relationship can be understood in terms of cross-bridge turnover during isometric contraction, an energy-consuming reaction that accounts for the "tension-time" heat, and the $f(P,t)$ term in Eq. 6.5 and 6.6. Because energy expenditure during maintained tension is proportional to the rate of myosin cross-bridge turnover, it is not surprising that preferential expression of the gene encoding the slow myosin isoform improves efficiency by decreasing tension-time heat.

As this energy-sparing effect of the preferential synthesis of the slow myosin isoform occurs at the expense of reduced myocardial contractility, due to a decreased V_{max} of the force-velocity curve, the effects of this isoform shift are most marked when the myocardium contracts against a low afterload. Conversely, preferential synthesis of the fast α-myosin heavy chain increases V_{max}, which accelerates emptying of the ventricle, especially when the heart ejects against a low afterload. This effect, however, reduces efficiency and so wastes energy, especially when high levels of tension are developed by the walls of the heart.

> The functional significance of these differences in myosins first became apparent when the energetics of fast and slow skeletal muscles were compared. When shortening against heavy loads, slow muscles use less ATP than fast muscles, whereas fast muscles perform more efficiently during lightly loaded contractions. These represent long-term functional adaptations made possible by the third paradigm in Table 14.1, as differences in *gene* expression allow each muscle type to contract most efficiently under the mechanical conditions it normally encounters: fast muscles during sprinting, slow muscles during sustained work (Chapter 3).

Myosin Heavy-Chain Isoform Shifts in the Heart

Expression of different members of the family of genes that encode the myosin heavy chain has been studied most extensively in the rat ventricle, where a V1 (α) myosin heavy-chain isoform determines a high myosin ATPase activity and rapid shortening velocity, and a V_3 (β) myosin heavy chain isoform determines low myo-

TABLE 14.4. *Myosin heavy-chain isoform switches in the rat ventricle*

Stimulus	Isoform expressed
Normal	α (fast) and β (slow)
Endocrinopathies	
Hyperthyroidism	α (fast)
Hypothyroidism	β (slow)
Diabetes mellitus	β (slow)
Adrenal insufficiency	β (slow)
Hypertrophy	
Overload-induced (pathological) hypertrophy	β (slow)
Exercise-induced (physiological) hypertrophy	α (fast)
Aging	β (slow)

sin ATPase activity and slow shortening velocity. The normal rat ventricle also contains smaller amounts of V_2 myosin, which is the αβ heterodimer. Replacement of one isoform with another occurs in response to several different stimuli (Table 14.4). The slow, β-isoform is synthesized preferentially in hypothyroidism and other abnormalities in endocrine balance, in response to chronic pressure overload (Chapter 25), and in the aging heart. Conversely, in hyperthyroidism and exercise-induced hypertrophy, the opposite change occurs and expression of the fast, α-isoform is increased.

Regulation by altered synthesis of myosin heavy chains illustrates how cardiac muscle function is adapted to the needs of the body. In the hearts of elderly rats, in hypothyroidism, and in rats with a chronic pressure overload, preferential expression of low ATPase myosin has an energy-sparing effect that, while reducing contractility, may be adaptive. In the hyperthyroid state, on the other hand, replacement of the normal myosin with a high-ATPase myosin aids in the adaptation to the rapid heart rate and low peripheral resistance. In this endocrinopathy, unlike most other types of heart failure, the burden on the heart is an abnormally high ejection rate with a low afterload, both being necessary to meet the abnormally high oxygen needs of the body seen in hyperthyroidism.

Exercise is, in some ways, similar to hyperthyroidism in that the major hemodynamic changes are a decrease in peripheral resistance and a more rapid heart rate, which together increase cardiac output (Chapter 16). Furthermore, the physiological overloading that occurs during exercise differs from that of most pathological states, such as a valve abnormality or hypertension, where the stimulus to cell growth continues without pause. In exercise, however, the overload is intermittent. It is not totally unexpected, therefore, that the myosin isoform shifts induced by a physiological overload like exercise differ from those caused by pathological overloading (Chapter 25).

The human ventricle, unlike that of the rat, synthesizes only a slow myosin isoform. However, changes similar to those described above for the rat ventricle are seen in human atria, where a decreased proportion of fast (α) atrial myosin heavy chain parallels the extent of atrial overloading. The significance of these, and other abnormalities in gene expression in the overloaded human heart are only now coming into focus (Katz, 1990; Wankerl et al., 1990).

In the following two chapters, the mechanisms that regulate myocardial contractility, which rely on the second and third paradigms described in Table 14.1 (*cell* and *gene*), are integrated with the first paradigm: the function of the heart as an *organ*. This is, after all, how most physicians view the heart. Using the discussion in this and earlier chapters as a basis, Chapters 15 and 16 describe how the first two paradigms operate to regulate the performance of the intact heart.

REFERENCES

De la Bastie D, Levitsky D, Rappaport L, Mercadier J-J, Marotte F, Wisnewsky C, Brokovich V, Schwartz K, Lompré A-M. (1990). Function of the sarcoplasmic reticulum and expression of its Ca^{2+} ATPase gene in pressure-overloaded cardiac hypertrophy in the rat. *Circ Res* 66;554–564.

Edman KAP, Lou F. (1990). Changes in force and stiffness induced by fatigue and intracellular acidification in frog muscle fibers. *J Physiol (Lond)* 424:133–149.

Gwathmey JK, Hajjar RJ. (1990). Effect of protein kinase C activation on sarcoplasmic reticulum function and apparent myofibrillar Ca^{2+} sensitivity in intact and skinned muscles from normal and diseased human myocardium. *Circ Res* 67:744–752.

Hoh JFY, Rossmanith GH, Kwan LJ, Hamilton AM. (1988). Adrenaline increases the rate of cycling of crossbridges in rat cardiac muscle as measured by pseudo-random binary noise-modulated perturbation analysis. *Circ Res* 62:452–461.

Katz AM. (1976). Tonic and phasic mechanisms in the regulation of myocardial contractility. *Basic Res Cardiol* 71:447–455.

Katz AM. (1988). Molecular biology in cardiology, a paradigmatic shift. *J Mol Cell Cardiol* 20:355–366.

Katz AM. (1990). Cardiomyopathy of overload. A major determinant of prognosis in congestive heart failure. *N Engl J Med* 322:100–110.

Kim D, Smith TW. (1986). Effects of amiloride and ouabain on contractile state, Ca and Na fluxes, and Na content in cultured chick heart cells. *Mol Pharmacol* 29:363–371.

Lee CO, Abete P, Pecker M, Sonn JK, Vasalle M. (1985). Strophanthidin inotropy: role of intracellular sodium ion activity and sodium-calcium exchange. *J Mol Cell Cardiol* 17:1043–1053.

Maciel LMZ, Polikar R, Rohrer D, Popovich BK, Dillmann WH. (1990). Age-induced decreases in the messenger RNA coding for the sarcoplasmic reticulum Ca^{2+}-ATPase of the rat heart. *Circ Res* 67:230–234.

McAulliffe JJ, Gao L, Solaro RF. (1990). Changes in myofibrillar activation and troponin T Ca^{2+} binding associated with troponin T isoform switching in developing rabbit heart. *Circ Res* 66:1204–1216.

Puceat M, Clement O, Lechene P, Pelosin JM, Ventura-Clapier R, Vassort G. (1990). Neurohumoral control of calcium sensitivity of myofilaments in rat single heart cells. *Circ Res* 67:517–524.

Rogers TB, Gaa ST, Massey C, Dösemci A. (1990). Protein kinase C inhibits Ca^{2+} accumulation in cardiac sarcoplasmic reticulum. *J Biol Chem* 265:4302–4308.

Wankerl M, Böhn M, Morano I, Rüegg JC, Eichhorn M, Erdmann E. (1990). Calcium sensitivity and myosin light chain pattern of atrial and ventricular skinned cardiac fibers from patients with various kinds of cardiac disease. *J Mol Cell Cardiol* 22:1425–1438.

Wood EH, Hepner RL, Weidmann S. (1969). Inotropic effects of electrical currents. *Circ Res* 24:409–445.

Woodworth RS. (1902). Maximal contraction, "staircase" contraction, refractory period, and compensatory pause of the heart. *Am J Physiol* 8:213–249.

BIBLIOGRAPHY

Bugaisky L, Zak R. (1986). Biological mechanisms of hypertrophy. In: Fozzard H, Haber E, Katz AM, Jennings R, Morgan HE, eds. *The heart and cardiovascular system*. New York: Raven Press; 1491–1506.

Endoh M, Blinks JR. (1988). Action of sympathomimetic amines on the Ca^{2+} transients and contractions of rabbit myocardium: reciprocal changes in myofibrillar responsiveness to Ca^{2+} mediated through α- and β-adrenoceptors. *Circ Res* 62:247–265.

Hamrell BB, Alpert NR. (1986). Cellular basis of the mechanical properties of hypertrophied myocardium. In: Fozzard H, Haber E, Katz AM, Jennings R, Morgan HE, eds. *The heart and cardiovascular system*. New York: Raven Press; 1507–1524.

Katz AM. (1990). Interplay between inotropic and lusitropic effects of cyclic adenosine monophosphate on the myocardial cell. *Circulation* 82(Suppl 1):I7–I11.

Lakatta E. (1987). Do hypertension and aging have a similar effect on the myocardium? *Circulation* 75(Suppl I):I69–I77.

van der Leyen H, Schmitz W, Scholz H, Scholz J. (1989). New positive inotropic agents acting by phosphodiesterase inhibition or alpha₁-adrenergic stimulation. *Pharmacol Res* 21:329–337.

15

The Heart as a Muscular Pump

At this point, we turn from our analysis of the physiology of the heart in terms of the two most primitive of the three paradigms set out in Table 14.1, *cell* biochemistry and biophysics, and *gene* expression, to examine the pumping action of the heart as an *organ*. Although this paradigm emphasizes such clinically important variables as stroke volume, cardiac output, and blood pressure, it should be kept in mind that these hemodynamic parameters are manifestations of the fundamental processes of muscular contraction that have been the focus of our earlier chapters.

The fact that the heart is a hollow, rather than linear muscle requires that we use a new terminology to describe the work of the atria and ventricles. The contractile behavior of skeletal muscles, and linear cardiac preparations such as trabeculae carneae and papillary muscles is described in terms of tension development and changes in length. Although the muscle fibers in the walls of the ventricles also develop tension and shorten during the pumping of the heart, as an organ the heart generates *pressure* not *tension*; and shortening of its muscular fibers causes the ejection of a *volume* of blood rather than a reduction in *length*. In the intact heart, therefore, changes in force and muscle length are transformed into changes in pressure and volume (Fig. 15.1).

VOLUME AND LENGTH: A GEOMETRIC RELATIONSHIP

In the ventricle, the relationship between length and volume is determined by the laws of geometry. In a sphere, for example, volume is defined by the equation:

$$V = \frac{4}{3}\pi R^3 \qquad [15.1]$$

where V = volume and R = radius. Because circumference is equal to $2\pi R$, volume is also related to the third power of circumference. For this reason, a 50% reduction of the circumference of a sphere reduces volume to one-eighth its original value.

The complex architecture of the ventricles, and especially that of the left ventricle, can be represented as an ellipsoid in which the three axes, D_A, D_L, and L_M are the anterior-

351

linear muscle

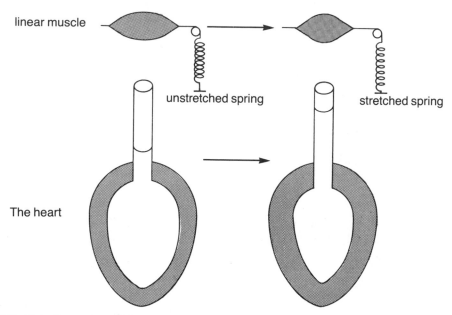

unstretched spring   stretched spring

The heart

FIG. 15.1. Comparison of the mechanical achievements of a linear muscle, which shortens and develops tension, and the heart, in which cavity volume is reduced and pressure increases.

posterior diameter, lateral diameter, and maximal length, respectively (Fig. 15.2). This is, of course, a simplification as the left ventricle is not truly ellipsoidal; however, measurements of D_A, D_L, and L_M can be used to estimate left ventricular volume in the following equation for the volume of an ellipse:

$$V = \frac{4}{3}\pi \left(\frac{D_A}{2}\right) \times \left(\frac{D_L}{2}\right) \times \left(\frac{L_M}{2}\right).$$

[15.2]

More elaborate methods for determining left ventricular volume are beyond the scope of this text.

anteroposterior
projection   lateral
                              projection

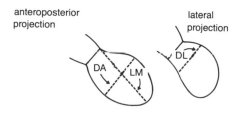

FIG. 15.2. Outline of the cavity of the left ventricle during diastole viewed in antero-posterior and lateral projections. The volume of the ventricle can be approximated by assuming the cavity to be an ellipse whose long axis is L_M, and whose short axes are D_A and D_L.

PRESSURE, STRESS, AND TENSION: LAW OF LAPLACE

The relationships between wall tension, wall stress, and the pressure within the ventricular cavity are as complex as the relationship between the circumference of the ventricle and its volume.

> The term *tension* is commonly used instead of *stress* in referring to the forces that are exerted around the circumference of the ventricle. This is not, however, strictly correct. Because tension is a force exerted along a line (e.g., dynes/cm) whereas stress is a force exerted across an area (e.g., dynes/cm^2), contraction of the muscular fibers of the ventricle generates a stress. Only if we ignore cross-sectional area is it correct to speak of the development of tension. Having defined these terms, this text reverts to common usage and speaks of tension in the walls of the heart, rather than the more correct term, stress.

In the intact heart, tension developed in the walls of the ventricle generates a pressure that is readily measured within its cavity. Pressure, like stress, is a force exerted across an area, and so has the same units: dynes/cm^2. Wall stress, however, is a shear force exerted around the circumference of the ventricle, whereas pressure is a distending force exerted at right angles to the ventricular walls. Pressures in cardiovascular hemodynamics are usually quantified in millimeters of mercury or centimeters of water, which represent the height of a column of mercury or water that exerts the corresponding force per unit of surface area. The conversions of these hemodynamic terms to gram-centimeter-second units are given in Table 15.1.

Like the relationship between length and volume, that between wall stress (or tension) and pressure is influenced by the size and shape of the ventricle. These relationships are defined by the law of Laplace, which takes into account the radius of curvature of the ventricular walls in the interconversions of pressure, stress, and tension. In its simplest form, as applied to a cylinder having infinitely thin walls (where wall stress really is tension), the law of Laplace states that wall tension is equal to the pressure within the cylinder times the radius of the curvature of the wall:

$$T = P \times R \qquad\qquad [15.3]$$

where T = wall tension (dynes/cm), P = pressure (dynes/cm^2), and R = radius (cm) (Fig. 15.3). The law of Laplace thus states that wall tension at any given pressure is increased as the radius of the cylinder increases, and vice versa. One application of the law of Laplace is seen in the tank trucks used to transport fluids and gases under pressure (Fig. 15.4). To minimize the hazard of bursting, tanks subject to high

TABLE 15.1. *Units of pressure*

Unit	Dynes/cm^2
1mm Hg	1,330
1 cm H$_2$O	980

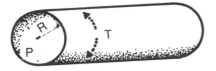

FIG. 15.3. The law of Laplace describes the tension on the walls of a thin-walled cylinder (*T*), which is equal to the pressure within the cylinder (*P*) times its radius of curvature (*R*).

internal pressures are constructed with smaller radii of curvature than are tanks that carry material at low pressures. The fact that the tension on the walls of the ventricle increases as chamber volume increases, even when the intraventricular pressure remains constant, is of considerable importance in the diseased heart, especially in those conditions that cause the heart to dilate.

The tendency of a tank to burst can also be reduced by increasing the thickness of its walls. In the thick-walled left ventricle as well, a greater number of muscle fibers reduces the tension on each fiber. The equation defining the operation of the law of Laplace in a thick-walled cylinder is:

$$T = \frac{P \times R}{h} \qquad\qquad [15.4]$$

where h = wall thickness. (The term T in Eq. 15.4 is actually a stress, i.e., the force exerted across an area.) The geometry of the ventricles is, of course, more complex than that of a cylinder (see, for example, Fig. 15.2) so that wall tension cannot be measured with precision. A number of formulae used to approximate this parameter are beyond the scope of this text.

The complexity of the relationship between the geometry of the ventricular cavity and the tension on its muscular walls should not obscure two fundamental facts. The first is that dilation of the ventricles leads directly to an increase in the tension on each muscle fiber in its walls. This follows both from the law of Laplace (Eq. 15.3), which defines a direct relationship between the diameter of a hollow organ and the

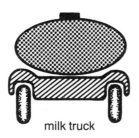

milk truck

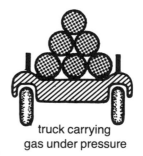

truck carrying
gas under pressure

FIG. 15.4. A practical application of the law of Laplace. In a truck carrying gas under high pressure (*right*) several cylindrical tanks, each having a short radius of curvature, are used. A single tank with a large radius of curvature is used in a milk truck, where the pressure in the tank is low (*left*).

tension on its walls at any given pressure, and from the thinning of the walls of the ventricle as the heart dilates. This is apparent in Eq. 15.4, where it is seen that ventricular dilation increases wall tension (T), even when intraventricular pressure P is constant, both by increasing radius (R) and decreasing wall thickness (h). The second major consequence of these geometric considerations is that an increase in wall thickness reduces the tension that must be developed during systole by any individual muscle fiber. Hence, by distributing tension among a greater number of active sarcomeres in the overloaded heart, ventricular hypertrophy reduces the load on each muscle fiber. Both of these considerations are important in understanding the impact of disease on the heart (Chapter 25).

DISTRIBUTION OF TENSION ACROSS THE WALLS OF THE HEART

Tension is not distributed uniformly in all layers of the muscular walls of the heart. Instead, analyses of the properties of a series of concentric spheres enclosing a cavity under pressure show that tension is highest near the inner surface. These regional differences in tension become especially marked when the thick-walled left ventricle becomes hypertrophied.

At first glance, this might appear to contradict the law of Laplace, which states that for an infinitely thin sphere, tension is greater as diameter increases. There is, however, no contradiction, as the present discussion is concerned with the *distribution* of tension across the layers of a thick-walled hollow organ, rather than absolute tension on individual thin-walled organs having different radii of curvature.

Although different methods to calculate the distribution of tension across the walls of the ventricle do not all give the same results, it is generally agreed that the endocardial regions of the ventricular walls develop higher tension than the epicardial regions. This accounts, at least in part, for the greater vulnerability of the left ventricular endocardium to the detrimental effects of a rapid increase in intraventricular pressure, as can occur in malignant hypertension. The higher tensions developed in the endocardial region of the ventricle also make this region especially vulnerable to a reduction in coronary flow. This accounts for the common occurrence of subendocardial myocardial infarction in patients in whom a coronary artery occlusion severely reduces, but does not totally interrupt, the flow of blood to a part of the left ventricle.

The greater vulnerability of the endocardium to an imbalance between energy demands and energy supply is exacerbated by its relatively low coronary flow. This is due to the fact that the coronary arteries penetrate the ventricles from the epicardium, and so must traverse a greater distance of contracting myocardium before they can supply the endocardial portion of the ventricles (Chapter 1).

WORK DIAGRAM

During each cardiac cycle, the walls of the ventricle undergo a sequence of changes in tension and length. These changes can be readily understood by first

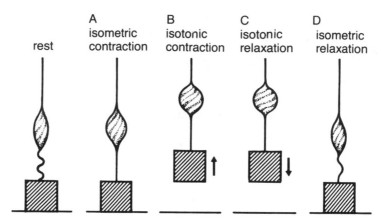

FIG. 15.5. Cycle of contraction and relaxation in an afterloaded skeletal muscle. At rest the load is not borne by the muscle, but rests on a support. During isometric contraction (*A*) the tension developed by the muscle rises until it equals the load, after which the load is lifted during an isotonic contraction (*B*). Relaxation is initially isotonic, during which the load is lowered to the support (*C*). When the load rests on the support, isometric relaxation (*D*) begins and continues until muscle tension falls to zero.

examining the changing mechanical state during the contraction of an afterloaded skeletal muscle, i.e., a muscle in which the load is not initially borne by the resting muscle. Such an afterloaded contraction can be divided into four phases (Fig. 15.5).

At *rest*, the muscle does not bear the load that rests on a support such as a table top. During *isometric contraction* (A in Fig. 15.5) the activated muscle begins to develop tension, although not enough to lift the load; as a result, the muscle does not shorten. Shortening can begin only after active tension equals the load, at which time the muscle lifts the load during the second phase of *isotonic contraction* (B in Fig. 15.5). When the muscle begins to relax, it initially lengthens while still bearing the load during the phase of *isotonic relaxation* (C in Fig. 15.5). After the load is

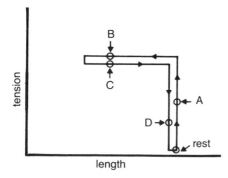

FIG. 15.6. Work diagram of the contraction-relaxation cycle depicted in Fig. 15.5: isometric contraction (*A*); isotonic contraction (*B*); isotonic relaxation (*C*); and isometric relaxation (*D*). The curves for contraction and relaxation, which should be superimposed, have been separated for clarity.

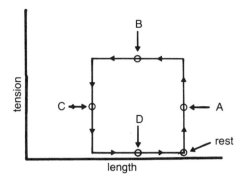

FIG. 15.7. Work diagram of a muscle from which the load is disengaged just prior to relaxation. Isometric contraction (A) and isotonic contraction (B) occur as in the afterloaded contraction depicted in Figs. 15.5 and 15.6. However, as the load is removed from the muscle before it begins to relax, muscle tension is zero during isotonic relaxation (C), after which the muscle lengthens (isometric relaxation; D) at zero load.

returned to its original position on the tabletop, the muscle dissipates its tension without further lengthening during *isometric relaxation* (D in Fig. 15.5).

A "work diagram" that defines the changes in force and length during the contraction cycle just described is shown in Fig. 15.6. This work diagram shows the four phases described in the preceding paragraph: two of contraction (A, isometric contraction; and B, isotonic contraction) and two of relaxation (C, isotonic relaxation; and D, isometric relaxation). Because contraction and relaxation take place under identical conditions of loading, the curves for contraction and relaxation in Fig. 15.6 should be superimposed.

If, instead of relaxing under the same loading conditions as were present during contraction, the muscle was relieved of its load at the end of its contraction (B in Fig. 15.5), muscle tension would fall to zero prior to lengthening. As a result, the phase of isometric relaxation would precede the return to initial length, so that the muscle would lengthen at zero load. The resulting work diagram (Fig. 15.7) is similar to that of the heart (Fig. 15.8), which normally relaxes under very low tensions because closure of the semilunar (aortic and pulmonic) valves disengages the load (pressure in the aorta and pulmonary artery) from the ventricles.

THE PRESSURE-VOLUME LOOP

The work diagram of the heart, shown in Fig. 15.8 for the left ventricle, is referred to as the pressure-volume loop. Although generally similar to that for the muscle shown in Fig. 15.7, there are several important differences (Fig. 15.1). The first is that the ordinate and abscissa represent pressure and volume in the ventricle, as described earlier in this chapter, although analogous to tension and length, they are not the same. The second difference between the work diagrams of skeletal muscle and the left ventricle is in the preload, the extent of loading at the start of contraction. Unlike the skeletal muscle shown in Fig. 15.5, the left ventricle does not begin its contraction at zero load; instead, there is normally a measurable end-

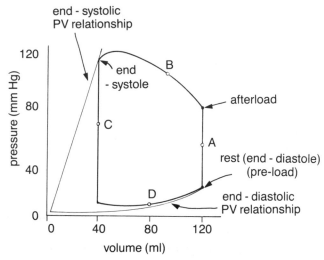

FIG. 15.8. Work diagram of the left ventricle. Unlike the skeletal muscle contraction depicted in Fig. 15.7, a small preload in the resting heart determines the point along the end-diastolic pressure-volume (PV) relationship at which systole begins. After the mitral valve closes, isovolumic contraction (*A*) proceeds until the ventricle encounters its afterload, the aortic pressure. After the aortic valve opens pressure first rises and then falls during ejection (*B*). When systole ends, ventricular pressure and volume come to lie on the end-systolic pressure-volume (PV) relationship. After aortic valve closure removes the load (aortic pressure) from the ventricle, relaxation begins under isovolumic conditions (*C*) because blood can neither enter nor leave the ventricle. When left ventricular pressure falls below that in the left atrium, the mitral valve opens and the atrium empties into the ventricle during the phase of filling (*D*). The cycle is completed when ventricular relaxation is completed and ventricular pressure and volume again lie on the end-diastolic PV relationship.

diastolic pressure, so that ventricular contraction is to a small, but significant, extent preloaded.

Analysis of the Pressure-Volume Loop of the Left Ventricle

The pressure-volume loop shown in Fig. 15.8 is constrained by two independently determined interactions between the heart and circulation. The first, which occurs at *end-diastole*, defines the interplay between the fully relaxed heart and the circulatory forces that tend to fill the ventricle just before the beginning of systole. The second interaction occurs at *end-systole*, just before the ventricle begins to relax. Each reflects a different property of the heart. End-diastolic conditions are influenced by the *lusitropic* properties of the relaxed heart, whereas the end-systolic pressure-volume relationship conditions provide an excellent index of the *inotropic* properties of the contracting heart, that is, of myocardial contractility.

End-Diastolic and End-Systolic Pressure-Volume Relationships

When preload and afterload are varied, intraventricular pressure and volume shift along two lines: one defines the conditions at the end of diastole, the other at end-systole. These lines thus reflect the lusitropic and inotropic states of the ventricle, respectively. The two pressure-volume (PV) relationships define the limits of the work diagram of the ventricle. Although the PV relationships themselves are determined by the properties of the ventricle, the positions of the end-diastolic and end-systolic points that lie along these lines for any given cardiac cycle are determined largely by the circulatory hemodynamics (preload and afterload, respectively).

At the end of diastole, interventricular pressure and volume are determined by preload (largely the venous return) and the lusitropic state of the relaxed ventricle. The latter, in turn, reflects all of the variables that influence the ability of the heart to fill; these include the extent to which the contractile proteins have been dissociated by the removal of activator calcium from the troponin complex, which in turn reflects the amount of calcium initially released during systole, the rate and extent of calcium uptake into the sarcoplasmic reticulum, and the ease with which calcium dissociates from troponin (i.e., the calcium affinity of troponin). Ventricular relaxation and filling are also influenced by the heart's connective tissue skeleton, the pericardium, and the geometry and thickness of the ventricular walls.

End-systolic pressure and volume, as noted above, are also determined by interactions between the circulation and the heart. The circulatory contribution is the afterload, mainly impedance (Chapter 13), which for the left ventricle reflects both peripheral resistance and the compliance of the aorta. The heart's contribution is the end-systolic PV relationship, which is determined mainly by the inotropic state of the ventricle. In fact, the end-systolic PV relationship probably provides the best definition of a term that gave us much difficulty in Chapter 14; this, of course, is *myocardial contractility*. The contractility of the ventricles, which encompasses *all* of the determinants of the heart's ability to perform work, is thus reflected in the end-systolic PV relationship.

Inscription of the Pressure-Volume Loop

The pressure-volume loop (Fig. 15.8), by convention viewed as beginning at the end-diastole, is inscribed in a counterclockwise direction. Four phases analogous to those described for the skeletal muscle in Fig. 15.5 are readily identified; as already noted, for the ventricle we are dealing with volume and not length, and pressure rather than tension.

The first phase, analogous to *isometric contraction* of the skeletal muscle (Fig. 15.5), begins when tension develops in the wall of the left ventricle. The rising intraventricular pressure closes the mitral valve so that blood can neither enter nor leave the ventricle until the aortic valve opens. Because pressure rises at constant volume, the loop begins with an upward deflection. The term *isometric contraction* applied to this phase of systole is, however, a misnomer as the left ventricular shape changes: the apex-base diameter shortens and the circumference increases, giving a more rounded contour to the cavity. For this reason, this phase is more appropriately called *isovolumic contraction*.

The second phase, analogous to *isotonic contraction*, begins when left ventricular pressure exceeds that in the aorta and the aortic valve opens. This allows *ejection* to begin, which causes the pressure-volume loop to turn to the left. Although aortic pressure rises and then falls, tension on the walls of the left ventricle actually decreases throughout ejection owing to the operation of the law of Laplace (Chapter 16). Systole ends at a point along the end-systolic PV relationship, which as already noted defines the inotropic state of the ventricle.

The third phase, analogous to *isometric relaxation*, begins after the end of ejection. At the beginning of diastole, when the ventricular myocardium starts to relax, the aortic valve closes. Because ventricular volume cannot change, due to the closed valves, the initial fall of the pressure-volume loop represents *isovolumic relaxation*. As was true for isovolumic contraction, isovolumic relaxation is accompanied by shape changes in the ventricle and so is not isometric. Ventricular relaxation, like that of the skeletal muscle shown in Fig. 15.7, is unloaded because aortic valve closure, by disconnecting the load (aortic pressure) from the relaxing left ventricle, relieves the ventricular myocardium of its afterload during all subsequent phases of relaxation.

> This last statement is, in fact, oversimplified because the coronary distending pressure contributes to sarcomere lengthening through a mechanism called "the garden-hose effect" (Chapter 16).

The final phase of the cardiac cycle, which is analogous to *isotonic relaxation*, begins when pressure in the left ventricle falls below that in the left atrium, allowing the mitral valve to open, and *filling* to begin. Left ventricular pressure and volume then rise gradually to end at a point along the end-diastolic PV relationship, which defines the state of the fully relaxed ventricle. The blood that enters the ventricle from the left atrium generates the preload for the next contraction.

Although the pressure-volume loop provides a useful visualization of the changing pressures and volumes during a cardiac cycle, these depictions of cardiac function provide no information regarding rates, as they have no time scale.

CARDIAC CYCLE

Each time the heart contracts, a series of electrical and mechanical events takes place. These in turn govern the flow of blood into and out of the heart. They determine the opening and closing of the cardiac valves and thus account for the characteristic timing of the heart sounds. This sequence of events is also manifest at the body surfaces as changes in electrical potential: the electrocardiogram, which is discussed in Chapter 20. All together, this sequence of events is called the *cardiac cycle*.

The description that follows, including Fig. 15.9, are modified only slightly from the last edition of the late Dr. Carl J. Wiggers's classic text *Physiology in Health and Disease*. This eloquent description and the "Wiggers diagram," once of interest mainly to the basic scientist, are now an integral part of modern cardiology and must be understood fully by all who wish to know the basis for the pumping action of the heart.

The series of superimposed curves which are reproduced in Fig. 15.9 unfold at a glance the story of cardiodynamic events which may be briefly summarized as follows:

At the onset of ventricular systole (I) the pressures are approximately equal in the atrium and ventricle, and the atrioventricular (AV) valves are in the act of floating into apposition. After the pressure has risen slightly within the ventricle, the AV valves close completely giving rise to the first heart sound [encircled I]. Since the semilunar valves are still closed, the ventricle contracts isovolumically, and the intraventricular pressure rises rapidly (I–II). The abrupt elevation of pressure causes a bulging of both the semilunar and AV valves, which accounts for the small positive oscillations in the aorta and atrium during this period. The descent of the ventricular base and the consequent traction on the aorta and atria cause the sharp oscillations—which are not, however, synchronous. The semilunar valves open at II, i.e., when the ventricular pressure exceeds the aortic. As a result, aorta and ventricle become a common cavity, and the two pressure curves follow one another closely.

With the rapid expulsion of blood during early moments of ejection—indicated by volume changes of the ventricles—the pressures in the left ventricle and aorta rise to a summit (III), because the rate at which blood is expelled into the aorta exceeds that at which it flows from its branches through the arterioles. As seen in Fig. 15.9 the rise is rounded (II–III) chiefly because, with rather constant ejection rate, the runoff increases gradually with progressive rise of aortic pressure. The rounded summit (III) is reached when ejection and runoff become equal. Since the rate of ejection diminishes during the latter part of systole (III–IV) while the flow from aortic branches continues high, aortic and ventricular pressures gradually decline. On the basis of pressure curves, it is therefore possible to separate the period of ejection into two phases, viz., maximum ejection (II–III) and reduced ejection (III–IV). Summarizing, the rise and fall of aortic and ventricular pressures always represent a balance between the rate at which blood is ejected into the aorta and the rate at which it leaves by its branches. However, the changes in rate of ventricular ejection normally dominate the shape of the curves during ejection.

At the onset of ventricular diastole (IV), aorta and ventricle are still in communication. The first effect of relaxation consists in a sharp drop in pressure in the ventricle and aorta, the latter being quickly terminated by the closure of the semilunar valves at V, after which a few vibrations occur, and the aortic curve declines very gradually for the remainder of diastole. The closure of the semilunar valves is associated with the second heart sound [encircled II]. The rate of diastolic decline is determined chiefly by the rate at which blood flows out of the aorta, but is affected to a variable extent by the increasing distensibility of arteries at different pressure levels.

Within the ventricle, the decline continues rapidly until VI, at which point the AV valves open, and the phase of isovolumic relaxation terminates. During this phase of ventricular relaxation the intra-atrial pressure continues to rise slowly; occasionally, however, a more marked positive elevation occurs, which must be assigned to a compression effect produced by the upward movement of the ventricular base. As soon as intraventricular pressure has declined to a level lower than that in the atrium (VI), the AV valves are opened again by the difference of pressure and a rapid inflow of blood into the ventricle begins. While this continues (VI–VII), pressures in the atrium and

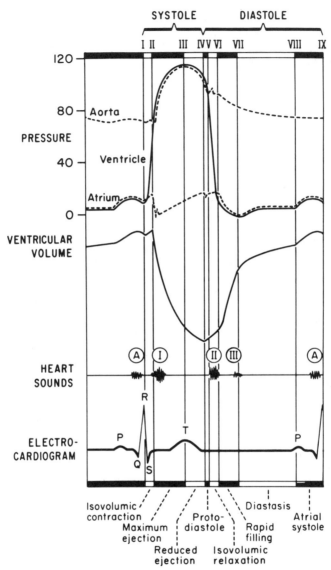

FIG. 15.9. The cardiac cycle (Wiggers diagram) showing eight phases. The top three *curves* represent aortic pressure (*upper dashed line*), left ventricular pressure (*solid line*), and left atrial pressure (*lower dashed line*). The units of pressure are millimeters of mercury. The middle *curve* (*solid line*) represents left ventricular volume, below which is a representation of the heart sounds. The latter are depicted as vibrations: Ⓐ, atrial (or fourth) sound; Ⓘ first heart sound; Ⓘ, second heart sound; Ⓘ, third heart sound. The *bottom line* represents the ECG with its P wave, QRS complex, and T wave.

ventricle decline together, but the atrial pressure remains a trifle higher than the ventricular. In long cycles this is followed by a diastasis phase (VII–VIII), during which ventricular inflow is exceedingly slow, and the pressure rises very gradually both in the atrium and ventricle. In young normal individuals, and in some pathological states, the rapid inflow of blood into the ventricle is associated with an audible sound, the third heart sound [encircled III]. Occasionally, atrial systole also produces a sound [encircled A] sometimes called the fourth heart sound.

The Phases of the Cardiac Cycle. The succession of atrial and ventricular events constitutes the cardiac cycle. Since ventricular contraction is dynamically the most important it is fitting to start the cycle with this event. Accordingly, the cardiac cycle can be divided advantageously into ventricular systole and diastole, but each of these periods must be further subdivided. For the sake of clarity these subdivisions are designated as phases of systole and diastole. The vertical lines of Fig. 15.9 serve to demarcate the successive periods and phases of systole and diastole. I–IV indicates the period of *systole*, V–IX the period of *diastole*. The first phase of systole, I–II, is called the *isovolumic contraction phase*, for the ventricle contracts essentially in this manner with all valves closed. The second phase, II–IV, is best referred to as the *ejection phase*. It can be further subdivided by reference to the aortic pressure curve alone or with the aid of the ventricular volume curve into the phase of *maximum ejection*, II–III, and the phase of *reduced ejection*, III–IV.

The *protodiastolic phase*, IV–V, which constitutes the first interval of diastole, ends with closure of the semilunar valves. It is followed by the *isovolumic relaxation* phase, V–VI, which ends as soon as atrial pressure exceeds that in the ventricle, viz., at VI. With opening of the AV valves at VI, the *rapid filling phase* supervenes, VI–VII, and this is followed by a variable phase of *diastasis*, VII–VIII. Finally, *atrial systole*, VIII–IX, terminates the period of ventricular diastole.

The durations of these successive phases have been repeatedly studied but with varying degrees of accuracy. The average values in seconds (Table 15.2) derived from an analysis of many pressure pulses, are sufficient to give an idea as to the relative duration in man of the most commonly used phases.

A schematic electrocardiographic recording of the changing electrical potential differences at the body surface and their relation to the cardiac cycle is also shown in Fig. 15.9. As is discussed at length in Chapter 20, the P wave reflects the electrical depolarization of the atria; the QRS complex that of the ventricles. The T wave is produced by potential differences set up within the ventricle during repolarization.

In attempting to understand the biochemical and biophysical bases of the mechanical and electrical events that produce the cardiac cycle, the reader should always keep the

TABLE 15.2. *Durations (in seconds) of the phases of the cardiac cycle in adult man*

Isovolumic contraction	0.05
Maximum ejection	0.09
Reduced ejection	0.13
Total systole	0.27
Protodiastole	0.04
Isovolumic relaxation	0.08
Rapid inflow	0.11
Diastasis	0.19
Atrial systole	0.11
Total diastole	0.53

"Wiggers diagram" in mind, for this classic view of the electrical and mechanical properties of the heart remains the focal point of modern cardiology.

The first and second heart sounds, although related to valve closure, probably do not arise from the valves themselves. Instead, vibrations involving the heart and great vessels, set up by rapid acceleration and deceleration of the moving stream of blood, contribute importantly to the genesis of "lub" and "dup."

END-DIASTOLIC VOLUME AS A DETERMINANT OF VENTRICULAR FUNCTION: THE FRANK-STARLING RELATIONSHIP AND STARLING'S LAW OF THE HEART

The relationship between the volume of blood in ventricles at the moment they begin to contract (end-diastolic volume) and the systolic pressure developed by the ventricle was first described in 1895 by Frank and later for the working mammalian heart by Starling in 1914. This relationship, which is a manifestation of the length-tension relationship described in Chapter 9, is referred to either as the Frank-Starling relationship or Starling's law of the heart.

The operation of this physiological law is seen clearly when a balloon placed within the left ventricle is filled with increasing volumes of an incompressible fluid such as saline. As the volume of the balloon is increased, diastolic pressure increases as shown in Fig. 15.10. The curve relating the changing pressures and volumes at the end of the diastole is, of course, the end-diastolic PV relationship described earlier in this chapter (Fig. 15.8).

Systolic pressure is also modified when the balloon in the ventricle is filled. Over the normal range of end-diastolic volume, the pressures developed during systole increase with increasing diastolic pressures in the balloon. Arrows can be drawn to connect each end-diastolic pressure with the corresponding pressure at the end of systole (Fig. 15.10). These arrows, which represent developed or "active" pressure, are vertical because the volume in the balloon filled with incompressible fluid cannot change; i.e., the ventricle is contracting under isovolumic conditions. When the net pressures developed during systole (i.e., systolic pressure minus diastolic pressure) are plotted as a function of the end-diastolic volume, a curve (often called the

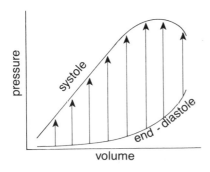

FIG. 15.10. The Frank-Starling relationship (Starling's law of the heart). The systolic pressure (*vertical lines*) developed in a series of isovolumic contractions increases with increasing end-diastolic volume. At very high end-diastolic volumes, systolic pressure can decline with increasing volume. The *lower line* is the end-diastolic pressure-volume (PV) relationship; the *upper line* the end-systolic PV relationship.

Starling curve) is obtained (Fig. 15.11). This curve is, of course, analogous to the length-tension relationship of a skeletal muscle. The ventricles normally operate on the left-hand portion of the Starling curve, called the *ascending limb*. Only at very high filling pressures does the ventricle enter the descending limb. This is very important because, as described below, the ventricle cannot function at a steady state on the descending limb.

The curves shown in Figs. 15.10 and 15.11 differ from the length-tension diagrams of skeletal muscle in two important respects: First, as already emphasized in this chapter, the relationships in Figs. 15.10 and 15.11 are between volume and pressure, not length and tension. Second, as the ventricles become distended, the resting pressure-volume curve rises sharply, leading to the development of high end-diastolic pressures that impede further filling (Fig. 15.10). This resistance to filling represents the low diastolic compliance of cardiac muscle also seen in simpler papillary muscle preparations (Chapter 9). The stiffness of cardiac muscle, along with the noncompliant pericardium, helps to protect the ventricle from the serious consequences of overfilling.

It is unlikely that the normal ventricle ever dilates to the point where it enters on the "descending limb" of the Starling curve (Fig. 15.11). In fact, were this to occur the heart would quickly dilate to the maximum volume allowed by the low compliance of the myocardium and pericardium. This follows because a negative feedback would develop in a ventricle that operates on the descending limb, where any additional increment in filling, by adding to the already excessive end-diastolic volume, would further reduce the pumping ability of the ventricle. Because increased venous return to a heart operating on the descending limb of the Starling curve would cause a further decrease in work performance, this represents a highly unstable state simply because more filling reduces the ability to empty. Thus, any intervention that decreases ejection or increases preload in such a heart would, by reducing ejection, increase preload and so further impair the ventricle's ability to empty. For this reason, operation of the ventricle in the face of the negative feedback of the descending limb can establish a vicious cycle from which the heart has no simple means of recovery; were it not for its low compliance, such a heart would burst like an overfilled balloon.

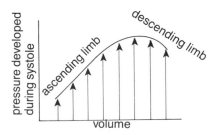

FIG. 15.11. The ascending and descending limbs of the Starling curve. The rise of systolic pressure that results from increased end-diastolic volume constitutes the ascending limb of the Starling curve; a fall in developed pressure as the ventricle dilates to very high volumes is the descending limb of this curve.

This situation is quite different from that in a skeletal muscle, which, even if it is forced onto the descending limb of its length-tension curve, is attached to bones where it is influenced by other muscles that could reverse any negative feedback. Furthermore, unlike the heart, a skeletal muscle does not determine its own preload, so that functioning of a skeletal muscle on the descending limb of its length-tension curve does not necessarily increase the load on the muscle at the start of the next contraction.

By operating on the ascending limb of the Starling curve (Fig. 15.11), the normal heart is able to avoid this situation. Instead, as described in Chapter 13, increased load normally enhances the ability of the ventricle to do work, and thus promotes emptying. In this way, the ascending limb of the Starling curve allows the heart to respond to increased end-diastolic volume by increasing ejection pressure, stroke volume, or both.

THE PERICARDIUM

The pericardium, along with the low compliance of the ventricular walls, plays an important role in limiting ventricular filling. In conditions where the pericardium fills with fluid (pericardial effusion) or shrinks due to chronic inflammation (constrictive pericarditis), inability of the heart to fill can become disabling and even fatal. Filling of the thin-walled right ventricle is generally impaired before that of the left ventricle in these conditions.

The pericardium also limits acute dilatation of the heart. However, when chronically stretched, the pericardial sac itself enlarges, probably due to addition of new fibrous tissue. For this reason, the pericardium plays little role in limiting the slow dilatation of the failing heart.

THE ATRIUM AS A PRIMER PUMP

The role of end-diastolic volume in determining the contractile properties of the ventricles provides a useful starting point for understanding the role of atrial systole in the regulation of cardiac performance. The fact that atrial systole normally occurs immediately before ventricular systole allows atrial contraction to augment the volume of blood in the ventricles at that instant (end-diastole) when ventricular volume determines the strength of ventricular contraction, without requiring the circulation to pay the price of high filling pressures throughout diastole (see below).

Loss of the atrial "kick," as commonly occurs when effective atrial contraction ceases in atrial fibrillation (Chapter 23), has two hemodynamic consequences, both bad. These are a rise in *mean* atrial pressure and a fall in ventricular *end-diastolic* pressure (Fig. 15.12). The rise in mean atrial pressure impedes the return of blood to the heart and so increases venous pressure, whereas the fall in end-diastolic volume reduces ejection, and so decreases cardiac output. Although well-tolerated in most individuals who have a normal heart (except for a very important risk of emboli due to clot formation in the fibrillating atria), atrial fibrillation can seriously

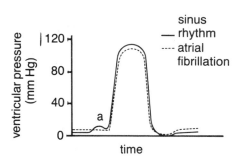

FIG. 15.12. Effects of loss of atrial systole. In the normal cardiac cycle (*solid line*) atrial contraction (*a*) increases left ventricular end-diastolic pressure to a level higher than that during the earlier phases of diastole. Loss of atrial systole (*dashed line*) is generally accompanied by a decline in left ventricular end-diastolic pressure. Because the ventricle loses the ability, provided by atrial systole, to elevate end-diastolic pressure only at the end of diastole, mean left atrial pressure becomes abnormally high even though end-diastolic pressure is abnormally low. The former impedes venous return, the latter reduces ventricular performance.

worsen the clinical symptoms of heart failure in patients whose cardiac function has already been compromised (Chapter 25).

The effects of losing the atrial primer pump are readily understood by viewing atrial systole as a mechanism for increasing diastolic volume *at that instant (end-diastole) when diastolic volume determines ventricular performance.* Atrial systole (a in Fig. 15.12) thus allows the ventricle the "luxury" of a high end-diastolic pressure without the need to "pay the price" of high atrial pressure throughout diastole; the latter, of course, would both reduce venous return and increase venous pressures. In order for ventricular end-diastolic pressure (and end-diastolic volume) to approach the normal level that existed before loss of effective atrial contraction, atrial pressure would have to remain high throughout diastole. This means that loss of atrial systole has two detrimental consequences: ventricular end-diastolic volume decreases, which reduces cardiac performance; and the ventricle ceases to enjoy the beneficial effects of a high end-diastolic volume without the cost of high pressures throughout diastole. Although both generally occur when atrial systole is lost, the extent to which one or the other predominates depends on the individual circulatory compensations.

> The important timing of atrial systole is made possible by the normal delay between atrial and ventricular systole, which is caused by slow conduction through the atrioventricular node (Chapter 20). Atrial systole is especially important in older patients, who often have noncompliant left ventricles. In patients whose atria contract either too weakly or not at all because of conduction or other electrophysiological disturbances (Chapter 22), electronic pacemakers have been developed to stimulate the atria immediately before the ventricles so as to provide a normal atrial "kick."

In this chapter we have seen how two laws operate to govern the relationship between ventricular volume and the hemodynamic characteristics of cardiac contraction. The first, the law of Laplace, is a physical law, which states that when the ventricle dilates, the tension on its walls needed to achieve a given intraventricular pressure is increased. The second, the Frank-Starling relationship, is a physiological law, which states that when the ventricle dilates, the ability to perform work

increases. Within limits (i.e., in the normal range of ventricular volumes) the operation of the physiological law is predominant, so that when the ventricle dilates, the
increased capacity to generate tension more than compensates for the increased wall
tension. As becomes apparent in the next chapter, these consequences of ventricular
dilation modify the energy cost of cardiac contraction, so that in the failing heart,
the detrimental effects of ventricular dilation can assume greater importance than
the beneficial effects.

BIBLIOGRAPHY

Brutsaert DL, Rademakers FE, Sys SU, Gillebert TC, Housmans PR. (1985). Analysis of relaxation in
    the evaluation of ventricular function of the heart. *Prog Cardiovasc Dis* 28:143–163.
Burton AC. (1962). Physical principles of circulatory phenomena: the physical equilibria of the heart and
    blood vessels. In: Hamilton WF, Dow P, eds. *Handbook of physiology, section 2: Circulation*, vol 1.
    Washington, DC: American Physiology Society, 85–106.
Fifer MA, Grossman W. (1991). Measurement of ventricular volumes, ejection fraction, mass, wall
    stress, and regional wall motion. In: Grossman WG, Baim DS, eds. *Cardiac catheterization, an-
    giography, and intervention*. Philadelphia: Lea & Febiger; 300–318.
Freeman GL, LeWinter MM. (1984). Pericardial adaptations during chronic cardiac dilation in dogs.
    Circ Res 54:294–300.
Katz AM. (1965). The descending limb of the Starling curve and the failing heart. *Circulation* 32:871–
    875.
Katz AM. (1988) Influence of altered inotropy and lusitropy on ventricular pressure-volume loops. *J Am
    Coll Cardiol* 11:438–445.
Katz LN. (1960). The performance of the heart. *Circulation* 21:483–498.
Luisada AA, Portaluppi F. (1983). The main heart sounds as vibrations of the cardiohemic system: old
    controversy and new facts. *Am J Cardiol* 52:1133–1136.
Smith VE, Katz AM (1983). Inotropic and lusitropic abnormalities in the genesis of heart failure. *Eur
    Heart J* 4(Suppl A):7–17.
Spadaro J, Bing OHL, Gaasch WH, Weintraub RM. (1981). Pericardial modulation of right and left
    ventricular diastolic interaction. *Circ Res* 48:233–238.
Yin FCP. (1981). Ventricular wall stress. *Circ Res* 49:829–842.

16

The Working Heart

Our description of cardiac function in Chapter 15 highlighted the muscular basis for the pumping action of the heart. The laws that govern the relationship between length and volume, tension and pressure, and the response of the heart to changing preload (i.e., end-diastolic volume) were discussed in terms of the left ventricle contracting on a fluid-filled balloon under isovolumic conditions. This preparation, however, represents a highly artificial model of the working heart. Although useful in defining the operation of the law of Laplace and the Frank-Starling relationship, the isovolumic heart fails to eject blood under pressure, which is the physiological function of the heart.

The ejection of a volume of blood under pressure represents *work*, and the product *pressure* × *volume* has the correct units for work (dynes/cm^2 × cm^3 = dynes cm). Thus, the work of the heart during each beat (stroke work) can be calculated by multiplying the volume of blood ejected during each stroke (the stroke volume, usually abbreviated *SV*) by the pressure (*P*) at which the blood is ejected.

$$\text{Stroke work} = P \times SV. \qquad [16.1]$$

Because pressure changes during the phase of ejection (Fig. 15.8), stroke work is more accurately the integral of pressure and volume change:

$$\text{Stroke work} = \int P dV \qquad [16.2]$$

where *P* is the pressure under which each increment (*dV*) of the stroke volume is ejected. For most practical purposes, however, the product $P \times SV$ is sufficiently accurate to characterize stroke work.

Stroke volume, the blood ejected during each stroke of the cardiac cycle, is equal to end-diastolic volume (*EDV*) minus end-systolic volume (*ESV*), the volume remaining in the ventricle at the end of systole, so that Eq. 16.1 can be rewritten:

$$\text{Stroke work} = P \times (EDV - ESV). \qquad [16.3]$$

Equation 16.3 tells us that three variables determine stroke work: *EDV*, *ESV*, and ejection pressure. As emphasized later in this chapter, these mechanisms have different energetic implications in the working heart.

369

Equation 16.3 provides the key to understanding a concept stressed in earlier chapters, that when the cardiac contractile proteins are activated, and so develop the capacity to perform work, the expression of this capacity in terms of pressure and flow is significantly influenced by loading. Afterload (which is related to peripheral and pulmonary resistances, or more accurately impedances) is a major determinant of pressure and end-systolic volume in Eq. 16.3, whereas preload (mainly the venous return) is a major determinant of end-diastolic volume. As we have seen in Chapter 15, the interactions between the contracting heart and afterload determine the point along the end-systolic pressure-volume (PV) relationship at which ejection ends, whereas interactions between the relaxed heart and preload determine where end-diastolic volume lies along the end-diastolic PV relationship.

EXTERNAL AND INTERNAL WORK

Two types of work must be considered in evaluating the energetics of cardiac contraction. The first is the *external work* that appears when blood leaves the ventricles and moves into the great vessels; this is relatively simple to measure in experimental preparations, and excellent indices are available for clinical use. Accurate measurement of the total work of the heart must, however, include the work done within the walls of the contracting ventricles: the *internal work* needed to stretch muscle elasticities and lengthen viscous elements. As the internal work is degraded to heat when the heart relaxes, it contributes an inefficiency to the performance of the heart.

External Work: Pressure-Volume Work

The external work of the heart can be approximated as the product $P \times SV$, or more accurately as the integral $\int PdV$, which is the *pressure-volume work* of the heart; that is, the work performed in moving blood under pressure from the left ventricle to the aorta, and from the right ventricle to the pulmonary artery. Under most conditions pressure-volume work represents the great majority of the useful work of the heart.

The work of the atria, which transports blood into the ventricles, usually makes only a negligible contribution to the pressure-volume work in that atrial systole normally generates only a low pressure; furthermore, most ventricular filling occurs before the atria contract. It should not be forgotten, however, that even though atrial systole makes little direct contribution to the energy output of the heart, it is important as a primer pump that determines ventricular end-diastolic volume (Chapter 15).

The stroke volumes of the two ventricles must, at steady state, be identical, whereas pulmonary artery pressure is approximately one-fifth that of aortic pressure. For this reason the pressure-volume work of the right ventricle is approximately one-fifth that of the left ventricle.

External Work: Kinetic Work

In addition to the pressure-volume work, the ventricles perform work in accelerating the stream of blood as it passes into the aorta and pulmonary artery. The acceleration of blood leaving the ventricles represents kinetic work, which according to the laws of physics is proportional to the square of the velocity at which the blood is ejected from the ventricle:

$$\text{Kinetic work } = \frac{1}{2} mv^2 \qquad [16.4]$$

where m is the mass of blood moving from the left ventricle to the aorta or from the right ventricle to the pulmonary artery, and v is the velocity at which this blood passes through the aortic and pulmonic valves.

The kinetic work of the left ventricle is normally a small fraction of the pressure-volume work, usually less than 5% of the latter. Because kinetic work increases as the square of the velocity at which blood leaves the ventricle, and since velocity increases when stroke volume increases, kinetic work is roughly proportional to the cube of stroke volume because the volume of blood ejected contributes to both the terms m and v^2 of Eq. 16.4. For this reason, in diseases where stroke volume is abnormally high (e.g., aortic insufficiency or severe anemia), kinetic work can represent a significant portion (although rarely more than 10%) of the work of the left ventricle. In the right ventricle, where systolic pressure is low, kinetic work represents a greater proportion of total work.

The kinetic energy imparted to the blood leaving the ventricles is converted to pressure when blood flow slows in the great vessels. Thus, kinetic work, along with pressure-volume work, represent the useful work that propels blood through the aorta and pulmonary artery.

Internal Work

In addition to performing the external work necessary for the circulation of the blood through the vascular system, during each cardiac cycle the heart expends a significant amount of energy performing internal work. This internal work stretches the series elasticity (Chapter 9), elongates viscous elements, and rearranges the spiral bundles that make up the muscular architecture of the ventricle (Figs. 1.5 and 1.6). The spiral bundles account for shape changes during isovolumic contraction, which require the expenditure of rather large amounts of energy that do not contribute to the pumping of blood under pressure into the aorta and pulmonary artery. Instead, much as relaxation of a loaded skeletal muscle generates recovery heat (Chapter 6), the energy expended to do internal work is degraded into heat at the end of the cardiac cycle. Because the internal work of the heart is proportional to wall tension (see below), the energy wasted in this manner is especially significant when the heart dilates or must eject against a high pressure.

ARCHITECTURE OF THE VENTRICLES

As noted in Chapter 1, the right ventricle functions primarily as a low-pressure volume pump, whereas the left ventricle is a pressure pump. The architecture of the two ventricles (Fig. 1.4) is adapted to these functional specializations, the radius of curvature of the walls of the more elongated left ventricle being less than in the right ventricle; furthermore, the left ventricular wall is thicker. According to the law of Laplace (Eq. 15.4), these adaptations allow the left ventricle to generate high intraventricular pressures with relatively low wall tensions.

> The first application of the law of Laplace to the heart was published one hundred years ago, when Woods (1892) observed that "the thickness of the heart at any place bears a direct proportion to the relative tension at that place." Using measurements of wall thickness and radii of curvature, Woods correctly predicted that left ventricular pressure was much higher than that in the right ventricle, and that these differences were less in the neonatal heart.

The operation of the law of Laplace is clearly seen in the adaptation of cardiac structure to different levels of intraventricular pressure (Fig. 16.1). In the giraffe, where left ventricular systolic pressures often exceed 300 mm Hg, this adaptation of structure to function explains the long, narrow, thick-walled ventricle. In contrast, the thin-walled amphibian left ventricle, which generates low pressures, is almost spherical. The human right ventricle, which ejects the same stroke volume as the left ventricle, but at a lower pressure, has a crescentic cross-sectional shape, and the right ventricular free wall is relatively thin (Fig. 16.2). The interventricular septum, which normally functions as part of the left ventricle, is thick-walled.

> The septum normally functions as part of the left ventricle because it compresses the left ventricular cavity during systole. However, in patients with severely elevated right ventricular pressure (as occurs, for example, in pulmonary hypertension), the septum contracts "paradoxically" by moving away from the left ventricular cavity so as to function as part of the right ventricle.

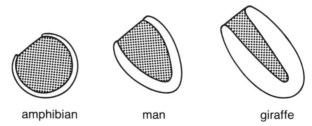

amphibian   man   giraffe

FIG. 16.1. Relationship between ventricular pressure and the shape of its cavity. The thin-walled left ventricle of the amphibian heart, which develops low pressures, is almost spherical, whereas that of the thicker human left ventricle, which develops a much higher pressure, is more elongated. In the heart of the giraffe, where left ventricular systolic pressure is extremely high, the cavity of the thick-walled ventricle is almost tubular.

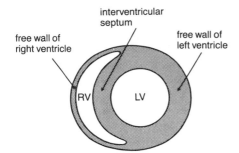

FIG. 16.2. Cross section of the human heart showing the thin-walled, crescentic right ventricle (RV) in which systolic pressure is approximately one-fifth that of the thick-walled, narrower left ventricle (LV).

STROKE WORK

The pressure-volume work that is performed during each cardiac cycle is the *stroke work* which, as noted above, represents most of the external work of the ventricle. Stroke work, which can be calculated as the integral $\int PdV$ (Eq. 16.2), is also the area of the pressure-volume loop depicted in Fig. 15.8.

The total work performed by the heart during each cardiac cycle is somewhat greater than the area of the pressure volume loop (Fig. 16.3). Thus, the entire shaded area in Fig. 16.3, including the darkly shaded area B beneath the pressure-volume loop, represents the integral $\int PdV$ viewed as the blood crosses the aortic valve. An additional small amount of work that fills the left ventricle, the darkly shaded area beneath the pressure-volume loop in Fig. 16.3, arises in part from atrial systole, and partly from the return of blood through the pulmonary veins, both of which contribute to the preload on the ventricle. The latter, of course, represents energy originally imparted to the blood by the right ventricle.

In estimating the work of the ventricle, it is customary to subtract the work done to fill the left ventricle during diastole, i.e., the work of atrial systole and the momentum of the venous return. Usually this is only a small adjustment, however, as the majority of left ventricular work (area A in Fig. 16.3) is the direct consequence of ventricular systole.

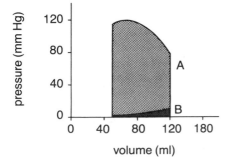

FIG. 16.3. Work of the left ventricle. Most useful work performed during each beat is equal to the area *A* (the pressure-volume loop, which represents the integral $\int PdV$) + *B*, which represents work contributed by atrial contraction and the inertia of the venous return.

Stroke work is readily estimated as the product $P \times SV$. Mean ejection pressure is normally ~105 mm Hg, whereas normal stroke volume is ~70 ml, so that normal stroke work is $\sim7,000$ mm Hg ml. In centimeter-gram-second units, this corresponds to $\sim9.3 \times 10^6$ dyne cm.

MINUTE WORK

Cardiac work performance is commonly related to a fixed period of time, generally defined as minute work, i.e., the work performed per minute. Minute work, or power, can be estimated by multiplying the work per beat (stroke work) by the number of beats per minute (HR = heart rate):

$$\text{Minute work} = HR \times SV \times P. \qquad [16.5]$$

Equation 16.5 contains another important term, *cardiac output* (*CO*), which is the product of $HR \times SV$. Thus, minute work can also be calculated as the product of pressure and cardiac output:

$$\text{Minute work} = P \times CO. \qquad [16.6]$$

In humans, cardiac output is normally ~5 liters per minute.

Determinants of Minute Work

Each of the variables in Eq. 16.5 makes an independent contribution to the minute work of the heart; for example, work can be increased by increasing systemic blood pressure, heart rate, stroke volume, or any combination.

Because stroke volume = $EDV - ESV$, there are actually four determinants of minute work:

$$\text{Minute work} = P \times HR \times (EDV - ESV). \qquad [16.7]$$

Thus, the work of the heart can be increased when end-diastolic volume is increased, end-systolic volume is decreased, or both.

As discussed later in this chapter, each of the four variables that contribute to minute work has a different impact on the energetics of cardiac contraction. For this reason, minute work itself is not a precise index of the energy needs of the heart.

WORK PERFORMED BY AN ISOLATED HEART

The influence of each of the variables that determine minute work can be evaluated in an isolated heart preparation, where each can be varied independently. The isolated heart preparation illustrated in Fig. 16.4 (which is similar to a turtle heart preparation used by the author as a medical student in 1953) considers only the work of the left ventricle. This preparation allows filling pressure (preload) to be varied

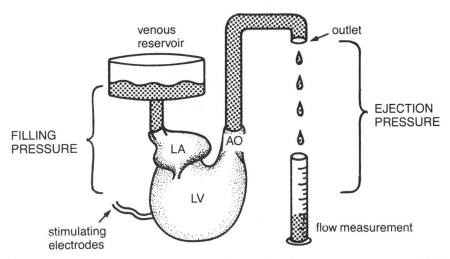

FIG. 16.4. Isolated left heart preparation. Blood flowing from the venous reservoir enters the left atrium (LA) at a pressure determined by the height of the reservoir relative to that of the atrium; this is the preload. The left ventricle (LV), when stimulated to contract, pumps the blood through the aorta (AO) into a tube; the height of its outlet constitutes the ejection pressure, which is the afterload. Stroke volume is the amount of blood ejected during each beat.

by adjusting the height of the venous reservoir, whereas ejection pressure (after-load) can be varied by raising or lowering the outlet connected to the aorta. Both pressures are related to a "zero" level at the center of the ventricle. Heart rate is controlled by stimulating electrodes. In the following discussion, we examine the effects of independent alterations in stroke volume, ejection pressure, and heart rate, keeping constant the other two determinants of minute work.

Variations in Stroke Volume

The stroke volume of the preparation illustrated in Fig. 16.4 can be varied by altering the height of the venous reservoir at constant stimulation rate and ejection pressure. Raising the venous reservoir increases ventricular end-diastolic pressure, thereby causing the heart to dilate. A series of graded changes in the level of the venous reservoir is therefore translated into a series of changes in end-diastolic volume. The resulting effects on cardiac performance are predicted by the Frank-Starling relationship; stroke volume increases with increasing filling pressure as long as the heart is functioning on the ascending limb of the Starling curve (Fig. 15.11). The manifestations of the Frank-Starling relationship under conditions where only stroke volume is allowed to vary are shown in Fig. 16.5. Because stroke work equals stroke volume times ejection pressure (Eq. 16.1), stroke work can be substituted for stroke volume on the ordinate in Fig. 16.5. Furthermore, as minute work is the product of stroke work and heart rate (Eq. 16.5), at constant heart rate

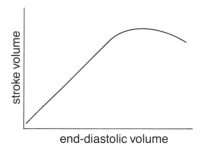

FIG. 16.5. Operation of the Frank-Starling relationship under conditions where only stroke volume is allowed to vary. At constant heart rate and ejection pressure, stroke volume rises with increasing end-diastolic pressure. The descending limb shown at high end-diastolic volumes is not always seen and is probably absent in the normal mammalian heart.

the ordinate in Fig. 16.5 also represents minute work. (Kinetic work, normally less than 5% of total external work, has been ignored.) The Frank-Starling relationship thus allows us to predict the effects of changing end-diastolic volume on stroke work and minute work.

Variations in Ejection Pressure

In the experimental preparation shown in Fig. 16.4, ejection pressure can be varied by raising or lowering the outlet of the tube connected to the aorta. If the rate of stimulation is unchanged, heart rate remains constant. However, stroke volume will change as outflow pressure is altered; increased afterload tends to decrease stroke volume, whereas reduced afterload facilitates ejection. To satisfy the design of our experiment, where only one variable at a time can change, the level of the venous reservoir must be adjusted to maintain constant stroke volume. Thus, when increased afterload impairs the ability of the ventricle to empty, the venous reservoir must be raised to maintain stroke volume; conversely, when reduced ejection pressure allows stroke volume to increase, the venous reservoir must be lowered. Because the pressure in the venous reservoir determines end-diastolic volume, our adjustments to the changing afterload increase end-diastolic volume when ejection pressure is elevated, and reduce it when ejection pressure is lowered (Fig. 16.6).

Figure 16.6, like Fig. 16.5, is a manifestation of the Frank-Starling relationship. As both stroke volume and heart rate are kept constant in this experiment, stroke

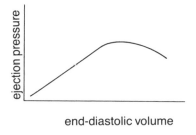

FIG. 16.6. Operation of the Frank-Starling relationship under conditions where only ejection pressure is allowed to vary. To maintain constant stroke volume, end-diastolic pressure must be increased when ejection pressure is increased.

work or minute work can be substituted for ejection pressure on the ordinate in Fig. 16.6.

Effect of Coronary Perfusion Pressure on Ventricular Function: The "Garden-Hose Effect"

Many years ago, changes in aortic pressure were found to influence work performance, even when the ventricle is drained of blood. This odd result is explained by the fact that coronary artery pressure itself influences ventricular function by distending the heart from within its walls. In other words, much as internal pressure distends a garden hose, the turgor of the coronary vasculature distends the heart, and so invokes Starling's law of the heart. Changing perfusion pressure has been recently shown also to modify calcium release during excitation-contraction coupling (Kitakaze and Marban, 1989).

Variations in Heart Rate

In the experimental model described in Fig. 16.4, heart rate can be varied at constant ejection pressure and venous pressure. Under these conditions, stroke volume remains constant as long as filling can increase to compensate for low heart rates, and diastole lasts long enough to allow adequate filling of the ventricle at rapid rates. In the model, therefore, minute work should, within limits, be directly proportional to heart rate as predicted by Eq. 16.5.

At this point, however, the dynamics of our isolated heart preparation differ from those of the intact circulation. This is because venous pressure in the model is determined by the height of a large reservoir, so that increasing heart rate does not affect venous return as long as diastole allows sufficient time for the heart to fill. However, this is not true in the intact animal because, at steady state, cardiac output can neither exceed nor fall below the venous return. For this reason, cardiac output is normally determined by the needs of the body, and not by the heart (Warner and Toronto, 1960). Thus when venous return is kept constant, the operation of Starling's law of the heart causes end-diastolic volume to fall when heart rate is increased, which decreases stroke volume. Conversely, Starling's law increases stroke volume when slowing of the heart increases filling.

At extremes of heart rate, however, changes in stroke volume are no longer able to maintain cardiac output at a level appropriate for the needs of the body (Fig. 16.7). At very rapid heart rates, diastole shortens to a point where ventricular filling cannot be completed, due both to limitations in flow across the mitral valve and the time available for the myocardium to relax completely (Chapter 11). As a result, stroke volume decreases at very rapid heart rates, causing cardiac output to fall. Conversely when heart rate is extremely slow, as in patients with complete heart block (where heart rates can be as low as 20/min), the heart cannot compensate by increasing stroke volume because the ventricles reach the peak of the Starling curve.

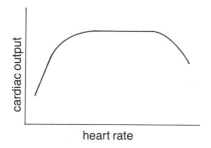

FIG. 16.7. Effects of varying heart rate on the minute work of the left ventricle *in the intact animal* where cardiac output is determined largely by the needs of the body, so that stroke volume tends to vary inversely with heart rate. Minute work is decreased only at rates too low to allow sufficient dilatation to maintain cardiac output, and at very high heart rates, where abbreviation of diastole does not allow the ventricle to fill completely.

Under these conditions, although left ventricular end-diastolic pressure increases, it cannot compensate for the slow rate of beating because of the low compliance of the myocardium. In these patients, where the slow heart rate has become the limiting determinant of cardiac work (Fig. 16.7), implantation of an electronic pacemaker can bring about a remarkable relief of the symptoms associated with the low cardiac output and high venous pressure.

INTERPLAY BETWEEN VENOUS RETURN AND CARDIAC OUTPUT

Because blood flows through our bodies in a circle, at steady state venous return has to equal cardiac output; this means that the circulation must be provided with mechanisms that can match cardiac output to venous return, and venous return to cardiac output. This text, which focuses on the heart, has emphasized the former: the influence of venous return on the output of the heart. This is, of course, the length-tension relationship and its expression as Starling's law of the heart. The other aspect of this interplay—the regulation of venous return—is, however, equally important in determining cardiac output.

Viewed from the heart, the balance between venous return and cardiac output is maintained by Starling's law of the heart, which increases stroke volume when more blood returns to the heart, and vice versa. The other side of this interaction is the ability of a decrease in stroke work to reduce venous return, and vice versa. The latter effects, in which the heart regulates the circulation, are not, however, brought about by any complex law of physiology. Instead, the output of the heart regulates venous return for the simple reason that when the heart cannot eject a given venous return, blood accumulating in the veins leading to the heart increases venous pressure. This, in turn, "pushes back" the column of blood that is flowing toward the heart, and so reduces venous return. Conversely, when an increase in the minute work of the heart allows more blood to be ejected, the resulting fall in venous pressure speeds the venous return. Key to understanding this interplay are the curves in Figure 16.8, which describe the two components of the relationship between atrial pressure (in this case on the right side of the heart) and the flow of blood around the circulation (venous return and its equivalent, cardiac output). Thus, Fig. 16.8 views the circulation from two vantage points: the heart and the periphery.

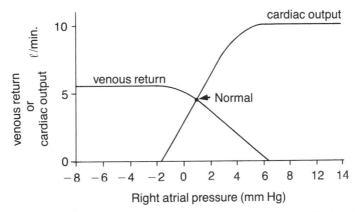

FIG. 16.8. Venous return and cardiac output are matched by opposing effects of right atrial pressure. For example, increasing right atrial pressure increases cardiac output (Starling's law of the heart) but decreases venous return. This defines a single steady state, where the point of intersection of these curves matches flow into and out of the heart.

Viewed from the heart, Starling's law tells us that an increase in venous pressure increases the ejection of blood *from* the right ventricle. Viewed from the circulation, however, an increase in venous pressure reduces the flow of blood *toward* the heart. The two curves that reflect these two relationships (Fig. 16.8) are therefore opposite in direction; one falls with increasing right atrial pressure, the other rises as right atrial pressure increases. This means that the two curves have a single intersection at any steady state involving the heart and circulation. This steady state defines both venous return and cardiac output, as well as the level of right atrial pressure. Shifts in the steady state depicted in Fig. 16.8, which can result from changes in either the heart or the circulation, are described later in this chapter.

The curve relating cardiac output to right atrial pressure in Fig. 16.8 is readily identified as the Starling curve in Fig. 16.5. The other curve, which relates venous return to right atrial pressure, rises to a plateau when the latter falls to negative pressures; this plateau is reached when the great veins collapse and so are no longer influenced by right atrial pressure. The maximal right atrial pressure is the mean circulatory pressure, which is recorded when the heart is stopped and all pressures in the cardiovascular system come to equilibrium.

ENERGY COST OF THE WORK OF THE HEART

The efficient pathways of oxidative metabolism (Chapter 5) allow the heart to meet its unremitting demand for adenosine triphosphate (ATP) almost entirely by oxidizing fat, carbohydrates, and, to a very minor extent, protein. As virtually all chemical energy used during cardiac contraction is generated by oxidative phosphorylation, and because energy production equals energy consumption in the normal heart, the utilization of chemical energy by the working heart is readily estimated by measurements of cardiac oxygen consumption.

The amount of chemical energy made available when a given amount of oxygen is consumed is virtually independent of the substrate oxidized. Even though oxidation of each gram of fat yields ~9 calories, whereas that of carbohydrate and proteins yields only ~4 calories/g of substrate, a greater amount of oxygen is consumed during the oxidation of each gram of fat (Chapter 3). Thus when the release of chemical energy is expressed per liter of oxygen consumed in metabolizing each of these foodstuffs, the average value is 4.8 ± 0.2 calories liberated per liter of oxygen consumed, regardless of the substrate oxidized. For this reason, cardiac oxygen consumption provides a valid index of the rate at which chemical energy is used during cardiac contraction.

Cardiac efficiency can be estimated by dividing the external work of the heart by the energy equivalent of the oxygen consumed. Both numerator and denominator can be expressed either per beat or per unit of time. The resulting quotient provides a useful index of cardiac efficiency.

$$\text{Cardiac efficiency} = \frac{\text{useful work}}{\text{energy equivalent of oxygen consumption}} . \qquad [16.8]$$

The overall efficiency of the working heart calculated in this manner is generally between 5 and 20%, the exact value depending on the nature and amount of work performed.

Influence of Work on Cardiac Efficiency

The importance of total work performed in determining cardiac efficiency is apparent if one recognizes that isovolumic contraction by the heart requires the expenditure of a significant amount of energy. This is because energy is consumed to perform internal work, even during a systole in which developed pressure is insufficient to open the aortic valve. Under these conditions, of course, no external work is done so that the external efficiency of the heart is zero. When left ventricular pressure exceeds aortic pressure and blood is ejected from the left ventricle, external work is performed; thus, both the numerator in the equation defining cardiac efficiency (Eq. 16.8) and efficiency become finite. Even though extra energy is required when the heart performs external work, efficiency initially increases with increasing external work simply because the energy wasted in performing internal work becomes a decreasing proportion of total energy expenditure.

Evans and Matsuoka, who in 1915 first showed the dependence of cardiac oxygen consumption and efficiency on increasing work (Fig. 16.9), found that oxygen consumption increases in a monotonic fashion as external work increases, whereas efficiency first rises then falls. The direct relationship between work performance and oxygen consumption is an expression of the Fenn effect described in Chapter 6. The origin of the biphasic curve relating efficiency to work is more complex, however, and depends on the nature of the work performed.

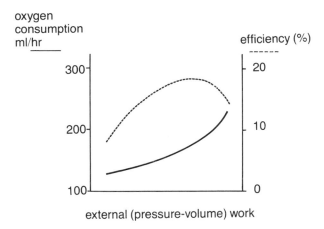

FIG. 16.9. Relationship between the amount of external work performed and the energetics of left ventricular contraction. Oxygen consumption (*solid line*) increases monotonically with increasing work, whereas efficiency (*dashed line*) first rises and then falls.

Pressure Work and Flow Work

In addition to defining the existence of a direct relationship between cardiac work and the liberation of chemical energy (the Fenn effect), Evans and Matsuoka described a clinically important difference in the energy costs of increasing work by increasing either aortic pressure (P) or cardiac output (CO) (Fig. 16.10). In either case, although increased work is associated with extra oxygen consumption (solid lines) and an initial gain in efficiency (dotted lines), at moderate levels of work (vertical line W_2) energy expenditure is greater when the heart is faced with a high aortic pressure (P) than when it is ejecting a larger volume of blood against a lower pressure (CO) *even though the level of work is the same.* This observation means that a given increment in work is performed more efficiently when brought about by raising cardiac output than when it results from increased aortic pressure. Stated simply, pressure generation by the myocardium is energetically more costly than ejection.

These differences in the energetics of "pressure work" and "flow work" are due mainly to different amounts of internal work performed by the heart. Even though the product of pressure × cardiac output provides an excellent index of the *external* work expended in moving blood from the venous system to the high-pressure arterial circuit, pressure and output have quite different effects on the energy expended in doing *internal* work. The latter, mainly energy absorbed by shape changes and elasticities in the ventricular walls during isovolumic contraction, is much greater when the ventricle develops pressure than when it ejects.

To understand why internal work increases disproportionately at high ejection pressures, compared to the much smaller increment of internal work that accompanies a similar increase in external work when cardiac output is increased, it is

oxygen
consumption
ml/hr   efficiency (%)
—   ----------

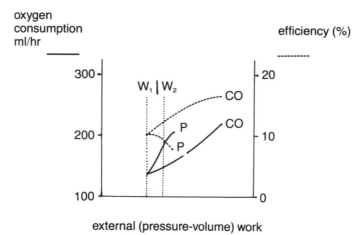

FIG. 16.10. Influence of the nature of the external work on ventricular oxygen consumption (*solid lines*) and efficiency (*dashed lines*). When cardiac work is increased from W_1 to W_2 by increasing cardiac output (CO) or ejection pressure (P), the resulting effects on oxygen consumption and efficiency differ strikingly. Cardiac efficiency at the higher level of work is much greater when cardiac output is increased than when ejection pressure is increased because of the lower energy requirements of flow work compared to pressure work.

useful to refer back to the load-energy curves discused in Chapter 6 (Fig. 6.6). In a frog sartorius muscle the curve relating total energy release to load parallels the curve that relates external work to load (Fig. 16.11); this is because the amount of heat liberated is essentially independent of load. In his early studies on the energetics of muscle, Fenn noted that curves in experiments like those shown in Fig. 16.11 are quite different for muscles other than the frog sartorius. In the frog gastrocnemius, for example, total energy expenditure does not decline appreciably with increasing load when the load is high (Fig. 16.12); instead, heat liberation increases at the high loads. These differences between the frog sartorius and gastrocnemius muscles are attributable to differences in internal work related to the arrangement of

energy
released
per
contraction

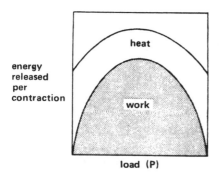

FIG. 16.11. Relationship between load, work, and total energy liberated by a frog sartorius muscle. Work and total energy liberation are maximal at intermediate loads, but heat production is relatively independent of load.

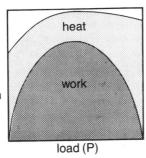

energy
released
per
contraction

load (P)

FIG. 16.12. Relationship between load, work, and total energy liberated by the myocardium. In contrast to the frog sartorius muscle (Fig. 16.11), heat production increases disproportionately at high loads.

the fiber bundles in the two muscles (Fig. 16.13). The fibers in the sartorius are arranged in a parallel fashion, whereas those in the gastrocnemius muscle have an asymmetrical bipennate arrangement that causes significant shape changes during contraction, even when the ends of the muscle are fixed under isometric conditions. This causes an energetically expensive rearrangement of the fibers when the gastrocnemius contracts at high loads, even under isometric conditions where external work is zero (Martin, 1928).

Although the extent of fiber shortening responsible for these shape changes is small, high forces are developed during isometric contraction. Thus, even small length changes are associated with high levels of internal work, which explains the excess energy expenditure when tension is increased (Fig. 16.12). In the sartorius muscle, where the parallel arrangement of fibers allows much less shape change during con-

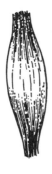

sartorius

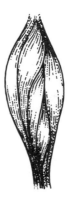

gastrocnemius

FIG. 16.13. Arrangement of muscle fibers in two skeletal muscles. In sartorius muscle, the fibers are parallel and oriented longitudinally. In gastrocnemius, which energetically is more like the myocardium, many of the fibers are oriented in directions not parallel to the long axis of the muscle. As a result, when the gastrocnemius lifts a heavy load, internal work is much higher than when the sartorius lifts the same load.

traction, internal work and energy wastage are less at the higher loads (Fig. 16.11). This is probably why the frog sartorius has become the standard preparation for studies of muscle energetics. In the heart, in which branching fiber bundles are arranged in interwoven spiral structures (Chapter 1), the energetics of contraction resemble those of the gastrocnemius muscle more than the sartorius. This explains why Evans and Matsuoka (and many others who came later, including the author in 1953) found that pressure work is more costly than flow work. The expenditure of energy in performing internal work, which increases directly with ejection pressure, and the eventual dissipation of this internal work as heat, thus accounts for the reduced mechanical efficiency when wall tension is increased.

Relationship Between Afterload and Efficiency

The high energy cost of pressure work helps us to understand an important detrimental effect of vasoconstriction, one of the body's key defenses to decreased cardiac output. Under these conditions, a drastic fall in blood pressure is prevented by neurohumoral reflexes that increase peripheral resistance. This maintains blood pressure and ensures perfusion of vital organs, mainly the brain and the heart, which are especially sensitive to ischemia (reduced blood flow). Reflex vasoconstriction, which plays a vital role in survival of such calamities as massive hemorrhage, is mediated largely by α-adrenergic responses in perhipheral resistance vessels, mainly arterioles. The resulting ability to survive hemorrhage must have been especially important to our species as it allowed our ancestors to survive the blood loss that often befalls the aggressive hunter, the mother during childbirth, and the defender of hearth and home.

Although vasoconstriction is vital as a short-term means to sustain cognitive and cardiac function in the face of a fall in cardiac output, the loss of cardiac efficiency associated with the increased afterload can, when sustained, prove harmful, especially when the heart is diseased. For this reason, careful administration of vasodilators to patients with heart failure, in whom a fall in cardiac output has led to excessive vasoconstriction, can both increase cardiac output and cardiac efficiency. Afterload reduction can be of considerable clinical benefit in these patients (Chapter 25).

Loss of Efficiency in the Dilated Heart

Energy wastage due to high internal work is significant not only when aortic pressure is increased, but also when the left ventricle becomes dilated. It follows from the law of Laplace that, even when intraventricular pressure remains constant, ventricular dilation increases the tension developed by its muscular walls (Chapter 15). By increasing the tension on the walls of the ventricles, cardiac dilation therefore increases internal work and decreases mechanical efficiency.

The inefficiency of the dilated heart is augmented by loss of the normal "unloading" of the myocardium during ejection. Normally, a marked decrease in the radius of the ventricle during ejection reduces wall tension for any level of intraventricular pressure. In the dilated heart, however, ejection of the same stroke volume is associated with a much smaller change in ventricular dimensions, so that the decrease in wall tension is less. These relationships are seen in Table 16.1, which provides volumes, radii, circumferences, and wall tensions for a normal and a dilated ventricle, calculated by assuming the ventricle to be a thin-walled sphere that ejects at a constant pressure. These assumptions, although simplifications that facilitate calculations of dimensions and wall tension, do not influence the validity of the following analysis.

At the start of ejection, the effect of ventricular dilation to increase wall tension is already apparent (Table 16.1); wall tension is almost twice of the normal at any intraventricular pressure owing to operation of the law of Laplace. If we assume stroke volume to be 70 cm^3, and use the resulting end-systolic volume to calculate dimensions and wall tension, ejection by the normal ventricle reduces wall tension by almost half (from 3.72×10^5 to 2.26×10^5 dynes/cm), whereas in the dilated ventricle wall tension decreases only ~10% during systole (from 5.98×10^5 to 5.59×10^5 dynes/cm). Although external work is the same for both ventricles, as the same volume of blood is ejected at the same pressure, the conditions under which this work is performed are quite different. In the dilated ventricle, the change in circumference is much less than in the normal ventricle because there is only a 5% reduction in circumference during systole. This is in contrast to the much greater (almost 40%) reduction in circumference, and thus of wall tension, as the normal ventricle ejects its stroke volume.

The significance of these differences is readily understood in terms of the differ-

TABLE 16.1. *Ventricular dimensions*

Parameter	Normal ventricle	Dilated ventricle
At start of ejection		
Pressure (mm Hg)	100[a]	100[a]
Volume (cm^3)	92	380
Radius (cm)	2.8	4.5
Circumference (cm)	17.5	28
Wall tension (dynes/cm)	3.72×10^5	5.98×10^5
Stroke volume (cm^3)	70	70
At end of ejection		
Pressure (mm Hg)	100[a]	100[a]
Volume (cm^3)	22	310
Radius (cm)	1.7	4.2
Circumference (cm)	11	26.5
Wall tension (dynes/cm)	2.26×10^5	5.59×10^5
External stroke work (dyne cm)	9.3×10^6	9.3×10^6
Conditions of external work		
Average wall tension (dynes/cm)	2.99×10^5	5.79×10^5
Change in circumference (cm)	6.5	1.5
As % of end-diastolic circumference	~40	~5

[a]Equals 1.33×10^5 dynes/cm^2.

ent energetics of pressure and flow work discussed above. From the data in Table 16.1 it can be seen that to do the same amount of work, the dilated ventricle must contract under conditions of sustained high wall tension with little wall shortening (analogous to pressure work), whereas the normal ventricle contracts against a lower, and decreasing, wall tension while undergoing significant fiber shortening (analogous to flow work). Thus, it is not difficult to understand why the cardiac efficiency is reduced in the dilated ventricle.

> The energetic disadvantages of dilatation are partially offset by hypertrophy when an overload becomes chronic; this follows because the increase in wall thickness reduces the tension that must be developed by each fiber. However, hypertrophy also creates a new set of problems (Chapter 25), and so is far from a perfect compensation in the overloaded heart.

Energetic Implications of Changes in Heart Rate

The high energy costs of internal work are also apparent when heart rate is increased. Because high levels of internal work accompany the development of pressure within the ventricle, and because this work is converted to heat during relaxation, a significant amount of energy is wasted during each systole. In addition, energy must be expended during each cardiac cycle to restore ion gradients across the plasma membrane and to pump calcium into the sarcoplasmic reticulum. In terms of the energetics of muscular contraction (Chapter 6), more activation energy (A) and more internal work (W) are expended when heart rate increases. Rapid heart rate increases the energy cost of cardiac work simply by increasing the frequency at which the ventricle must be activated and stretches its elastic walls, and so is an energetically costly way to increase the minute work of the heart.

Clinical Estimates of the Energy Requirements of Cardiac Work

Two indices have been found empirically to provide useful estimates of energy expenditure by the working heart in intact animals. The simplest is the product of aortic pressure and heart rate, which correlates closely with cardiac oxygen consumption. This product includes two of the three terms of the equation for minute work (Eq. 16.5), but omits stroke volume, which is the most difficult to measure. However, as noted above, stroke volume is also the least important determinant of the energy costs of cardiac contraction. For this reason the "double product," as this index is called, has gained wide acceptance as a measure of cardiac energy consumption, for example, during routine treadmill exercise testing.

A somewhat more elaborate index of myocardial oxygen consumption is the tension-time index, in which average ejection pressure is multiplied by the duration of ejection (Fig. 16.14); a better term for this area would be pressure-time index. It is not clear that this provides more useful clinical information than the double product; the requirement for direct arterial pressure recordings makes it inconvenient for routine use.

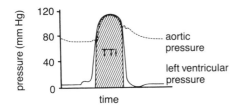

FIG. 16.14. Tension-time index (TTI). The oxygen consumption of the heart is roughly proportional to the area under the ejection phase of the left ventricular pressure curve, which represents the "tension-time index."

Although both of these indices correlate well with cardiac oxygen consumption, neither takes into account the effects of the law of Laplace and changing contractility. In the clinical setting, where blood pressure and heart rate are easily measured, these two indices do provide a reasonably accurate, and useful, index of the energy demands of the heart.

CHANGES IN MYOCARDIAL CONTRACTILITY AS A FAMILY OF STARLING CURVES

The importance of changes in myocardial contractility in the adjustment of the heart to a variety of physiological, pharmacological, and pathological interventions was emphasized in Chapters 13 and 14. Although it is difficult to quantify the *absolute level of myocardial contractility*, especially in a clinical setting (Chapter 17), it is much easier to document a *change in myocardial contractility*. Since myocardial contractility is, by definition, the ability of the cardiac muscle to do work *at constant end-diastolic fiber length*, a Starling curve obtained under control conditions defines a baseline of contractility. More importantly, a change in contractility shifts the Starling curve, so that any intervention that alters this basic property of the heart generates a new Starling curve, which is the same as saying there is a new end-systolic PV relationship (Chapter 15). This means that, as shown in Fig. 16.15, there is a "family of Starling curves," each of which represents a different level of contractility.

The ability of Starling's law to regulate cardiac work is readily apparent in Fig. 16.15, in which points A, B, and C lie along a control Starling curve. Thus, at a constant level of contractility, operation of Starling's law increases pressure-volume work (A→B) when end-diastolic volume rises and, conversely, work decreases (A→C) when end-diastolic volume falls. A positive inotropic intervention, which by definition increases work capacity at any given end-diastolic volume (or fiber length), does not abolish the Frank-Starling relationship. Instead, a new Starling curve is inscribed in which work at each end-diastolic volume is increased (curve containing D). Conversely, a negative inotropic intervention, by causing a downward shift in the Starling curve (to the curve containing E), reduces the work of the heart.

There are therefore two ways by which the heart can increase its stroke work: (a) by increasing end-diastolic volume (A→B, Fig. 16.15), and (b) by increasing contractility (A→D, Fig. 16.15). If one considers minute work, an increased heart rate

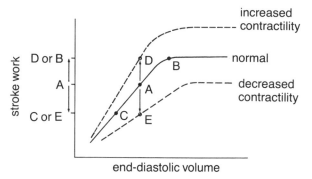

FIG. 16.15. Family of Starling curves. The *solid curve* (*C-A-B*) is an end-systolic PV relationship that describes the "normal" myocardial contractility, and point *A* represents a "basal" state along this curve. The work of the heart (*ordinate*) varies with changing end-diastolic volume (*abscissa*) according to the Frank-Starling relationship. These length-dependent changes in the work of the heart are described by the three curves, which represent a family of Starling curves. Stroke work can also be varied by changes in contractility, which by definition increase or decrease cardiac work at constant end-diastolic volume. Thus, changing contractility shifts the heart to a new Starling curve. Changes in venous return, by altering end-diastolic volume (not shown) shift the end-systolic point along the normal Starling curve, which allows cardiac work to increase from *A* to *B* when venous return increases, or to decrease from *A* to *C* when venous return is reduced. These changes in cardiac work are not associated with a change in contractility. The work of the heart can also be changed by interventions that modify myocardial contractility. A positive ino-tropic agent increases cardiac work from *A* to *D*, whereas cardiac work is decreased from *A* to *E* by a negative inotropic agent. Points *D* and *E* fall on different Starling curves (*dashed lines*), allowing a change in contractility to modify the work of the heart with no change in end-diastolic volume. Note that is not possible to define the mechanism responsible for a change in myocar-dial function simply by measuring either stroke work or end-diastolic volume alone. Instead, these analyses require sufficient data to define the relationship between changing cardiac work and end-diastolic volume in terms of the family of Starling curves.

represents a third independent means for increasing the amount of work performed per unit of time. These three mechanisms are independently controlled and so are not mutually exclusive. Nor need they all move in the same direction, as contrac-tility, end-diastolic volume, and heart rate can change discordantly.

ENERGY COST OF INCREASING CARDIAC WORK

The energetic implications of these mechanisms for altering cardiac work are quite different. By increasing end-diastolic volume the heart increases its work per-formance via a mechanism (Starling's law of the heart) that relies on an increase in the size of the ventricular cavity which, by altering the geometry and leverage of the walls of the heart (the law of Laplace), increases wall tension and so tends to reduce cardiac efficiency (see above). This costly effect of dilatation is avoided by an increase in contractility because this mechanism increases ejection and so reduces ventricular cavity volume. These differences are apparent when it is remembered that stroke work equals $P \times (EDV - ESV)$ (Eq. 16.3). The Frank-Starling relationship increases work by increasing *EDV*, whereas increased contractility increases work by decreasing *ESV*. An increase in heart rate is an energetically costly way to increase minute work [which equals $P \times HR \times (EDV - ESV)$; Eq. 16.7] because energy is wasted during isovolumic contraction.

As discussed in Chapter 13, Starling's law of the heart and changes in myocardial contractility serve different regulatory roles in the intact animal. The Frank-Starling relationship is most important in beat-to-beat adjustments to changes in circulatory dynamics, such as balancing the outputs of the right and left ventricles and in mediating responses to changing venous pressure such as occur when body position is changed. The heart's response to more drastic changes in circulatory dynamics, notably those that accompany exercise, is mediated largely by changes in contractility. In fact, the human heart normally becomes smaller during exercise in a standing position, even though cardiac work is markedly increased. To a large extent, therefore, increased contractility allows the normal heart to meet the increased hemodynamic needs of the body while avoiding the inefficiency that accompanies dilation.

INTERPLAY BETWEEN CHANGES IN THE INOTROPIC (CONTRACTILE) AND LUSITROPIC (RELAXATION) PROPERTIES OF THE HEART

Changes in contractility have already been described in terms of the Starling curves, which are, in fact, end-systolic PV relationships. As shown in Fig. 16.15 the points A, B, and C, which lie along one such curve, define a given level of myocardial contractility. The two points D and E illustrate changes in contractility that have shifted the end-systolic PV relationship, and so define new Starling curves.

Changes in the lusitropic (relaxation) properties of the ventricle involve another family of curves; these are the end-diastolic PV relationships that describe the filling characteristics of the ventricle. The latter are added to a family of Starling curves in Fig. 16.16, which shows two sets of PV relationships: one that defines the ability of the heart to empty, the other its ability to fill.

Changes in the peripheral circulation can move both the end-systolic and end-diastolic points along each of these two PV relationships; these changes are different from those that result from changing the inotropic and lusitropic properties of the heart, which shift the end-systolic and end-diastolic PV relationships themselves.

To illustrate the interplay between the heart's ability to fill and its ability to empty in response to changing circulatory hemodynamics, we return to the pressure-volume diagram which describes the external work performed during each cardiac cycle. Responses to four separate interventions are examined; two involve changes in contractile (inotropic) properties, and two involve altered relaxation (lusitropic) characteristics.

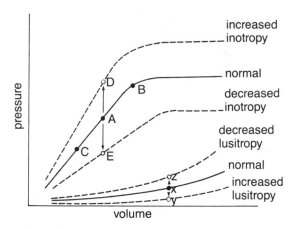

FIG. 16.16. Two end-diastolic pressure-volume curves are shown along with a control end-diastolic PV relationship containing point *x* to illustrate a family of filling curves. (Three end-systolic curves are included) A positive lusitropic intervention (*y*) improves the ability of the ventricle to fill by shifting the end-diastolic PV relationship to the right and downward, whereas a negative lusitropic intervention (*z*) reduces ventricular filling by shifting this relationship to the left and upward.

Effects of a Negative Inotropic Intervention

As already noted, a decrease in contractility shifts the end-systolic PV relationship (the Starling curve) to the right and downward (Fig. 16.17), which depending on the response of the peripheral circulation, can reduce ejection, aortic pressure, or both.

Usually, depression of ventricular function causes blood pressure to fall at the expense of cardiac output because reflex vasoconstriction tends to maintain perfusion pressure (Chapter 25). For the sake of illustration, however, the examples in this section assume that stroke volume does not change.

When contractility falls suddenly, as when a region of the left ventricle loses its blood supply in acute myocardial infarction, reduced ejection increases end-systolic (residual) volume. If for this illustration it is assumed that venous return does not change, addition of the constant venous return to the increased end-systolic volume increases end-diastolic volume (Fig. 16.17).

In real life, of course, acute heart failure decreases venous return because the increased end-diastolic volume increases diastolic pressures (Fig. 16.8). In addition, as noted above, reflex peripheral arteriolar vasoconstriction tends to maintain pressure rather than cardiac output, so that stroke volume generally falls as a result of a decrease in myocardial contractility.

As this example assumes that stroke volume does not change, the fall in the end-systolic point to a depressed Starling curve decreases aortic pressure (Fig. 16.17). Furthermore, although ejection is initially impaired (not shown), the constant

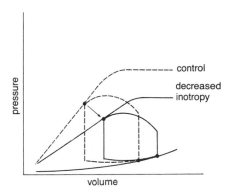

FIG. 16.17. A negative inotropic intervention shifts the end-systolic PV relationship to the right and downward (*arrow*); if stroke volume is assumed to remain constant, the pressure-volume loop shifts to the right (*dashed line*), end-diastolic pressure increases, and end-systolic pressure falls to the new Starling curve.

venous return assumed in this example shifts the end-diastolic point of the pressure-volume loop to higher volumes along the unchanged end-diastolic PV relationship. The obviously decreased area of the pressure-volume loop, as noted in Chapter 15, means that stroke work has decreased.

Effects of a Positive Inotropic Intervention

When contractility is increased, the end-systolic PV relationship shifts to the left and upward (Fig. 16.18). This increases the ability of the ventricle to eject so that, if for the sake of this illustration we again assume that venous return does not change, addition of the constant venous return to the decreased end-systolic volume shifts the pressure-volume loop to the left. As a result, end-diastolic volume is reduced along the unchanged end-diastolic PV relationship and the end-systolic points shifts to a smaller volume along the new Starling curve shown in Fig. 16.18. The increased area of the pressure-volume loop means that stroke work has also been increased.

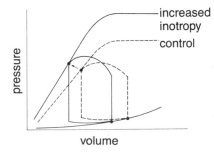

FIG. 16.18. A positive inotropic intervention shifts the end-systolic PV relationship to the left and upward (*arrow*); if stroke volume is assumed to remain constant, the pressure-volume loop shifts to the left (*dashed line*), end-diastolic pressure decreases, and end-systolic pressure rises to the new Starling curve.

Effects of a Negative Lusitropic Intervention

An intervention that impairs ventricular filling shifts the end-diastolic PV relationship to the left and upward, and so raises the pressure needed to achieve a given
increment in diastolic volume (Fig. 16.19). If, as in the preceding examples, stroke
volume is assumed to remain constant, the increased resistance to filling elevates
end-diastolic pressure while at the same time decreasing end-diastolic volume. The
leftward shift in the origin of the pressure-volume loop decreases heart size, even
though diastolic pressures are increased, so that according to Starling's law of the
heart, the work of the heart is decreased. As our model assumes that a constant
stroke volume is ejected by the smaller ventricle, less pressure is developed, which
moves the end-systolic point of the cardiac cycle to a lower point on the unchanged
end-systolic PV relationship. The net result is that a smaller heart operates at higher
diastolic pressures to eject the same stroke volume at lower systolic pressures.

> It must be emphasized that this example ignores important circulatory adjustments,
> most important of which is reflex vasoconstriction caused by the fall in aortic pressure.
> This normally increases afterload and so moves the end-systolic point to the right and
> upward along the unchanged end-systolic PV relationship so as to decrease stroke
> volume while maintaining aortic pressure (Fig. 25.8B).

Effects of a Positive Lusitropic Intervention

Interventions that facilitate ventricular filling shift the end-diastolic PV relationship to the right and downward (Fig. 16.20), so that end-diastolic pressure decreases in the dilated ventricle. If, as in all of these examples, stroke volume does
not change, the heart develops a higher pressure, due to Starling's law, so that
systole ends at a higher point to the right along the unchanged end-systolic PV
relationship. This means that the larger heart does more work, but at reduced diastolic pressures. Once again, the model ignores reflex changes in the peripheral
circulation, in this case vasodilatation that, in response to the increased aortic pressure, would increase cardiac output while reducing systolic pressure.

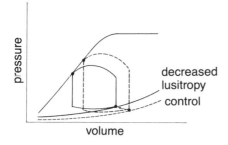

decreased
lusitropy

control

FIG. 16.19. A negative lusitropic intervention
shifts the end-diastolic PV relationship to the
left and upward (*arrow*); if stroke volume is assumed to remain constant, the pressure-vol
ume loop shifts to the left (*dashed line*), end-
diastolic pressure increases, and developed
pressure falls along the control end-systolic
PV relationship.

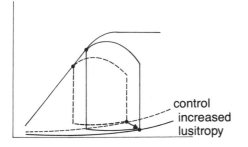

control

increased

lusitropy

FIG. 16.20. A positive lusitropic intervention shifts the end-diastolic PV relationship to the right and downward (*arrow*); if stroke volume is assumed to remain constant, the pressure-volume loop shifts to the right (*dashed line*), end-diastolic pressure decreases, and developed pressure rises along the control end-systolic PV relationship.

CHANGES IN THE INTERPLAY BETWEEN VENOUS RETURN AND CARDIAC OUTPUT

This chapter has attempted to apply concepts of regulation at the *cell* and *gene* levels to the heart working as an *organ*. At the same time we have examined the interplay between the heart and the circulation. Although these complex interactions can be clarified by focusing on specific components of interactive systems, it is an inescapable fact that blood flows in a circle. For this reason, the circulation is more complex than has been depicted in many of our illustrations. For example, filling of the heart influences its ability to empty, and vice versa, whereas changing arterial pressure causes vasomotor changes that affect cardiac output. At this point, we return to the two interactions between the heart and the periphery that keep the circulation operating at a steady state (Fig. 16.8). One of these interactions, Star-

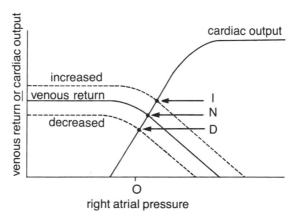

FIG. 16.21. Curves relating venous return and cardiac output (Fig. 16.8) showing effects of changes in venous return. Increased venous return increases right atrial pressure and cardiac output (Starling's law of the heart); conversely, a decreased venous return, by lowering atrial pressure, reduces cardiac output. Each interaction between the heart and periphery achieves a unique steady state. N, normal; I, increased venous return; D, decreased venous return.

ling's law of the heart, adjusts ejection to filling. The other, discussed briefly at an earlier point in this chapter, is the relationship between atrial pressure and venous return that equalizes the latter with cardiac output.

As already noted, the balance between venous return and cardiac output is maintained by the interplay depicted in Fig. 16.8, in which a change in one brings about a corresponding adjustment in the other so as to equalize the flow of blood into and out of the heart. Viewed in terms of the effects of the periphery on the heart, changing venous return causes a corresponding adjustment of cardiac output through the operation of Starling's law of the heart (Fig. 16.21). Viewed in terms of effects of the heart on the circulation, changing cardiac output caused by altered contractility, which shifts the heart to a new Starling curve, modifies the pressure behind the heart (atrial pressure) so as to vary the resistance to venous return (Fig. 16.22). Thus, increased contractility, by facilitating ejection, lowers atrial pressure and so shifts the equilibrium point to the left and upward; the reduced filling pressure, of course, increases venous return. Conversely, a negative inotropic intervention reduces ejection and so decreases cardiac output; this leads to an opposite shift in the equilibrium point that increases atrial pressure and so reduces venous return. In this way, the interplay between the heart and the periphery (Figs. 16.21 and 16.22) defines a series of equilibrium points that match venous return to cardiac output.

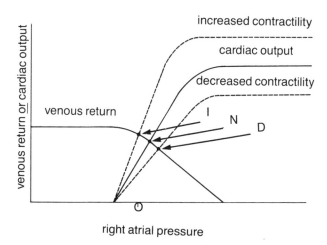

FIG. 16.22. Curves relating venous return and cardiac output (Fig. 16.8) showing effects of changing the inotropic state of the heart. An increase in contractility decreases right atrial pressure, which allows venous return to increase. Conversely, a decrease in contractility raises atrial pressure and so lowers venous return. N, normal; I, increased contractility; D, decreased contractility.

REFERENCES

Evans DC, Matsuoka Y. (1915). The effect of various mechanical conditions on the gaseous metabolism and efficiency of the mammalian heart. *J Physiol (Lond)* 49:378–405.

Kitakaze M, Marban E. (1989). Cellular mechanism of the modulation of contractile function by coronary perfusion pressure in ferret hearts. *J Physiol (Lond)* 414:455–472.

Martin DS. (1928). The relation between work performed and heat liberated by the isolated gastrocnemius, semitendinosus and tibialis anticus muscles of the frog. *Am J Physiol* 33:543–547.

Warner HR, Toronto AF. (1960). Regulation of cardiac output through stroke volume. *Circ Res* 8:549–552.

Woods RH. (1892). A few applications of a physical theorem to membranes in a state of tension in the human body. *J Anat Physiol* 26:362–370.

BIBLIOGRAPHY

Fenton TR, Cherry JM, Klassen GA. (1978). Transmural myocardial deformation in the canine left ventricular wall. *Am J Physiol* 235:H523–H530.

Hawthorne EW. (1966). Dynamic geometry of the left ventricle. *Am J Cardiol* 18:566–573.

Sagawa K. (1981). Editorial: The end-systolic pressure-volume relation of the left ventricle: definition, modifications and clinical use. *Circulation* 63:1223–1227.

Salisbury PF, Cross CA, Rieben PA. (1960). Influence of coronary artery pressure upon myocardial elasticity. *Circ Res* 8:794–800.

Sarnoff SJ, Braunwald E, Welch GH Jr, Base RB, Stainsby WN, Macruz R. (1958). Hemodynamic determinants of oxygen consumption of the heart with special reference to the tension-time index. *Am J Physiol* 192:148–156.

Weber KT, Janicki JS, Shroff SV, Fishman AP. (1981). Contractile mechanics and interaction of the right and left ventricles. *Am J Cardiol* 47:686–695.

Wong AYK, Rautaharju PM. (1968). Stress distribution within the left ventricular wall approximated as a thick ellipsoidal shell. *Am Heart J* 75:649–662.

See also Bibliography to Chapter 15.

17

Indices of Myocardial Contractility and Relaxation

Accurate assessment of cardiac function is essential in managing patients with heart disease. It is relatively simple to quantify the pumping of the heart as an *organ;* however, characterization of the *cellular* and *genetic* properties of the myocardium, which often impair the pumping action of the heart, remains a daunting task. This is due in part to the interplay between the heart and the circulation, which requires that alterations in the heart muscle be distinguished from the many circulatory abnormalities that occur in patients with depressed cardiac function.

The large number of indices used to assess cardiac performance are of two general types; measurements of contractile (inotropic) performance, and methods to define the relaxation (lusitropic) properties of the heart. All are designed to define the state of the myocardium in the face of complex circulatory abnormalities, and most attempt to separate abnormalities of the myocardium from those of the heart as an organ, such as leaky (insufficient or regurgitant) and narrowed (stenotic) valves. None is perfect, which of course explains why there are so many of them.

It is difficult, even on theoretical grounds, to separate abnormalities of contraction from those of relaxation. Because blood flows in a circle, reduced emptying eventually reduces filling; furthermore, because failure of the ventricle to empty (an inotropic abnormality) increases residual (end-systolic) volume, it also impairs filling. Similarly, a ventricle that does not fill adequately cannot eject normally, so that lusitropic abnormalities impair contractile performance. In spite of these and other obvious difficulties, attempts to quantify the inotropic and lusitropic state of the myocardium can provide important data that are invaluable in the care of the cardiac patient.

Most of the indices of ventricular function described in this chapter are for the left ventricle. Although primary abnormalities of the right ventricle do occur, they are not common; in addition, the ease with which right atrial pressures can be estimated—by simple inspection of the jugular veins—has focused attention on the more difficult evaluation of the frequently encountered abnormalities of left ventricular function. Unless otherwise stated, therefore, the indices described in this chapter are of left ventricular contraction and relaxation. The abbreviation *P* in this chapter refers to pressure and not, as in earlier chapters, to tension.

GLOBAL MYOCARDIAL CONTRACTILITY

It is often vital to know the contractile state of the myocardium; for example, timing of palliative surgery in a patient with valvular heart disease is often determined by the state of the overloaded myocardium rather than the severity of symptoms. If surgery is performed too soon in the natural history of a patient with valvular disease, such as mitral insufficiency, the patient is subject to needless prolongation of the hazards that accompany valve replacement, including embolism, infection, and deterioration of the prosthetic valve. On the other hand, if surgery is delayed too long, the benefits of even a technically perfect operation can be outweighed if the myocardium has been irreversibly damaged by the long-standing overload (Chapter 25). This can lead to the tragic situation of a superb valve repair in an operation that, because the myocardium has been so badly damaged by the heart's response to chronic overload caused by the abnormal valve, ends with the death of the patient.

A variety of approaches are used to estimate myocardial contractility. Although none provides a precise measure of the cellular and molecular state of the heart muscle, many are of considerable value in patient management.

Clinical Indices

A simple means for evaluating left ventricular function is to elicit signs and symptoms associated with impaired left ventricular failure (Chapter 25). Although providing the keystone for the clinical evaluation of any patient with heart disease, these are quite nonspecific. The *subjective symptoms* of left ventricular failure, including dyspnea (difficulty breathing), orthopnea (difficulty breathing when reclining), and weakness are invaluable in gaining an overall clinical impression of the patient's condition. However, the severity of symptoms gives only a rough estimate of left ventricular performance, and in many conditions provides essentially no useful information by which to quantify the state of the left ventricular myocardium. There are, unfortunately, few *objective signs* of left ventricular failure. Abnormalities such as low systemic blood pressure (which falls only when heart failure is severe), weak peripheral pulses, elevated systemic venous pressure (measured by observing the jugular veins), a loud pulmonary valve closure sound, and an audible left ventricular filling sound (S_3, Fig. 15.8, which in patients with heart failure is called a gallop) are either indirect measurements or very crude indices of left ventricular function. An atrial filling sound (S_4 or A, Fig. 15.8) is less specific as this indicates that the left ventricle is stiff, and not necessarily that contractility is reduced.

More than 30 years ago, the great English cardiologist Paul Wood observed that one of the first signs of heart failure was loss of the normal sinus arrhythmia, speeding of the heart with inspiration and slowing during expiration (Chapter 22). Recently rediscovered, this sign identifies patients in whom the delicate interplay between the heart, the circulation, and central reflexes has been blunted or lost, as occurs very early in the development of heart failure.

Systolic Time Intervals

The simple bedside techniques of external carotid pulse recording, phonocardiography, and electrocardiography allow the events during the cardiac cycle to be timed and related to the mechanical state of the left ventricle by the calculation of *systolic time intervals* (Fig. 17.1). The carotid pulse tracing, which can be recorded from arterial pulsations in the neck, allows *left ventricular ejection time (LVET)* to be measured from the upstroke of the carotid pulse (the beginning of left ventricular ejection) to the dicrotic notch (the closure of the aortic valve at the end of protodiastole). The phonocardiogram defines the interval between the onset of mechanical systole, which occurs shortly before the first heart sound (S_1, associated with

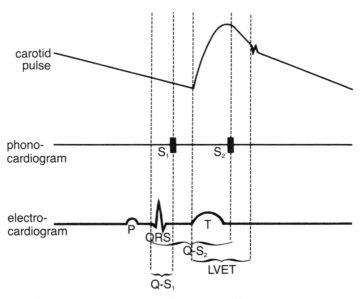

FIG. 17.1. Estimation of systolic time intervals from the carotid pulse (*upper*), phonocardiogram (*middle*), and electrocardiogram (*lower*). The left ventricular ejection time (LVET) is measured from the upstroke of the carotid pulse to the dicrotic notch. The Q-S_2 interval represents the total duration of electromechanical systole. Subtraction of the LVET from the Q-S_2 interval yields the preejection period (PEP).

mitral valve closure) and the end of protodiastole which is marked by the second heart sound (S_2). Although the second heart sound corresponds to the dicrotic notch on the carotid pulse at the end of protodiastole, they are not recorded simultaneously because transmission of the pulse wave from the root of the aorta to the carotid artery is delayed. The initial deflection of the QRS complex is produced by left ventricular depolarization (Chapter 20), so that the electrocardiogram can identify the onset of electrical systole in the left ventricle.

Commonly used systolic time intervals are listed in Table 17.1. The Q-S_2 interval defines the duration of electromechanical systole from the beginning of ventricular depolarization to the end of protodiastole. This can be subdivided into three phases: the *Q-S_1 interval,* from the onset of depolarization to mitral valve closure, the *isovolumic contraction time* between S_1 and aortic valve opening, and *left ventricular ejection time* (see above).

> Isovolumic contraction time cannot be measured directly in Fig. 17.1. Because transmission of the pulse wave from the aortic root to the carotid artery is delayed, the interval between S_1 and the start of the carotid upstroke must be corrected. The delay, called the *pulse transmission time,* can be estimated from the recordings in Fig. 17.1 by measuring the time elapsed between the second sound (S_2) on the phonocardiogram and the dicrotic notch on the carotid pulse tracing, which are virtually simultaneous events. Thus, to measure isovolumic contraction time, the interval between S_2 and the dicrotic notch must be subtracted from the interval between S_1 and the onset of the rise in aortic pressure.

The Q-S_1 interval, which is the period between the onset of left ventricular depolarization and the time that left ventricular pressure rises sufficiently to cause mitral valve closure, provides an index of the speed of excitation-contraction coupling. Isovolumic contraction time, which corresponds to the duration of isovolumic systole, is related to the rate of pressure rise during isovolumic contraction in the left ventricle, and provides a useful index of left ventricular contractility (see below). Ejection time includes the phases of maximum ejection, reduced ejection, and protodiastole (Fig. 15.8).

TABLE 17.1. *Systolic time intervals*

Interval	Measurement	Physiological correlation
Q-S_2	*From* beginning of QRS *to* first high frequency vibration of S_2	Total electromechanical systole
Q-S_1	*From* beginning of QRS *to* beginning of S_1	Velocity of excitation-contraction coupling
Isovolumic contraction time	*From* S_1 *to* onset of rise in aortic pressure	Velocity of muscle shortening
LVET (left ventricular ejection time)	*From* onset of carotid upstroke *to* the dicrotic notch	Total ejection (plus protodiastole)
PEP (preejection period)	Q-S_2 *minus* LVET	Isovolumic contraction time plus Q–S, interval

TABLE 17.2. *Normal values for systolic time intervals*

	Normal value (msec)	At heart rate = 72
Q-S$_2$	546 − (2 × heart rate)	402
PEP	132 − (0.4 × heart rate)	103
LVET	415 − (1.6 × heart rate)	300

The *preejection period (PEP)*, another index obtained by subtraction of the LVET from the Q-S$_2$ interval, is the interval between the onset of electrical depolarization of the ventricles and the beginning of ejection. The PEP is thus a rough means of assessing the rapidity of excitation-contraction coupling. In patients with reduced myocardial contractility, PEP is prolonged and LVET is shortened, so that the ratio PEP/LVET can be used to identify patients with depressed myocardial contractility. In normal individuals, this ratio is 0.35 ± 0.04.

Because the durations of the phases of cardiac systole are related to the heart rate (see Chapter 19), estimates of left ventricular contractile function based on systolic time intervals must be corrected for heart rate; otherwise, the systolic time intervals would be shortened when heart rate increases. Normal systolic time intervals, and corrections for heart rate, are given in Table 17.2. The systolic time intervals are influenced by preload and afterload, and by abnormalities in conduction of the wave of depolarization over the left ventricle. The latter, by prolonging the QRS complex (Chapter 22), prolongs the PEP.

Hemodynamic Indices

A more accurate picture of the left ventricle as a pump can be provided by measurements of cardiac output and left atrial pressure. The latter is commonly estimated by "wedging" an end-hole catheter passed from a systemic vein into a small pulmonary artery so as to detect pulmonary venous pressure, which is generally the same as left atrial pressure. Bedside catheters can also be used to measure cardiac output, so that along with readily available measurements of systemic arterial blood pressure, cardiac work can be calculated. These hemodynamic measurements, however, are influenced not only by the state of the heart, but also by its interaction with the circulation. For example, cardiac output can be reduced by loss of circulating blood volume, which is a common occurrence following vigorous diuretic therapy to relieve fluid retention in patients with heart failure or excessive blood loss during surgery. Stenosis (narrowing) of one of the cardiac valves, obliteration of the pulmonary vessels in pulmonary hypertension, and excessive afterload can also reduce cardiac output at any level of contractility. Similarly, pulmonary wedge (left atrial) pressure can be reduced when the body is depleted of salt and water by excessive diuresis, which can normalize end-diastolic pressure even in patients with severe left ventricular failure. (Unfortunately, when this occurs, it is often accompanied by a marked fall in cardiac output that can cause renal and hepatic failure.)

Although these and other circulatory effects limit the value of direct hemo-dynamic measurements in assessing left ventricular contractility, hemodynamic measurements are clinically useful. They are especially valuable in defining patho-physiology and the overall state of the circulation in patients with heart failure, especially when the failure is acute.

Starling Curves

As described in the preceding chapter, Starling curves are readily constructed from measurements of aortic pressure, stroke volume, and end-diastolic volume in isolated heart preparations, where concurrent determinations of cardiac oxygen con-sumption allow cardiac energetics to be evaluated. Clinical measurements of end-diastolic volume, however, are difficult, as is concurrent control and determination of left ventricular pressure, stroke volume, and heart rate. For this reason, Starling curves in patients are usually plotted as the dependence of minute work on end-diastolic pressure (Fig. 17.2).

Although Starling curves generated in patients can yield elegant data, their practi-cal use is limited. These curves can change from moment to moment because of variable neurohumoral influences that alter preload, afterload, and heart rate. Mea-surements of minute work do not accurately reflect energetics because, as described in Chapter 16, an increase in work brought about by increased heart rate or aortic pressure is energetically more costly than a comparable increase brought about by an increased stroke volume. Even when stroke work, instead of minute work, is used to construct the Starling curves, the different effects of pressure and flow in determining the energy cost of contraction make it difficult to attach precise mean-ing to these curves. Furthermore, hypertrophy changes cardiac thickness so that additional data are needed to estimate wall tension (stress), a better measure of the actual load on the muscular walls of the heart. Finally, regional wall motion abnor-malities, as are seen in ischemic heart disease where some parts of the left ventricle are destroyed by infarction while other regions perform increased amounts of work, make quantitative interpretations of these curves impossible.

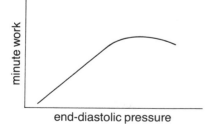

FIG. 17.2. Starling curves as usually recorded in humans. The *ordinate* is minute work because neither blood pressure nor cardiac output are readily controlled. The *abscissa* is end-diastolic pressure, which is more readily measured than end-diastolic volume.

Concurrent measurements of left ventricular work and left ventricular end-diastolic volume, which define a single point on the Starling curve, are of little value in estimating myocardial contractility. A measured point which falls below that expected in normals suggests a depressed Starling curve, and thus that left ventricular contractility is reduced. However, both end-diastolic pressure and volume can be shifted dramatically by structural changes in hypertrophied hearts (Fig. 25.10).

Acute Heart Failure

Hemodynamic measurements are extremely useful in patients in whom heart failure is of sudden onset (as in cardiogenic shock after myocardial infarction), or in states of circulatory collapse such as in septic shock or after a large pulmonary embolus. Hemodynamic data are also essential when heart failure is changing rapidly, as can occur following major changes in therapy, or when an additional variable such as the need for surgery is encountered. Under these conditions, hemodynamic measurements provide invaluable data both to define pathophysiology and to monitor the response to therapy.

Left ventricular diastolic pressures, either measured directly through a catheter in the left heart, or more commonly from pulmonary "wedge" pressures, can be obtained by bedside catheterization (using Swan-Ganz catheters). When coupled with determinations of arterial blood pressure and cardiac output, these measurements can be used to evaluate left ventricular function in acutely ill patients. Although invaluable in following hemodynamic abnormalities that, in a coronary or intensive care unit, can evolve quite rapidly and so require immediate attention, these measurements are less useful as indices of contractility in chronic heart disease.

Isovolumic Indices

A number of indices of myocardial contractility are based on analyses of pressure measurements obtained during isovolumic contraction. The major advantage of the isovolumic indices is that they are independent of afterload because data are collected before the aortic valve opens; however, these are invasive determinations, which limits their use.

Measurements of the rate of isovolumic pressure rise, when processed by mathematical treatments using arbitrary or measured elastic constants, can describe ventricular function in terms of the Hill equations (Chapter 6). In spite of the often impressive appearance of some of these calculations, the data generated by these indices cannot be interpreted in the same manner as data obtained using tetanized frog sartorius muscle.

Maximum dP/dt

The simplest index of myocardial contractility that can be derived from pressure measurements during isovolumic contraction is maximum dP/dt, the maximal rate of pressure rise. Although a useful index of myocardial contractility that is clearly depressed in the failing heart, maximum *dP/dt* is influenced by changes in ventricular end-diastolic volume (preload), and so cannot distinguish length-dependent properties (Starling's law) from those arising from altered contractility. Maximum *dP/dt* is also influenced by cavity size, muscle mass, and valve abnormalities. Furthermore, like all indices of global left ventricular function, maximum *dP/dt* measures only average contractility so that its use is limited in patients with regional left ventricular damage, as generally occurs after myocardial infarction.

Maximum (dP/dt)/P

Dividing the ratio *dP/dt* continuously by instantaneous pressure in the left ventricle yields a quotient, *(dP/dt)/P,* that provides an index of contractility whose units are reciprocal seconds. Although less influenced by preload than maximum *dP/dt,* maximum *(dP/dt)/P* is subject to most of its other limitations. Unfortunately, maximum *(dP/dt)/P* is relatively insensitive to changes in myocardial contractility, and so has not proven to be of much practical value in the clinical assessment of left ventricular function.

Shortening Velocity (V_{CE})

Fiber shortening velocity during isovolumic contraction can be estimated from pressure measurements by either assuming or measuring a stiffness constant (K) that describes the increment in tension that accompanies each increment in the length of a nonlinear elasticity in series with the contractile elements in the ventricular wall. The velocity of fiber shortening, V_{CE}, is:

$$V_{CE} = \frac{dT/dt}{KT} + C \qquad [17.1]$$

where *T* is the tension developed by the contractile element, *t* is time, *dT/dt* is the rate of rise of wall tension calculated according to the law of Laplace, and K is the stiffness constant of the series elasticity. The value *C,* which represents a small stiffness extrapolated for zero load, is generally ignored in calculating V_{CE}. Because K has the units *dT/dl,* V_{CE} is expressed in terms of changing muscle length.

Estimates of K require that assumptions be made to account for the geometric relationship between parallel and series elasticities and the contractile element. These commonly use one of two models, named after Maxwell and Voigt, to describe the relationship between the series elasticity, parallel elasticity and contractile element (Fig. 17.3). According to the Maxwell model, only the parallel elasticity supports resting tension, whereas the Voigt model allows resting tension to be supported by both series and parallel elasticities. As the series elasticity plays a significant role in determining the relationship between contractile element shortening and the appearance of tension at the ends of the muscle (Chapter 9), the high resting tension of cardiac muscle makes it important to chose the correct model. The location of the contractile element relative

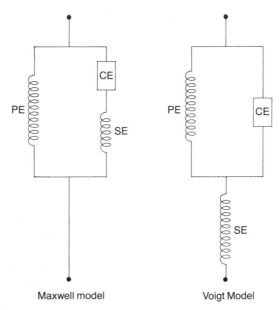

Maxwell model   Voigt Model

FIG. 17.3. Alternative models that relate the series elasticity (SE) to the contractile element (CE) in the myocardium. In both, the parallel elasticity (PE) is in parallel to the contractile element.

to the series elasticity also influences the relationship between the cross-bridge cycle and the tension developed at the ends of the muscle. For example, shortening of the parallel elasticity in the Voigt model, but not the Maxwell model, helps the contractile element to stretch the series elasticity. Because of the high elasticity of the resting myocardium, parallel elasticity must be correctly subtracted in calculating series elasticity; for this reason, the choice between these models influences calculated values of V_{CE}.

The Maxwell model is generally used in estimating V_{CE} in papillary muscle preparations. In the intact left ventricle, however, the Voigt model also applies because ballooning of the mitral and aortic valves adds elasticities that influence the rate at which left ventricular pressure rises during isovolumic contraction.

Clinical estimates of V_{CE} derived from left ventricular pressure measurements during isovolumic contraction often assume K to be a constant with a value of 28. This value is based on data obtained in isolated papillary muscles and corrected for such factors as the ballooning of the mitral valve (which would decrease apparent stiffness) and the low compliance of excised papillary muscles (which would artifactually increase this constant when applied to the entire ventricle). As usually calculated, $V_{CE} = (dP/dt)/28P$; in other words, V_{CE} is simply one twenty-eighth of $(dP/dt)/P$. Thus, although V_{CE} is presented in terms reminiscent of the elegant analyses of the frog sartorius muscle by Hill and Fenn, this index of contractility differs little from the simpler $(dP/dt)/P$. Thus, V_{CE} is subject to the assumptions and simplifications described above for dP/dt and $(dP/dt)/P$. If attempts are made to estimate wall tensions instead of intraventricular pressures, difficulties in defining the radius of curvature and wall thickness, both of which are heterogeneous in the left ventricle, complicate the clinical use of this index.

V_{pm} and V_{max}

Two additional indices of myocardial contractility are generated when changing values of instantaneous V_{CE} plotted as a function of developed pressure throughout isovolumic contraction. As shown in Fig. 17.4, V_{CE} rapidly increases after the beginning of systole, and then slowly declines as intraventricular pressure rises. The highest value of instantaneous V_{CE} calculated during isovolumic contraction is V_{pm}, whereas extrapolation of instantaneous V_{CE} back to zero pressure provides an estimate of V_{max}. Because the latter is based on an extrapolation to zero intraventricular pressure, V_{max} is sometimes assumed to be the V_{CE} of the unloaded ventricle. Although values for V_{max} obtained as shown in Fig. 17.4 are reminiscent of V_{max} of the force-velocity curve of the frog sartorius muscle, these estimates of the true V_{max} of the ventricle are, at best, only rough approximations of the maximal shortening velocity of the walls of the heart at zero load. This is because V_{max} is derived from measurements of V_{CE}, whose limitations have already been described.

Both V_{pm} and V_{max} are relatively insensitive to changing afterload, but are influenced by preload, decreasing with increasing left ventricular end-diastolic pressure. As used clinically, these indices are only partially successful in separating patients with other clinical evidence of left ventricular dysfunction from those with normal ventricles. For this reason, these indices of myocardial contractility have not found wide acceptance.

Volume and Dimension Measurements

The contractile state of the left ventricle, as well as myocardial contractility, can be evaluated by evaluating left ventricular volume and wall motion. Volume

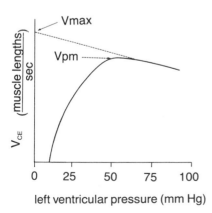

FIG. 17.4. Plot of instantaneous V_{CE} as a function of developed left ventricular pressure during isovolumic contraction. The curve begins at the *left* (end-diastolic pressure) from which V_{CE} rises to a maximum (V_{pm}) and then falls. Extrapolation of V_{CE} to zero pressure provides an index of the maximal V_{CE} in the unloaded heart (V_{max}).

changes during ejection can be recorded by both invasive and noninvasive methods; the latter, which utilize echocardiographic and nuclear measurements, are especially useful as they allow serial determinations in an individual patient. Another important advantage of many volume measurements is that they can identify the regional wall motion abnormalities that occur in patients with coronary disease.

The most precise measurements of left ventricular volume use planimetry of the silhouette of the irregularly shaped left ventricular cavity filled with a radiopaque contrast material injected through a catheter in the left ventricle. Calculation of ventricular volumes by frame-to-frame analyses of images recorded by biplane cineangiography is tedious when done by hand, but can be simplified by computer measurements. As these are "invasive" data that must be obtained by cardiac catheterization, they are expensive and not readily repeated.

Over the last decade, two noninvasive methods have gained wide acceptance: echocardiography and nuclear cardiology. Both allow repeated measurements at virtually no risk to the patient, and at much lower cost than cardiac catheterization. Echocardiography uses reflected sound waves to determine left ventricular dimensions; these can be supplemented with Doppler flow measurements which, along with two-dimensional echocardiograms, provide totally safe means for the serial analysis of left ventricular dimensions and flow in humans. Various equations can be used to calculate ventricular volumes from measurements of several dimensions. Nuclear methods for the evaluation of ventricular function generally analyze the volume of the blood pool in the left ventricle using red blood cells "tagged" with a short-lived radionuclide. Counting of radioactivity over the chest provides good estimates of left ventricular volume changes throughout the cardiac cycle, and special cameras that define the outlines of the radioactive blood pool can detect regional wall motion abnormalities. Neither method allows accurate measurements of intraventricular pressure.

Like the pressure-derived indices described above, these noninvasive methods provide valuable information about the function of the ventricle as an *organ*, but tell us little regarding myocardial contractility, which reflects the properties of heart muscle at the level of *cell* and *gene*.

Global Ventricular Function

The simplest, and now most commonly used index of global left ventricular function during the entire period of ejection, is the *ejection fraction* (EF). More elaborate determinations can be employed to obtain two additional indices: *mean normalized systolic ejection rate (MNSER)* and *mean velocity of circumferential fiber shortening (mean V_{CF})*.

Ejection Fraction

Ejection fraction, generally expressed as a percent, is the ratio of stroke volume to end-diastolic volume, which is defined in the following equations:

$$\text{Ejection fraction} = \frac{EDV - ESV}{EDV} = \frac{SV}{EDV}.$$ [17.2]

Thus EF is simply the percent of the end-diastolic volume that is ejected as the stroke volume.

End-diastolic and end-systolic volumes can be estimated by left ventricular cineangiography, radionuclide imaging, or echocardiography (see above). Normal ejection fractions range between 55 and 75%, whereas ejection fractions in patients with heart failure can fall below 20%. As discussed later, low ejection fractions occur in patients with depressed contractility, whereas in patients with relaxation abnormalities ejection fraction can be normal or, when the left ventricle has hypertrophied so as to reduce cavity volume, increased.

Measurements of ejection fraction can be misleading in the evaluation of the state of the left ventricle in patients with valve abnormalities. In mitral insufficiency, for example, ejection fraction can be normal, even when contractility is severely depressed, because regurgitation of blood into the low-pressure left atrium allows the ventricle to empty in spite of reduced contractility. Mitral valve replacement in such patients, by eliminating the ability of the ventricle to "vent" into the atrium, reveals a depressed ejection fraction. (The sudden increase in afterload can also worsen symptoms, and may prove fatal, even when the valve repair is, itself, excellent, because of the detrimental effects of elevated afterload described in Chapter 16.) In aortic stenosis, on the other hand, hypertrophy tends to reduce cavity size (as in the giraffe—Fig. 16.1). For this reason, ejection fraction can be normal even when the hypertrophied left ventricular myocardium is severely damaged by chronic pressure overload.

It is clear that ejection fraction is really a measure of pump function, rather than of contractility, as it is influenced by a variety of hemodynamic variables, including preload, afterload, and heart rate. In spite of these limitations, ejection fraction readily distinguishes between the two major types of heart failure: impaired contractility, where ejection fraction is low (Fig. 16.17), and impaired relaxation, where ejection fraction is normal or even increased (Fig. 16.19). Even more important, the extent to which ejection fraction is reduced in patients with some forms of heart disease, notably coronary occlusive disease, has proved to be a remarkably useful predictor of clinical outcome. For these reasons, and because of the relatively simple measurements needed for its estimation, ejection fraction has become a standard means for assessing left ventricular function in humans.

Mean Normalized Systolic Ejection Rate

Mean normalized systolic ejection rate, sometimes abbreviated MNSER, represents an index of myocardial contractility that provides some information as to the velocity of muscle shortening. This index is calculated by dividing the ejection fraction by the duration of ejection:

$$\text{MNSER} = \frac{\text{Ejection fraction}}{\text{Ejection time}} \ . \qquad [17.3]$$

MNSER, therefore, simply represents the percent of the end diastolic volume ejected per unit of time averaged throughout the ejection period.

Although division of ejection fraction by the ejection time offers theoretical advantages in terms of relating ejection fraction to muscle shortening velocity, MNSER is more cumbersome to calculate and has proven less useful than ejection fraction as a clinical index of cardiac performance.

Mean V_{CF}

The mean velocity of circumferential fiber shortening, mean V_{CF}, is similar to MNSER, except that V_{CF} is calculated by dividing a ventricular diameter change during systole [end-diastolic diameter (*dED*) minus end-systolic diameter (*dES*)] by the product of *dED* and ejection time:

$$\text{Mean } V_{CF} = \frac{dED - dES}{dED \times \text{ejection time}} \ . \qquad [17.4]$$

Thus, V_{CF} can be calculated using simple echocardiographic determination of a left ventricular diameter change, rather than a volume change.

The use of a single left ventricular diameter means that V_{CF} can be calculated from M-mode echocardiograms, which utilize a narrow beam of sound waves to provide an "ice pick" view of the ventricle. Although lacking the elegant display of two-dimensional echocardiography, this method allows much more rapid sampling of images and so provides useful data regarding time-dependent changes in ventricular dimensions.

Mean V_{CF}, which has the units of reciprocal time, like MNSER, is sensitive to changing rates of ejection and can be related conceptually to velocity of fiber shortening. Like ejection fraction, V_{CF} is influenced by preload, afterload, and heart rate, and so does not really measure left ventricular contractility as defined earlier in this text.

Regional Left Ventricular Function

Recognition and evaluation of localized, or regional, left ventricular wall motion abnormalities are especially important in patients with ischemic heart disease (Chapter 24), and can allow regional wall motion abnormalities to be related to occlusive lesions in specific coronary arteries.

Methods to evaluate regional left ventricular function depend on measurements of the changing blood pool within the ventricle, or the motion of its walls. These include simple visual inspection of ventriculograms, echocardiograms, and radionuclide images. In our current world of computers, more elaborate means are often used to evaluate regional contractility; for example, V_{CF} for several diameters in the left ventricle, including both normal and damaged regions of the myocardium, can be calculated and compared. Cross-sectional representations of left ventricular wall motion recorded by two-dimensional echocardiography can also be analyzed to quantify regional abnormalities in left ventricular function.

The extent of impairment of regional left ventricular contractility is often described using terms that define the severity of a localized wall motion abnormality. Mild impairment of ventricular contractility causes *asyneresis,* which is reduced inward movement, or *asynchrony,* a disordered temporal sequence of contraction. More severe impairment of function causes *akinesis,* or failure of a damaged segment of the left ventricular wall to participate in ejection. Akinesis generally occurs when the pressure generated by the undamaged regions of the left ventricle matches the tension developed by the damaged region. Most severe is *dyskinesis,* in which the damaged region bulges outward during systole because it is unable to overcome the pressure generated by the normal myocardium, and so is stretched during systole. When a large region of the left ventricle exhibits *dyskinesia,* it is called an *aneurysm.* Many aneurysms consist simply of a thin layer of fibrous scar.

Clinical Value of Contractility Indices

It is apparent that, in spite of extensive basic knowledge of myocardial function reviewed in this text, clinical evaluation of myocardial contractility is not a precise science. To some extent, uncertainties in the quantification of contractility in the human heart reflect the difficulty of defining contractility in simple cardiac muscle preparations. In addition, there is no "gold standard" by which to evaluate clinical indices of myocardial contractility, so that all such indices are largely empirical. This means that the many indices of contractility must be evaluated in terms of the clinical questions they are designed to answer. Most clinical problems involve prognosis; for example, as noted at the beginning of this chapter, the extent to which left ventricular contractility is depressed may define the optimal time for surgical therapy in a patient with valvular heart disease. In patients with angina pectoris (the symptom caused when the energy demands of the heart exceed energy supply, which as described in Chapter 24 is commonly seen when coronary artery disease reduces coronary flow), the extent to which coronary bypass surgery can be expected to prolong life is predictable from the ejection fraction; in general, patients with the lowest ejection fraction obtain the greatest benefit. Thus, although we still—and may always—lack precise means to quantify myocardial contractility, even simple methods are of proven value in clinical decision-making.

QUANTIFICATION OF THE DIASTOLIC PROPERTIES OF THE HEART

Contraction and relaxation are, in fact, quite different processes, as was emphasized in the early chapters of this text. Both require energy, both are highly regulated, and they can change independently of each other. However, until recently, cardiologists have tended to focus on abnormalities of contraction. This probably reflects the widespread application of pressure-derived methods made possible by cardiac catheterization, and the seeming elegance of efforts to analyze isovolumic pressure data in terms of muscle mechanics. It also seemed to make sense that heart failure was due largely to impaired contraction.

As so often happens in medicine, principles that made sense intuitively turned out to be oversimplifications. In the case of impaired cardiac pumping, noninvasive studies of ventricular wall motion and volume now make it clear not only that relaxation and contraction abnormalities can appear independently, but that impaired relaxation is, in fact, at least as important as impaired contractility in producing clinical disability.

Four phases of diastole are commonly evaluated in patients with heart disease (Fig. 17.5). The first is *isovolumic relaxation,* which begins immediately after the aortic valve closes (Fig. 15.8); this is followed by ventricular *filling,* which follows mitral valve opening. The third occurs later in diastole, after filling has slowed during the period of *diastasis.* Finally, ventricular diastole ends with *atrial systole.* Different methods are used to evaluate the lusitropic properties of the ventricle during each of these four phases, which reflect the operation of quite different mechanisms.

Clinical Indices

Diastolic function can be evaluated clinically by such simple methods as auscultation of a third or fourth heart sound, which implies that the ventricle has become more stiff and does not fill normally. However, bedside quantification of diastolic function, like that of contractility, is imprecise.

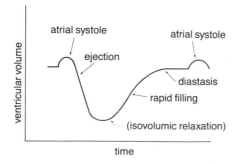

FIG. 17.5. Phases of the cardiac cycle as seen in changing left ventricular volume. Isovolumic relaxation cannot be quantified from volume curves, but instead requires measurement of intraventricular pressure.

Diastolic Time Intervals

Diastolic time intervals can be derived from apexcardiography (measurements of low-frequency movements of the ventricular apex through the chest wall) and phonocardiography. These older methods, now supplemented by M-mode and two-dimensional echocardiography, readily measure the durations of the four diastolic phases of the cardiac cycle described above. Most intervals are derived from simultaneous heart sound recordings and M-mode echocardiograms.

Isovolumic relaxation time is the interval from aortic valve closure (A_2) or end-systole (minimal end-systolic dimension) to the time of mitral value opening. While providing an index of the properties of the ventricle that determine the speed of isovolumic relaxation, isovolumic relaxation is influenced by preload and afterload.

Volume Measurements

Left ventricular volumes can be estimated by echocardiography, which provides a safe and easily repeated means to evaluate ventricular filling. Somewhat more cumbersome, but also somewhat more quantitative, are measurements of the volume of a radioactive blood pool in the left ventricle using radionuclide techniques (see above). A number of indices based on events during the rapid filling period have provided useful means to quantify diastolic function. These include *filling fraction,* which is the percentage of end-diastolic filling that occurs during the first third of diastolic interval, *average rapid filling rate, peak filling rate,* and the *time to peak filling rate.* Although these determinations provide information regarding the filling phase of the cardiac cycle that identify patients with abnormal diastolic function, it should not be difficult to appreciate that these indices are all preload-dependent.

Flow Measurements

Doppler flow measurements provide useful noninvasive indices of diastolic function that are not very different from the volume measurements described above. The most useful indices are based on flow across the mitral valve. One currently popular index is the *E/A ratio,* which measures the ratio between early and late maxima of flow velocity; the former is related to rapid filling, whereas the latter is, of course, due to atrial systole. These indices, however, are significantly affected by left atrial pressure (preload) as well as heart rate. They are quite useful in patients with rheumatic heart disease when used, along with echocardiographic images, to assess possible obstruction to flow across the mitral valve, as occurs in patients with mitral stenosis.

Hemodynamic Indices

As already pointed out, early attempts to quantify the diastolic properties of the left ventricle used pressure, rather than volume data. Most indices derived from pressure data are based on measurements of the rate of fall of left ventricular pressure during isovolumic relaxation (maximum negative dP/dt). Because maximum negative dP/dt is highly dependent on aortic pressure, a correction must be made to obtain a pressure-independent index. If it is assumed that the decline in left ventricular pressure is exponential with time, negative dP/dt can be expressed as an exponential function that allows time constants, called τ to be calculated. For example, τ can be estimated as the time required for ventricular pressure to decline to either $\frac{1}{2}$ or $\frac{1}{e}$ of its peak value, beginning at the time of aortic valve closure. As the fall of left ventricular pressure during isovolumic relaxation is not usually exponential, elaborate calculations are often used to calculate τ. The complexity of these determinations generally limits these measurements to the research laboratory.

Stiffness and Compliance

Diastolic *stiffness* is most simply estimated as dP/dV; *compliance* (dV/dP) is the reciprocal of stiffness. Because the relationship between diastolic pressure and volume is curvilinear, more complex calculations are often used to characterize stiffness. The *modulus of ventricular stiffness* is a measure of the slope of the relation between dP/dV and P during diastole. As the relationships between pressure and tension, and between volume and length, are complex geometric functions in the intact ventricle (Chapter 15), these measurements are very difficult to use in determining the lusitropic properties of the myocardium itself.

Measurements of stiffness are generally made late in diastole, during diastasis, and so reflect the properties of the myocardium at a time when calcium uptake by the sarcoplasmic reticulum and the dissociation of calcium from troponin have slowed. Thus, stiffness provides little information regarding the *rates* of these processes, which are better estimated during isovolumic relaxation and filling. Stiffness does, however, provide an index as to the completeness of calcium removal from troponin, and so—at least on theoretical grounds—may provide some information as to the calcium sensitivities of the sarcoplasmic reticulum and troponin. However, stiffness is also influenced by the geometry of the ventricle and changes in the fibrous skeleton of the heart.

Significance of Relaxation Measurements

As noted above, different processes operate at different times during diastole, so that the mechanisms responsible for the decrease in pressure during *isovolumic relaxation* (negative dP/dt) differ from those responsible for the volume changes that occur later, during *filling*. It is likely that the negative *dP/dt* (the fall in pressure during early diastole) is influenced by the rate at which calcium is removed from the contractile proteins by the calcium pump of the sarcoplasmic reticulum. Early filling is probably also influenced by calcium transport into the sarcoplasmic reticulum, but the extent of relaxation later during *diastasis* is probably more closely dependent on the nadir of cytosolic Ca^{2+} concentration. Diastolic pressure and volume are also influenced by the passive properties of the ventricle and the pericardium. The flow and volume changes that occur during *atrial systole* are, of course, determined by the strength of atrial contraction. Thus, like measurements of contractility, those of relaxation are really clinical indices, rather than determinations of one or another of the fundamental properties of heart muscle.

CONCLUSIONS

The reader who has toiled through this chapter and attempted to relate the many indices of myocardial function to the fundamental properties of contraction and relaxation discussed in earlier chapters should not, at this point, conclude that application of modern technology to clinical problems is useless. In fact, the opposite is the case. Today we are able to learn more about the heart of the living cardiac patient by the judicious use of science and technology than could be determined a generation ago at autopsy.

The real problem in our efforts to identify reliable indices to define the state of the myocardium in our patients is that we expect too much from technology and science. In fact, it may be that hemodynamic and other data regarding cardiac contraction and relaxation will never provide unequivocal indices to quantify either the inotropic or lusitropic state of the diseased heart. This rather bleak conclusion must not, however, be taken to mean that these measurements are not without value. On the contrary, they are of enormous use for the management of cardiac patients. Our mistake is that we continue to search for a measurement, or an index, that will provide *answers* to the many vital questions asked by clinicians, whereas all that we can really expect are *data*. It thus remains the task of the expert clinician to select and evaluate these data so as to arrive at appropriate answers to the challenges posed by each patient. On reviewing the rapidly developing science of cardiology, it appears that solutions to the infinite variety of clinical questions posed by our patients are best achieved by integration of the bedside evaluation with appropriate laboratory data, all weighed in terms of normal and abnormal physiology.

BIBLIOGRAPHY

Hugenholtz PG, Rutishauser W, eds. (1974). Symposium: assessment of left ventricular function. *Eur J Cardiol* 1:229–334.
Katz AM, Smith VE, Weisfeldt ML. (1986). Relaxation and diastolic properties of the heart. In: Fozzard

H, Haber E, Katz A, Jennings R, Morgan HE, eds. *The heart and cardiovascular system.* New York: Raven Press, 803–818.

Krayenbuehl HP, Hess CM, Turina J. (1978). Assessment of left ventricular function. *Cardiovasc Med* 2:883–910.

Levine RA, Gillam LD, Weyman AE. (1986). Echocardiography in cardiac research. In: Fozzard H, Haber E, Katz A, Jennings R, Morgan HE, eds. *The heart and cardiovascular system.* New York: Raven Press, 369–452.

Mirsky I. (1984). Assessment of diastolic function: suggested methods and future considerations. *Circulation* 69:834–841.

Pasipoularidies A. (1990). Clinical assessment of ventricular ejection dynamics with and without outflow obstruction. *JACC* 15:859–892.

Ross J Jr, Covell JW, Sonnenblick EH, Braunwald E. (1966). Contractile state of the heart characterized by force-velocity relations in variably afterloaded and isovolumic beats. *Circ Res* 18:149–163.

Smith V-E, Zile M. (1991). Relaxation and diastolic properties of the heart. In: Fozzard H, Haber E, Katz A, Jennings R, Morgan HE eds. *The heart and cardiovascular system,* 2nd ed. New York: Raven Press. In Press

Weissler AM, Garrard CL Jr. (1971). Systolic time intervals in cardiac disease. *Mod Conc Cardiovasc Dis* 40:1–8.

18

Ion Channels of the Heart

This chapter marks a major shift in the focus of our discussion, from the mechanical function of the heart to the origins, regulation, and pathophysiology of its electrical activity. In discussing contractility, our focus was on calcium, which plays the central role in excitation-contraction coupling. Positively charged calcium ions, although also important in the electrical activity of the heart, are but one of several ions that, at different times during the action potential, occupy center stage in determining the membrane voltage changes that generate the cardiac action potential.

MEMBRANE POTENTIAL

Before the molecular basis for the cardiac action potential is discussed, several terms must be defined. An action potential, whether described by electrophysiologists or electrocardiographers, is a sequence of changes in the potential difference across the plasma membrane. These potential differences, generally referred to as the *membrane potential* (E_m), represent voltage differences between the interior of the cell and the surrounding extracellular space.

In the resting cell, a microelectrode inserted through the plasma membrane records an intracellular potential more negative than that of the extracellular fluid (Fig. 18.1). However, the polarity assigned to this potential difference is a matter of convention. If the resting potential difference is viewed from within the cell, it will be negative relative to the surrounding medium. If, on the other hand, we define resting potential as the potential at the outside of the cell, resting potential will be positive, relative to the cell interior. It is a source of no small confusion that both conventions are used in cardiac electrophysiology!

The first convention is employed by membrane electrophysiologists, who describe a negative resting potential because they place electrodes inside the cell and measure the potential of the cell interior relative to that in the surrounding medium. Electrocardiographers, on the other hand, place electrodes on the body surface and so view the electrical events of the heart in terms of changing potentials outside the cell. For the electrocardiographer, therefore, the resting cell is viewed from the outside, which is positively charged. In this and the next chapter, we don the cloak of the electro-

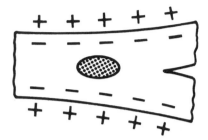

FIG. 18.1. Cardiac muscle cell at rest. The polarity of the normal resting potential is negative inside and positive at the cell exterior.

physiologist and so view resting cells as negatively charged. When we assume the role of the electrocardiographer, in Chapters 20–23, we turn our cloaks to view the resting cell as positively charged.

According to the conventions of electrophysiology, an increase in resting potential, called *hyperpolarization,* represents increased electronegativity inside the cell (Fig. 18.2). Conversely, a decrease in resting potential, called *depolarization,* represents a decrease in the electronegativity of the interior of the resting cell. *Repolarization,* like hyperpolarization, describes an increased electronegativity within the cell. The term hyperpolarization generally refers to an increase in the resting potential of an unexcited cell, whereas repolarization describes the return of membrane potential to its resting negative value after depolarization, at the end of the action potential (Fig. 18.2). The *amplitude* of the action potential defines the extent to which cellular electronegativity decreases from its resting level, including any reversal to electropositivity.

MEMBRANE CURRENTS

The terminology used to describe the different types of electrical *currents* that cross the cell membrane is even more complex than that which describes membrane

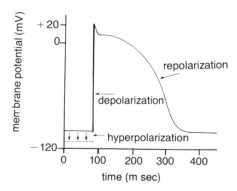

FIG. 18.2. The cardiac action potential as conventionally represented with the interior of the resting cell depicted as negatively charged. Hyperpolarization is an increase in resting potential, depolarization is the decrease (and reversal) of the resting potential, and repolarization is the return of membrane potential to its resting level at the end of the action potential.

potential. Because the ionic (or ohmic) currents caused by the flux of cations are the most important, the accepted terminology in electrophysiology describes these currents as if they were carried across the cell membrane by positively charged ions. This convention holds even when the currents are carried by negatively charged ions or represent the discharge of membrane capacitance.

Inward and Outward Currents

An *inward current,* according to electrophysiological convention, represents the flux of charge that would result if positive ions moved into the cell. Most inward currents are generated when positively charged sodium and calcium enter the cell. Because the outward movement of a negative ion like chloride has the same effect on membrane potential as the inward movement of positive ions, the efflux of negative ions also gives rise to an inward current. As the interior of the resting cell is negatively charged (Fig. 18.1), inward ionic currents cause *depolarization.*

An *outward current* can result either from the movement of positively charged ions out of the cell interior to the surrounding medium, or from the flux of negatively charged ions into the cell interior. Outward ionic currents therefore increase electronegativity in the cell interior. In the resting cell, mechanisms that increase outward currents cause *hyperpolarization.* Outward currents that occur after depolarization tend to restore the resting potential to its original negative value and so cause *repolarization* (Fig. 18.2).

Ionic and Capacitive Currents

There are two fundamentally different types of *membrane current*: *ionic currents,* which are the major subject of this and the following chapters, and *capacitive currents,* which arise because biological membranes act as capacitors.

Capacitive currents are readily understood because, as pointed out in Chapter 2, phospholipid bilayers contain a central lipid region that acts as an insulator between two differently charged polar solutions. The heart's plasma membrane, which separates regions having different electrical potentials, therefore acts as a capacitor. In the resting cell, where the extracellular surface of the plasma membrane is positively charged (Fig. 18.1), a cathode placed outside the cell draws positive charge from its external surface (Fig. 18.3A). This cathode could be a stimulating electrode or the normal approaching wave of depolarization described in Chapter 19. The resulting decrease in positive charge at the outer side of the plasma membrane discharges part of the membrane capacitance; by reducing the negative charge on the intracellular surface of the membrane, this capacitive discharge causes the resting cell to depolarize. As described in Chapter 19, cardiac action potentials are normally initiated when a cathodal current outside the cell, accompanied by an anodal current inside the cell, discharges the membrane capacitance and opens channels that carry inward currents that, together, reduce membrane potential.

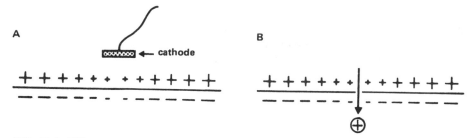

FIG. 18.3. Differences between capacitive and ionic currents. A: Discharge of the membrane potential by a cathode outside the cell draws positive charge from the extracellular surface of the plasma membrane and so causes negative charge to move away from the inner surface. This generates a capacitive current that resembles the inward ionic current shown in B, where the flux of cations from the outside to the inside of the cell causes a similar change in membrane potential.

Ionic currents represent the charge movements that occur when ions cross the insulating lipids in the center of the bilayer. These ionic currents are quite different from the capacitive currents described in the preceding paragraph. Inward ionic currents, because they bring positively charged ions into the electronegative interior of the resting cell, are depolarizing (Fig. 18.3B). When depolarization reaches a threshold (defined in Chapter 19), opening of voltage-dependent sodium and/or calcium channels allows these positively charged ions to cross the plasma membrane. Because both Na^+ and Ca^{2+} concentrations are much higher outside than inside the cells, the resulting ionic current is inward. This leads to further depolarization that opens still more channels that carry inward current, thereby initiating a regenerative action potential in which a complex series of ion channel openings and closings orchestrate a sequence of ionic currents across the plasma membrane (Chapter 19).

MEMBRANE RESISTANCE

The ratio between membrane potential and current flow, which is *membrane resistance,* follows Ohm's law: $R = E/I$, where R is resistance, E is potential, and I is current flow. *Membrane conductance,* usually designated g, is the reciprocal of membrane resistance, so that $g = I/E$.

Permeability and Conductance

The terms *permeability* and *conductance,* both of which reflect the ability of substances to cross membranes, are not, in fact, the same. *Permeability* (P) is a measure of the ability of a membrane to allow the movement (flux) of molecules from one side to the other, whereas *conductance* (g) describes charge movements across the membrane. Both conductance and permeability have the dimensions of a velocity (centimeters per second); however, permeability characterizes molecular fluxes that can be in both directions across the membrane at any time, whereas conductance describes an electrical current that can flow in only one direction at any time.

Permeability (P): The flux of an uncharged molecule (e.g., sucrose) in either direction is defined by the relationship:

$$\text{Sucrose flux} = P_{\text{sucrose}} \times [\text{sucrose}]. \qquad [18.1]$$

In the case of a charged molecule, the relation of flux to concentration is more complex than that described in Eq. 18.1 because ion movements are modified when there is a membrane potential.

Conductance (g): Ionic conductance provides an index of the ability of a membrane to carry the current (i) that accompanies the transfer of charge when an ion moves from one side of a membrane to the other. This current flow is determined by the corresponding conductance and the difference between the equilibrium potential across the membrane (E_{ion} in the Nernst equation; see Chapter 19) and the actual transmembrane potential (E_m). In the case of potassium, for example:

$$i_K - g_K \times (E_m - E_K) \qquad [18.2]$$

where i_K is the current carried by potassium ions and g_K is the potassium conductance. Even though Eq. 18.2 does not contain a term equivalent to the ion concentration, the latter contributes to E_K in the Nernst equation (see Chapter 19). Depending on the difference between E_K and E_m, current can flow in either direction, although not in both directions at any given time. Conductance, although intended to describe current flow, provides a valid index of the ability of the membrane to allow an ion to move from one side to the other when that ion is the sole carrier of the current.

CHANGING MEMBRANE CONDUCTANCES AND THE ACTION POTENTIAL

At the turn of this century, there was already evidence that mammalian cells contained a high concentration of potassium. As early as 1902, Julius Bernstein had proposed that the plasma membrane was selectively permeable to potassium ions, and that fixed negative charge inside the cell created a Donnan equilibrium, which caused the cell to resemble a battery in which the interior was negatively charged. However, aside from its postulated selective permeability for potassium, little was known of the properties of the membrane, and how its permeabilities changed in the excited cell.

In the early decades of this century, before electrodes could be introduced into cells, membrane conductance was studied by measuring the impedance to currents applied across intact cells. In the 1930s, whole-cell impedance was observed to decrease when cells were excited, which provided indirect evidence that membrane conductance had increased. However, definitive data did not appear until shortly before the outbreak of World War II, when Hodgkin and Huxley in England, and Curtis and Cole in the United States were able to insert microelectrodes into squid giant axons to record the potential differences across the plasma membrane.

The observation of resting electronegativity within the cell, and loss of this negativity during the action potential, was in accord with earlier theories that resting potential was determined largely by the Nernst potential for potassium (Chapter 19), and that this potential difference was dissipated when the cell was excited. The intracellular recordings, however, did provide a surprise: During excitation, membrane potential did not simply decrease to zero as would be expected if changing potassium permeability alone was responsible for activation. Instead, membrane potential actually reversed during excitation, and the cell interior became positive. This meant that the action potential must have been generated by processes other than the simple dissipation of a potential difference created by the potassium gradient.

THE VOLTAGE CLAMP

After World War II, Hodgkin, Huxley, and Katz returned to this question in a now classical series of experiments designed to characterize the ionic basis for the action potential of the squid giant axon. Conceptually, their approach was simple. Instead of measuring membrane potential changes during an action potential, when unknown ionic currents depolarized and repolarized the membrane, they held voltage constant (the "clamp") and measured the currents. This was accomplished when they placed microelectrodes in the squid axon that allowed them to pass currents across the membrane so as to hold membrane potential constant at any desired level. Membrane potential could be "clamped" only when the applied currents *exactly matched the ionic currents that would have otherwise caused membrane potential to change*. Thus, by measuring the small currents they applied across the membrane to maintain a constant membrane potential, Hodgkin and Huxley were able to quantify both the timing and strength of the actual ionic currents that were crossing the membrane (of course in the opposite direction). This allowed simple interventions like changing Na^+ and K^+ concentrations in the medium bathing the axon to define the ionic currents responsible for the action potential. These ionic currents, and how they generate the cardiac action potential, are discussed in the next chapter.

GENERAL PROPERTIES OF PLASMA MEMBRANE IONIC CURRENTS

The ionic currents responsible for membrane depolarization and repolarization share a number of important properties. Like the calcium fluxes that initiate excitation-contraction coupling, these ionic currents are passive, in that the ions move down their electrochemical gradients. This means that, like calcium delivery to the contractile apparatus, the ion fluxes that depolarize and repolarize the heart do not require the expenditure of energy. On the other hand, energy is required by the ion pumps and ion exchangers that maintain the ionic gradients responsible for these passive fluxes; in the heart, these include the plasma membrane sodium and calcium pumps and the sodium/calcium exchanger described in Chapter 10.

A second important feature of these ionic currents is that each ion moves through its own channel. In fact, as described later in this and the next chapter, there are many different molecular structures through which a given ion species can cross the plasma membrane.

It is obvious that for an ion channel to serve a physiological function, it must be able to shift between at least two states: open and closed. In fact, physiological ion channels exhibit much more complex behavior. Until recently, membrane channels were viewed as existing in *three* functional states: one open and two closed. The latter differ because in one closed state (often called the *resting* state), the channel readily opens in response to an appropriate stimulus, whereas in the other closed state (often called the *inactivated* or *refractory* state), the channel cannot be made to open. It is now apparent, however, that there can be more than one of each of these three states (see below).

Membrane channels are generally viewed as cycling through the three functional states according to the following general scheme:

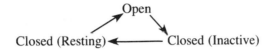

The transitions between these three states are normally controlled by changes in membrane potential, which initiate time-dependent processes that alter the probability that the channels shift from one to another of these states. The states and their transitions are also influenced by chemical factors, notably phosphorylations, by the G-proteins, and by a variety of drugs, most of which appear to modify channel behavior after first dissolving in the membrane bilayer (Chapter 2).

GATING OF ION CHANNELS

In their initial description of the ionic currents responsible for the squid axon action potential, Hodgkin and Huxley (1952) developed a model that postulated that special regulatory systems, called gating mechanisms, control the opening and closing of distinct entities ("gates") in both sodium and potassium channels. According to this model, the action potential begins when, in response to an appropriate stimulus like depolarization, sodium ions carry a positive charge into the cell. The inward sodium current begins when an activation mechanism, by opening "*m*" *gates*, causes the sodium channels to change from the closed (resting) to the open state. This gating response was postulated to depend on a cooperative interaction between three m gates, located near the outside of the membrane, that controlled sodium channel opening. Closing of the sodium channel was postulated to be under the control of a different gating mechanism, called the "*h*" *gate*, located at the intracellular surface of the plasma membrane. In order for sodium ions to pass through the channel, both sets of gates must be open, whereas closure of either suffices to close the channel. As each gate has two positions, there are three possible combina-

TABLE 18.1. *Gating of the squid axon sodium channel*

State of the channel	State of the m gate	State of the h gate
Closed (resting)	Closed	Open
Open	Open	Open
Closed (inactive)	Open	Closed

tions that define the three states of the channel listed in Table 18.1. In one, where both gates are open, the sodium channel is *open;* the other two define the different closed states: *closed (resting),* when the m gates are closed and the h gate open, and *closed (inactive),* when the h gate is closed and the m gates open (Table 18.1).

The Hodgkin-Huxley Equations

Hodgkin and Huxley developed a series of elegant equations to describe time- and voltage-dependent properties of the gating mechanisms that open and close the sodium and potassium channels of the squid axon. Although a full discussion of these equations is beyond the scope of this text, they contain two important terms, m and h (often used to designate "gates" that close the channel), which define key functional aspects of sodium channel structure. The term m appeared in the Hodgkin-Huxley equations as an *activation* coefficient that defines the probability that the sodium channel is in the open state, whereas h is an *inactivation* coefficient that defines the probability that the sodium channel is closed by a separate structure.

According to the Hodgkin-Huxley equations, the magnitude of the sodium current i_{Na}, which reflects the probability that the sodium channel is in the open state, is determined by these two coefficients and maximal channel conductance. Because m is a coefficient of channel opening whereas h is a coefficient of channel closing, i_{Na} increases with increasing m and decreasing h. Thus, the sodium current is maximal when m is 1 (100% probability of being open) and h is 0 (0% probability of being closed). As described in Eq. 18.2, the sodium current also depends on membrane voltage, so that the Hodgkin-Huxley equation for the sodium channel is:

$$i_{Na} = m^3 \, h \, \bar{g}_{Na} \, (E_m - E_{Na}). \qquad [18.3]$$

The opening coefficient is cubed in accord with data that suggest a cooperative interaction involving three m gates control sodium channel opening.

Voltage-Dependent Properties

Equation 18.3 states that the sodium current is a function (determined by m and h) of the maximal sodium conductance ($\bar{g}$) and the difference between actual membrane potential (E_m) and the sodium equilibrium potential (E_{Na}). The latter, which is the potential that would be recorded if the membrane were permeable only to sodium ions, is generally about + 70 mV (Chapter 19).

The *voltage dependence* of sodium channel opening means that depolarization from the normal resting potential (approximately -80 mV) has two opposing effects. The first effect of increasing $(E_m - E_{Na})$ is to increase the probability of an *open* channel, in proportion to the cube of the *activation* coefficient for opening of the m gate (m^3). At the same time, however, depolarization also increases the probability of a *closed* channel, in proportion to the *inactivation* coefficient for closing of the h gate. If m and h, both of which increase when the membrane depolarizes, had similar time-dependent properties, depolarization would have little effect on i_{Na} because if the m gates opened and h gates closed at the same rates, the sodium channel would remain closed.

Time-Dependent Properties

The key to understanding how Eq. 18.3 predicts the transient depolarization observed by Hodgkin and Huxley lies in the fact that m and h have different *time-dependent properties;* m gates open much faster than h gates close after the plasma membrane is depolarized. For this reason, the initial response to depolarization is opening of the m gates that *activates* (opens) the channel. However, sodium channel opening is brief because, even when the membrane remains depolarized, the slower increase in the other coefficient, h, eventually *inactivates* (closes) the channel.

Reactivation (Recovery) of the Channel

In order for the cell to return to the resting state, and for sodium channels to *reactivate*, the cell must be repolarized. Although closing of the sodium channels contributes to repolarization, outward potassium currents through an entirely different class of ion channels are the most important cause for the return to resting potential (see below). Once the cell has repolarized, the m gates close and the h gate reopens; because the m gates close more rapidly than the h gates open, the sodium channel does not reopen during recovery.

Other Relationships

Hodgkin and Huxley developed additional equations to describe the time-dependence of changes in the m and h gates, as well as the kinetics of the potassium channels, whose activation gate is designated n. The equation for the potassium current uses the fourth power of n to describe potassium channel gating:

$$i_K = n^4 \, \bar{g}_K \, (E_m - E_K). \qquad [18.4]$$

Overall, the Hodgkin-Huxley equations described the basis for the ionic currents that generate squid axon action potentials in terms of two types of channel, one selective for sodium, the other for potassium. The cardiac action potential, however, is more complex (Chapter 19) in that a third plasma membrane channel plays a major role in both the electrical activity and mechanical response of cardiac muscle; this third channel is, of course, the calcium channel described in Chapter 10.

Although the properties of plasma membrane ion channels are much more complex than could have been foreseen 40 years ago, and channel structure more diverse, the Hodgkin and Huxley equations remain a landmark in electrophysiology. Much as the elegant concepts of A. V. Hill served as the watershed in the physiology and biochemistry of muscle (Chapter 6), even today the Hodgkin-Huxley model explains functional correlates of newly discovered aspects of channel structure (see below).

Gating Currents

To explain the ability of changing membrane potential to open and close voltage-sensitive ion channels, Hodgkin and Huxley postulated that the channels contained charged regions that underwent conformational changes in response to depolarization and repolarization of the membrane. This led to the prediction that careful measurements of membrane currents, recorded under conditions that eliminated or corrected for the contributions of membranes capacitance and ion fluxes, might detect small currents arising from the movements of these charged gating regions of the channel.

In the 1960s, small currents believed to arise from charge movements within membrane structures were recorded. These small currents, called gating currents, exhibit the properties expected of the activation (m) gates. As noted below, these charge movements can now be attributed to the movement of positively charged membrane-spanning helices that are part of the channel protein molecules.

It is of interest that, even though inactivation abolishes most of the gating current attributable to activation, no gating current has been found to correlate with inactivation. This has been interpreted to mean that the h gate closes when an inactivating "particle" moves only a small distance to enter and block the open channel. This has

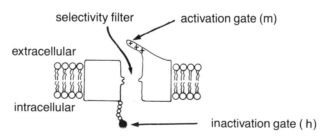

FIG. 18.4. Old-style "imaginary" model of an ion channel showing a positively charged activation (m) gate at the extracellular surface of the bilayer, and a "ball and chain" to represent the inactivation (h) gate. A "selectivity filter" within the channel determines the ion species that the channel allows to cross the membrane.

been called a "ball and chain" or "foot in the door" mechanism, in which a part of the cytoplasmic domain of the channel binds to and plugs the intracellular side of the pore (Fig. 18.4).

Structural Correlates to the Hodgkin-Huxley Gates

In the past 5 years, remarkable discoveries regarding channel structure have tentatively equated both the m and h gates to specific regions of the channel proteins whose structures are described in detail in the following pages. At this point it seems appropriate to anticipate this discussion by stating that the m gates postulated by Hodgkin and Huxley almost a half-century ago correspond to the positively charged S_4 membrane-spanning helix common to all known voltage-regulated plasma membrane ion channels (Noda et al., 1986). In 1989, analysis of altered sodium channel proteins produced by site-directed mutagenesis tentatively located the h gate exactly where Hodgkin and Huxley predicted it must lie, on a peptide loop within the cytosol (Aldrich, 1989; Stümer et al., 1989). This remarkable history clearly illustrates the essential interplay between classical physiology and modern molecular biology in advancing our knowledge of biological function, and ultimately, of human disease.

STRUCTURES OF PLASMA MEMBRANE ION CHANNELS

The most logical mechanism by which an ion could cross the hydrophobic region of a membrane is through a water-filled pore that spans its fatty acyl chain layer (Chapter 2). Until recently, such pores were imaginary structures (Fig. 18.4) that allowed electrophysiologists to explain a growing body of data regarding ion fluxes across membranes. As has so often been the case, the explosive growth of molecular biology has transformed imagination into reality, and at a pace more rapid than could have been anticipated even 5 years ago. We now know the complete amino acid sequences of many of the huge and complex proteins that contain the ion channels responsible for the changing conductances during the cardiac action potential. Data are also beginning to appear that tell us how these channels differ, and how they are regulated. Most exciting, and in accord with a motif that has already been highlighted in our discussions of other proteins, we are encountering a new type of regulation—or more accurately, we have come to recognize a very primitive regulatory mechanism—that allows cells to respond to a changing environment (Chapter 14). As we begin to appreciate the variabilities and similarities in channel structure, we are learning that cells can select from a number of amino acid sequences in synthesizing the ion channel structure needed to meet a given set of functional requirements. Once again, we are seeing how *organ* function, in this case activation of the heart by membrane depolarization, is regulated by *cellular* processes (channel openings and closings) that are, in turn, subject to control by selective *gene* expression.

TABLE 18.2. *Major calcium channels in the heart*

Property	L-type calcium channel	T-type calcium channel
Threshold	Low ($-$ 40 mV)	High ($-$ 70 mV)
Inactivation	Slow (L = long-lasting)	Fast (T = transient)
Response to β-adrenergic stimulation	Stimulated	None
Response to calcium channel blockers	Blocked	None
Size	Large (15–25 pS)[a]	Small (7–9 pS)
Found in	All cardiac cells	Conducting and nodal cells

[a]pS (picosiemens) are single channel conductances.

DIVERSITY OF CHANNEL STRUCTURE

Several converging lines of evidence have made it clear that ion channels are a remarkably diverse group of related structures. Even before the detailed molecular characterizations described below revealed the basis for what is really a "micro-regulation" of channel structure, functional studies had demonstrated the existence of several distinct types of calcium channel. Salient differences between the two major cardiac calcium channels are listed in Table 18.2. Most important is the L-type channel, which is the calcium channel described in this and subsequent chapters. The T-type calcium channel, found in nodal and specialized conducting tissue, probably contributes to spontaneous pacemaker depolarization and possibly to the long-lasting depolarizations of the His-Purkinje system; overall, its functional significance appears to be less than that of the L-type calcium channel. Unless otherwise specified, the term *calcium channel* as used in this text refers to L-type channels.

ION CHANNEL STRUCTURE

Voltage-dependent ion channels are glycosylated proteins composed of several channel peptides[1] (Table 18.3). The large carbohydrate content of these proteins, which can make up as much as one-third of their mass, is located at the extracellular surface of the plasma membrane. The most important proteins are the large α- and α_1-channel peptides of the sodium and calcium channels, respectively. Each channel peptide is made up of four similar subunits that surround the water-filled pore through which ions cross the phospholipid bilayer. The potassium channels are probably tetramers of similar subunits that are *not* covalently linked (Table 18.3).

---

[1]In this discussion, a confusing terminology is organized as follows: The larger channel proteins listed in Table 18.3 are referred to as *channel peptides*. The four covalently linked components of the α- and α_1-peptides of the sodium and calcium channel, numbered I–IV, are *channel subunits*. These subunits, which are similar to the corresponding free subunits of the potassium channel, all contain six *membrane-spanning* α-helices, designated S_1–S_6.

TABLE 18.3. *Peptide components of voltage-dependent ion channels*

Ion selectivity	Subunit	Number	Approximate mol. weight	Possible function
Sodium	α	1	260,000	Pore, PK-A[b] substrate
	β	0–2	30,000–40,000	
Calcium	α_1 (212)	1	212,000	Pore, PK-A substrate
	α_1 (175)	1	175,000	"Voltage sensor"
	α_2	1	140,000	PK-A substrate
	β	1	54,000	PK-A substrate
	γ	1	30,000	
	Δ	1	27,000	
Potassium		4	70,000–80,000	Pore

[b]PK-A: protein kinase A.

Thus, the major peptides of the different channels all appear to contain four channel subunits as depicted below in Fig. 18.7.

The evolutionary development of the ion channel peptides is remarkably similar to that proposed for the calcium-binding proteins (Chapter 7). Both are families of proteins, the most advanced members of which are tetramers derived from a primitive monomeric ancestor. In the case of the ion channel peptides, the ancestor appears to have been similar to the channel subunit shown in Figure 18.5. Reduplication of the genes that encode these subunits, as for the E-F hand proteins described in Chapter 7, has occurred in the genes encoding the sodium and calcium channels, giving rise to the four covalently linked channel subunits in each α- and α_1-peptide. As noted above, the functional potassium channel is probably also a tetramer of the

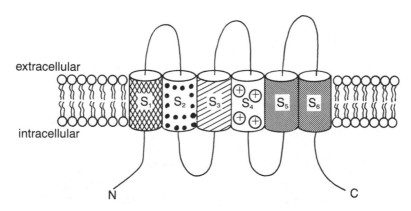

FIG. 18.5. The ion channel subunit contains six α-helical membrane-spanning α-helices. Each channel peptide is made up of four of these basic subunits. One of these, S_4, is rich in positively charged amino acids and appears to represent the voltage sensor of the m gate that opens the channel when the membrane is depolarized. The membrane-spanning helices S_1, S_2, and S_3 all contain charged amino acid residues and so are proposed to line the water-filled pore within the channel, whereas the more hydrophobic S_5 and S_6 helices probably interact with the bilayer lipids.

channel subunits, but in this highly variable channel the subunits are not covalently linked.

It is likely that the potassium channels are the more primitive of these structures because they are the smallest and, like the ancestral E-F hand proteins described in Chapter 7, do not exhibit evidence for gene reduplication. Potassium channels, along with the calcium channels that probably evolved next, are present in such simple organisms as protozoa, coelenterates, and ctenophores. The most recent addition to this family appears to be the sodium channels which, because they generate the largest and most rapidly rising action potentials, generate impulses that conduct far more rapidly than calcium-dependent action potentials (Chapter 19). It should be no surprise, therefore, that the sodium channels, which provide for the fastest conduction, have been found only in multicellular organisms that require means for speedy communication between different regions of their bodies.

Channel Subunit Structure

The subunits (as defined above) of all ion channels are made up of six putative membrane-spanning helices that share several important features (Figs. 18.5 and 18.6). Two of these helices, S_5 and S_6, are hydrophobic and so are likely to interact with the hydrophobic core of the bilayer that surrounds the channel. The S_1 and S_3 membrane-spanning helices, which contain negatively charged amino acids, and the S_2 helix, which contains both positively and negatively charged amino acids, probably surround the water-filled pore. Most interesting is S_4, which because it contains

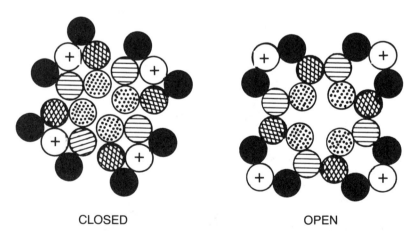

CLOSED   OPEN

FIG. 18.6. Ion channel viewed from above the plane of the membrane. Each voltage-sensitive ion channel is a tetramer made up of four of the basic subunits shown in Fig. 18.5. Shading of the membrane-spanning helices is as in Fig. 18.5. Movement of the S_4 membrane-spanning domain is believed to initiate a rearrangement of the channel subunits that opens a water-filled pore through which ions can cross the bilayer. (Modified from Noda et al., 1986.)

a "ribbon" of positively charged arginine and lysine residues around the membrane-spanning α-helix, has the properties expected of the "voltage sensor" that moves within the bilayer in response to changing transmembrane potential. As already noted, the S_4 membrane-spanning helix has been postulated to represent the m gate whose movements in the membrane give rise to the gating currents (see above) associated with the actual conformational change that opens the sodium channel.

A likely candidate for the h gate has also been identified (Fig. 18.7); as mentioned earlier, this is the cytoplasmic loop connecting the S_6 membrane spanning helix of subunit III, and the S_1 membrane-spanning helix of subunit IV. This short

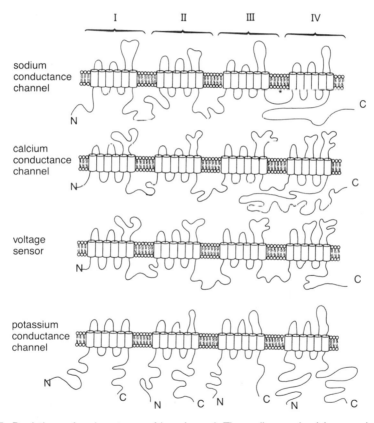

FIG. 18.7. Depictions of various types of ion channel. The sodium and calcium conductance channels are tetramers made up of the subunits shown in Fig. 18.5, which are numbered I–IV. The cytoplasmic loop linking subunits III and IV in the sodium channel (✳) is likely to represent the inactivation gate. The voltage sensor of the dyad may be a proteolytic product derived from the calcium conductance channel that has lost a large portion of its C-terminal amino acid sequence. The potassium conductance channel is also made up of four of the subunits, but in this channel these are not linked to each other through a continuous peptide chain. (Modified from Catterall, 1988.)

cytoplasmic peptide chain may represent the "ball" or "foot" that inactivates the channel, possibly by plugging the open channel (Fig. 18.4).

Channel Peptide Structure

The α-subunit of the sodium channel and the α_1-subunit of the calcium channel each contain four channel subunits linked together by peptide bonds that surround the water-filled channel pore (Figs. 18.6 and 18.7). The functional potassium channel also appears to consist of four channel subunits, but as already pointed out, these are not covalently bound to each other (Fig. 18.7). The α_1-peptide of the calcium channel binds to all three classes of calcium channel blocking drugs (dihydropyridines, benzothiazepines, and phenylakylamines), whereas the α-peptide of the sodium channel contains the binding site for tetrodotoxin. In both, these peptides also are substrates for adenosine $3'$, $5'$-cyclic monophosphate (cyclic AMP)–dependent protein kinases (Table 18.3).

Two forms of the large calcium channel α-peptide are found in muscle. A larger, 212,000 Da molecule, which contains sites for protein kinase A–catalyzed phosphorylation, is almost certainly the L-type channel responsible for the depolarizing inward calcium currents during the cardiac action potential (De Jongh et al., 1989). A smaller form of this molecule, which is similar to the larger peptide except that it lacks ~ 320 amino acids at the C-terminal end and so has a molecular weight of $\sim 175,000$, may represent the "voltage sensor" of the dyad that opens the calcium release channels of the sarcoplasmic reticulum (Chapter 11).

Less well understood are the many smaller peptides that are associated with, and appear to regulate, many of these channels (Table 18.3). Not all of these small peptides are expressed in the many channels found in nature; for example, functional sodium channels may contain zero, one or two β-peptides. Although the function of the β-peptides associated with the sodium channels is not yet known, many smaller channel peptides associated with the calcium channel appear to mediate a variety of signals. The β-peptide, like the α_2-peptide, is a substrate for protein kinase A, and when phosphorylated, activates the channel (Nunoki et al., 1989; Ruth et al., 1989). The Δ-peptide, which is encoded by the same gene as the α_2 peptide, is linked to the latter by disulfide bonds, which suggests that, like insulin and several other proteins that are derived from "proproteins," the Δ-peptide may be produced from a larger peptide by proteolysis during posttranslational processing (DeJongh et al., 1990). Yet another level of regulation is probably reflected in the ability of most of these peptides to be modified by posttranslational glycosylation.

REGULATION OF CHANNEL FUNCTION BY VARIABLE GENE EXPRESSION

Most of the remainder of this chapter and Chapter 19 follow the traditional *cell* approach to understanding the control of ion fluxes in the myocardium, and Chapter

20 centers on an analysis of the heart as an *organ*. However, it is likely that altered *gene* expression, the third paradigm of regulation, probably plays an important role in the "tonic" regulation of cardiac function described in Chapter 14. It is becoming apparent that the variability of ion channel structure described above is another example of the operation of the third paradigm listed in Table 14.1 because all of the ion-selective channels are members of multigene families, and most are made of several peptides that can be modified extensively at a posttranscriptional level by alternate splicing. As we have seen in many other systems, therefore, myocardial cells can select from among a number of different gene products in synthesizing each type of ion-specific channel.

The significance of so many different forms of these channels is just now coming into focus. Many are tissue-specific; for example, sodium channels differ in the brain and various muscle types. Others change during growth and development as in muscles that express different sodium channels at different times during ontogeny (Kallen et al., 1990). Most striking is the plasticity of the potassium channels which, as pointed out above, appear to be made up of many different combinations of four of the basic channel subunits. Although all functional potassium channels are tetramers made up of different combinations of these basic subunits, the four subunits of the potassium channel are *not* linked covalently.

The variability of potassium channels has been studied most extensively in a number of mutants in *Drosophila,* where potassium channels can be both homo- and heterotetramers assembled from a vast family of channel subunits that are derived from alternate splicing (Timpe et al., 1988). Furthermore, it now appears that a large variety of heteromultimeric potassium channels can be synthesized by "mixing and matching" different members of this large family of genetically variable basic subunits (Agnew, 1988; Aldrich, 1990). The result is a capacity for functional diversity in the potassium channels that could allow for the existence of hundreds, indeed thousands, of potassium channel subtypes! This remarkable plasticity of potassium channels may explain why there has been so much difficulty in characterizing the repolarizing currents in the heart (Chapter 19).

Synthesis of abnormal potassium channels in the response of the heart to stress may explain several puzzling electrocardiographic T-wave abnormalities (the T waves, as described in Chapter 20, are generated by potential differences that appear during ventricular repolarization). These abnormalities include "posttachycardia T-wave changes" and "T-wave evolution" after an acute myocardial infarction (heart attack). In both, a prolonged sequence of T-wave changes follows a transient event that lasts a few hours. In the case of the posttachycardia T-wave changes, the stimulus is an episode of rapid beating that ends when rhythm is restored to normal, whereas T-wave evolution follows a period of cell injury that ends when the injured cells either die or begin to heal. Both are commonly followed by repolarization abnormalities that not only can evolve clinically over several days, or even weeks, but can, before beginning their slow return toward normal, become more pronounced for several days after the termination of the precipitating event. Although long-lasting biochemical changes could explain the slow appearance and disappearance of these repolarization abnormalities, it is possible that they might, instead, appear when abnormal potassium channels are synthesized as part of the heart's response to stress (Chapter 25).

SINGLE CHANNEL RECORDINGS

Techniques for the study of the opening and closing of single channels have revolutionized our understanding of the control of ion fluxes across biological membranes. The ability to record the behavior of *single ion channel molecules,* both in natural membranes and after they have been reconstituted into synthetic bilayers, has revealed a complexity unimaginable when the first edition of this text was written in 1977.

A typical recording from a single calcium channel, depicted in Fig. 18.8, shows that shortly after the application of a current that depolarizes the membrane from -20 mV to $+50$ mV, the channel quickly flickers into and out of its open state. As shown in Fig. 18.8, channel opening and closing are extremely rapid events; as a result, the more languid appearance and decline in the ion currents thus gives us no information whatsoever about the rates of these transitions among channel states. Instead, as described below, the ionic currents—which simply represent the sum of all channel openings at any moment—are determined by the probability of finding individual channels in their open state.

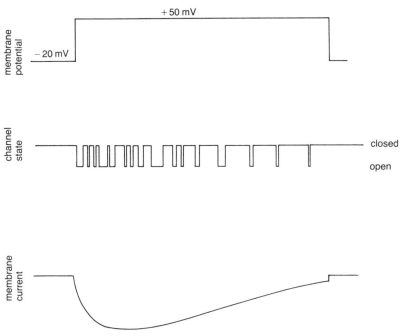

FIG. 18.8. Response of a single calcium channel to membrane depolarization. When the membrane (*upper tracing*) is depolarized from -20 to $+50$ mV, the channel begins to alternate between its closed and open states (*middle tracing*). Later, during the period of continued depolarization, the channel tends to open less frequently so that membrane current (*lower tracing*), after its initial increase (downward deflection), begins to fall even though membrane potential remains the same.

When cells are stimulated by prolonged depolarizing currents, with time the channel openings become less frequent and eventually cease. Stated another way, immediately after the membrane is depolarized, the *probability* that the channel will be in an open state initially increases, but with prolonged depolarization this probability decreases. These changes in probability explain why the membrane current associated with these channel openings, after quickly increasing to a maximum, slowly subsides.

STATES OF AN ION CHANNEL

Studies of single channel conductances have greatly added to our understanding of the relationship between the open and closed states of the ion channels (see above) and the resulting properties of the ionic currents responsible for the cardiac action potential. As already pointed out, the slow appearance of an ionic current (lower tracing in Fig. 18.8) does not tell us much about the rate of channel openings, which are actually very rapid (middle tracing). Changes in the magnitude and time course of an ionic current are, in fact, generally not due to changes in the magnitude or speed of channel openings, but instead reflect changes in the *probability* that the channel will be found in an open state. An increase in any ionic current can occur if the channels begin their openings sooner after the stimulus, open more frequently, or continue to open for a longer period before they are inactivated. The molecular mechanisms responsible for these probability changes, and what structure(s) determine this property of the channel, are still not known.

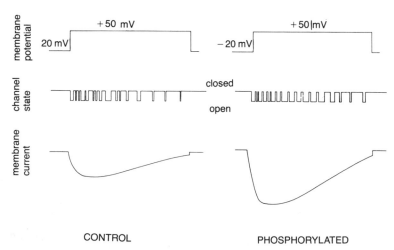

FIG. 18.9. Response of a single calcium channel to phosphorylation by a cyclic AMP–dependent protein kinase. In response to the same depolarization (*upper tracing*), the calcium channel spends more time in its open state (*middle tracing*) so that membrane current (*lower tracing*) is increased.

Changes in the probability of channel opening are of considerable physiological importance. For example, phosphorylation of the calcium channel, which as noted in Chapter 14 plays a vital role in the response to exercise, promotes calcium entry not by increasing the rate of channel opening or the current that it carries when open, but instead by increasing the probability that the channel will be in an open state after the membrane is depolarized (Fig. 18.9).

The earlier concept that voltage-sensitive ion channels could exist in three functional states—open, closed (resting), and closed (inactivated) (see above)—has been modified on the basis of analyses of single channel recordings. For example, different members of one class of calcium channel blocking drugs, the dihydropridines, can either activate or inhibit calcium channel opening. Actually, many of these drugs do both, and at the same time! These puzzling responses are now known to reflect the ability of the drugs to modify differently the transitions among three states of the calcium channel (Hess et al., 1984). In addition to the closed state (mode 0) described earlier in this chapter, there are two ways the channel can flicker in the open state: brief openings (mode 1), and long-lasting openings (mode 2) (Fig. 18.10). As the transition from mode 1 to mode 2 can also occur spontaneously, in the absence of any drugs (Bean, 1990; Mazzanti and DeFelice, 1990), it is evident that these two modes of opening are, in fact, natural states of the channels. The effects of the drugs, therefore, are to modify the probability that the channels will be in one or another of these states.

Another recently discovered property of single channels is their ability to exist in open states that differ not in the duration of opening as described above, but in the amplitude of the current that they allow to cross the membrane. These different

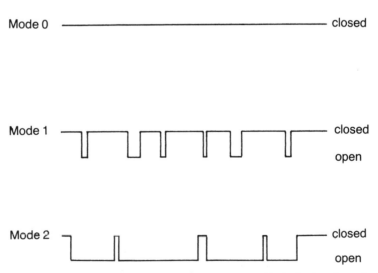

FIG. 18.10. Different modes of opening of a calcium channel. Mode 0: closed; mode 1: brief openings; mode 2: long-lasting openings.

conductance states may arise from graded interactions among the channel subunits. Although different conductance states of a single channel have, so far, been identified only in two types of the intracellular calcium release channel described in Chapter 11 (Smith et al., 1988; Watras et al., 1991), it may well be that varying current flux through different conductance states of open plasma membrane channels provides yet another means for regulating membrane voltage.

The transitions between opening modes, and probably also conductance states, provide an incredibly elaborate means by which ion currents can be controlled at the level of the *cell*. Thus, besides increasing the probability of channel opening, the phosphorylation reactions initiated by β-adrenergic agonists appear also to favor the appearance of long-lasting openings (mode 2) (Yue et al., 1990). This suggests that the opening of cardiac plasma membrane calcium channels, and so both the cardiac action potential and myocardial contractility, is regulated physiologically by transitions between these modes. In addition, evidence has been presented that the long-lasting openings are more likely in the response to strong depolarizations (Pietrobon and Hess, 1990); this observation, it should be noted, contradicts the "all-or-none" law discussed in Chapter 14.

ION PERMEATION THROUGH CHANNELS

One of the fundamental properties of membrane channels is their selectivity; that is, sodium channels conduct sodium ions, calcium channels conduct calcium ions, etc. Although this selectivity is not perfect, the preferences of different channels for one or another ion is strong. Thus, even though there is almost a 100-fold greater concentration of sodium than calcium ions in the extracellular fluid, the high selectivity of calcium channels allows them to conduct mainly calcium. Ion size cannot account for this selectivity because if size was the major determinant, all channels would be expected to select for the smallest ions. A more likely explanation is that the preferred ions bind specifically to sites within the channel in a manner that allows only those ions that interact with this site to enter the channel. One model is shown in Fig. 18.11, in which two ions are shown within a channel that is selective for the ion species shown. Because other types of ion cannot bind to the sites within the channel, they are unable to displace the preferred species. This model is in accord with other evidence that the preferred ions move in single file through the channel from the region of high concentration to that of low ion concentration. This direction of flux, of course, is favored because the ions that enter the channel from the side of the membrane containing the higher ion concentration are most likely to displace ions already bound within the channel. The model shown in Fig. 18.11 thus explains selectivity as arising from the requirement that each ion species bind to specific sites within the channel. The reason that other ions cannot use the channel is simply that the preferred ion bound specifically within the channel excludes other ions by electrostatic repulsion.

The relationships between channel structure and channel function described in

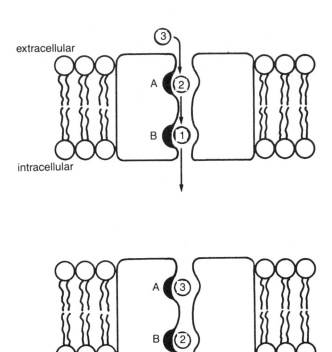

FIG. 18.11. Model to explain ion selectivity in a calcium channel. Calcium ions (*numbered circles*) move in single file through the channel while interacting with two calcium-binding sites (*A* and *B*). In order for a calcium ion to enter the channel (3, above), the ions bound within the channel (1 and 2) must be displaced as shown by the *arrows*.

this chapter are useful in understanding normal cardiac electrophysiology (Chapter 19) and pathophysiology (Chapters 21–23). This is apparent in the next chapter, when we refer to these ion channels as the basis for the currents that give rise to the cardiac action potential.

REFERENCES

Agnew WS. (1988). A Rosetta stone for K channels. *Nature* 331:114–115.

Aldrich RW. (1989). Ion channels. Mutating and gating. *Nature* 339:578–579.

Aldrich RW. (1990). Potassium channels. Mixing and Matching. *Nature* 345:475–476.

Bean B. (1990). Calcium channels. Gating for the physiologist. *Nature* 348:192–193.

Catterall WA. (1988). Structure and function of voltage-sensitive ion channels. *Science* 242:50–61.

De Jongh KS, Merrick DK, Catterall WA. (1989). Subunits of purified calcium channels. A 212-kDa form of α_1 and partial amino acid sequence of a phosphorylation site of an independent β subunit. *Proc Natl Acad Sci USA* 86:8585–8589.

De Jongh KS, Warner C, Catterall WA. (1990). Subunits of purified calcium channels. α_2 and Δ are encoded by the same gene. *J Biol Chem* 265:14738–14741.

Hess P, Lansman JB, Tsien RW. (1984). Different modes of Ca channel gating behaviour favoured by dihydropyridine calcium agonists and antagonists. *Nature* 311:538–544.

Hodgkin AL, Huxley AF (1952). A quantitative description of membrane current and its application to conduction and excitation in nerve. *J Physiol (Lond)* 117:500–544.

Kallen RG, Sheng Z-H, Yang J, Chen L, Rogart RB, Barchi RL. (1990). Primary structure and expression of a sodium channel characteristic of denervated and immature rat skeletal muscle. *Neuron* 4:233–242.

Mazzanti M, DeFelice LJ. (1990). Ca channel gating during cardiac action potentials. *Biophys J* 58:1059–1065.

Noda M, Ikeda T, Kayano T, Suzuki H, Takeshima H, Kurasaki M, Takahashi H, Numa S. (1986). Existence of distinct sodium channel messenger RNAs in rat brain. *Nature* 320:188–192.

Nunoki K, Florio V, Catterall WA. (1989). Activation of purified calcium channels by stoichiometric protein phosphorylation. *Proc Natl Acad Sci USA* 86:6816–6820.

Pietrobon D, Hess P. (1990). Novel mechanism of voltage-dependent gating of L-type calcium channels. *Nature* 346:651–655.

Ruth P, Röhrkasten A, Biel M, Bosse E, Regulla S, Meyer HE, Flockerzi V, Hoffman F. (1989). Primary structure of the β subunit of the DHP-sensitive calcium channel from skeletal muscle. *Science* 245:1115–1118.

Smith JS, Imagawa T, Ma J, Fill M, Campbell K, Coronado R. (1988). Purified ryanodine receptor from rabbit skeletal muscle is the calcium release channel of sarcoplasmic reticulum. *J Gen Physiol* 92:1–26.

Stümer W, Conti F, Suzuki H, Wang X, Noda M, Yahagi N, Kubo H, Numa S. (1989). Structural parts involved in activation and inactivation of the sodium channel. *Nature* 239:597–603.

Tlmpe LC, Schwartz TL, Tempel BL, Papazian DM, Jan YN, Jan LY. (1988). Expression of functional potassium channels from *Shaker* cDNA in *Xenopus* oocytes. *Nature* 331:143–145.

Watras J, Bczprozvanny I, Ehrlich BE. (1991). Inositol 1,4,5-trisphosphate-gated channels in cerebellum presence of multiple conductance states. *J Neurosci*, In Press.

Yue DT, Hertzig S, Marban E. (1990) β-adrenergic stimulation of Ca channels occurs by potentiation of high-activity gating modes. *Proc Natl Acad Sci USA* 87:753–757.

BIBLIOGRAPHY

Armstrong CM. (1981). Sodium channels and gating currents. *Physiol Rev* 61:644–683.

Barchi RL. (1988). Probing the molecular structure of the voltage-dependent sodium channel. *Annu Rev Neurosci* 11:455–495.

Hille B. (1984). *Ionic channels of excitable membranes.* Sunderland, MA: Sinauer Associates.

Mikami A, Imoto K, Tanabe T, Niidome T, Mori Y, Takeshima H, Narumiya S, Numa S. (1989). Primary structure and functional expression of the cardiac dihydropyridine-sensitive calcium channel. *Nature* 340:230–233.

Nilius B. (1989). Gating properties and modulation of Na channels. *News in Physiol Sci* 4:225–230.

Perez-Reyes E, Kim HS, Lacerda AE, Horne W, Wei X, Rampe D, Campbell K, Brown A, Birnbaumer L. (1989). Induction of calcium currents by the expression of the α_1-subunit of the dihydropyridine receptor from skeletal muscle. *Nature* 340:233–236.

Rehm H, Lazdunski M. (1988). Purification and subunit structure of a putative K^+ channel protein identified by its binding properties for dendrotoxin I. *Proc Natl Acad Sci USA* 85:4919–4923.

Tsien RW, Hess P, McClesky EW, Rosenberg RL. (1987). Calcium channels: mechanisms of selectivity, permeation and block. *Annu Rev Biophys Biophys Chem* 16:265–290.

19

The Cardiac Action Potential

The generalization that all processes in the heart are at least an order of magnitude more complex (and interesting) than the corresponding mechanisms in skeletal muscle is clearly illustrated when we examine the morphology and ionic basis of the cardiac action potential. In skeletal muscle, as in nerve, the action potential is a brief, biphasic event in which rapid depolarization is quickly followed by restoration of the resting potential (Fig. 19.1). With the exception of a low-amplitude afterpotential, this entire process requires no more than a few milliseconds. In the heart, on the other hand, the action potential lasts longer, consists of several phases, and varies in its characteristics from region to region. In Purkinje fibers, for example, large action potentials last over 300 msec and include at least five distinct phases (Fig. 19.2), whereas in nodal cells the action potential is smaller and often exhibits spontaneous diastolic depolarization.

The upstroke of the cardiac action potential (phase 0) is extremely rapid in the cells of the His-Purkinje system and the working cells of the atria and ventricles, as it is in nerve and skeletal muscle; however, depolarization is much slower in nodal cells. This difference, which is discussed later in this chapter, arises because different channels carry the initial inward depolarizing currents in these regions of the heart.

Depolarization of the His-Purkinje system and working cells of the atria and ventricles is followed by two phases that do not have clear counterparts in nerve and skeletal muscle. A brief phase of early repolarization (phase 1) is followed by a plateau (phase 2) that is largely responsible for the long duration of the cardiac action potential. Repolarization (phase 3) corresponds to the repolarization phase of the action potentials in nerve and skeletal muscle, and resting potential (phase 4) in all cardiac cells, as in other excitable cells, is determined mainly by the potassium equilibrium potential (see below). The ion fluxes responsible for the complex series of events during the cardiac action potentials are generally similar to those in nerve and skeletal muscle, but many significant differences exist. These specializations in the cardiac sarcolemma give rise to important clinical features of both normal and abnormal electrocardiograms.

Action potentials are generated by the opening and closing of ion channels in the

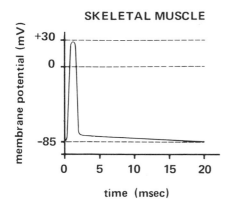

FIG. 19.1. The skeletal muscle action potential is a brief biphasic event in which rapid depolarization (upward deflection) is quickly followed by repolarization (downward deflection). A small positive afterpotential causes an approximately 10-msec delay prior to return of the membrane potential to its resting level of −85 mV.

heart's plasma membrane. During diastole, potassium channels are open, whereas channels that are selective for sodium, chloride, and calcium are closed. In other words, g_K is high and g_{Na}, g_{Cl}, and g_{Ca} are low. Sequential changes in these ion conductances (g), caused by changing states of the ion channels described in Chapter 18, are responsible for the complex characteristics of the cardiac action potential.

IONIC BASIS FOR RESTING MEMBRANE POTENTIAL (PHASE 4)

As pointed out in Chapter 18, the fact that intracellular K^+ concentration is higher than that in the extracellular fluid (Table 19.1) was known long before membrane potentials were first measured. Furthermore, the similarity between the electrical potential predicted on the basis of the potassium ion gradient across the plasma membrane and observed resting potentials was recognized in the earliest recordings of membrane potentials.

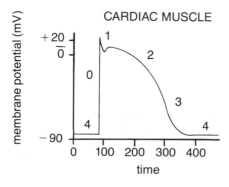

FIG. 19.2. The cardiac action potential (shown here for a Purkinje fiber) lasts over 300 msec and consists of five phases. Phase 0 (the upstroke) corresponds to depolarization, and phase 3 (repolarization) to repolarization in skeletal muscle. Phases 1 (early repolarization) and 2 (plateau) have no clear counterpart in skeletal muscle, and phase 4 (diastole) corresponds to the resting potential.

TABLE 19.1. *Ion activities inside and outside the mammalian heart*

Ion	Intracellular concentration	Intracellular activity	Extracellular concentration	Extracellular activity
Sodium	5–34	8	140	110
Potassium	104–180	100	5.4	4
Chloride	8–79	15	100	75
Calcium		0.0002	3	1

Values are in mM. Data for all intracellular values except calcium are selected from Walker (1986); calcium data are from Blinks (1986). The activities in this table are "averages" weighted arbitrarily by the author for use in various equations.

Donnan Equilibrium in the Resting Cell

The resting potential of the myocardial cell is directly related to the electrochemical gradient for potassium across the plasma membrane (Fig. 19.3), which is maintained largely by the Na-K-ATPase (Chapter 10), which pumps sodium out of the cell in exchange for the potassium that is concentrated within the cell.

Because many of the heart's potassium channels are in their open state at negative (intracellular) potentials, the resting plasma membrane is permeable to potassium; accordingly, potassium tends to move down its concentration gradient and so leaks out of the cell. However, as potassium ions leave the cell, they carry positive charge across the plasma membrane; this outward current (Chapter 18) creates an electrical potential difference across the plasma membrane in which the cytosol is negatively charged. Because the cytosol contains large anions to which the plasma membrane is impermeable, notably proteins and organic phosphates, a Donnan equilibrium is established. In this equilibrium, $[Cl^-]_i$ is lower than $[Cl^-]_o$, $[K^+]_o$ is higher than $[K^+]_i$, and the cytosol is negatively charged. This equilibrium establishes a balance between the potassium concentration gradient, which favors potassium efflux, and the electronegativity of the cell interior, which favors potassium influx.

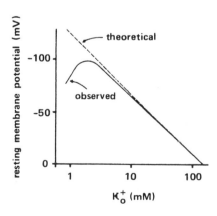

FIG. 19.3. Relationship between potassium concentration outside the myocardial cell (K^+_o) and resting membrane potential. Changing extracellular potassium at normal and high K^+_o levels causes membrane potential (*solid line*) to respond in a manner that closely approximates the predicitions of the Nernst equation for potassium (*dashed line*). However, at low K^+_o levels, reduced extracellular potassium causes an unexpected decrease in membrane potential because potassium permeability falls.

There are two important exceptions to the statement that the potential difference of the resting cell is due to the potassium ion gradient. The first is a small, but finite, permeability to sodium ion. Because Na^+ concentration is much higher outside the cell, any open sodium channels would favor a membrane potential opposite in polarity to that associated with the potassium gradient (see below). Second, two electrogenic ion exchanges described in Chapter 10 also contribute to the resting potential; these are the sodium pump and sodium/calcium exchange, both of which make a small contribution to resting potential. Interestingly, the currents that they create are opposite in direction. The sodium pump generates an outward current because three sodium ions move out of the cell in exchange for two potassium ions. The sodium/calcium exchanger, which exchanges one calcium ion for three sodium ions, generates a small inward current during diastole, when the electronegative cytosol favors sodium influx as described in Chapter 10.

The Nernst and Goldman-Hodgkin-Katz Equations

Both the Nernst equation and the Goldman-Hodgkin-Katz equation define the relationship between ion concentrations and membrane potential, so that they provide a basis for calculating the membrane potentials at steady states where there is no net flux of ions through the ion channels described in Chapter 18. These equations do not, therefore, apply when there are net ion fluxes across the membrane, as occurs during an action potential.

The Nernst Equation

The equilibrium between an ion concentration difference and the potential across a semipermeable membrane is given by the Nernst equation:

$$E_m = \frac{RT}{zF} \ln \frac{Pa_o}{Pa_i} \qquad [19.1]$$

where E_m is the membrane potential, R the gas constant, T the absolute temperature, z the valence of the ion, F the Faraday constant, P the permeability to the ion, and a_o and a_i the activities of the ion outside and inside the membrane. Activities rather than concentrations must be used in these equations as the latter include immobilized or bound ions.

In the case of the alkali metal ions, Na^+ and K^+, $z=1$, so that for a freely permeable membrane $(P=1)$ at 37°C, the constants in the Nernst equation can be written for ordinary (base 10) logarithms as

$$E_m = 61.5 \log a_o/a_i. \qquad [19.2]$$

Equation 19.2 states that a tenfold difference in the activity of a monovalent cation, where $a_o/a_i = 10$, produces a potential difference of $+61.5$ mV. If a_o/a_i is 0.1, E_m is -61.5 mV.

In resting cardiac muscle, where $[K^+]_o$ is ~5.4 mM and $[K^+]_i$ is ~120 mM, the corresponding potassium ion activities are approximately 4 and 100 mM (Table 19.1). Thus, if the resting myocardium were freely permeable to K^+ and impermeable to all other ions for which a concentration gradient exists between the inside and outside of the cell, E_m would equal E_K according to the following Nernst equation:

$$E_m = 61.5 \times \log \frac{4}{100} = -86 \text{ mV}. \qquad [19.3]$$

Because resting potential is close to that predicted by the Nernst equation for potassium in most regions of the heart, variations in extracellular potassium, according to Eq 19.3, directly influence resting potential. Increased extracellular potassium causes depolarization, whereas reduction in extracellular potassium tends to hyperpolarize the membrane. Resting potential does not, however, follow the Nernst equation for potassium when extracellular potassium is very low (Fig. 19.3). When extracellular potassium is less than ~3 mM, the extent of hyperpolarization is less than that predicted by the Nernst equation because hypokalemia reduces potassium permeability (P_K), which allows the limited permeability to other ions, notably sodium, and electrogenic ion pumps and exchangers to have a greater influence on membrane potential (see below).

The Goldman-Hodgkin-Katz Equation

Membrane potential is calculated more accurately by the Goldman-Hodgkin-Katz equation, which takes into account the permeabilities (P) and activities (a) of all ion species that could contribute to membrane potential. For a membrane permeable to sodium and chloride, as well as to potassium, this equation is:

$$E_m = \frac{RT}{zF} \ln \frac{P_K a_{K_o} + P_{Na} a_{Na_o} + P_{Cl} a_{Cl_i}}{P_K a_{K_i} + P_{Na} a_{Na_i} + P_{Cl} a_{Cl_o}}. \qquad [19.4]$$

This equation highlights two important facts. The first is that the contribution of any ion to the membrane potential is determined both by the activity gradient across the membrane, and by the permeability of the membrane to that ion. The second important feature of Eq. 19.4 is that it shows how membrane potential is determined both by activity gradients and permeability. This is obvious since either an absent activity gradient or zero permeability would cancel the contribution of any ion to E_m.

THE "TYPICAL" CARDIAC ACTION POTENTIAL .

Cardiac contraction is initiated by a regenerative action potential that is propagated throughout the heart. Some structures are specialized for rapid conduction, notably the Purkinje fibers in the bundle of His, the bundle branches, and their arborizations within the ventricular endocardium. It is essential to appreciate that *all impulses in the heart are transmitted between muscle cells.* The cardiac nerves, which arise from the sympathetic and parasympathetic nervous system (Chapter 1), serve only to modulate myocardial performance and do not participate in the propagation of the wave of excitation over the heart.

As action potentials differ in different regions of the heart, the following discussion focuses on the action potential of the Purkinje fiber, in which the ionic basis for the electrical events during depolarization has been studied most extensively.

The Upstroke (Phase 0)

The similarity between resting potential and the Nernst potential for potassium, along with the observation that activation decreases membrane potential, led early investigators to conclude that depolarization of excited cells was due mainly to a fall in potassium permeability. As described in Chapter 18, however, the first intracellular microelectrode recordings of membrane potential made it quite clear that changes other than a fall in potassium permeability excited the heart. These recordings showed that membrane potential did not simply decrease toward zero during the action potential, as would be expected if potassium permeability fell to a low value; but instead, membrane potential *reversed* at the height of the action potential (Figs. 19.1 and 19.2). The appearance of a positive intracellular potential at the peak of the action potential could only be explained if membrane potential came to be influenced by the transmembrane distribution of another ion, as described in the Goldman-Hodgkin-Katz equation (Eq. 19.4). This other ion is, of course, sodium.

The Nernst potential for sodium, which is present at higher concentration in the extracellular fluid than in the cell interior (Table 19.1), would cause membrane potentials opposite in polarity to those caused by that for potassium ion. Reversal of membrane potential at the peak of the action potential therefore occurs because potassium permeability becomes low and sodium permeability high. This is apparent in a simplified Goldman-Hodgkin-Katz equation that describes the dependence of membrane potential on both potassium and sodium:

$$E_m \sim \frac{P_K a_{K_o} + P_{Na} a_{Na_o}}{P_K a_{K_i} + P_{Na} a_{Na_i}}. \qquad [19.5]$$

Depolarization in most, but not all, regions of the heart is determined largely by inward sodium currents through ion channels that, when open, have a reversal potential that approaches the Nernst potential determined by the sodium gradient across the plasma membrane (Table 19.1). As extracellular Na^+ concentration is ~140 mM, which corresponds to an activity of ~110 mM, whereas intracellular sodium activity is ~8 mM, the Nernst equation for sodium predicts a positive membrane potential of +70 mV:

$$E_m = 61.5 \times \log \frac{110}{8} = +70 \text{ mV}. \qquad [19.6]$$

The fact that the action potential does not reach the high level of positivity predicted by Eq. 19.6 indicates that the sodium channel opening and potassium channel closing are not complete.

The increased sodium permeability in the depolarized cell means that the opening of the sodium channels is *voltage dependent*; that is, the extent of channel opening depends on membrane potential. Small subthreshold depolarizations cause only limited activation (opening) of the sodium channels. Greater depolarization, by opening more sodium channels, initiates an inward (depolarizing) current sufficiently large to overwhelm the potassium conductance, thereby causing the regenerative depolarization that is responsible for the upstroke (phase 0) of the action potential.

> As discussed later in this chapter, the cells of the sinoatrial and atrioventricular nodes either lack sodium channels, or, if present, they do not function under physiological conditions. In these more primitive cells (as defined in Chapter 18), the initial inward, depolarizing, currents are carried by calcium ions.

At this point a common misconception must be dismissed: that the concentration gradients for sodium and potassium across the plasma membrane are dissipated during the action potential. In fact, each depolarization causes only a very small fraction of cellular potassium to be exchanged for sodium. As a result, even when the Na-K-ATPase is poisoned, a number of action potentials can be generated before the cell gains a significant amount of sodium or loses a measurable amount of the intracellular potassium. Although rapid stimulation does produce a measurable gain of sodium in the cytosol, intracellular Na^+ activity increases only about 10% when sheep Purkinje fibers are stimulated at steady-state frequencies of 2 Hz (Cohen et al., 1982).

Threshold

The threshold for a regenerative response reflects the fact that small membrane depolarizations initiate only a limited opening of ion channels that carry inward (depolarizing) current (Fig. 19.4). The potential at which these inward currents suffice to initiate a regenerative action potential is the "threshold." When the extent of depolarization exceeds this threshold, the opening of enough sodium channels (or in nodal cells, calcium channels) brings the adjacent membrane to the threshold where further sodium channel opening continues membrane depolarization, even after the initial depolarizing stimulus has ended. In other words, once threshold is reached, inward ionic currents take over, allowing subsequent depolarization to become independent of the initial depolarizing stimulus (C in Fig. 19.4).

Levels of depolarization that fail to reach threshold (A and B in Fig. 19.4) do not initiate an action potential; instead, after a limited number of sodium channels open in the partially depolarized cell, these channels become inactivated (or refractory, see below). The resulting decrease in sodium permeability returns membrane potential to its resting level, so that no propagated wave of depolarization is initiated.

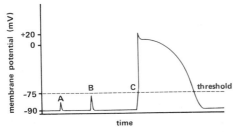

FIG. 19.4. Threshold for initiation of an action potential. Small depolarizing stimuli (*A* and *B*) that fail to reach threshold (*dashed line*) are unable to initiate an action potential, whereas a depolarization that reaches threshold (*C*) produces a regenerative action potential in which subsequent depolarization becomes independent of the intial stimulus.

Amplitude and Rate of Rise of the Action Potential

The rapidity of depolarization during the upstroke of the action potential (*dV/dt*) reflects the rate at which cations enter the cell through plasma membrane ion channels. The large inward current in the Purkinje fiber, which develops rapidly and so is often referred to as the fast inward current, depends on the influx of sodium ions through the sodium channels. Similarly, the large action potentials in the working cells of the atria and ventricles reflect the rapid and transient opening of sodium channels.

The fact that the fast inward current in these cells is carried by sodium ions is readily demonstrated by its disappearance when sodium in the medium bathing the myocardium is replaced by an impermeant ion like choline. Tetrodotoxin (TTX), a poison derived from a Japanese puffer fish, is useful for studying the ionic basis of the action potential because TTX, which binds to the α-peptide of the sodium channel, has a specific action that blocks the passage of sodium through this channel and so inhibits the fast inward current.

As nodal cells lack functional sodium channels, their depolarization depends on a much slower increase in the activation of the open state of the "smaller" (lower conductance) calcium channels (see below). These differences are of considerable clinical importance because, as discussed in Chapter 21, both the rate of rise and amplitude of the action potential are critical determinants of conduction velocity.

Inactivation of Sodium Channels

The closing and inactivation of the sodium channels in Purkinje cells, like their opening, are under the control of membrane potential. Thus, these channels are similar to the sodium channels of the squid axon, in which closure of inactivation (h) gates in the depolarized cell terminates the inward current (Chapter 18). As in the squid axon, when the cardiac channels close, they become inactivated, which means that they cannot be reopened until after the membrane is repolarized. Thus, the cell becomes refractory in that it is unable to respond to a stimulus that, in the fully rested cell, would produce a regenerative action potential (see below). Although sodium channels are rapidly inactivated by depolarization, return of their ability to reopen (called reactivation) is slow, even in the fully repolarized cell.

The inability of sodium channels to respond to a second stimulus during and immediately after depolarization is due initially to the long-lasting plateau of the cardiac action potential (Fig. 19.2), which prevents membrane potential from returning toward the resting levels at which the sodium channels reactivate. The slow recovery of the ability to transmit an action potential depends not only on the extent of repolarization, but also on the time elapsed since the preceding depolarization. The requirement that the heart repolarize before the sodium channels recover their ability to reopen means that reactivation is *voltage-dependent*. The additional requirement that sufficient time elapse to allow for the slow recovery of the channel means that reactivation is also *time-dependent*.

Voltage-Dependence of Inactivation

Because depolarization not only opens m gates (activation) but also closes h gates (inactivation), subthreshold depolarizing currents inhibit the subsequent ability of the sodium channels to generate a fast inward sodium current. Similar voltage-dependent inactivation is seen in cells whose depolarization depends on calcium channels, except that the latter require greater degrees of depolarization both to activate and inactivate (see below).

The fact that depolarization leads to closure of the h gates explains why the level of resting potential immediately prior to stimulation is an important determinant of the rate and extent of sodium channel opening. At highly polarized resting potentials, in the normal range between − 80 and − 90mV, stimuli that rapidly depolarize the membrane cause rapid opening of sodium channels. The result is an action potential with a rapid upstroke and a large amplitude (Fig. 19.5a). If, however, the cell is partially depolarized to potentials around − 70 mV, a similar depolarizing stimulus produces a smaller, more slowly rising action potential (Fig. 19.5b). This is because the prior subthreshold depolarization has inactivated some of the sodium channels by closing their h gates.

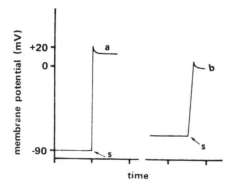

FIG. 19.5. The rate and extent of depolarization depend on the resting membrane potential prior to stimulation. A large, rapidly rising action potential is produced by a stimulus (S) when the resting membrane potential is high (a), whereas partial depolarization prior to stimulation (b) causes the same stimulus to produce a small, slowly rising action potential. These changes in the action potential upstroke reflect the voltage-dependent closing of the inactivation (h) gates of the sodium channels.

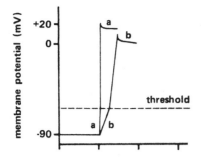

FIG. 19.6. The rate and extent of depolarization depend in part on the rate at which membrane potential approaches threshold. A large, rapidly rising action potential is produced when the stimulus reaches threshold rapidly (a), whereas a stimulus that slowly reaches threshold produces a small, slowly rising action potential (b). These changes in the rate of rise and size of the action potential reflect the voltage-dependent inactivation of the sodium channels.

Voltage-dependent sodium channel inactivation is also apparent when threshold is approached at a slow rate. If threshold is reached quickly, sodium conductance develops rapidly and completely so that the upstroke of the action potential is rapid and the amplitude high (Fig. 19.6a). If, however, threshold is approached very slowly, voltage-dependent closure of the h gates, by reducing both the rate and extent of the depolarizing sodium currents, gives rise to a smaller action potential with a slow upstroke (Fig. 19.6h).

These and other manifestations of the voltage-dependent inactivation of depolarizing currents can slow impulse propagation and produce conduction block in the intact heart; they are therefore of considerable importance in the genesis of clinical arrhythmias (Chapter 21).

Time-Dependence of Inactivation

Premature activation of the heart, before the sodium channels have had an opportunity to recover fully from the preceding depolarization, also produces small and slowly rising action potentials. This is because, unlike the rapid—almost explosive—opening of the m gates during the upstroke of the action potential, reopening of the h gates is slow shortly after repolarization, and can take up to 100 msec or more immediately after membrane potential has returned to its resting level. Some antiarrhythmic drugs reduce excitability by increasing this delay in sodium channel reactivation (Chapter 23).

Early Repolarization (Phase 1)

A brief phase of rapid repolarization that follows the peak of the cardiac action potential, often called phase 1, is due in part to the fall in sodium permeability discussed above. In addition to the decreased inward sodium current, two outward currents appear to contribute to early repolarization. One, the *transient outward current* or *positive dynamic current*, which is carried by potassium, is discussed later, along with other potassium currents. The second is a less well-defined *outward chloride current* caused by a transient increase in chloride permeability.

Because extracellular Cl^- activity is ~ 75 mM, which is about five times higher than that inside the cell (~ 15 mM) (Table 19.1), opening of chloride channels would allow this anion to flow into the cell and so generate an outward current (Chapter 20). A highly regulated chloride current has been found to be activated by β-adrenergic agonists and inhibited by the muscarinic agonist acetylcholine (Bahinski et al., 1989, Harvey et al., 1990). Although the role of this outward chloride current is still not clear, it is strategically timed so as to be able to influence action potential duration; for example, activation of this outward current by adenosine 3', 5'-cyclic monophosphate (cyclic AMP) would be able to accelerate repolarization and so could contribute to the well-known ability of sympathetic stimulation to abbreviate the cardiac action potential.

The Plateau (Phase 2)

The most distinctive feature of depolarization in heart muscle is the plateau, which is responsible for the prolonged cardiac action potential. The stability of membrane potential at or near zero for well over 100 msec (compare Fig. 19.2 with 19.1) could have two explanations: an overall decrease in the ionic currents flowing between the inside of the cell and the extracellular fluid, or a balance between inward and outward currents across the plasma membrane. In fact, both explanations apply.

More than 20 years ago Weidmann showed that membrane conductance was relatively high during the early portion of the plateau, but then fell toward the end of this phase of the action potential. This is now known to result from parallel declines in inward and outward currents, both of which are high at the beginning of the plateau but then decrease until another outward current completes repolarization. The inward current that is high early during the plateau is the calcium current described in the following paragraphs. The outward current that follows a similar time course, declining during the plateau, is a potassium current called the anomalous, or inward, rectifier (see below).

A depolarizing (inward) current that appears at the beginning of the plateau is carried by calcium ions that enter the cell through the calcium conductance channels described in Chapter 18. This current, often called the slow inward current, is activated at more depolarized membrane potentials than the sodium current; that is, the cell must be depolarized to a greater extent than needed to activate the inward sodium current (Table 19.2). Because the calcium channels are not inactivated by partial depolarizations that close the h gates of the sodium channels, this calcium current can generate slow action potentials in partially depolarized cells.

The distribution of calcium across the membrane, like that of sodium, causes an inward (depolarizing) current when the membrane becomes permeable to this cation because extracellular Ca^{2+} activity is ~ 1 mM, whereas during diastole cytosolic Ca^{2+} is ~ 0.2 μM (0.0002 mM). The 5,000-fold activity gradient for calcium, according to the Nernst equation, would generate an equilibrium potential of approximately $+114$ mV:

TABLE 19.2. *Comparison of sodium and calcium inward currents*

Property	Sodium channel	Calcium channel
Threshold (mV)	− 60	− 35
Activation time constant (msec)	~1	5–20
Inactivation time constant (msec)	2–10	30–300
Reactivation time constant (msec)	20–10	30–300

Modified from Gettes (1976).

$$E_m = \frac{61.5}{2} \log \frac{1}{0.0002} = +114 \text{ mV}. \qquad [19.5]$$

During systole, if intracellular Ca^{2+} concentration increases to 1 μM (0.001 mM), the calcium reversal potential would fall to +92 mV.

The cardiac calcium channel is regulated by β-adrenergic agonists, which increase calcium entry and contractility during sympathetic stimulation by increasing the probability of channel opening (Fig. 18.9). This response is mediated by G_s, which stimulates a cyclic AMP–dependent protein kinase that phosphorylates the channel and directly promotes channel opening (Chapter 12). These effects are attenuated by G_i, which is activated by acetylcholine and adenosine. A peptide hormone related to calcitonin and found in nerves supplying the heart may also activate the calcium channel (Ono et al., 1989).

The two important depolarizing currents in the heart are contrasted in Table 19.2. At the start of the normal action potential in a Purkinje fiber, threshold is reached when depolarization opens the sodium channels that, by carrying a large inward current, generate the rapid upstroke of the action potential. When the additional depolarization caused by sodium entry reaches the threshold of the calcium channels, the latter open and generate a second depolarizing current. The calcium current, which activates and inactivates much more slowly than the sodium current, provides the inward current that maintains the membrane in a depolarized state during the plateau.

The overall current flux during the Purkinje fiber action potential is depicted in Fig. 19.7, which shows a free-running action potential at the top and, below, the current flux when the membrane is depolarized in a voltage-clamp experiment. Although still controversial (see above), a small outward chloride current is included in Fig. 19.7 and in Fig. 19.8, which depict the four ion fluxes now believed to make the major contributions to the normal Purkinje fiber action potential. Figures 19.7 and 19.8 should be useful in following the complex discussion of the repolarizing potassium currents that follows.

Repolarization (Phase 3)

At this point we must still account for the outward currents that repolarize the heart. Except for the chloride current that may contribute to phase 1, these re-

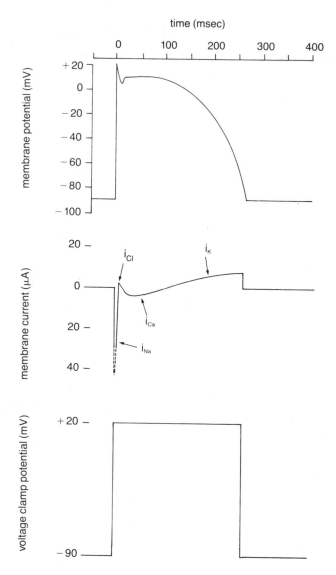

FIG. 19.7. Changing Purkinje fiber membrane currents (*middle tracing*) during a depolarization that is maintained by a voltage clamp (*lower tracing*). For reference, a normal action potential at the same time scale is shown in the *upper trace*. Four major ion species that contribute to the net current flux that generates the action potential are labeled.

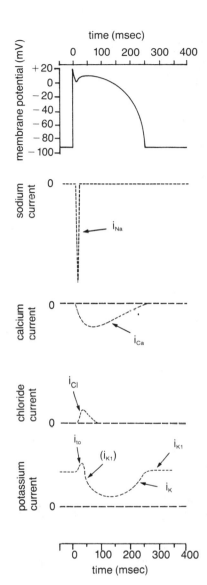

FIG. 19.8. Changing Ionic currents during the Purkinje fiber action potential. The action potential is shown at the top and currents generated by the four major ions that cross the plasma membrane are shown below. Inward currents are downward, outward currents are upward. Three potassium currents are shown: i_{to}, the transient outward current; i_K, the delayed rectifier; and i_{K1}, the inward (anomalous) rectifier. The fall in the last of these potassium currents during the plateau phase is labeled (i_{K1}). Repolarization is caused by an increase in i_K and the return of i_{K1} to its resting value.

polarizing currents are generated by the outward flux of potassium through a number of potassium-selective ion channels. The nomenclature of these potassium currents is, unfortunately, very confusing, which reflects both the complexity of the potassium channels described in Chapter 18 and the rapid growth of knowledge in this area.

Rectifying Currents

The high potassium permeability of the resting heart, which was highlighted at the beginning of this chapter, means that during diastole potassium channels are open. Immediately after the heart begins to depolarize, however, one class of potassium channels (called i_{K1}) begins to lose its ability to conduct an outward current. This causes the fall in membrane conductance early during the plateau that was described in the preceding section of this chapter. This decrease in outward current during depolarization is called *inward* or *anomalous rectification*. To understand the inward rectifier, as well as the other potassium currents in the heart, we must digress at this point to consider how a rectifier modifies current flow.

An *unrectified*, or *ohmic*, current (Fig. 19.9) is linearly dependent on voltage; thus an ohmic current, where resistance is independent of membrane potential, is described by Ohm's law: $I = E/R$. *Rectification* occurs when resistance is altered by a change in voltage. In an electronic circuit a rectifier is a device, usually used to convert alternating current to direct current, that passes current preferentially in one direction or another.

Outward rectification, as shown in Fig. 19.9, occurs when the membrane passes current most readily in the outward direction when membrane is depolarized. Outward rectification is important in the squid axon, where depolarization increases potassium permeability and so generates outward currents that return membrane potential to its resting level. In the heart, the most important outward rectifying current (called i_x, see below) is carried by potassium. Because outward rectifying currents are repolarizing, they tend to return membrane potential in the depolarized cell to its resting level.

The heart's plasma membrane also contains channels that pass inward current more readily than outward current (Fig. 19.7). These channels are responsible for a quite different rectifier current, called i_{K1}, that is referred to as *anomalous or inward rectification*. The potassium channels responsible for i_{K1}, although they dominate resting potential, are inactivated during depolarization and so contribute little to repolarization. The cardiac inward rectifier is anomalous because closure of these potassium channels during the action potential favors further depolarization, rather than repolarization.

Decreasing outward current through the anomalously rectifying potassium channels in the heart parallels inactivation of the inward calcium current during the plateau of the action potential. Together, the decreasing outward current and increasing inward current sustain the plateau of the cardiac action potential, and ex-

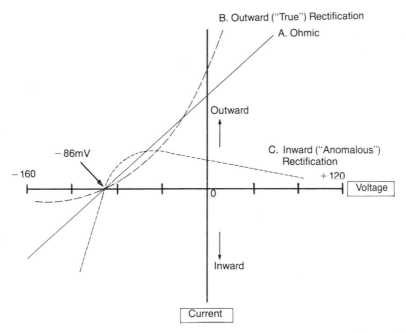

FIG. 19.9. Current-voltage relationships showing the effects of changing membrane potential (*abscissa*) on the ionic currents (*ordinate*) generated by three different types of potassium channel. Inward currents are downward, outward currents are upward. All potassium currents are zero at −86 mV, the Nernst potential for potassium. An ohmic current (*A*) is a linear function of membrane voltage because resistance is constant. Outward ("true") rectification (*B*) occurs when depolarization opens potassium channels and so increases outward current. Inward ("anomalous") rectification (*C*) occurs when depolarization causes potassium channels to close, thereby decreasing outward current. One way to understand these terms is to remember that outward rectification favors outward current, whereas inward rectification favors inward current.

plain the fall in membrane conductance during the plateau described many years ago by Weidmann.

From a functional standpoint, inward rectification in the heart is neither a mistake nor an anomaly. This response generates the long-lasting action potentials that, by maintaining a long refractory period, prevent the heart from being tetanized, allow ventricular filling, and help avoid disordered activation.

The *transient outward current* (i_{to}) discussed earlier in this chapter is an outward rectifying current that, as shown in Fig. 19.7, is turned on by depolarization and so helps the heart to repolarize during phase 1 of the action potential.

Yet another potassium current is responsible for repolarization at the end of the cardiac action potential. This third potassium current, called i_K (or i_x), is an *outward rectifier* analogous to the outwardly rectifying potassium current in nerve. The behavior of i_K is opposite to that of i_{K1}; instead of decreasing as the cell depolarizes, i_K increases with depolarization (Fig. 19.7). However, these two currents have different time courses; the outwardly rectifying i_K develops later, after attenuation of the inwardly rectifying i_{K1}. The fact that i_K appears at the end of the plateau explains why it is also referred to as the *delayed rectifier*. The increased potassium conductance caused by i_K is largely responsible for repolarizing the heart during phase 3 of the action potential (Fig. 19.7).

The delayed rectifier current (i_K) is highly regulated, being increased by both cyclic AMP and protein kinase C. The ability of protein kinase A to increase outward (repolarizing) currents probably contributes to the abbreviation of the action potential commonly seen when the heart is stimulated by β-adrenergic agonists. This effect plays an important role in maintaining excitability in the face of the tachycardia that accompanies sympathetic stimulation.

Other Repolarizing Currents

Additional repolarizing currents that do not involve potassium channels can be generated by an outward chloride current (see above), the electrogenic sodium pump, and sodium/calcium exchange. The ATP-dependent sodium pump, as discussed in Chapter 10, transports three potassium ions out of the cell in exchange for only two sodium ions; the resulting transfer of positive charge out of the cell generates a small outward ionic current that contributes to resting potential. The sodium/calcium exchanger is also electrogenic because it transports one calcium ion across the plasma membrane in exchange for three sodium ions. As noted in Chapter 10, the sodium/calcium exchanger appears to contribute a small outward current during the plateau; however, this current probably makes only a minor contribution to repolarization.

Regenerative Aspects of Repolarization

Because the inwardly rectifying potassium channels (i_{K1}) are reactivated by a fall in membrane potential (Fig. 19.9C), repolarization itself increases outward potassium currents that return the cell to its resting potential (Toyoshima and Burgess, 1978). In other words, repolarization favors further repolarization. Insofar as regions of the heart that have begun to repolarize tend to reduce membrane potential in nearby depolarized areas, repolarization is regenerative.

The Family of Potassium Channels

The advent of single channel recordings has provided evidence for a number of different potassium channels. This diversity has been underscored by rapid advances in molecular biology which, as noted in Chapter 18, have documented the existence of a remarkably heterogeneous family of potassium channels. Like other ion channels, potassium channels are tetramers; however, because the four potassium channel peptides are not covalently linked (Fig. 18.7), there can be considerable variability in potassium channel assembly. Although it is not possible at this time to provide an authoritative summary of the many different types of potassium channels, a tentative list is given in Table 19.3, which is based on measured currents supplemented by data from single channel recordings.

The three potassium currents described in the preceding paragraphs are attributed to *inward (anomalous) rectifying channels* (i_{K1}), channels responsible for the *transient outward current* (i_{to}), and channels that give rise to *delayed (outward) rectification* (i_K). In addition to the channels responsible for i_{K1}, i_{to}, and i_K, responses to a variety of regulatory agents have defined other functionally important potassium channels, some of which are listed in Table 19.3. However this field is moving so rapidly that one has the sense of writing on the surface of a swiftly flowing stream.

Calcium-Activated Potassium Channels

Calcium-activated potassium channels, which open in response to increased cytosolic calcium, probably contribute to the delayed rectifier current (i_K). The ability of calcium to "turn off" the action potential by opening these repolarizing channels is yet another example of the many mechanisms that prevent runaway signaling (see Chapter 14). In this case, a rise in cytosolic calcium, the major intracellular activator, activates outward potassium currents that terminate the action potential.

ATP-Inhibited Potassium Channels

The ATP-inhibited potassium channels are relatively insensitive to membrane potential. Because opening is inhibited by normal levels of cytosolic ATP, this channel, like a contented house cat asleep before the hearth, appears to spend most

TABLE 19.3. *Potassium channels and their functional roles*

Current	Functional role
Inward (anomalous) rectifier (i_{K1})	Maintains resting potential; closed by depolarization and so prolongs the plateau
Transient outward current (i_{to})	Opens briefly after depolarization, and so contributes to early repolarization
Outward (delayed) rectifier (i_K)	Opens at end of plateau, largely responsible for repolarization
Calcium-activated potassium channel	Activated by high cytosolic calcium, opens during calcium overload
ATP-inhibited potassium channel	Normally inhibited by ATP, opens in the energy-starved heart
Acetylcholine-activated potassium channel ($i_{K.Ach}$)	Activated by vagal stimulation, hyperpolarizes resting heart, shortens plateau

of its life in a dormant state. However, if the cell becomes depleted of ATP, these channels activate and, by carrying a repolarizing current, help to turn off activation signals that would otherwise promote energy-depleting cellular processes. In the heart, of course, the most important of the latter is contraction. Thus, activation of these channels after coronary artery occlusion may contribute to the early pump failure in the ischemic heart. The ability of these channels to attenuate activation in skeletal muscle is enhanced at acid pH (Davies, 1990); if this effect is also present in the heart, it would contribute to the well-known negative inotropic effect of acidosis.

   ATP-inhibited potassium channels appear to be more sensitive to ATP generated by glycolysis than generated by oxidative phosphorylation. This effect may reflect the local production of ATP by glycolytic enzymes bound to the adjacent plasma membrane or cytoskeleton (Weiss and Lamp, 1987).

In the pancreas, ATP-inhibited potassium channels play an important role in the regulation of insulin secretion. In the heart, as in the pancreas, these channels are inhibited by sulfonylureas, drugs commonly used to treat mild diabetes. Other ATP-inhibited potassium channels are regulated by peptide hormones, suggesting that these channels might have additional functional roles in the heart.

Acetylcholine-Activated Potassium Channels

Vagal stimulation has an important effect of hyperpolarizing resting cells and shortening the atrial action potential. These effects appear to arise not from stimulation of i_{K1}, the inward rectifier, but instead from the opening of *acetylcholine-activated potassium channels* ($i_{K.Ach}$). As noted in Chapter 12, this effect is mediated by G_i, the inhibitory G protein.

Other Potassium Channels

There is evidence for at least two additional types of outwardly rectifying potassium channel. One, which is activated by phospholipids and fatty acids (Kim and Clapham, 1989), may hasten repolarization in the ischemic heart. A potassium channel activated by intracellular sodium has also been described (Kameyama et al., 1984).

Ion Fluxes During The Action Potential

The major ion fluxes responsible for both depolarizing and repolarizing currents during the action potential (Table 19.4) share two salient features. The first is that they are "downhill" in that the ions move down an electrochemical gradient. Secondly, none is accompanied by the flux of a counter-ion, which is, of course why they are electrogenic.

The ion pumps and ion exchangers discussed in Chapter 10 have a fundamentally

TABLE 19.4. *Major ion fluxes during the cardiac action potential*

Name	Ion	Movement	Current	Phase of action potential
i_{Na}	Na^+	In	Inward	0 (depolarization)
i_{Cl}	Cl^-	In	Outward	1 (early repolarization)
i_{to}	K^+	Out	Outward	1 (early repolarization)
i_{Ca}	Ca^{2+}	In	Inward	2 (plateau)
i_{K1}[a]	K^+	Out	Outward	2 (plateau)
i_k	K^+	Out	Outward	3 (repolarization)
i_f	Na^+	In	Inward	4 (pacemaker depolarization)

[a]Open i_{K1} channels in resting cells are the major contributor to the equilibrium responsible for the Nernst potential during phase 4 (resting potential).

different *modus operandi* than these ion channels. This is because active ion transport, which in a manner of speaking cleans up the mess left behind after the action potential, involves uphill ion movements. Thus, after an action potential has passed along the plasma membrane, the chemical composition of the cardiac cell has changed slightly; sodium, calcium, and chloride have entered the cell, and potassium has been lost. To return the ions listed in Table 19.4 to their original locations, therefore, sodium, calcium, and chloride must be eliminated, and the cell must regain potassium. This requires the expenditure of energy by ion pumps and exchangers.

The electrochemical work that must be done by ion transport mechanisms to restore the resting composition of the heart is generally reduced by the coupled flux of a counter-ion in the opposite direction. For example, unlike the sodium influx responsible for the upstroke of the action potential, which is not accompanied by the movement of a counter-ion, most of the sodium pumped out the cell is exchanged for potassium, which cancels most net movement of electrical charge. By coupling two cation fluxes—sodium efflux and potassium influx—the sodium pump not only reduces the electrical work required to transport positively charged sodium ions out of the electronegative cell interior, but at the same time restores the potassium content of the cell interior. Similarly, the electrochemical work involved in the transport of calcium out of the cell is reduced by an exchange for sodium.

In the case of the sarcoplasmic reticulum calcium pump (Chapter 11), electrical work is reduced by the cotransport of anions through anion channels in this intracellular membrane, rather than countertransport of a cation.

From the standpoint of energy expenditure by the cell, the counter-ion fluxes that accompany the active ion fluxes that restore the composition of excited cells, by reducing electrochemical work, are energy-sparing.

REFRACTORY AND SUPERNORMAL PERIODS

The delayed reactivation of the sodium channels described earlier in this chapter accounts for the heart's refractoriness, which means that the heart cannot be reexcited during and immediately after the passage of an action potential. Although able to generate a local response, the heart cannot develop a propagated action potential during its refractory period. The nonconducted local responses in the refractory heart can, however, play an important role in the genesis of arrhythmias (see below).

Two degrees of refractoriness are commonly described in nerve and skeletal muscle (Fig. 19.10). During the *absolute*, or *effective refractory period*, which begins with depolarization, no stimulus, whatever its magnitude, can produce a propagated response. The *relative refractory period*, which begins after the end of the absolute refractory period, is an interval when only stimuli that exceed the normal threshold can initiate a propagated response.

Although propagated action potentials may not be initiated during the heart's refractory periods, electrical stimuli may elicit local responses that can contribute to reentrant arrhythmias (Chapter 21) and a phenomenon called concealed conduction (Chapter 23). Furthermore, even though abnormally strong stimuli can initiate propagated action potentials during the heart's relative refractory period, these responses are not normal. Unlike the large action potentials that appear in fully rested cells, they are generally slow-rising and of low amplitude (Fig. 19.5). As these small action potentials conduct slowly, they are of considerable importance in the arrhythmias associated with reentry (Chapter 21).

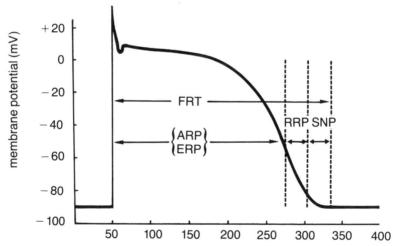

FIG. 19.10. Excitability during the cardiac action potential. The absolute, or effective refractory period (ARP or ERP), during which no stimulus regardless of its strength is able to initiate a propagated action potential, is followed by the relative refractory period (RRP) during which only stimuli that exceed the normal threshold can cause a propagated action potential. The latter is followed by the supernormal period (SNP), during which stimuli slightly less than those which normally reach threshold can generate a propagated action potential. The action potentials generated during both the RRP and SNP propagate slowly, so that full recovery time (FRT) is the interval following depolarization which ends when threshold returns to normal and stimulation produces a normally propagated action potential. (Modified from Hoffman and Cranefield, 1960, with permission of McGraw-Hill.)

A "supernormal period," which can follow the relative refractory period, is characterized by the ability of stimuli slightly below the normal threshold to produce propagated action potentials. Although excitability is thus supernormal, the action potentials generated during this period are not unusually large; on the contrary, the action potentials elicited during the supernormal phase are usually of low amplitude. This apparent discrepancy reflects the fact that whereas threshold is low during the supernormal period, the sodium channels, although able to produce a propagated impulse, remain partially inactivated.

Supernormality, although apparent in isolated His-Purkinje cells, is probably absent in the cells of the atrioventricular (AV) node, atria and ventricles (Spear and Moore, 1980) and appears to be of only minor clinical importance. Supernormality occurs at approximately the same time as the "vulnerable period," which is described in Chapter 23, but vulnerability and supernormality describe different properties. Whereas supernormality is simply a lowered threshold, vulnerability represents an increased susceptibility to ventricular fibrillation.

The interval between the onset of depolarization and the return of normal, resting excitability is the "full-recovery time," which encompasses the effective and relative refractory periods, as well as the supernormal period. At the end of the full-recovery time, therefore, threshold returns to normal.

Recovery of the ability to generate a full-sized action potential usually occurs well after membrane potential has returned to its resting level. As already pointed out, this delay reflects the fact that reactivation of sodium channels is not only voltage-dependent, but also time-dependent. In other words, even when membrane voltage has returned to its normal resting level, time must elapse before the h gates return to their open conformation and the channel recovers fully. The delay between repolarization and the dissapation of refractoriness can be markedly increased by a number of antiarrhythmic drugs.

Afterdepolarizations and Triggered Activity

Afterdepolarizations, which are spontaneous oscillations of membrane potential that appear during and after repolarization, can give rise to one or more premature responses that are called *triggered depolarizations*. There are two general types of afterdepolarization: early afterdepolarizations and delayed afterdepolarizations (Fig. 19.11). The former appear at relatively high membrane potentials, in the range between -10 and -30 mV, whereas the latter occur after membrane potential has returned almost to resting level. Neither depends on external stimuli.

Early Afterdepolarizations

Early afterdepolarizations are caused by abnormalities in the ionic currents that flow across the plasma membrane during early repolarization (phase 3), but their ionic basis is not well understood. As repolarization is brought about by a fall in the inward calcium current and an increase in outward potassium currents, abnor-

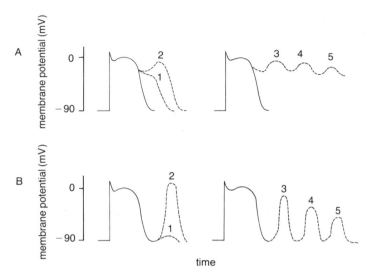

FIG. 19.11. Different types of afterdepolarization. *A*: Early afterdepolarizations showing a sub-threshold afterdepolarization that does not reach threshold (1), and larger afterdepolarizations cause a single (2) and repetitive (3–4–5) triggered depolarizations. *B*: Late afterdepolarizations showing a subthreshold afterdepolarization that does not reach threshold (1) and afterdepolarizations that reach threshold so as to produce one (2) or a series (3–4–5) of triggered depolarizations. (Modified from Wit and Rosen, 1981.)

malities in either of these currents, as well as reactivation of the sodium current and an inward current due to sodium/calcium exchange (see below), have been suggested to contribute to early afterdepolarizations. Early afterdepolarizations can be initiated by hypokalemia, hypoxia, ischemia, β-adrenergic agonsits, and some anti-arrhythmic drugs. They may also contribute to repetitive impulse formation seen in a group of conditions characterized by abnormal action potential prolongation, the "long Q-T syndomes."

Delayed Afterdepolarizations

Delayed afterdepolarizations, which arise from inward currents that appear spontaneously after the cell has repolarized, are generally seen in calcium-overloaded hearts. This explains the tendency of inotropic drugs like digitalis and epinephrine to cause delayed afterdepolarizations. The mechanism by which calcium overload induces late inward currents is related to calcium release from the sarcoplasmic reticulum, which becomes oscillatory when the cell becomes overloaded with calcium. The mechanism responsible for this behavior is not well understood, but may reflect partial reversal of the calcium pump described in Chapter 11.

Unlike most arrhythmias, which are suppressed when the heart is paced rapidly (called "overdrive suppression"), premature systoles due to delayed afterdepolarizations become more severe when heart rate is increased. This may be related to the ability of accelerated calcium uptake by the sarcoplasmic reticulum to promote oscillations in the calcium pump (Katz et al., 1977).

Delayed afterdepolarizations are caused by an inward current called the *transient inward current* (i_{ti}). The appearance of this current during calcium overload was initially interpreted to mean that i_{ti} was an inward calcium current; however, it is now clear that although calcium induces this current, the ion that enters the cells is mainly sodium. It is still not certain if i_{ti} represents an inward sodium current that passes through a special class of plasma membrane ion channels, or if i_{ti} is due to sodium/calcium exchange. The latter hypothesis is attractive because, as discussed in Chapter 10, calcium overload increases the exchange of three sodium ions for one intracellular calcium ion, which generates an inward (depolarizing) current.

Reperfusion of ischemic myocardium is a major cause of calcium overload (Chapter 24), so that the widespread use of thrombolytic therapy after acute myocardial infarction has probably increased the clinical importance of arrhythmias caused by delayed afterdepolarizations.

INTERVAL-DURATION RELATIONSHIP

The duration of each cardiac action potential is determined in part by the preceding diastolic interval, so that when rapid heart rates shorten cycle length, the duration of the action potential is also reduced (Fig. 19.12A,B). This influence of preceding cycle length on action potential duration is also seen when cardiac rhythm is irregular (Fig. 19.12C).

The *interval-duration relationship* is an essential physiological adjustment that allows adequate time for the rapidly beating ventricles to fill. Its importance is

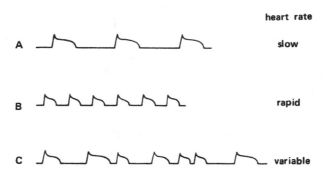

FIG. 19.12. Interval-duration relationship. At slow heart rates (*A*), where diastolic intervals are long, action potential duration is long. Where the diastolic interval is short, action potential duration is also short (*B*). When cycle length varies (*C*), action potential duration is directly proportional to the duration of the preceding diastolic interval. The lengths of the refractory periods in these beats are correlated with the durations of these action potentials.

apparent from a simple calculation. As the normal action potential duration is ~0.3 sec at a heart rate of 75 beats/min (cycle length 0.8 sec), an increase in heart rate to 200 beats/min, which reduces cycle length to 0.3 sec, could not occur unless action potential duration shortens. As heart rates of ~200/min are readily achieved by trained athletes, and abnormal tachycardias at rates approaching 200/min can be tolerated for hours, or even days in patients with otherwise normal hearts, accelerated heart rate clearly reduces action potential duration.

The direct relationship between action potential duration and the length of the preceding diastolic interval arises from several factors. Abbreviation of the action potential at fast heart rates is due in part to a gain in cytosolic calcium caused by the increased number of calcium channel openings. In addition to causing the positive staircase described in Chapter 14, increased intracellular Ca^{2+} concentration accelerates repolarization by opening calcium-activated potassium channels (see above). Increased heart rate also increases cytosolic sodium, again due to more frequent channel openings; because the sodium pump extrudes three sodium ions in exchange for only two potassium ions (Chapter 10), sodium overload increases this outward current and so accelerates repolarization.

Two time-dependent decreases in inward current at rapid heart rates also contribute to the interval-duration relationship. The first is incomplete recovery of calcium channels at rapid heart rates, which promotes repolarization by decreasing depolarizing calcium currents and so shortens the plateau. At the same time, incomplete decay of the delayed rectifier (i_{K1}) also shortens the action potential at fast heart rates.

The interval-duration relationship defines a clinically important effect of prolonged cycle length to increase refractoriness. Prolongation of the refractory period after a long diastole means that short cycles which follow long cycles tend to find the heart in a partially refractory state. This dependence of the refractory period on the preceding cycle length is most marked in the His-Purkinje system, which has the longest action potentials in the heart, and accounts for the frequent occurrence of intraventricular conduction abnormalities (Chapter 20) when short cycles follow long cycles (called the "Ashman phenomenon"). For example, the third action potential in Fig. 19.12C, where a short cycle follows a long cycle, may be conducted abnormally due to incomplete recovery from the long refractory period following the second action potential. We return to this subject in Chapter 23 when we discuss the phenomenon of *aberrant conduction*.

ACTION POTENTIALS IN DIFFERENT REGIONS OF THE HEART

The preceding description of the cardiac action potential focused on the Purkinje fiber, as this is the most extensively studied heart tissue. At this point, we examine the action potentials in other regions of the heart (Fig. 19.13) where distinctive features are related to, and in many cases account for, specialized electrophysiological roles.

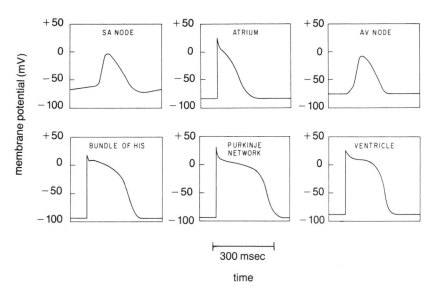

FIG. 19.13. Action potential configurations in different regions of the mammalian heart.

Sinoatrial Node

The sinoatrial (SA) node is derived embryologically from the right sinus venosus, which as the most rapidly beating chamber of the embryonic heart provides the "pacemaker" that initiates contraction in all its chambers (Chapter 20). In the adult heart the SA node is a band of specialized myocardial tissue located in the wall of the right atrium near its junction with the superior vena cava (Chapter 1), that serves as the normal pacemaker. *Spontaneous diastolic depolarization* in the SA node, also called *phase 4 depolarization* or the *pacemaker potential*, thus sets up the propagated wave of depolarization that initiates systole in all regions of the heart (Chapter 20).

The action potentials of the SA node are small and have a slow upstroke (Fig. 19.13), which reflects the lack of functioning sodium channels. The absence of an inward sodium current is due in part to the high resting potential of the SA node, which as noted earlier in this chapter, inactivates sodium channels. As a result, the upstroke of the SA node action potential is due largely to an inward calcium current.

Pacemaker Activity

The hallmark of a pacemaker cell is its ability to depolarize spontaneously, so that pacemaker activity can be defined as an instability of diastolic (resting) potential that initiates a propagated action potential. This means that the plasma membrane ion channels in a pacemaker cell cause membrane potential to depolarize

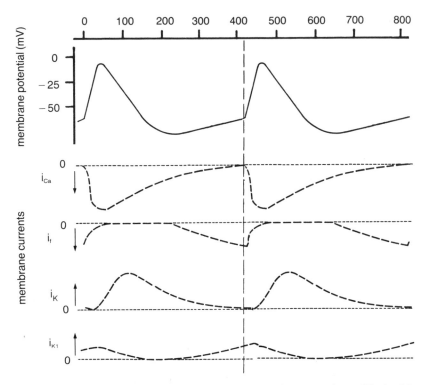

FIG. 19.14. Changing ionic currents during depolarization of a pacemaker cell in the SA node. Inward currents are downward, outward currents are upward. Action potentials are shown above for reference. Changes in four currents probably contribute to spontaneous diastolic depolarization. Two are increasing inward currents: the inward pacemaker current (i_f) and the inward calcium current I_{Ca}, the latter is largely responsible for the upstroke of the action potential. Two are decreasing outward currents: the delayed rectifier i_x, and the inward (anomalous) rectifier i_{K1}.

spontaneously during diastole. Diastolic depolarization, in turn, arises from both decreasing outward currents and increasing inward currents (Fig. 19.14).

Decreasing Outward Currents

Pacemaker activity is due in part to decay of the delayed rectifier current (i_K), which in the Purkinje fiber is an outward current that appears during the plateau and then inactivates after the cell repolarizes. Slow decay of i_K in the SA node, which reduces outward current in early diastole, is mainly permissive in allowing other currents to depolarize the pacemaker.

The anomalous rectifier (i_{K1}) makes an additional permissive contribution to pacemaker activity. Although not primarily responsible for pacemaker activity, once the pacemaker begins to fire, the normal decay of i_{K1} helps it along. This is simply because the normal property of the anomalous rectifier, which attenuates outward currents as the cell depolarizes, is to promote depolarization.

A special outward pacemaker current, called i_{K2}, whose decay was postulated to allow background inward currents to depolarize pacemaker cells, must be mentioned at this point. This current, once thought to be a major cause for pacemaker activity in Purkinje cells, now appears to be artifactual.

Increasing Inward Currents

Set against the background of the declining outward currents associated with the decay of i_K and the inward rectifier i_{K1} are two inward currents. The first is our old friend i_{Ca}, the slow inward calcium current discussed earlier in this chapter and, in terms of its role in regulating myocardial contractility, in Chapter 14. Although i_{Ca} is mainly responsible for the action potential upstroke in pacemaker cells, its continuation into diastole may contribute to early diastolic depolarization. The most important pacemaker current (i_f), which is an inward sodium current, probably plays a major role in mediating the control of heart rate by the autonomic nervous system. Together, these two inward currents operate throughout diastole; i_{Ca} mainly earlier, at the end of repolarization, and i_f later during spontaneous diastolic depolarization.

Control of Heart Rate

Three general mechanisms are traditionally stated to modify the discharge frequency of the SA node pacemaker (Fig. 19.15). In terms of mechanisms that would cause slowing, these are (a) a decreased rate of diastolic depolarization, (b) diastolic hyperpolarization, and (c) an increase in threshold (Fig. 19.15). Although useful

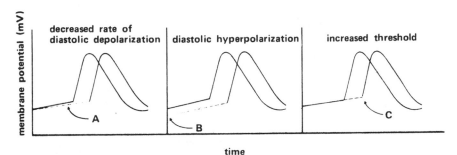

FIG. 19.15. Three possible mechanisms that can slow the SA node pacemaker (*solid line*, control; *dashed line*, slowed): decreased rate of diastolic depolarization (*arrow A*), diastolic hyperpolarization (*arrow B*), and increased threshold (*arrow C*). More than one of these changes may be induced by a given intervention. Pacemaker discharge can be accelerated by opposite changes in any or all of these parameters (increased rate of diastolic depolarization, diastolic depolarization, lowered threshold).

conceptually, it is likely that this paradigm will soon be replaced by analyses of changes in the membrane currents described above.

The physiological control of heart rate, which is mediated by the autonomic nervous system, is due mainly to changes in the slope of diastolic depolarization (Fig. 19.15A). The latter is slowed by vagal stimulation and increased by β-adrenergic agonists. These effects are mediated largely by direct effects of G_i and G_s on the channels that carry the pacemaker current i_f (Yatani et al., 1990). The effects of the inhibitory G_i appear to be more potent than those of G_s, which may explain the fact that vagal slowing of the heart normally predominates over sympathetic acceleration.

Changes in diastolic potential also play an important role in the control of heart rate. As the diastolic potential of SA node pacemaker cells, even at its maximum, is less than that estimated from the Nernst equation for potassium, these cells do not become freely permeable to potassium during diastole. Thus, opening of acetylcholine-activated potassium channels by vagal stimulation, which hyperpolarizes the SA node, probably contributes to parasympathetic slowing of heart rate.

As noted in Chapter 1, the SA node is not simply a small nest of cells, but instead is a band of cells that surrounds the right atrial-superior vena caval junction. Pacemaker activity appears to arise within this rather extensive structure by a "democratic" process in which a "consensus" is reached among the hundreds of cells whose coordinated interactions determine when the SA node actually fires (Michaels et al., 1987).

Atrium

Atrial action potentials are generally similar to the "typical" action potential of the Purkinje fibers except that their durations are shorter (Fig. 19.13). Although most atrial cells lack pacemaker activity, latent pacemaker cells are found in several regions of the atria. Depolarization (phase 0) is rapid and is followed by a phase of rapid repolarization (phase 1) and a brief plateau (phase 2) that merges into the phase of repolarization (phase 3); thus, separate phases 2 and 3 often cannot be identified. The terminal portions of phase 3 tend to return more slowly to the diastolic level than do those in the ventricle or Purkinje fibers.

The relatively brief duration of the action potential in atrial cells is due to a rapidly rising potassium permeability. The atrial potassium channels are under autonomic control, and vagal stimulation gives rise to clinically important shortening of both action potential duration and refractory period in the atria.

Atrioventricular Node

The AV node, which is derived from the left sinus venosus, is a region of slow conduction that delays atrioventricular conduction so as to allow the ventricles time to accept the blood delivered by the atrial "primer pump" (Chapter 15). Resting potential is approximately -80 mV, and membrane voltage during depolarization (overshoot) does not usually exceed $+5$ to $+10$ mV. Action potential duration in the AV node is longer than in the atrium, but less than in the Purkinje fibers.

The AV node can be divided functionally into three regions (Fig. 19.16): the AN region (upper or atrionodal portion), the N region (middle or nodal portion), and the NH region (lower or nodal-His bundle portion). Resting potential is lowest in the N region and duration is shortest in the AN region, increasing progressively through the N region to the NH region. Spontaneous pacemaker activity is found in all regions of the AV node, being more prominent in the lower H and NH regions. The slowest rate of spontaneous diastolic depolarization is found in the N region. Both the rate of AV nodal pacemaker activity and the rate and amplitude of the upstroke are under autonomic control.

The atrioventricular conduction delay is due in part to the properties of the action potentials in this region of the heart, which are slowly rising and low in amplitude (Fig. 19.13). As in the SA node, slow depolarization in the AV node reflects the absence of functional sodium channels. Thus, AV node depolarization is due primarily to a slow inward calcium current. Control of this current by sympathetic and parasympathetic neurotransmitters plays an important role in regulating the slow conduction velocity in this key segment of the heart's conduction system.

Slow conduction in the AV node is also due to the small size of the AV nodal cells, especially in the N region where the smallest and most slowly rising action potentials are found. The relatively small number of gap junctions, which is responsible for a high internal resistance, also contributes to slow conduction in this region of the heart (see Chapter 21).

It is surprising that even though the AV node normally provides the only electrical connection between the atria and the ventricles, conduction through this structure is precarious. This explains the frequent clinical occurrence of conduction failure, called *atrioventricular block* (see Chapter 22). Because the currents generated during depolarization are barely sufficient to maintain a propagated action potential along this structure, the AV node is said to have a low *safety factor*.

Even though the AV node is a relatively narrow strand of specialized cardiac muscle, it can be divided longitudinally into more than one functional conducting

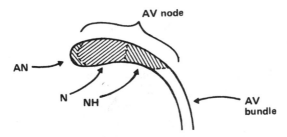

FIG. 19.16. Atrioventricular conduction system. The AV node can be divided functionally into three regions: AN (upper, or atrionodal), N (middle, or nodal), and NH (lower, or nodal-His bundle).

pathway. Thus, this structure can be viewed as a cable containing parallel wires that can conduct independently of each other. It is well established that multiple conduction pathways in the AV node are the most common cause for supraventricular tachycardias (Chapter 21).

His-Purkinje System

The "typical" Purkinje fiber action potential has served as the basis for our earlier discussion of the ionic currents during the cardiac action potential. The cells of the His-Purkinje system have a prominent phase of early repolarization (phase 1), and normally exhibit slow pacemaker activity that can be accelerated by pharmacological or pathological influences. These cells, which are specialized for rapid conduction, have very large action potentials; resting potentials are nearly -90mV and the overshoot may reach $+30$ mV, so that action potential amplitudes can be greater than $+120$ mV (Fig. 19.13). Along with a high rate of depolarization during phase 0 and low internal resistance, these features favor rapid conduction and so provide the Purkinje cells with a very high safety factor.

The cells of the His-Purkinje system have very long action potentials; in fact, the action potentials in the distal fibers of the His-Purkinje system and their arborizations in the ventricular endocardium are the longest found in the mammalian heart. These long action potentials contribute a property called "gating" (not to be confused with the gating of a single ion channel) that, by preventing impulses from reentering the Purkinje system after they have activated the ventricles (Myerburg et al. 1970), provides an important safeguard against potentially fatal disorganization of ventricular depolarization.

Ventricles

The ventricular action potential is similar to that already described for the Purkinje fibers; it is of large amplitude, although smaller than the latter (Fig. 19.13). Its duration is longer than that of the atria and shorter than that of the His-Purkinje system. Spontaneous diastolic depolarization is not seen normally, but can appear under abnormal conditions to give rise to rhythms called "parasystole" (Chapter 23) or the usually benign accelerated ventricular rhythms often seen 1 to 2 days after an acute myocardial infarction (Chapter 24).

Action potential configurations differ markedly in the epicardium and endocardium of the canine ventricle. Most striking is a prominent transient outward current in the epicardium, which may contribute to heterogeneities in the responses of action potential duration and refractoriness to changes in heart rate (Litovsky and Antzelevitch, 1988).

PROPERTIES OF THE INTERCALATED DISC

The permeability and conductivity properties of the ion channels in the intercalated disc, which separates the interiors of adjacent myocardial cells, are quite different from the plasma membrane channels described above. As described in Chapter 1, the channels of the nexus are large and freely permeable to charged molecules. Radioactive potassium injected at one end of a bundle of myocardial cells, for example, diffuses freely across the intercalated discs from cell to cell almost as rapidly as this ion would diffuse in an aqueous medium. Because the nexus provides a low electrical resistance pathway between adjacent cells, rapid conduction across the intercalated discs facilitates excitation by allowing electrical activity to spread rapidly from one cell to the next (Fig. 19.17). For this reason, the number of gap junctions between adjacent cells is a major determinant of conduction velocity, and factors that close these channels notably acidosis and high cytosolic Ca^{2+} concentration, cause electrical uncoupling of adjacent heart cells.

Closure of the channels in the intercalated disc is essential in limiting cell death when one region of the heart is damaged, as occurs clinically after myocardial infarction. Like the bulkhead doors in a ship, the intercalated discs close when cells fill with calcium (which in excess is as lethal to the heart as flooding is to an ocean liner), and so demarcate necrotic from viable myocardium.

Both ATP (Sugiura et al., 1990) and cyclic AMP–dependent protein kinases increase the permeability of the cardiac gap junction (DeMello, 1989). The first of

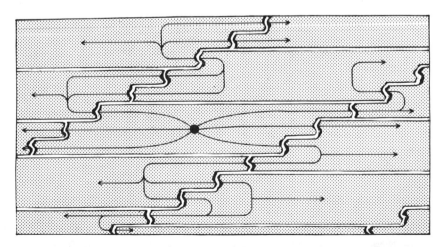

FIG. 19.17. Distribution of current flow in the myocardium (*shaded*, intracellular space; *unshaded*, extracellular spaces). *Straight lines* represent the plasma membrane, which has a high electrical resistance. *Curved heavy lines* represent the intercalated discs, which have lower electrical resistance. The flow of current (*thin arrows*) from an intracellular electrode (*dot* in center) is transmitted through the intercalated discs primarily in a longitudinal direction, but current also flows laterally through the branching myocardial syncytium, as shown. However, very little current flows transversely across the plasma membranes. (Modified from Woodbury, 1962.)

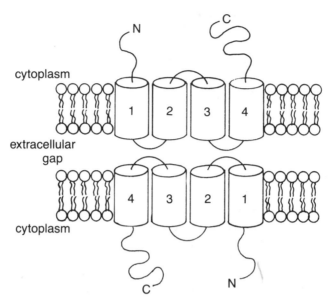

FIG. 19.18. Two connexin molecules, each of which contains four membrane-spanning helices, as located in the membranes of two cells at the nexus of an intercalated disc. Hexamers made up of connexin in the two plasma membranes surround a channel that crosses the extracellular gap between the cells. The membrane-spanning subunit labeled 3, which contains several amphipathic amino acids, probably lines the channel.

these effects appears to be another example of the regulatory effect of ATP, whereas the effect of cyclic AMP may help to speed conduction in the heart after sympathetic stimulation.

The channels in the intercalated disc are composed of *connexon*, which is made up of six subunits. Two connexon hexamers, one from each adjacent cell, contribute to the functional channel shown in Fig. 1.25. The subunits of connexon are, in turn, called *connexins*. Although connexins can have different molecular weights, all appear to contain four membrane-spanning helices (Fig. 19.18). Connexin43, found in the heart, has a molecular weight of 43,000.

In concluding this long and complex chapter, it should be emphasized that the many details regarding the cardiac action potential represent more than "facts to be memorized." This is because, as highlighted in Chapter 20, the clinical electrocardiogram records potential differences at the body surface that arise from the ionic currents described in this chapter. Furthermore, most cardiac arrhythmias arise from abnormalities in these ion currents. For these reasons, the descriptive material in the preceding pages provides a basis for understanding many features of the electrocardiogram, as well as the clinical arrhythmias and antiarrhythmic drugs discussed in the following chapters.

REFERENCES

Bahinski A, Nairn AC, Greengard P, Gadsbey DC. (1989). Chloride conductance regulated by cyclic AMP–dependent protein kinase in cardiac myocytes. *Nature* 340:718–721.

Blinks JR. (1986). Intracellular Ca^{2+} measurements. In: Fozzard H, Haber E, Katz A, Jennings R, Morgan HE, eds. *The heart and cardiovascular system*. New York: Raven Press; 671–701.

Cohen CJ, Fozzard HA, Sheu S-S. (1982). Increase in intracellular sodium ion activity during stimulation in mammalian cardiac muscle. *Circ Res* 50:651–662.

Davies NW. (1990). Modulation of ATP-sensitive K^+ channels in skeletal muscle by intracellular protons. *Nature* 343:375–377.

DeMello WC. (1989). Effect of isoproterenol and 3-isobutyl-1-methyxanthine on junctional conductance in heart cell pairs. *Biochim Biophys Acta* 1012:291–298.

Gettes LS. (1976). Possible role of ionic changes in the appearance of arrhythmias *Pharmacol Ther B* 2:787–810.

Harvey RD, Clark GD, Hume JR. (1990). Chloride current in mammalian cardiac myocytes. Novel mechanism for autonomic regulation of action potential duration and resting membrane potential. *J Gen Physiol* 95:1077–1102.

Hoffman BF, Cranefield P. (1960). *Electrophysiology of the heart*. New York. McGraw-Hill.

Kameyama M, Kakei M, Sato R, Shibaski T, Matsuda H, Irisawa H. (1984). Intracellular Na^+ activates a K^+ channel in mammalian cardiac cells. *Nature* 309:354–356.

Katz AM, Repke DI, Dunnett J, Hasselbach W. (1977). Dependence of calcium permeability of sarcoplasmic reticulum vesicles on external and internal calcium ion concentrations. *J Biol Chem* 252:1950–1956.

Kim D, Clapham DE. (1989). Potassium channels in cardiac cells activated by arachidonic acid and its metabolites. *Science* 244:1174–1176.

Litovsky SH, Antzelevitch C. (1988). Transient outward current prominent in canine ventricular epicardium but not endocardium. *Circ Res* 62:116 126.

Michaels DC, Matyas EP, Jalife J. (1987). Mechanisms of sinoatrial pacemaker synchronization: a new hypothesis. *Circ Res* 61:704–714.

Myerburg RJ, Stewart JW, Hoffman BF. (1970). Electrophysiological properties of the canine peripheral A-V conducting system. *Circ Res* 26:361–378.

Ono K, Delay M, Nakajima T, Irisawa H, Giles W. (1989). Calcitonin gene-related peptide regulated calcium current in heart muscle. *Nature* 340:721–724.

Spear JF, Moore EN. (1980). Supernormal conduction in the canine bundle of His and proximal bundle branches. *Am J Physiol* 238:H300–H306.

Sugiura H, Toyama J, Tsuboi N, Kamiya K, Kodama I. (1990). ATP directly affects junctional conductance between paired ventricular myocytes isolated from guinea pig heart. *Circ Res* 66:1095–1102.

Toyoshima H, Burgess MJ. (1978). Electrotonic interaction during canine ventricular repolarization. *Circ Res* 43:348–356.

Walker J. (1986). Intracellular inorganic ions in cardiac tissue. In: Fozzard H, Haber E, Katz A, Jennings R, Morgan HE, eds. *The heart and cardiovascular system*. New York: Raven Press; 561–572.

Weiss JN, Lamp ST. (1987). Glycolysis preferentially inhibits ATP-sensitive K^+ channels in isolated guinea pig cardiac myocytes. *Science* 238:67–69.

Wit AL, Rosen MR. (1981). Cellular electrophysiology of cardiac arrhythmias. Part I. Arrhythmias caused by abnormal impulse generation. *Mod Conc Cardiovasc Dis* 50 (1):1–8.

Woodbury JW. (1962). Cellular electrophysiology of the heart. In: Hamilton WF, Dow P, eds. *Handbook of physiology. Section 2: Circulation*, vol 1. Washington, DC: American Physiological Society; 237–286.

Yatani A, Okabe K, Codina J, Birnbaumer L, Brown AM. (1990). Heart rate regulation by G proteins acting on the cardiac pacemaker channel. *Nature* 249:1163–1165.

BIBLIOGRAPHY

Baumgarten CM, Fozzard HA. (1986). The resting and pacemaker potentials. In: Fozzard H, Haber E, Katz A, Jennings R, Morgan HE, eds. *The heart and cardiovascular system*. New York: Raven Press; 601–626.

Boyett MR, Jewell BR. (1978). A study of the factors responsible for rate-dependent shortening of the action potential in mammalian ventricular muscle. *J Physiol (Lond)* 285:359–380.

Campbell DL, Rasmusson RL, Strauss HC. (1992). Ionic current mechanisms generating vertebrate primary cardiac pacemaker activity at the single cell level: an integrative view. *Annu Rev Physiol*, in press.

Cohen IS, Datyner NB, Gintant GA, Kline RP. (1986) Time-dependent outward currents in the heart. In: Fozzard H, Haber E, Katz A, Jennings R, Morgan HE, eds. *The heart and cardiovascular system.* New York: Raven Press; 637–669.

deWeille JR, Lazdunski M. (1990). Regulation of the ATP-sensitive potassium channel. In: Narahashi T, ed. *Ion channels*, vol 2. New York: Plenum; 205–220.

Fozzard HA, Arnsdorf MF. (1986). Cardiac electrophysiology. In: Fozzard H, Haber E, Katz A, Jennings R, Morgan HE, eds. *The heart and cardiovascular system.* New York: Raven Press; 1–30.

Hartzell HC. (1988). Regulation of cardiac ion channels by catecholamines, acetylcholine and second messenger systems. *Prog Biophys Mol Biol* 52:165–247.

Hille B. (1984). *Ionic channels of excitable membranes.* Sunderland MA: Sinauer Associates.

Jongsma HJ, Gros D. (1991). The cardiac connection. *News Int. Physiol. Sci.* 6:34–40.

Katz B. (1966). *Nerve, muscle and synapse.* New York: McGraw-Hill.

Noble D. (1979). *The initiation of the heartbeat,* 2nd ed. Oxford: Clarendon Press.

Walsh KB, Begenisch TB, Kass RS. (1989). β-adrenergic modulation of cardiac ion channels. Differential sensitivity of potassium and calcium currents. *J Gen Physiol* 93:841–854.

Wit AL, Rosen MR. (1986). Afterdepolarizations and triggered activity. In: Fozzard H, Haber E, Katz A, Jennings R, Morgan HE, eds. *The heart and cardiovascular system.* New York: Raven Press; 1449–1490.

20

The Electrocardiogram

Cardiac muscle can possess at least four major properties: *automaticity* (chronotropy), which is the ability to initiate an electrical impulse; *conductivity* (dromotropy), the ability to conduct electrical impulses; *contractility* (inotropy), the ability to shorten and to do work; and *lusitropy*, the ability to relax and to fill. All are found in primitive myocardial cells, but some may be lost when the heart differentiates. All cells of the adult heart retain the property of conductivity. The *working myocardial cells* of the atria and ventricles are able to contract and relax, but under normal conditions generally lack automaticity. Conversely, *pacemaker cells* are specialized for the ability to initiate an electrical impulse, but contain only a few contractile filaments. The most important pacemaker cells are concentrated in the sinoatrial (SA) node; however, other normally dormant pacemaker cells are found in the atrioventricular (AV) node and in the His-Purkinje system. The *atrioventricular nodal cells* conduct impulses very slowly, and so delay the wave of depolarization as it passes from atria to ventricles. In contrast, the *His-Purkinje cells*, which are specialized for rapid conduction, propagate the excitatory wave of depolarization rapidly over the ventricles and so synchronize contraction of the walls of the ventricles.

PACEMAKERS AND IMPULSE FORMATION

The primary pacemaker of the heart is the SA node, which normally initiates the wave of depolarization that is transmitted through the myocardium to activate all regions of the heart. In the adult human, action potentials are normally generated in the SA node 60 to 100 times each minute. The SA node, located in the sulcus formed where the superior vena cava joins the right atrium (Fig. 1.8), is derived from the sinus venosus, the most rapidly beating portion of the tubular embryonic heart. The latter, like the adult hearts of primitive metazoans, can be divided into four regions: the sinus venosus, atria, ventricles, and truncus arteriosus (Fig. 20.1). All regions beat in response to an impulse initiated in pacemaker cells of the sinus venosus. Although contraction in the atria, ventricles, and truncus arteriosus is normally controlled by impulses transmitted from the sinus venosus, several of these

473

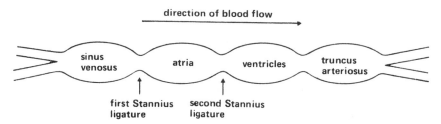

FIG. 20.1. Embryonic or primitive heart. The flow of blood in this tubular heart is from left to right. The intrinsic rates of the pacemaker activity of each chamber also decreases from left to right, as first demonstrated by Stannius, who placed ligatures at the sinoatrial junction (first Stannius ligature) and AV junction (second Stannius ligature) in a frog heart, which has a functional anatomy similar to that shown here.

regions contain pacemaker cells. As the intrinsic rates of pacemaker depolarization decrease as one proceeds from the "higher" venous end to the "lower" arterial end of the tubular embryonic heart (i.e., from left to right in Fig. 20.1), the less rapid lower pacemaker cells do not have time to initiate a propagated wave of depolarization unless they are isolated from the more rapidly firing sinus venosus pacemaker.

> The existence of a hierarchy of pacemakers in different regions of the heart was clearly demonstrated in 1852 by Stannius, who placed tight ligatures between different regions in primitive hearts. This allowed Stannius to show that when the influence of the more rapid higher pacemakers is removed, the previously hidden activity of lower pacemakers was able to initiate slower beating of the distal regions.

A similar hierarchy of pacemaker activity exists in the adult human heart, where impulses conducted from the rapid SA node pacemaker normally obscure the intrinsic pacemaker activity in lower regions. This is simply because the rate of diastolic depolarization in the lower pacemakers is too slow to reach threshold before they are discharged by the wave of depolarization propagated from the more rapid SA node pacemaker. In pathological conditions, such as depression of the SA node pacemaker or blocked impulse propagation in the AV node, the activity of the lower pacemakers can become apparent.

The most rapid of the lower pacemakers, which are generally in the lower (NH) region of the AV node (Fig. 19.16) have an intrinsic rate of ~40 to 55 beats/min. If this lower pacemaker also fails, or if disease of the conduction system blocks transmission of the wave of depolarization through the AV bundle into the ventricles, latent pacemaker activity in Purkinje fibers within the ventricles can initiate propagated action potentials at rates of ~25 to 40 beats/min.

> Although a large number of potential pacemaker cells is found throughout the heart, these do not always exhibit active pacemaker function when cut off from the normally dominant influence of the SA node pacemaker. The resulting cessation of ventricular contraction represents an important cause for sudden cardiac death (Chapter 22).

IMPULSE PROPAGATION THROUGH THE HEART

The normal activation sequence, which is initiated by impulses that arise in the SA node, is shown in Table 20.1. As would be predicted from the heart's anatomy and embryology, the impulse that originates in the SA node first activates the atria and then the ventricles; the last regions of the ventricles to be activated being the areas surrounding the outflow tracts.

Although the wave of activation is transmitted only through cardiac muscle, the conduction velocities in all regions of the heart are not the same (Table 20.1). Propagation of the wave of depolarization is fastest in the Purkinje fibers of the bundle branches and the network of His-Purkinje cells in the endocardial regions of the ventricles.

Conduction is less rapid in the AV bundle and atrial and ventricular myocardium, whereas conduction velocity in the AV and SA nodes is extremely slow. Although the AV node is a small structure, conduction is so slow that it causes a significant delay in transmitting the wave of depolarization from the atria to the ventricles (Chapter 19).

Atrial Depolarization

The wave of depolarization that originates in the SA node spreads into the adjacent right atrium and then to the left atrium and AV node. Propagation of this impulse over the atria follows a complex path that can be modified by changing heart rate and by autonomic influences (Boineau et al., 1978). The variability of the

TABLE 20.1. *Normal activation sequence*

Normal sequence of activation	Conduction velocity (meters/sec)	Time for impulse to traverse structure (sec)	Rate of pacemaker discharge (min^{-1})
SA node	<0.01	~0.15	60–100
↓			
Atrial myocardium	1.0–1.2		None
↓			
AV node	0.02–0.05	~0.08	Most rapid in lower fibers:
↓			40–55
AV bundle	1.2–2.0		
↓			
Bundle branches	2.0–4.0		25–40
↓			
Purkinje network			
↓			
Ventricular myocardium	0.3–1.0	~0.08	None

pathways of atrial depolarization explains changes in the morphology of the P waves, which arise from atrial depolarization (see below).

Internodal Tracts

Rapidly conducting pathways in the atria, called internodal tracts (Fig. 20.2), have been proposed to represent preferred conduction pathways between the SA and AV nodes (Scherf and James, 1979). However, the nature—and even the existence—of these tracts remains controversial because the internodal tracts are defined on a functional, rather than an anatomical, basis. Many electrophysiological studies have provided evidence for rapid internodal conduction along specialized pathways in the atria, but most histological studies have failed to demonstrate clearly demarcated bundles of cells to explain the rapid conduction observed physiologically. This discrepancy may be explained if accelerated impulse conduction involves the thick pectinate muscles (Fig. 1.3), rather than special tracts, or if rapid

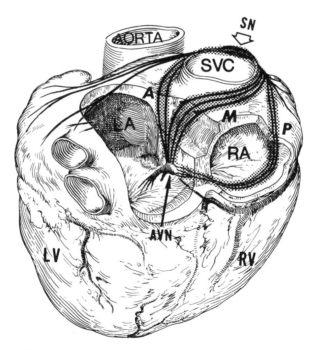

FIG. 20.2. Internodal tracts as seen in a posterior view of the heart in which the right ventricle (RV) is to the *right* and the left ventricle (LV) to the *left* on the figure. The three internodal tracts are anterior (A), middle (M), and posterior (P). Each provides a preferential pathway for conduction between the SA node (SN), located in the wall of the right atrium (RA) near the superior vena cava (SVC), and the AV node (AVN). The anterior internodal tract also provides a conduction pathway to the left atrium (LA). (Modified from James, 1967.)

transmission in the atrial wall occurs in regions that, although lacking clearly demarcated tracts, are enriched in rapidly conducting Purkinje-like cells.

Three internodal tracts are generally described. The *anterior* internodal tract has two branches: one provides a pathway between the SA and AV nodes, and the other passes through the atrial septum where it is presumed to transmit impulses from the right atrium (which is the first to be activated) to the left atrium. The latter pathway, called *Bachmann's bundle*, has been postulated to synchronize contraction of the two atria, and there is evidence that interruption of Bachmann's bundle can cause a characteristic P wave abnormality ("left atrial abnormality") in which left atrial depolarization is delayed relative to that in the right atrium. The *middle* and *posterior* internodal tracts (named after *Wenckebach* and *Thorel*, respectively) represent preferential conduction pathways between the SA and AV nodes.

Atrioventricular Conduction

The connective tissue of the fibrous skeleton of the heart, which separates the atria and ventricles, serves as an electrical insulator. As a result, impulse propagation between these chambers normally depends on a single strand of specialized muscle tissue, the *AV bundle*. Impulses arriving from the SA node normally enter the AV bundle only by way of the *AV node*, a small mass of specialized cardiac muscle located above the coronary sinus on the posterior wall of the right atrium. Together, the AV node and AV bundle normally provide the only electrical connection that links the atria and ventricles (Fig. 20.3).

Accessory Pathways

Additional strands of cardiac muscle linking the atria and ventricles are sometimes found in human hearts (Fig. 20.4). Although generally dormant, they can give rise to abnormal rhythms in patients in whom these conduction pathways become functionally active. Most important of the abnormal pathways linking the atria and ventricles are accessory pathways (also called a bypass tract or a *bundle of Kent*)

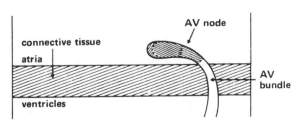

FIG. 20.3. The AV node and AV bundle provide the major conduction pathway traversing the connective tissue barrier between the atria (*above*) and ventricles (*below*).

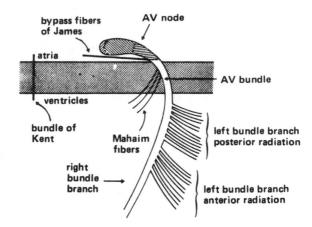

FIG. 20.4. Additional conduction pathways sometimes found to link the atria and ventricles. These include accessory pathways ("bundle of Kent"), which are variably located; the bypass fibers of James, which connect the atrial myocardium to the upper portion of the AV bundle; and the Mahaim fibers, which carry impulses from the AV bundle (or bundle branches) to abnormal sites in the ventricles. These additional pathways do not function in the normal human heart.

which is simply any strand of muscle tissue that crosses the central fibrous body to provide an abnormal electrical connection between the atria and ventricles. An accessory pathway can be found at various locations around the junction between the atria and ventricles. By creating a "short circuit" that bypasses the conduction delay in the AV node, rapid conduction in these pathways allows inappropriate impulse transmission between the atria and ventricles. These structures, which can be responsible for important, and sometimes life-threatening arrhythmias, represent the anatomical substrate for an arrhythmia called *preexcitation*, or the *Wolff-Parkinson-White (WPW) syndrome* (Chapter 21).

Another conduction pathway, the *bypass fibers of James*, by linking the atria to the upper portion of the AV bundle, can also bypass the normal conduction delay in the AV node. The *Mahaim fibers* represent another pathway that can transmit impulses from the AV node or AV bundle to the ventricles (Gallagher et al., 1981). In some patients, conduction through Mahaim fibers that link the AV node to the ventricle can participate in reentrant arrhythmias.

Ventricular Activation

Ventricular systole is normally initiated by impulses propagated from the SA node pacemaker via the AV node. The impulse is then transmitted into the ventricles through the *AV bundle* (also called the *His bundle* or *common bundle*), which as noted above represents the only conduction pathway between the atria and ventricles in normal individuals. The AV bundle divides at the top of the interventricular septum into the *right* and *left bundle branches* (Fig. 1.8). The right bundle branch

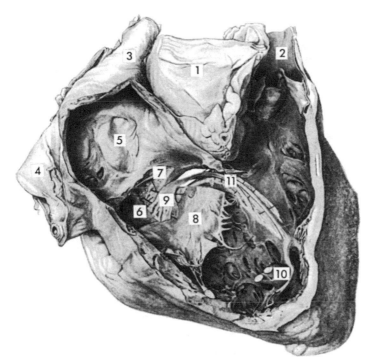

FIG. 20.5. Conduction system of the human right ventricle viewed from the right after removal of a portion of the right atrial and ventricular walls. Note the aorta (1); pulmonary artery (2); superior vena cava (3); inferior vena cava (4); fossa ovale of the interatrial septum (5); thebesian valve overlying the coronary sinus (6); false tendon (7); medial leaflet of the tricuspid valve, which has been separated from its point of insertion (8); AV node, dissected free, with finger-like branches radiating proximally toward the coronary sinus (9). The AV bundle is seen to arise from the AV node and, at the top of the membranous septum (which has been partially opened in this preparation) divides into the right and left bundle branches. The right bundle branch (11) runs along the right side of the interventricular septum and continues, usually without branching, toward the anterior papillary muscle (10), which it usually reaches within the moderator band. (Modified from Wenckebach and Winterberg, 1927.)

(Fig. 20.5) is generally a distinct strand of conducting tissue that activates the right ventricle, often reaching the right ventricular free wall within a structure called the *moderator band*. The left bundle branch, in contrast, does not continue as a distinct bundle, but instead fans out over the endocardium of the left ventricle.

Electrocardiographers view the left bundle branch as dividing into two branches, the *anterior* and *posterior fascicles*, in which the anterior radiations arise more distally (Fig. 20.6). Interruption of either fascicle can delay conduction to portions of the left ventricle, and so give rise to abnormalities in the mean QRS vector described later in this chapter. Delayed activation of the anterior radiations produces an electrocardiographic abnormality called *left anterior fascicular block*, or *left anterior hemiblock*, whereas conduction block in the posterior radiations is respon-

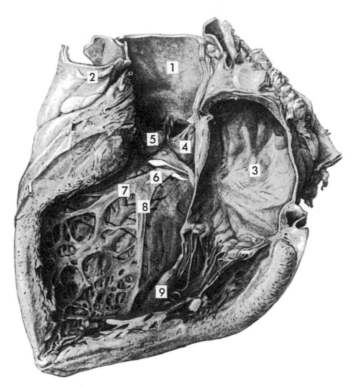

FIG. 20.6. The same heart shown in Fig. 20.5, viewed from the left after removal of a portion of the left atrial and ventricular walls. Note the aorta (1); pulmonary artery (2); left atrium (3); and two cusps of the aortic valve (4, 5). The left bundle branch, which emerges through an opening made by removal of a portion of the membranous septum, originates as a wide, flat band (6). The left bundle branch then fans out into anterior (7) and posterior (8) fascicles, which run toward the anterior (not shown) and posterior (9) papillary muscles of the left ventricle. (Modified from Wenckebach and Winterberg, 1927.)

sible for *left posterior fascicular block*, or *left posterior hemiblock*. Although the fascicular blocks are well-defined electrocardiographic entities, their anatomic basis is tenuous because division of the left bundle branch is highly variable (Fig. 20.7). Even though discrete anterior and posterior fascicles appear to be uncommon, fascicular block is a well-established concept that is useful clinically in electrocardiographic interpretation.

The working myocardial cells of the ventricles are depolarized by impulses conducted via the *Purkinje network*, a system of rapidly conducting His-Purkinje cells that arise from the bundle branches and course within the inner third of the ventricular walls. Rapid conduction in this structure, by coordinating the electrical activation of the ventricles, provides an essential synchrony to ventricular systole.

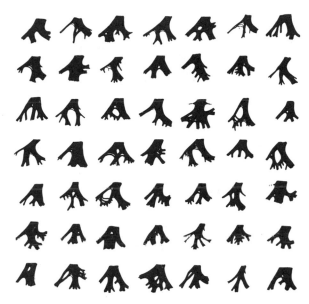

FIG. 20.7. Diagrammatic sketches of the division of the left bundle branch viewed from the left in 49 human hearts showing that simple bifurcation into anterior and posterior fascicles is uncommon. (From Demoulin J-C, Thesis)

THE ELECTROCARDIOGRAM

The *electrocardiogram* (ECG), which provides a record of electrical events occurring within the heart, is obtained from electrodes placed on the surface of the body. An ECG is thus a plot of the time-dependence of changing potential differences between electrodes on the body surface (Fig. 20.8). Electrical potentials can also be recorded from catheters placed in the cavities of the atrial and ventricles. If a bipolar electrode catheter is placed in the right atrium adjacent to the tricuspid valve so that the two recording electrodes are on either side of the AV bundle, the resulting *intracardiac electrogram*, or His bundle electrogram, records not only the spread of the wave of depolarization over the atria (A) and ventricles (V), but also the passage of the wave of depolarization through the bundle of His (Fig. 20.8).

The P Wave: Atrial Depolarization

The waves of the ECG were named at the beginning of this century by Einthoven, who chose to start in the middle of the alphabet with the letter P. Thus the first deflection of the ECG, which represents atrial depolarization, is the P wave. Although depolarization of the SA node precedes atrial depolarization (Table 20.1; Fig. 20.9), no manifestations of this pacemaker activity are seen in the ECG. This is simply because the SA node is too small to generate electrical potential differences

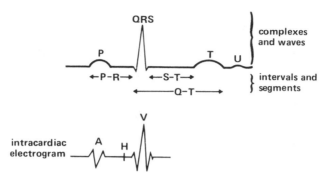

FIG. 20.8. *Top:* ECG recorded from the body surface. *Bottom:* Intracardiac electrogram.

great enough to be recorded from the body surface. The width (or duration) of the P wave, which reflects the time taken for the wave of depolarization to spread over the atria, can be prolonged by either atrial enlargement or a conduction delay in Bachmann's bundle (see above).

The P-R Interval: Atrioventricular Conduction

After inscription of the P wave, the ECG returns to its baseline because changing potential differences within the heart are no longer recorded at the body surface. However, during this "silent" interval between atrial depolarization (the P wave) and ventricular depolarization (the QRS complex described below), the wave of depolarization is, in fact, being propagated through the AV node, the AV bundle, bundle branches, and Purkinje network (Fig. 20.9). The absence of any influence of these electrical events on the body surface ECG, like the failure to record the activity of the SA node, is due to the small mass of the tissues involved in these important aspects of atrioventricular conduction.

The interval between the P wave and the QRS complex represents an important index of impulse propagation through the AV node, AV bundle, and bundle branches (Fig. 20.9). The time needed for the impulse to pass from the atria to the ventricles can be estimated from the *P-R interval* (Fig. 20.8), which extends from the beginning of the P wave to the first deflection of the QRS complex (whether this deflection is a Q wave or an R wave, as defined below). Additional information regarding the passage of the wave of depolarization through the AV bundle can be obtained by timing the His deflection recorded on intracardiac electrograms (Fig. 20.10).

The QRS Complex: Ventricular Depolarization

The *QRS complex* records potentials at the body surface generated when the wave of depolarization passes through the ventricular myocardium (Fig. 20.11). The am-

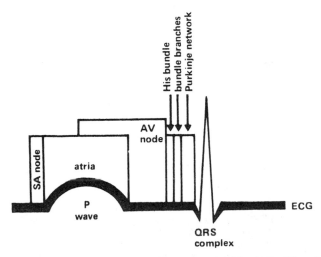

FIG. 20.9. Tissues depolarized by a wave of activation commencing in the SA node are shown in a series of blocks superimposed on the deflections of the ECG. Depolarization of many important structures does not generate potential differences sufficiently large to be recorded at the body surface.

plitude of the QRS complex is greater than that of the P wave because the ventricular mass is greater than that of the atria; the fact that the duration of the QRS complex is about the same as that of the P wave is readily explained by rapid propagation of the wave of depolarization through the ventricle by the specialized conducting cells of the Purkinje network (Table 20.1).

Confusion is sometimes engendered by attempts to define the mechanical behavior of the heart from the ECG, which of course is a recording of electrical activity.

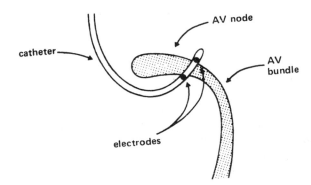

FIG. 20.10. The intracardiac electrogram (See Fig. 20.8) measures the potential difference between two electrodes on a catheter introduced into the right atrium and placed over the proximal portion of the AV bundle.

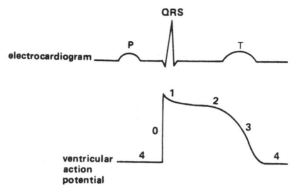

FIG. 20.11. Temporal relationships between the ECG (*top*) and a representative cardiac action potential (*bottom*). The QRS complex is produced by the upstrokes (phase 0) of all of the action potentials throughout the ventricles; the isoelectric S-T segment corresponds to the plateaus (phase 2), whereas the T wave is inscribed during repolarization (phase 3) of the ventricular mass. The isoelectric segment which comes after the T wave corresponds to ventricular diastole (phase 4).

Although there is a very rough correlation between such parameters as QRS amplitude and the force of ventricular contraction, these relationships are much too indirect to be of any practical value.

> The conventions followed in naming the "waves," or deflections, of the QRS complex are as follows. Q: any initial downward deflection followed by an upward deflection (if there is only a downward deflection, it is called QS). R: any upward deflection whether or not it is preceded by a Q wave. S: any downward deflection preceded by an R wave. Additional upward deflections after S waves are called R', R", etc.; additional downward deflections after S waves are S', S", etc.

The S-T Segment: Plateau of the Ventricular Action Potential

Following the inscription of the QRS complex, the ECG normally returns to, or very nearly to, its baseline, where it remains until the inscription of the T wave. This isoelectric phase, the *S-T segment*, occurs when all regions of the ventricle are in a depolarized state, during the plateau (phase 2) of the ventricular action potential (Fig. 20.11). The duration of the S-T segment thus reflects the normally long plateau of the cardiac action potential (Chapter 19).

The fact that the potential difference recorded by the ECG during the S-T segment is normally the same as that during the interval after the T wave and before the P wave (the T-P segment), when the ventricles are fully repolarized, reflects the absence of potential differences within the ventricles. An isoelectric segment on the ECG therefore provides no information regarding the polarity of the ventricular myocardium; when *all* regions of the ventricles are depolarized, as when *all* regions are at resting potential, the ECG records no potential differences.

The preceding discussion emphasizes the fact that although the ECG records the changing potential differences between different parts of the body surface, there is no way of determining the true zero potential of an ECG. It is for this reason that we cannot distinguish between two causes of an altered relation between the S-T segment and the T-P segment: an abnormal potential difference during the S-T segment (ventricular systole) and an abnormal potential difference during the T-P segment (ventricular diastole). By convention, the T-P segment is assumed to represent the baseline (zero potential), so that both abnormalities are viewed as S-T segment shifts (See Chapter 24).

The T Wave: Ventricular Repolarization

Repolarization of the ventricles generates the T wave, which corresponds to the end of phase 2 and phase 3 of the cardiac action potential (Fig. 20.11). The duration of the T wave is considerably longer than that of the QRS complex because, unlike ventricular depolarization, repolarization does not spread as a rapidly propagated wave. The T waves, which are very labile, are therefore determined largely by local factors that influence the outward currents that end the action potentials in the various regions of the ventricle. Thus, although the narrow QRS complex arises from the rapidly conducted wave of depolarization conducted through the ventricles by the Purkinje network, the broader T wave reflects the less synchronous repolarization of the ventricles. (As described later in this chapter, the sequence of ventricular repolarization also differs from that during depolarization.)

The influence of local factors on the T waves is readily demonstrated in a simple experiment. If one rapidly drinks several glasses of ice water, cooling of the inferior surface of the ventricles can lead to marked T-wave abnormalities.

The U Wave

In some normal ECGs a small deflection is seen after the T wave. This is the U wave, whose origin remains uncertain. The U wave may be related to repolarization of the Purkinje network, in which the action potential duration is greater than that of the ventricular myocardium (Chapter 19); however, this explanation is not fully substantiated.

Relationship Between the ECG and Ventricular Action Potentials

The QRS complex, S-T segment, and T waves are all generated by action potentials in the ventricle (Fig. 20.11). As a first approximation, the QRS complex corresponds to the upstroke of the action potential (phase 0), the S-T segment to the plateau (phase 2), and the T wave to repolarization (phase 3). The relationship between electrical events in the ventricles and the potential differences recorded at the body surface is, however, more complex than that shown in Fig. 20.11. This is because the QRS complex and T wave represent the *sum* of *all* of the action potentials in the millions of ventricular cells that are depolarized during the time that action potentials are propagated throughout the ventricles. The rapidly changing potential differences that give rise to the sharp deflections of the QRS complex reflect the high velocity at which the wave of depolarization is conducted over the ventricles, whereas the broader T wave reflects the more disperse nature of ventricular repolarization.

> The atria, like the ventricles, generate a potential difference during their repolarization. A T_P wave (i.e., the "T" of the P) is not usually seen, however, because its amplitude is small and it is "buried" in the much larger QRS complex. On occasion, such as when P waves are not followed by QRS complexes (heart block; Chapter 22), T_P waves may be seen on the ECG.

The *Q-T interval*, which is the time that elapses between the onset of the QRS complex and the end of the T wave, provides a useful index of the ventricular action potential duration (Fig. 20.8). As already pointed out, however, there is only a rough correlation as both the QRS complex and T wave represent the sum of the potential differences produced by all of the cells of the ventricular myocardium. In spite of this limitation, measurements of the Q-T interval, along with determinations of the duration of the QRS complex, allow clinical evaluation of the effects of drugs and diseases on the time-dependent properties of the ion channels responsible for ventricular depolarization and repolarization (Surawicz and Knoebel, 1984).

Normal Intervals and Durations in the Clinical ECG

Table 20.2 provides approximate values for the durations of various waves and intervals in the normal adult ECG. Many are age-dependent and can vary with heart rate; furthermore, the normal Q-T interval differs in men and women. Although

TABLE 20.2. *Durations of waves and intervals in normal adult human heart*

Parameter	Duration (sec)
Intervals	
P-R	0.12–0.20
P-H	0.080–0.140
P-A	0.025–0.045
A-H	0.050–0.120
H-V	0.035–0.055
Q-T	0.30–0.40[a]
Waves	
P	0.08–0.10
QRS	0.06–0.10

[a]Highly dependent on the heart rate, to which the Q-T interval is inversely related.

several formulae have been devised to define the relationship between the Q-T interval and heart rate, in the author's opinion none is very successful. A table that gives the range of Q-T intervals for a large normal population at various heart rates is probably the best way to define normal values.

THE HEART AS A DIPOLE IN A VOLUME CONDUCTOR

Any electrocardiographic recording provides a one-dimensional view of the potential differences in the heart generated during the cardiac cycle. As each electrocardiographic lead records time-dependent changes in electrical potential between only two points on the body surface, the pioneers in electrocardiography recognized that the shape and directions of the waves inscribed during the cardiac cycle depended on where recording electrodes were placed on the body surface. To understand how the spread of the wave of depolarization over the atria and ventricles produces the potential changes depicted in the ECG, we first examine the much simpler model of the heart as a *dipole* in a *volume conductor* (Fig. 20.12).

A *dipole* is an electrical source consisting of an asymmetrically distributed electrical charge. Thus, at any instant during the spread of a wave of depolarization, the heart can be depicted as a dipole because one portion of the myocardium is depolarized while the remaining regions are still in their resting state. In the resting myocardium, the outside of the cell is positively charged relative to the cytosol (Chapter 18), whereas in depolarized regions the outside of the cell is negatively charged relative to the cytosol. For this reason Fig. 20.12, which is analogous to a single frame in a motion picture, shows the ventricles at one instant during depolarization; that is, when the partially depolarized heart is an electrical dipole that consists of a resting (positive) region and a depolarized (negative) region.

To generate potentials that can be recorded at a distance, the dipole must be placed in a conducting medium called a *volume conductor*; in Fig. 20.12 this is provided by placing the dipole in a dish of salt water. In electrocardiography, the tissues of the body provide the volume conductor that transmits the potentials generated by the heart to the electrodes on the body surface.

The model of the heart as a dipole in the center of a volume conductor is of course greatly oversimplified. The heart is not a simple dipole in that the complex pathways of impulse conduction allow multiple dipoles to coexist during depolarization of the ventricles. For the sake of this illustration, however, it is not incorrect—only oversimplified—to consider the partially depolarized ventricles as a single dipole. A more serious oversimplification arises because the body is not a homogeneous volume conductor. For example, the lungs represent a region of high electrical resistance, so that in patients with emphysema or a pneumothorax, serious distortions can appear in the ECG. In spite of these limitations, the model shown in Fig. 20.12 remains useful in understanding the physical principles that govern the genesis of the ECG.

Lines of equal potential, along which no potential differences exist, can be drawn in the model of the dipole in a homogeneous volume conductor (Fig. 20.12). Those lines in the half of the volume conductor occupied by the negative pole define

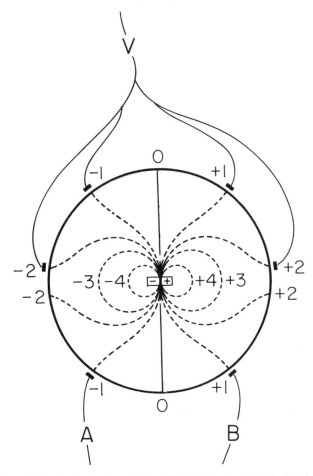

FIG. 20.12. The partially depolarized ventricles within the body can be depicted as an electrical dipole in a volume conductor. The dipole is the *rectangle* in the center of the figure, which is positively charged to the right and negatively charged to the left. The volume conductor is shown as a *circle* (*solid line*) within which are drawn isopotential lines (*dashed lines*). Potentials (indicated in millivolts) can be recorded from the surface of the volume conductor via electrodes such as *A* and *B*, which face regions of the surface where potentials are −1 and +1 mV, respectively. Also shown is an indifferent electrode, or central terminal (V), which records zero potential because it is connected to several electrodes placed on the surface of the volume conductor in such a way that the sum of the recorded potentials is zero.

negative potentials, and those in the other half positive potentials. The lines of equal potential in Fig. 20.12 illustrate the effects of two simple variables on potentials recorded within the volume conductor. First, the amplitude of the potentials decreases in proportion to the square of the distance from the dipole; second, potential falls as one moves away from the axis of the dipole. Distance, the first variable, is largely ignored in clinical electrocardiography so that the potential differences measured at various points on the body surface arise from the second variable. In other words, *the amplitude of the deflections of the ECG are due largely to the angle between the leads on the body surface and that of the cardiac dipole.* For this reason, the lead systems used in electrocardiography were chosen to sample the cardiac dipole from a number of different angles.

Electrocardiographic Lead Systems

The potential difference in the dipole illustrated in Fig. 20.12, like those in the partially depolarized heart, can be sampled using either of two types of lead systems. A *bipolar lead*, in which both electrodes are influenced by the dipole (A and B in Fig. 20.12), records the potential difference between the two electrodes. In the example shown in Fig. 20.12, the potential difference between leads A and B is 2 mV. Whether the recorded potential is $+2$ mV or -2 mV depends on the conventions chosen by the observer: if electrode A is defined as zero, then B records $+2$ mV; if B is chosen as zero, then A is -2 mV. Because of their simplicity, bipolar lead systems were the first to be used in clinical electrocardiography.

Attempts to define the true zero potential in the human body led to the introduction of so-called *unipolar leads* in which one electrode (the *exploring* electrode) is influenced by the dipole, whereas the other (the *indifferent* electrode) is considered to be recording zero potential at all times, i.e., not influenced by the dipole. Theoretically an indifferent electrode can be achieved by one of two means. The first involves placing the electrode so far from the dipole that it records virtually no potential simply because potential declines with increasing distance. One can, for example, place an individual in one corner of a salt water swimming pool and record from the opposite corner; however, this approach is not very practical for clinical electrocardiography. The second solution is to connect a number of electrodes, all of which are influenced by the dipole, to each other in a manner that cancels out the potential differences generated by the dipole. This second type of indifferent electrode, called *V* in clinical electrocardiography, is assumed to be at or near zero because the potentials recorded by the many electrodes, although each is influenced by the dipole, cancel each other.

The V electrode shown at the top of Fig. 20.12 has been constructed according to the second of these assumptions, that by connecting several exploring electrodes together, zero potential is recorded. As before, electrodes A and B are the exploring electrodes. Thus, the unipolar lead VA, which detects the absolute potential at the point of placement of electrode A, records a potential of -1 mV. This potential is negative because V is conventionally assigned a value of zero. Similarly, the unipolar lead VB detects a potential of $+1$ mV because electrode B is located in a region where potential is $+1$ mV relative to zero.

The V leads used in clinical electrocardiography are not, in fact, true unipolar leads (see below), which presents some theoretical drawbacks. However, for all practical purposes, the fact that the V leads do not provide true unipolar recordings is of no real clinical significance. This is because most interpretations of electrocardiographic contour are empirical rather than absolute.

THE DIPOLE GENERATED DURING VENTRICULAR DEPOLARIZATION

The example of the dipole in a volume conductor depicted in Fig. 20.12 describes the distribution of electrical potential at one instant during depolarization of the ventricles. Yet during each cardiac cycle, the potentials produced by ventricular depolarization change from moment to moment. To understand the genesis of the QRS complex, which records the time-dependence of the changing electrical potential differences during ventricular depolarization, it is useful to consider first the data obtained when a simple bipolar lead is used to record the potential differences generated by an activated rectangular strip of cardiac muscle (Figs. 20.13–20.17).

> As pointed out in Chapter 18, electrophysiologists put electrodes into cells and so focus mainly on *intracellular* potentials, which at rest are obtained from the electronegative cytosol. In contrast, electrocardiographers view the myocardium from the body surface, and so see the resting potentials recorded from *outside the heart* as positive in polarity.

Resting

In the resting strip (Fig. 20.13), where all of the cell surfaces are positively charged, no differences in potential are recorded, so that bipolar "ECG" remains at the baseline (zero potential).

During Depolarization

When the strip of myocardium shown in Fig. 20.13 is stimulated at its left-hand end, a wave of depolarization propagates from left to right. As this wave of depolarization advances over the surface of the strip, a potential difference appears between electrodes A and B (Fig. 20.14). If electrode A is chosen to represent zero potential, electrode B records a positive potential relative to electrode A. In this situation, the convention in electrocardiography is to set the polarity of the recording device so that when B (the recording electrode) is positive relative to A (the indifferent electrode), an upright deflection is written. For this reason, the wave of depolarization

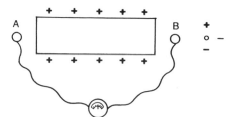

FIG. 20.13. The entire surface of a strip of resting myocardium is positively charged (relative to the interior of the cells); as a result, no potential difference is recorded between electrodes *A* and *B*. A strip chart recording of the bipolar lead *AB* (*right*) records no potential difference and so remains at its baseline.

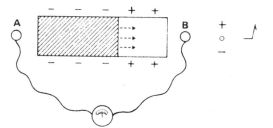

FIG. 20.14. The strip of myocardium depicted in Fig. 20.13 has been stimulated at its left side and is now slightly more than half depolarized (*shaded area*). The surface of the depolarized area is negatively charged (relative to the interior of the cells of the fiber) so that electrode B is facing a region of greater positivity than is electrode A. The strip chart recorder at the *right*, which has been wired so that an upward deflection is written when electrode B is more positive than A, thus inscribes an upward deflection. The deflection of this bipolar lead reaches its maximum when exactly half of the myocardial strip is depolarized. Note that the partially depolarized strip of myocardium is similar to the dipole shown in Fig. 20.12.

approaching the recording electrode B records an upright deflection in the ECG. As the wave of depolarization comes to include a greater fraction of the strip of myo-cardium, the potential difference increases, reaching its peak when half of the strip is depolarized.

Depolarized

The potential difference between electrodes A and B returns to zero when the entire strip is depolarized (Fig. 20.15) because both electrodes face a similar degree of electronegativity. Thus, the deflection returns to baseline. Note that a zero potential difference between A and B cannot distinguish between a fully depolarized and a fully repolarized strip of myocardium as neither generates a *potential difference*.

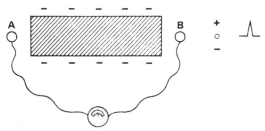

FIG. 20.15. The strip of myocardium depicted in Figs. 20.13 and 20.14 is now fully depolarized. When the action potentials of all cells are in phase 2, their external surfaces are negative relative to their interiors. Because no potential differences exist between the external surfaces of the cells in the strip of myocardium, electrodes A and B both face a similar degree of negativity. The deflection in the bipolar lead (*right*) thus returns to the baseline.

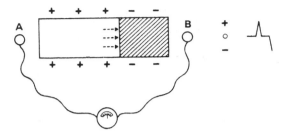

FIG. 20.16. Strip of myocardium depicted in Figs. 20.13–20.15 in which repolarization has begun in the same region that was first to be depolarized, i.e., at the *left*. Because the cell exteriors in the repolarized region of the strip (*left*) have returned to their normal, resting positivity, electrode *B* is facing a region of greater negativity than is electrode *A*. The bipolar lead at the right thus inscribes a downward deflection (see legend to Fig. 20.14).

During Repolarization

If repolarization begins at the same point on the strip of myocardium at which the propagated wave of depolarization began, a potential difference opposite in polarity to that seen during depolarization is created (Fig. 20.16). Thus, electrode B faces an area of electronegativity (relative to A) so that according to the conventions described above, a downward deflection is recorded in the ECG.

Repolarized (Resting)

At the end of the phase of repolarization, the entire strip is once again fully repolarized (Fig. 20.17) so that, as in Fig. 20.13, no potential differences are recorded. Thus, the ECG record returns to baseline.

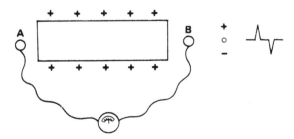

FIG. 20.17. Strip of myocardium depicted in Figs. 20.13–20.16 in its fully repolarized state. The situation is as shown in Fig. 20.13, so that the bipolar lead (*right*) returns to its baseline.

Conventions

A simple rule, which should be memorized, is that a recording electrode (lead) facing an *approaching* wave of depolarization records a *positive* potential, which inscribes an *upright* deflection in the ECG because positive potentials are conventionally recorded as upward deflections. When a wave of depolarization recedes from a recording electrode (as would have occurred if B, rather than A, had been chosen to represent zero in the example just given in Figs. 20.13–20.17), a downward deflection is written.

ELECTRICAL VECTORS

The potential differences at any instant during ventricular depolarization can be represented as a dipole that has both magnitude and direction. The directionality (axis) of the cardiac dipole in the body is determined by the orientation of the positive and negative poles. If the dipole is oriented transversely in the chest as shown in Fig. 20.18, an electrode on the right arm (A) records a negative potential and an electrode on the left arm (B) records a positive potential.

The cardiac dipole can be represented as a vector having both magnitude and direction. By convention, when the cardiac dipole is depicted by an arrow, the head points to the positive pole, as shown in Fig. 20.19. This is a useful convention because the arrow points in the direction of propagation of the wave of depolarization, and toward the lead that inscribes an upright deflection. It is thus easy to remember that vector arrows point in the direction followed by the wave of depolarization as it passes through the ventricles, and their length indicates the magnitude of the potential difference.

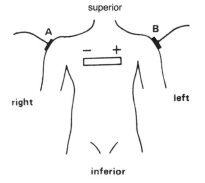

FIG. 20.18. A cardiac dipole in the human body. The partially depolarized ventricles are analogous to the strip of myocardial tissue shown in Fig. 20.14, which establishes a dipole similar to that shown in Fig. 20.12. This figure is obviously an oversimplification as the heart does not lie in the center of the chest, nor are electrical resistances the same throughout the chest. The analogy remains useful, however, as it simplifies understanding the electrical potential differences recorded between ECG electrodes on the right (*A*) and left (*B*) arms.

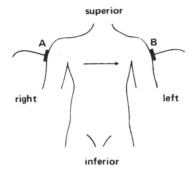

FIG. 20.19. The dipole shown in Fig. 20.18 is conventionally represented as an *arrow* oriented in the direction of the dipole axis. Also by convention, the head of the *arrow* points to the positive pole of the dipole, and so points in the direction of the propagated wave of depolarization.

QRS Vectors

Because of the complex geometry of the ventricular mass and the fact that the wave of electrical depolarization normally enters both ventricles at almost the same time (by way of the right and left bundle branches), many regions of the ventricles are activated simultaneously during the inscription of the QRS complex. Thus, at any instant during the spread of the wave of depolarization over the ventricles, many electrical vectors can be drawn over the surface of the ventricles. The *mean instantaneous QRS vector* is the sum of *all* vectors generated at *any moment* during depolarization. Depending on where the recording electrodes are placed on the body surface, this vector can describe deflections that are upright, inverted, or absent (see below).

The sequential appearance of a series of mean instantaneous QRS vectors throughout the period of ventricular depolarization is recorded by the ECG as the QRS complex. Thus, the changing deflections of the QRS complex are due simply to the changing direction and magnitude of the mean instantaneous QRS vector as the wave of depolarization sweeps over the ventricles. The sum of *all* of the mean instantaneous QRS vectors inscribed during ventricular activation is the *mean QRS vector*, which thus represents the mean electrical vector generated by ventricular depolarization.

Normal Sequence of Ventricular Activation

Normal activation of the ventricles can be divided *arbitrarily* into three phases, each of which can be viewed as generating a mean instantaneous QRS vector. The first phase is septal activation, the second activation of the apex, and the third activation of the base of the heart. Although these three events merge into each other and do not represent three distinct events, for purposes of illustration they are considered separately.

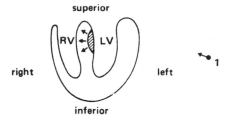

FIG. 20.20. Genesis of the QRS vector: septal activation. The initial portion of the QRS complex is produced by depolarization of the interventricular septum. Activation begins at the left ventricular surface of the septum and produces an initial QRS vector (*right*) that in the frontal plane is directed to the right and superiorly.

Septal Activation

The interventricular septum and anterior regions of the base represent the first regions of the ventricular mass to be depolarized during normal ventricular activation. As septal activation begins in the endocardium of the left ventricle, the initial deflection on the normal QRS is a small electrical vector directed to the right. This septal vector, which gives rise to a small downward deflection in leads facing the left ventricle (the normal "septal Q wave"), is depicted in the frontal plane of the body in Fig. 20.20.

Activation of the Apex

Activation of both ventricles proceeds from the endocardial surface toward the epicardium because the rapidly conducting Purkinje network is located in the endocardium. The much larger mass of the left ventricle causes leftward electrical forces to predominate over those directed to the right, so that the second arbitrarily defined frontal plane vector is directed inferiorly and to the left, as shown in Fig. 20.21.

Activation of the Base

The last portions of the ventricles to be depolarized are the left and right ventricular bases. Again, because activation proceeds from endocardium to epicardium and left ventricular forces dominate, the third vector is directed superiorly and to the left as shown in Fig. 20.22.

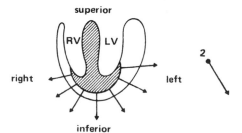

FIG. 20.21. Genesis of the QRS vector: activation of the apex. The midportions of the QRS complex are produced when depolarization of the apex of the heart is activated. Activation begins at the endocardial surfaces of the ventricles that, because left ventricular forces are dominant, generates a frontal vector plane (*right*) that is directed to the left and inferiorly.

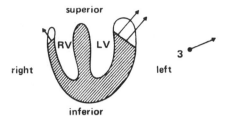

FIG. 20.22. Genesis of the QRS complex: activation of the base. The terminal portions of the QRS complex are produced by depolarization of the base of the heart. Activation begins at the endocardial surfaces and, because left ventricular forces are dominant, generates a frontal plane vector (*right*) that is directed to the left and superiorly.

The Vector Loop

All three of the mean instantaneous QRS vectors depicted by arrows in Figs. 20.20 to 20.22 share a common origin at zero potential, whereas the arrowheads that project from this common origin define both the magnitude and direction of the three arbitrarily defined vectors. As the tails of all three arrows correspond to the same zero potential, they can be superimposed in a single figure that depicts these three mean instantaneous QRS vectors (Fig. 20.23). If one now imagines *all* of the instantaneous vectors recorded during the inscription of the QRS complex, the heads of the many vector arrows generated during ventricular depolarization inscribe a "vector loop," as shown in Fig. 20.24A. This loop, which is zero when the QRS complex begins and returns to zero when the QRS has ended, thus links the heads of all of the mean instantaneous QRS vectors generated during ventricular depolarization.

The Mean QRS Vector

The *mean QRS vector* (Fig. 20.24B), which is made up of all electrical vectors generated at all times in all regions of the ventricles during the inscription of the QRS complex, is also the sum of all of the vectors that contribute to the vector loop shown in Fig. 20.24A. Measurement of the angle of this vector in the body provides an important part of clinical electrocardiographic analyses.

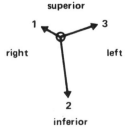

FIG. 20.23. Because the tails of the three frontal plane QRS vectors shown in Figs. 20.20–20.22 all represent zero potential, they have been superimposed. This allows the vectors produced by septal activation (1), activation of the apex (2), and activation of the base (3) to be projected in a single figure.

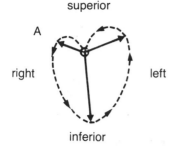

superior

A

right

left

inferior

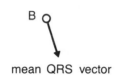

B

mean QRS vector

FIG. 20.24. QRS vector loop and mean QRS vector. The *vector arrows* in Fig. 20.23, which are reproduced in *A*, represent only three of the instantaneous QRS vectors generated during ventricular depolarization. When the heads of all of these instantaneous vectors are connected (*dashed line*), a loop is formed (*A*). The mean QRS vector (*B*) is the sum of all of the instantaneous vectors generated at all times and in all regions of the ventricles during their depolarization.

RECORDING THE ELECTROCARDIOGRAM

Bipolar Limb Leads and the Einthoven Triangle

The first systematic approach to evaluating the potential differences set up at the body surface by the cardiac dipole was made possible by Einthoven, whose invention of the string galvanometer provided the earliest high-fidelity recording of the ECG. Einthoven utilized three electrodes placed on the left arm, right arm, and left leg, which he assumed to be at the corners of an equilateral triangle, the *Einthoven triangle*. For simplicity he also assumed that the heart lay at the center of this triangle (Fig. 20.25).

In using these electrodes to construct the three standard limb leads Einthoven defined the potentials at the right arm electrode as zero in leads I and II, and the left arm electrode was chosen as zero in lead III (Table 20.3). This convention causes positive deflections to be recorded in lead I when the left arm is positive relative to the right arm, in lead II when the left leg is positive to the right arm, and in lead III when the left leg is positive to the left arm. Each of these limb leads is of course a bipolar lead in that both electrodes are influenced by the cardiac dipole.

Einthoven's selection of the "zero" electrodes in his leads I, II, and III was based on his desire to obtain upright deflections in all three leads of the normal ECG (see below) rather than on mathematical considerations, which most logically would assign "zero" to electrodes proceeding in a sequence around the sides of the triangle in a single direction. For this reason the sum of the potential differences in leads I and III equal that recorded in lead II.

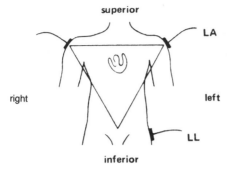

FIG. 20.25. Einthoven triangle. Einthoven simplified interpretation of the frontal plane ECG by assuming the heart to lie in the center of an equilateral triangle, the corners of which are in contact with electrodes placed on the left arm (LA), right arm (RA), and left leg (LL).

Determination of the Mean QRS Vector

The Einthoven triangle can be used to analyze the mean QRS vector by projecting the potential generated by the cardiac dipole in each of the bipolar leads onto its three sides as shown in Fig. 20.26, which is based on the normal ECG shown in Fig. 20.30. Key to this analysis is the fact that, as shown in Fig. 20.12, each bipolar lead records only that portion of the electrical vector that is parallel to the lead axis. The amplitudes of the deflections in leads I to III (shown along the bottom of Fig. 20.26), measured as the net potential differences in each lead, have thus been projected along the sides of the triangle, as shown by the three arrows in Fig. 20.26. Note that the greatest potential difference is recorded in lead II which, because its angle most nearly parallels the dipole axis, has the tallest QRS complex. In contrast, the least potential difference (and so the smallest QRS complex) is recorded in lead III, which is most nearly perpendicular to the dipole.

The smallest QRS complex, or a QRS complex in which upward and downward deflections are most nearly the same, is found in a lead that is oriented nearly at the right angles to the mean QRS axis. This is because no potential difference is recorded by electrodes that are perpendicular to a dipole. The small QRS in lead III, which is nearly perpendicular to the mean QRS vector, is called a *transitional* complex because it represents a transition between regions of electronegativity and electropositivity (see Fig. 20.12).

Figure 20.26 illustrates another important consequence of the conventions of electrocardiography, that an upright deflection is recorded in any lead when the recording electrode faces a wave of approaching depolarization. As shown in this

TABLE 20.3. *Standard limb leads*

Lead	Potential between	"Zero electrode"
I	Right and left arms	Right arm
II	Right arm and left leg	Right arm
III	Left arm and left leg	Left arm

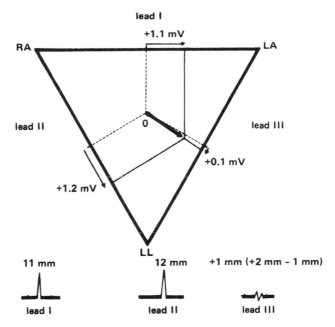

FIG. 20.26. A normal mean QRS vector projected on the Einthoven triangle, each side of which represents one of the three bipolar limb leads (I, II, III). The QRS deflections shown at the bottom of the figure are from the ECG in Fig. 20.30. The tail of this vector, which represents zero potential, is at the center of the triangle and is projected to the midpoints of the three sides (*dashed lines*). The projections of the mean QRS vector on each side of the triangle (i.e., in each lead) are determined by dropping perpendiculars (*thin lines*) from the sides of the triangle to the head of the mean QRS vector. According to the conventions introduced by Einthoven, upright deflections are produced by the projections of this vector in leads I and II. The QRS complex in lead III, which contains small upright and inverted deflections, is a transitional complex in that it is midway between being upright and inverted. Transitional complexes are found in leads that are perpendicular to the mean vector axis.

example, the mean QRS vector is directed inferiorly and toward the left so that, relative to the right arm, both the left arm (lead I) and left leg (lead II) are positive and inscribe upright deflections. As noted above, because the wave of depolarization is nearly perpendicular to lead III, this lead records only the small transitional QRS (the small upright deflection is about the same size as the small inverted deflection in this lead).

In clinical electrocardiography, the Einthoven triangle can be used to derive the mean QRS vector from the net deflections in each of the three standard limb leads (Fig. 20.26). These are determined for each lead by adding positive deflections and subtracting negative deflections. The resulting net QRS voltages, which represent the magnitude of the potential differences during ventricular depolarization recorded in each limb lead, are then used to locate the head of the mean QRS vector within the Einthoven triangle. The "tail" (zero) of the mean QRS vector is first placed at the center of the triangle, and projected as perpendiculars to the midpoint of each side of the triangle. The lengths of the arrows, defined by the net QRS voltage in each lead (see above), are then added to these zero points as shown in Fig. 20.26 and perpendiculars are drawn from the head of each arrow toward the center of the triangle. If placed precisely, these perpendiculars should intersect at a point that represents the head of the arrow generated by the mean QRS vector.

> In student laboratories, the projections of the three arrowheads calculated for the bipolar limb leads rarely meet at a single point as shown in Fig. 20.26; instead, due to inevitable imprecisions in measurement, they form a small triangle. The head of the mean QRS vector lies somewhere in this triangle, which represents a "triangle of uncertainty." This imprecision is generally of little importance in estimating the mean QRS vector; in fact, as noted by many student groups, any two of the perpendiculars drawn in Fig. 20.26 provide a reasonable estimate of this vector.

The Einthoven triangle provides only a rough estimate of the mean QRS vector in the frontal plane because the actual triangle defined by the limb leads is usually not equilateral, the heart is not in the center of the triangle, and the body is not a homogeneous volume conductor. More precise triangles for the analysis of the QRS vector can be drawn, but even these are not constant from one individual to the next. In spite of the fact that the Einthoven triangle is only an approximation, it is both clinically useful and clinically used.

Unipolar Limb Leads

Three unipolar limb leads are conventionally recorded in clinical electrocardiography along with the standard bipolar limb leads described above. Each unipolar lead is assumed to measure the potential difference between an exploring electrode that is influenced by the cardiac dipole, and an indifferent electrode that records zero potential. The indifferent electrode used in electrocardiography is the central terminal described by Wilson, which is constructed by connecting the three limb electrodes used for the bipolar leads I, II, and III (Fig. 20.27). High resistances (R in Fig. 20.27) are placed in each circuit to overcome the effects of variable resistances between the electrodes and the skin. The resulting terminal, called V, was initially assumed to record zero potential throughout the cardiac cycle. Although Wilson's central terminal does not, in fact, represent an indifferent electrode, the V leads have become an integral part of clinical electrocardiography.

The three unipolar limb leads recorded in the conventional 12-lead ECG are derived from leads VR, VL, and VF, which record the potential differences between V (Wilson's central terminal) and the right arm, left arm, and left leg (F = foot), respectively. In each of these leads, the central terminal is assumed to measure zero potential, so that an upright deflection is inscribed when the exploring electrode is positive relative to the central terminal. In lead VF, for example, an upright deflection is recorded when the left leg electrode faces an approaching wave of depolarization, i.e., when the electrical vector is directed inferiorly.

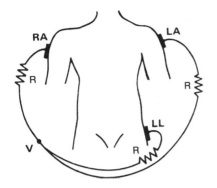

FIG. 20.27. Wilson's central terminal (V) is constructed by connecting the three limb electrodes. Resistances (R) are placed between each electrode and the central terminal to overcome effects of variable resistances between the electrodes and the skin.

Augmented Unipolar Limb Leads

The potentials recorded in VR, VL, and VF are often very small because one electrode in each lead is connected to both sides of the potentiometer. In lead VF, for example, the potential difference recorded is between the leg electrode and the central terminal, which is also connected to the leg electrode. To increase these small potential differences, Goldberger "augmented" the unipolar limb leads by disconnecting the lead that was on both sides of the circuit. For example, in aVF (augmented VF) the leg electrode is disconnected from the central terminal, which increases the potential differences recorded between the leg and the two arms that remain connected to the central terminal. Of course, "augmentation" of the unipolar limb leads invalidates the concept that V leads are unipolar; in aVF, for example, the terminal connected to the left and right arm electrodes clearly does not record zero potential throughout ventricular depolarization. This lack of adherence to theory in the recording of the unipolar limb leads, like the imprecision of the Einthoven triangle mentioned above, highlights the fact that interpretations of contour in electrocardiography are largely empirical.

Chest Leads

The six chest leads (V_1 to V_6) that make up the remainder of the conventional 12-lead ECG are unipolar leads that record the potential differences between Wilson's central terminal (V) and electrodes at each of six positions on the chest wall (Table 20.4). In the chest leads, as in the unipolar limb leads, the central terminal is assumed to record zero potential so that an upright deflection is recorded when the electrode on the chest wall is in an area of relative electropositivity, as would occur when a wave of depolarization approaches the exploring electrode.

The chest leads are useful in evaluating abnormalities arising in one or the other ventricle. This is because the chest electrodes are placed so that the QRS complexes recorded in leads V_1 and V_2 (over the anterior right chest wall) are influenced by the

TABLE 20.4. *Standard chest leads*

Lead	Position of exploring electrode
V_1	Fourth intercostal space just to the right of the sternum
V_2	Fourth intercostal space just to the left of the sternum
V_3	Midway between V_2 and V_4
V_4	Fifth intercostal space at the left midclavicular line
V_5	Left anterior axillary line horizontally to the left of V_4
V_6	Midaxillary line horizontally to the left of V_4 and V_5

spread of the wave of depolarization over the right ventricle, whereas V_5 and V_6 (over the left side of the chest) reflect left ventricular depolarization. In the normal ECG, however, the potentials generated by the left ventricle are so predominant that they overwhelm, and usually completely obscure, the potential differences caused by right ventricular depolarization. For this reason, although the normal QRS complexes in V_5 and V_6 are upright because they record the approaching wave of depolarization over the left ventricle, QRS complexes recorded in leads V_1 and V_2 are normally inverted because they are also generated almost entirely by the wave of depolarization in the left ventricle that moves away from the right side of the chest (see Fig. 20.30).

Clinical Estimation of the Mean QRS Vector

As the estimation of mean QRS vector in the frontal plane by the method illustrated in Fig. 20.27 is cumbersome, a simple method uses the six limb leads listed in Table 20.5. Each lead is assigned an angle that, although not precise, is useful in calculating the mean QRS vector that helps to distinguish normal from abnormal ECGs, and to characterize any abnormalities in the record. These angles are then used to search for a transitional complex, which has fixed relationships to the angle of the leads in which it is recorded. When a complex in any lead is transitional, only two mean vectors (axes) are possible (Table 20.5) because, as noted above, a transitional complex is perpendicular to the axis of the lead in which it is recorded. For

TABLE 20.5. *Angles conventionally assigned to the limb leads*

Lead	Angle	Axis of transitional QRS complex[a]
I	$0°$	$+ 90$ or $- 90°$
II	$+60°$	$- 30$ or $+ 150°$
III	$+120°$	$+ 30$ or $- 150°$
aVL	$-30°$	$+ 60$ or $-120°$
aVF	$+ 90°$	0 or $180°$
aVR	$- 150°$	$- 60$ or $+ 120°$

[a]As a transitional QRS complex is at right angles to the lead, these axes are equal to the lead axis $\pm90°$.

example, a transitional complex in lead I, which is assigned an angle of 0°, could only be generated by a vector having an angle of +90° or −90°.

Because there are two perpendiculars to any line, a mean vector cannot be estimated only by identifying a transitional complex; thus another lead must be examined to estimate the correct axis of a transitional complex. In Fig. 20.26, where the mean QRS is transitional in lead III (which is assigned an angle of +120° in Table 20.5), the mean QRS vector can be either +30° or −150° (120° ± 90°). Because the QRS is upright in lead I, the wave of depolarization must be directed to the left, which means that the correct vector is +30°.

Normal Mean QRS Vectors

The mean QRS vector in the frontal plane is normally between −30° and +110° (Fig. 20.28). These limits are somewhat arbitrary as this vector is quite variable, and depends on such factors as body habitus. Mean QRS vectors greater than +110° are said to represent *right axis deviation*; those less than −30° are designated as *left axis deviation*. Even though the normal range is broad, many individuals with normal hearts have an abnormal QRS axis, and unfortunately, the QRS axis is often normal in patients with severe heart disease.

The chest leads help to define the position of the cardiac dipole in the horizontal plane of the body, but electrical vectors are not usually calculated in this plane. Instead, the transitional lead (where upward and downward deflections are most nearly equal) is identified; this is usually V_3 or V_4.

Mean vectors for electrocardiographic deflections other than the QRS complex can be calculated, although only the QRS is routinely measured. For example, mean T-wave vectors, which are calculated exactly as the QRS vector, are useful because estimates of the QRS-T angle (the angle between the mean QRS and T-wave vectors) can be of help in determining whether a T wave is normal or abnormal. This is because, as discussed below, the T-wave vector is usually concordant with the mean QRS vector, so that a wide QRS-T wave angle implies that there is a primary T-wave abnormality.

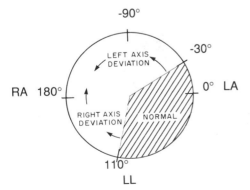

FIG. 20.28. The angle of an ECG vector in the frontal plane is assigned a value according to the convention shown here. A vector directed to the left is assigned an angle of 0°, one directed to the right is said to have an angle of 180°. A vector directed inferiorly has an angle of +90°, one directed superiorly has an angle of −90°. Normal mean QRS vectors range between −30° and +110°. Vectors with angles less than −30° exhibit left axis deviation, and those with angles greater than +110° exhibit right axis deviation.

MUTUAL CANCELLATION OF ELECTRICAL VECTORS IN THE HEART

One reason that analysis of electrocardiographic contour is empirical arises from the fact that the ECG normally records less than 10% of the total electrical activity of the heart. Failure to record most of electrical forces arising in the heart is due largely to mutual cancellation of vectors oriented in opposite directions. This cancellation occurs in part because different regions of the heart are activated at the same time (Figs. 20.21 and 20.22), and because the left and right ventricles are depolarized in opposite directions. The extent to which mutual cancellation reduces the voltage of the QRS recorded at the body surface is apparent when the amplitude of the large QRS complexes associated with ventricular premature systoles are compared with that of adjacent normal complexes (Chapter 23); this comparison shows that loss of synchrony during ventricular activation can dramatically augment the potential differences recorded on the ECG (See Fig. 23.11).

Cancellation of oppositely propagated waves of depolarization also stems from the fact that the rapidly conducting Purkinje fibers penetrate the inner third of the ventricular wall, which causes activation of the ventricular myocardium to begin deep within the wall of the ventricle (Fig. 20.29A). As long as the expanding sphere of depolarization remains within the ventricular wall, no potential differences are apparent outside the heart and no deflections can be recorded by electrodes at the body surface. It is only after the wave of depolarization breaks through the surface of the ventricles that a potential difference exists between electrodes outside the ventricle (Fig. 20.29B).

The resulting discrepancies between the electrical activity generated during ventricular depolarization and that recorded by electrodes at the body surface seriously undermine most attempts to put electrocardiographic interpretation on a solid scientific foundation.

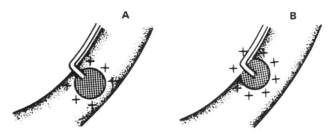

FIG. 20.29. A wave of depolarization that begins at the termination of a Purkinje fiber within the ventricular wall, where a depolarized sphere of muscle (*stippled circle*) is surrounded by resting tissue, does not generate a potential difference that can be recorded by electrodes outside the heart (*A*). A potential difference that can be recorded at the body surface appears only after the sphere of depolarized tissue has expanded to include one surface of the ventricular wall (*B*); this is usually the endocardial surface.

THE NORMAL ELECTROCARDIOGRAM

A normal 12-lead ECG is shown in Fig. 20.30; as noted above, this ECG served as the basis for the vector analysis in Fig. 20.26. Each large "box" in the horizontal direction (time) represents 0.20 sec and is divided into five small boxes of 0.04 sec each. In the normally standardized ECG, each large ventrical box (voltage) represents 0.5 mV and is divided into five small boxes of 0.1 mV each.

> This, and many other ECGs in this text, were obtained with an old-fashioned string galvanometer, which explains the thick line (it is the shadow of the string). Although almost all ECGs today are recorded by pens attached to electronic recorders, the old-fashioned ECGs used in this text are of superb fidelity and, most important, reproduce clearly. The reader should not be confused by the thick baseline, and should understand that when calculating amplitudes, measurements must be made between either the tops or bottoms of the deflections so as not to include the width of the shadow, which is almost 3 small "boxes" in Fig. 20.30.

The mean QRS vector of the ECG in Fig. 20.30 is approximately $+30°$, which as noted above is within normal limits. This axis was calculated from the Einthoven triangle using the three bipolar limb leads in Fig. 20.26. The frontal plane vector can also be estimated by identifying the transitional QRS in the six limb leads; as this is in lead III and the QRS in lead I is upright, reference to Table 20.5 defines an

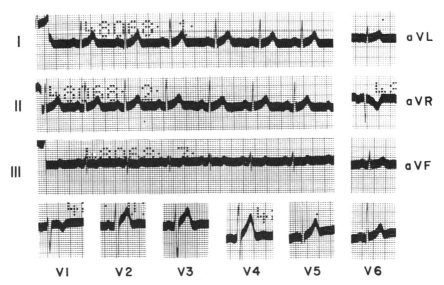

FIG. 20.30. Normal ECG. The mean QRS vector in the frontal plane derived from this ECG is analyzed in Fig. 20.26. Note the minor variations in QRS and T wave configuration in lead III, which are due to changes in the position of the heart within the chest that are related to respiration. (From Katz and Pick, 1956.)

axis of $+30°$. In the horizontal plane, the transitional QRS is in lead V_4, which is also normal.

This ECG also illustrates the normal finding that the T wave is broader than the QRS complex, and that T waves are inscribed in almost the same direction as the QRS complex. This concordance of QRS and T, which is in contrast to that shown in the simplified drawings in Figs. 20.13 to 20.17, is explained below.

Normal Concordance of the QRS Complex and T Wave

The fact that the polarity of the QRS complex is normally the same as that of the T wave (Fig. 20.30) indicates that the last areas of the ventricles to depolarize are the first to repolarize. This is shown in the strip of myocardium discussed earlier in this chapter where, because repolarization normally proceeds in a direction opposite to that of depolarization, the deflections recorded during depolarization and repolarization are concordant (Fig. 20.31). The normal concordance of QRS and T occurs largely because of heterogeneities in action potential duration. Most important is that the plateau (phase 2) of the action potential is longer in the endocardium, where ventricular depolarization begins, than in the epicardium. The relatively long action potentials of the endocardium, which reflect the prolonged action potentials in the cells of the His-Purkinje system (Chapter 19), make this the last region to repolarize.

THE ABNORMAL ELECTROCARDIOGRAM

A few simple examples of abnormal ECGs are provided at this point to illustrate the application of some of the principles discussed in this and earlier chapters. These examples are intended to show how certain electrocardiographic abnormalities can be understood in terms of altered physiology.

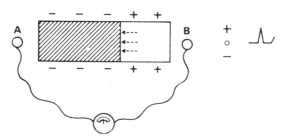

FIG. 20.31. Genesis of the normally concordant T waves. Repolarization of the depolarized strip of myocardium shown in Fig. 20.15 begins in those regions that were depolarized last. This figure, which should be compared with Fig. 20.16, shows that repolarization causes a deflection in the bipolar lead (*right*) that has the same polarity as that inscribed during depolarization.

Intraventricular Conduction Delay

The ventricles are normally activated when a wave of depolarization propagated through the His-Purkinje system spreads simultaneously through the right and left ventricles. The resulting synchrony of ventricular activation occurs because the impulse that emerges from the AV bundle is rapidly conducted through both right and left bundle branches. Interruption of the AV bundle before its bifurcation at the top of the interventricular septum (or less commonly of *both* bundle branches) produces a condition called *complete heart block*, in which the ventricles can no longer be activated by impulses propagated from the atria (Chapter 22).

If conduction in only one of the bundle branches is blocked, impulses from the atria still reach the ventricles; however, activation of the "blocked" ventricle occurs only after a delay, and the wave of depolarization conducted through the latter follows an abnormal pathway. The resulting intraventricular conduction delay causes characteristic ECG abnormalities called *bundle branch block*.

Impulses that depolarize the ventricle in patients with bundle branch block cannot reach the "blocked" ventricle by way of the rapidly conducting His-Purkinje system; instead, the impulse that activates the blocked ventricle is delayed because it must cross the interventricular septum through more slowly conducting ventricular myocardium (Table 20.1). This delay in the spread of the wave of depolarization over the ventricles prolongs the QRS complex, which is the salient abnormality in bundle branch block. The contour of the prolonged QRS complex in bundle branch block is also bizarre because of the altered activation sequence of the ventricles.

Right Bundle Branch Block

The abnormal features of the ECG in right bundle branch block arise from delayed conduction of the wave of depolarization over the right ventricle, which widens the QRS complex and generates a late wave of depolarization over the right ventricle (Fig. 20.32). In Fig. 20.32, for example, the QRS complex in lead II extends through 3.5 small boxes, which represents an abnormally long duration of 0.14 sec (Table 20.2). Because right bundle branch block delays activation of the right ventricle, a late wave of depolarization approaches the anterior, right side of the chest; this gives rise to a broad late R′ wave in lead V_1, which is the hallmark of right bundle branch block. The late R waves in the right precordial leads (V_1 and V_2) are accompanied by broad S waves over the left side of the chest (leads V_5 and V_6); the latter represent a *reciprocal* abnormality because the wave of depolarization approaching the right side of the chest (which generates R waves in V_1 and V_2) recedes from the left chest. The delayed wave of depolarization that spreads over the right ventricle also explains the broad, late R′ wave in lead aVR in Fig. 20.32. A rightward shift of the mean QRS vector is apparent in the frontal plane vector illustrated in Fig. 20.33.

These changes reflect the fact that the late portions of the wave of depolarization

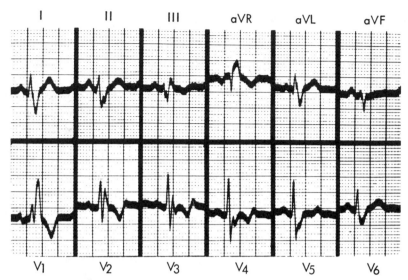

FIG. 20.32. ECG showing right bundle branch block. The broad, slurred, late S waves in leads I and II, and the late R wave in lead aVR, arise from a terminal QRS vector that is directed to the right. The late QRS forces, which dominate the main QRS vector, thus exhibit right axis deviation. The diagnosis of right bundle branch block is established by abnormal widening of the QRS complex in the limb leads to 0.14 sec, and by the rightward orientation of the QRS vector in the precordial leads that produces the prominent late R wave over the right ventricle recorded in lead V_1. (From Littman, 1972.)

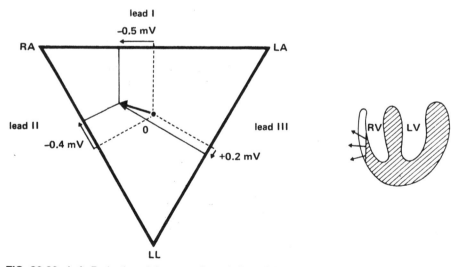

FIG. 20.33. *Left*: Projection of the mean frontal plane QRS vector of the ECG in Fig. 20.32 on the Einthoven triangle. *Right*: Late activation of the base of the right ventricle produces a mean QRS vector that, because it is directed to the right and slightly superiorly, exhibits right axis deviation.

that activates the ventricles are directed anteriorly and toward the right side of the chest, as would be expected because of the normal anatomical position of the right ventricle to the right and anterior to the left ventricle.

Other abnormal features of the ECG in right bundle branch block are apparent in Fig. 20.32. These include the discordance between the QRS complex and T wave, for example in lead V_1, which appears because the impulse is propagated slowly through an abnormally long conduction path in the right ventricle. The slow conduction and long path overcome the influence of the local determinants of action potential duration, and so cause the sequence of depolarization to dominate the sequence of repolarization. The reader is referred to standard electrocardiography texts for further details of this abnormality and its clinical significance.

Left Bundle Branch Block

Complete interruption of the left bundle branch delays activation of the left ventricle so that, as in right bundle branch block, the QRS complex is widened (Fig. 20.34). The orientation of the late QRS deflections in the precordial leads is opposite to that in right bundle branch block, so that tall R waves are seen in leads V_5 and V_6, which arise from delayed depolarization of the left ventricle. As the late wave of

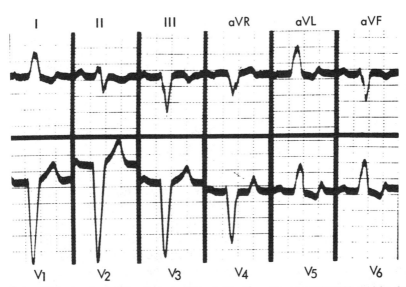

FIG. 20.34. ECG showing left bundle branch block. The broad R wave in lead V_6 and the deep S waves (or QS complexes) in leads V_{1-4} arise form a mean QRS vector that is directed to the left and posteriorly. The QRS forces that dominate the mean QRS vector also produce the tall R waves in leads I and aVL, and the deep S waves in leads III and aVF. The diagnosis of left bundle branch block is established by the widening of the QRS complex to 0.17 sec. (From Littman, 1972.)

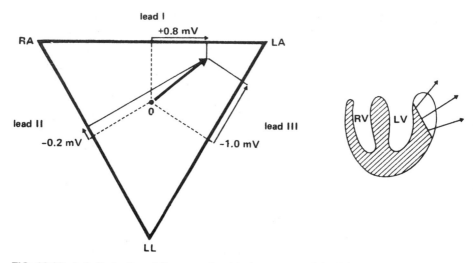

FIG. 20.35. *Left*: Projection of the mean frontal plane vector of the ECG in Fig. 20.34 on the Einthoven triangle shows that there is left axis deviation. *Right*: Late activation of the base of the left ventricle explains the orientation of the QRS vector to the left and superiorly.

depolarization that gives rise to the large R wave in leads V_5 and V_6 is, at the same time, receding from the right precordium, late inverted QRS deflections are seen in leads V_1 to V_4. This explains the inverted QRS deflections (here present as QS complexes) recorded in these "right-sided" leads. The late, unbalanced depolarization of the left ventricular mass also causes a leftward shift of the mean QRS vector in the frontal plane, so that broad, tall R waves appear in leads I and aVL, and deep, broad S waves are seen in leads III and aVF. The mean QRS vector in the frontal plane is shown in Fig. 20.35.

As in right bundle branch block, the long conduction path in left bundle branch block overcomes the effects of local determinants of T wave morphology, so that the T waves become discordant from the QRS complexes.

Fascicular Blocks (Hemiblocks)

Interruption of either the posterior or, as occurs more commonly, the anterior radiations of the left bundle branch gives rise to electrocardiographic findings attributable to fascicular block, or hemiblock. Even though the left bundle branch does not regularly bifurcate into anterior and posterior fascicles (Fig. 20.7), the concept of partial conduction delay over the left ventricle provides an important explanation for abnormalities in frontal plane QRS axis unaccompanied by either QRS prolongation or evidence for ventricular hypertrophy. In both left anterior and left posterior fascicular block, the QRS complex is ordinarily not abnormally widened because the left ventricle is initially activated by way of the Purkinje network. The

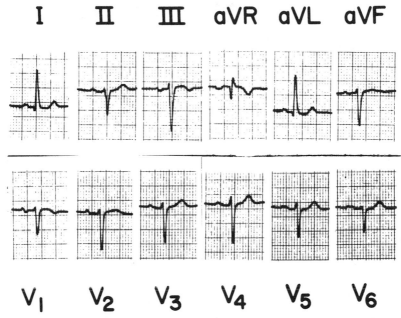

FIG. 20.36. ECG showing left anterior fascicular block. Delayed conduction through the anterior radiations of the left bundle branch causes prominent S waves in leads III and aVF and left axis deviation (mean QRS axis = $-50°$) without prolongation of the QRS complex. The abnormal leftward shift of the transitional QRS in the precordial leads (note that normal R waves do not appear even in V_6) can be seen in this condition. (Modified from Alpert and Flaker, 1984.)

fact that only the terminal phase of left ventricular depolarization is delayed explains why the abnormality is limited to a shift in the mean QRS vector, which reflects the abnormal direction in which the late wave of depolarization activates the left ventricle. In left anterior fascicular block these late electrical forces are deviated to the upward and to the left (Fig. 20.36)[1], toward the "blocked" region of the left ventricle. In left posterior fascicular block the late unbalanced forces are deviated inferiorly and toward the right (Fig. 20.37).

Ventricular Hypertrophy

As might be predicted, the alterations in the QRS complex produced by right (Fig. 20.38) and left ventricular hypertrophy (Fig. 20.39) tend to deviate the mean QRS axis to the right or to the left, respectively. However, changes in the frontal plane QRS vector are not the main criterion for the electrocardiographic diagnosis of ventricular hypertrophy. Instead, the most prominent abnormalities are in the

---

[1]No formal vector analyses are provided for these and other abnormal ECGs; the interested reader is advised to prepare his or her own.

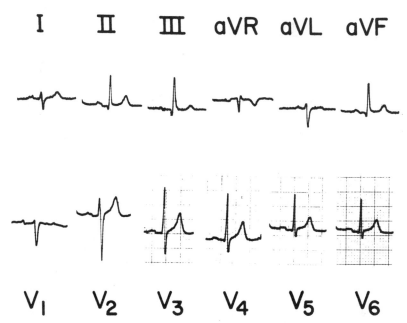

FIG. 20.37. ECG showing left posterior fascicular block. Delayed conduction through the posterior radiations of the left bundle branch causes prominent R waves in leads III and aVF and right axis deviation (mean QRS axis = +110°) without prolongation of the QRS complex. (Modified from Alpert and Flaker, 1984.)

chest leads, where voltage is generally increased in the leads that face the hypertrophied ventricle. Increased amplitude of the QRS complexes in the precordial leads over a hypertrophied ventricle is due in part to its increased mass and partly to delayed conduction. In fact, prolongation of the time required for the passage of the wave of depolarization over the enlarged hypertrophied ventricle, rather than the increased muscle mass, is probably the most important determinant of the large QRS complexes.

Prominent repolarization abnormalities are also seen in ventricular hypertrophy. Most striking is the discordance of the QRS complexes and T waves, which are similar to those seen in bundle branch block. These changes are due both to slowing of conduction, caused by fibrosis of the hypertrophied ventricle, and to the longer conduction pathway over the enlarged ventricle. It must be emphasized that the electrocardiographic diagnosis of ventricular hypertrophy is not very precise. This is because the ECG provides only an indirect index of the mass of the ventricles. Furthermore, as noted earlier in this chapter, the ECG provides virtually no information regarding myocardial contractility.

The abnormal ECGs shown in this chapter have been selected to illustrate the principles that underlie the electrocardiographic recording of the electrical activity of the normal heart and to demonstrate the type of information that can be obtained

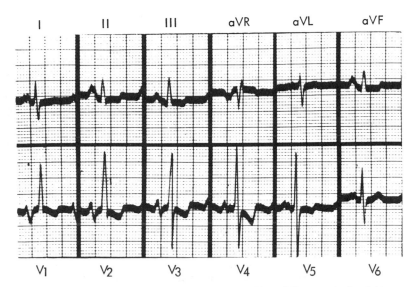

FIG. 20.38. ECG showing right ventricular hypertrophy. The tall R waves in the right precordial leads (V_1 and V_2) and prominent S waves in the left precordial leads (V_5 and V_6) indicate a predominance of electrical forces directed toward the right ventricle. There is also a slight right axis shift in the limb leads, but unlike bundle branch block (Fig. 20.32), the QRS complex is not prolonged. (From Littman, 1972.)

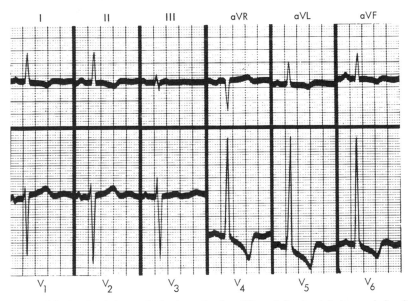

FIG. 20.39. ECG showing left ventricular hypertrophy. Although the frontal plane axis is within normal limits, there are very tall R waves in the left precordial leads (V_5 and V_6) and deep S waves in the right precordial leads (V_1 and V_2). These abnormalities, without prolongation of the QRS complex, indicate a predominance of electrical forces directed toward the left ventricle. Although the high voltage does not, itself, establish this diagnosis, the depressed ST segments and discordant T waves throughout this ECG are typical of this condition. (From Littman, 1972.)

from analysis of the QRS vector in the abnormal heart. No attempt has been made to provide a basis for the electrocardiographic diagnosis of cardiac disease, which is the goal of the many excellent textbooks of clinical cardiology and electrocardiography. The presentation of clinical ECGs in this text is intended, instead, to emphasize that analysis of an unknown ECG, although largely empirical, is based on the rapidly growing body of electrophysiological knowledge that has been described in this and the preceding chapters.

REFERENCES

Alpert MA, Flaker CG. (1984). Chronic fascicular block. Recognition, natural history, and clinical implications. *Arch Intern Med* 144:799–802.

Boineau JP, Schuessler RB, Mooney CR, Wylds AC, Miller CB, Hudson RD, Borremans JM, Brockus CW. (1978). Multicentric origin of the atrial depolarization wave: the pacemaker complex. Relation to dynamics of atrial conduction, P-wave changes and heart rate control. *Circulation* 58:1036–1048.

Gallagher JJ, Smith WM, Kasell JH, Benson DW, Sterba R, Grant AO. (1981). Role of Mahaim fibers in cardiac arrhythmias in man. *Circulation* 64:176–189.

James TN. (1967). Cardiac innervation: anatomic and pharmacologic relations. *Bull NY Acad Sci* 43:1041–1086.

Katz LN, Pick A. (1956). *Clinical electrocardiography. Part I. Arrhythmias.* Philadelphia: Lea and Febiger.

Littman D. (1972). *Textbook of electrocardiography.* New York: Harper and Row.

Scherf L, James TN. (1979). Fine structure of cells and their histologic organization within internodal pathways of the heart: clinical and electrocardiographic implications. *Am J Cardiol* 44:345–369.

Surawicz B, Knoebel SB. (1984). Long QT: good, bad or indifferent. *J Am Coll Cardiol* 4:398–413.

Wenckebach KF, Winterberg H. (1927). *Die Unregelmässige Herstätigkeit.* Leipzig: Verlag von Wilhelm Engelmann.

BIBLIOGRAPHY

A number of excellent teaching textbooks of electrocardiography have their strengths and weaknesses. No one of these texts can be recommended for all students because learning styles and tastes differ. However, an excellent and authoritative bibliography is found in:

Friedman HH. (1985). Diagnostic electrocardiography and vectorcardiography, 3rd ed. New York: McGraw-Hill.

21

The Arrhythmias

I. Introduction and Mechanisms

Our understanding of cardiac rhythm disorders, initially analyzed by recording the arterial and venous pulses, was greatly facilitated by the introduction of electrocardiography into clinical medicine at the beginning of the 20th century. Precise recordings of the spread of electrical activity through the atria and ventricles in both experimental animals and humans with cardiac arrhythmias led to dramatic advances in the understanding of the mechanisms responsible for these disorders. As clinical and experimental electrocardiography remain closely linked, the growth of basic knowledge of the electrophysiological properties of cardiac muscle has made it possible to understand a number of rules that govern the behavior of clinical arrhythmias.

Several important physiological principles that explain the origins of arrhythmias are described in this chapter, and the following chapters present examples of clinical arrhythmias that illustrate some applications of these basic principles. A simple classification of the clinical arrhythmias is presented, but this classification is neither rigorous nor complete. As emphasis is on the electrophysiological basis of the arrhythmias, the reader who wishes a comprehensive review of clinical arrhythmias is referred to the many excellent textbooks and reviews of clinical electrocardiography.

Although arrhythmias can be produced and studied in experimental models, it is extremely difficult, and sometimes impossible, to apply this knowledge to cardiac patients. Rapid advances in clinical electrophysiology, in which arrhythmias are produced and studied in patients, have demonstrated both similarities and unexpected differences between experimental and clinical arrhythmias. In addition, studies of natural history in patients with arrhythmias are uncovering valuable, but sometimes very surprising, information regarding the benefits and hazards of therapy; these findings, in turn, are adding to our knowledge of what may (and may not) be occurring in the hearts of patients who are at risk for the lethal arrhythmias that cause sudden cardiac death.

A GENERAL CLASSIFICATION OF ARRHYTHMIAS

Arrhythmias can be classified two ways: the *type* of arrhythmia, and the *cardiac structure* in which the arrhythmia is believed to originate. There are, in turn, two general types of arrhythmias: *tachycardias*, where the heart beats too rapidly, and *bradycardias*, where the heart rate is too slow; each of these, of course, includes a large number of specific arrhythmias. The normal heart rate is defined as 60 to 100/ min,[1] a range that was chosen to simplify ECG interpretation because these rates correspond to five and three large "boxes" in these recordings (Chapter 20). Brad-yarrhythmias (bradycardias) represent abnormally slow rates of ventricular beating and so are readily diagnosed by palpation of the peripheral pulse. Tachyarrhythmias (tachycardias) are more complex because rapid beating of the atria does not always accelerate the peripheral pulse, as, for example, when impulse propagation is blocked in the AV node.

Arrhythmias can originate in the sinoatrial (SA) node, atria, atrioventricular (AV) node, His-Purkinje system, and ventricles. All but the last two are generally grouped together as *supraventricular arrhythmias* (because they arise above the ventricles), whereas arrhythmias originating in the His-Purkinje system and ventricles are described as *ventricular arrhythmias*.

It would appear logical that the mechanisms responsible for the tachyarrhythmias that abnormally accelerate the heart are quite different from those that slow the heart; indeed, it seems almost obvious that an increased number of conducted impulses reflects mechanisms that are the opposite of those that reduce the number of conducted impulses. Yet, as is much too often the case in cardiology, what seems obvious is wrong! Thus, it is now clear that the same abnormalities of ion channel opening that cause the bradyarrhythmias discussed in Chapter 22 also produce many of the tachyarrhythmias described in Chapter 23. Although this overlapping of ar-rhythmogenic mechanisms complicates efforts to systematize their classification, a number of important principles in this didactic quagmire are readily understood. These are reviewed in the following section, which provides a simple, and, it is hoped, useful, approach to understanding the pathophysiology of arrhythmias.

MECHANISMS RESPONSIBLE FOR BRADYARRHYTHMIAS

There are two common causes for an abnormally slow pulse: (a) impaired impulse formation in the SA node pacemaker, and (b) a conduction abnormality, usually in the SA node, AV node, or AV bundle, that blocks transmission of normal pacemaker impulses to the ventricles. In other words, bradyarrhythmias can be caused by *depressed impulse formation* or *impaired impulse conduction* (the latter is called *block*).

---

[1]The denominator /*min* (per minute) is omitted in the subsequent discussion.

Depressed Impulse Formation

Slowing of the sinus pacemaker, which is by no means a reliable sign of heart disease, commonly occurs as the result of abnormal autonomic influences on this pacemaker, notably excessive parasympathetic (vagal) tone. The resulting *sinus bradycardia* (Chapter 22), which is seen in vasovagal syncope (the common "swoon"), arises from the effects of acetylcholine on resting potential and the pacemaker currents in the SA node (Chapter 18). Although heart rates below 60 are, by convention, abnormal, they are commonly seen in normal individuals, especially athletes in whom training has increased vagal tone. Sinus bradycardia can also be caused by disease of the SA node, a condition commonly seen in the elderly that has the sibilant name *sick sinus syndrome*.

Abnormal slowing of a "lower" pacemaker in the AV node or His-Purkinje system cannot itself cause a bradycardia, because these pacemakers are normally dormant and so do not cause ventricular beating to slow unless the sinus pacemaker has also failed. This does not mean that abnormal slowing of lower pacemakers is without clinical significance. In fact, failure of latent pacemakers to provide "escape rhythms" in patients with marked sinus bradyarrhythmias or block can cause severe symptoms, and if these pacemakers fail altogether, can lead to sudden cardiac death.

Impaired Impulse Conduction (Block)

Bradycardias can also occur in patients in whom, although pacemaker activity in the SA node is normal, there is failure, or *block*, of impulse conduction into the ventricles. As noted above, three areas in the heart are especially vulnerable to conduction block. Two are regions of normally slow conduction, where the safety factor (Chapter 18) is low; the other is a precarious strand of conducting tissue. The former are, of course, the SA node and AV node; the latter is the AV bundle (Table 21.1). Block in the SA node can be caused by either structural or functional abnormalities, whereas block in the AV node is usually functional. In contrast, conduction failure in the AV bundle usually occurs when this rapidly conducting structure, with its high safety factor, is damaged or destroyed (Chapter 22).

TABLE 21.1. *Major sites of conduction block*

Site of block	Usual cause
SA node	Structural and functional
AV node	Functional
AV bundle	Structural

Determinants of Conduction Velocity

Failure of impulse conduction, especially in the SA and AV nodes, is often an exaggeration of the same property that accounts for the normally slow propagation of action potentials through these structures. Understanding of the determinants of conduction velocity is therefore essential to appreciate the mechanisms that can block conduction.

Four physiological variables determine conduction velocity: (a) action potential amplitude, (b) the rate of rise of the action potential, (c) threshold, and (d) internal and external electrical resistances. These determinants are interrelated, and interventions that modify conduction velocity may act through more than one of these factors.

The determinants of conduction velocity are best understood in terms of the *cable properties* of the myocardium, which describe the passage of the regenerative action potential along both a copper wire and a strand of excitable tissue. The currents that propagate an impulse along these structures are *electrotonic*, and so are quite different from the ionic currents across the plasma membrane that generate the action potential. However, the fact that these electrotonic currents are initiated by regenerative action potentials provides the link between ion fluxes (through the channels described in Chapter 18) and the arrhythmias described in this and in the following two chapters.

The propagation of a wave of depolarization along a strand of cardiac muscle depends on the spread of depolarizing electrotonic currents that "reach ahead" from already activated regions of the strand to regions that are still in their resting state. Thus, electron flux from depolarized cells, where the outside of the membrane is negatively charged, to resting excitable cells, where membrane polarity is reversed, determines conduction velocity (Fig. 21.1).

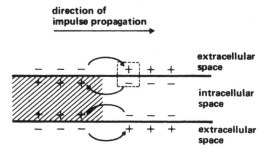

FIG. 21.1. Cable properties in a strand of cardiac muscle transmitting a propagated impulse from left to right. Currents between the depolarized tissue (*shaded, left*) and resting tissue (*unshaded, right*), viewed here as electron flux, are indicated by *arrows*. Current flows away from the depolarized tissue along the outside of the cell, and the circuit is completed when current returns toward the depolarized region inside the cell.

In discussing cable properties, electrotonic current flow is viewed as the transfer of negative charge. This convention, unfortunately, is the opposite of that used to describe transmembrane ionic currents, which are considered in terms of the transfer of positive charge (Chapter 18).

Local electrotonic currents set up during the propagation of a wave of depolarization along a strand of cardiac muscle are represented in Fig. 21.1 by arrows. The flow of electrons between depolarized and resting areas of the strand can occur only through a complete electrical circuit, which requires that current flow in *two* directions. The first is the electron flow toward the resting tissue along the *outside* of the cells; the second is the return of electrotonic current through the *interior* of the cells. This requirement for longitudinal current flow within adjacent cells in the strand explains the importance of the low-resistance gap junctions in the intercalated disc for rapid impulse propagation through the myocardium (Fig. 19.7).

An electrical analog of the strand is shown in Fig. 21.2, which corresponds to the region of the cell membrane enclosed within the small dotted rectangle in Fig. 21.1. This analog illustrates how the cable properties of the membrane arise from the resistive and capacitive characteristics of the circuit discussed above. Key determinants of conduction velocity along the cable are the magnitude and rate of development of the depolarizing currents (light arrows); as these currents increase, the unexcited regions of the strand are depolarized more rapidly. This relationship explains why large and rapidly depolarizing action potentials conduct rapidly: they simply induce large electrotonic currents that quickly depolarize the membranes of unexcited cells further along the strand to their threshold, thereby accelerating their participation in further propagation of the action potential. Other important determinants of conduction velocity are the resistance to longitudinal current flow, both inside and outside the fiber (Fig. 21.2), and threshold. To understand the effects of these variables on conduction velocity, it must be remembered that the spread of the electrotonic currents that initiate a regenerative action potential is *much* faster than the propagation of a wave of depolarization along a strand of cardiac muscle.

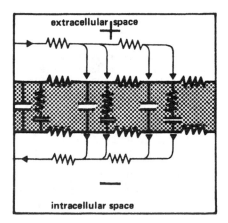

FIG. 21.2. Current flow along and across the cardiac cell membrane (*thin arrows*) shown in Fig. 21.1. Longitudinal currents are influenced by extra- and intracellular resistances, whereas current flow across the membrane (*shaded*) is determined by membrane capacitance and membrane resistance. Conduction is slowed when extracellular or intracellular resistance is increased, but is accelerated by increased membrane resistance.

The cable properties responsible for impulse propagation can be viewed in terms of four electrically different, but often physiologically interdependent, factors that, together, determine conduction velocity in the heart (Table 20.2). Two of these factors, *action potential amplitude* and *rate of depolarization*, are determined by the inward, depolarizing currents responsible for the upstroke of the action potential. *Threshold*, the third determinant of conduction velocity, reflects the time- and voltage-dependent ability of the channels that carry inward currents to respond to an approaching wave of depolarization. The *electrical resistances* of the tissues that transmit the electrotonic currents generated by the depolarizing ion currents represent the fourth determinant of conduction velocity. The latter can be confusing because diametrically opposite effects on conduction velocity are caused by increasing longitudinal resistance (in the extracellular space and within the cell) and increasing the transverse resistance across the sarcolemma (see below).

Action Potential Amplitude and Rate of Depolarization

The dependence of conduction velocity on action potential *amplitude* and *rate of depolarization* is readily understood in terms of the electrotonic spread of depolarizing currents in the cable described in Figs. 21.1 and 21.2. Action potential amplitude, because it determines the size of the depolarizing current, also determines the distance ahead that the depolarized tissue can initiate a propagated action potential. Increasing the amplitude of the action potential projects currents that exceed threshold, and thus are able to excite quiescent tissue, a greater distance ahead of the wave front. Viewed another way, the depolarizing effects of a large action potential "reach" further ahead and thus lead to more rapid impulse conduction than those of a smaller action potential. Similarly, conduction is accelerated by an increased rate of depolarization because of the more rapid spread of depolarizing currents into the excitable, resting tissue ahead of the wave front.

> Slow conduction in the cells of the SA and AV nodes reflects the fact that their action potentials are generated by calcium, rather than sodium currents. Because calcium currents are of low amplitude and develop slowly, calcium-dependent action potentials are also small and slowly rising, which provides the major explanation for the slow conduction in nodal tissue. The ability of parasympathetic stimulation to inhibit calcium channel opening, and of β-adrenergic agonists to increase these calcium currents, are the most important mechanisms for the autonomic control of nodal conduction velocity.

Threshold

The role of *threshold* in determining conduction velocity can also be understood in terms of the cable properties described above. Decreased threshold accelerates conduction by reducing the amount of current needed to initiate a propagated action potential in the resting tissue ahead of the wave front. In other words, reduction in threshold allows the depolarizing effects produced by the approaching wave of depolarization to generate propagated action potentials in the resting tissue at a greater distance ahead of the wave front.

Resistances

The effects of changing *electrical resistances* are less readily understood because changes in longitudinal and transverse resistances have opposite effects on conduction velocity. Decreased longitudinal resistance within the strand, as occurs when the channels in the intercalated disc are opened, accelerates conduction by increasing longitudinal current flow; this, in turn, increases the distance over which an action potential can depolarize unexcited myocardium ahead of an approaching wave of activation (Fig. 21.2). In contrast, decreased transverse resistance across the plasma membrane slows conduction because, by shunting depolarizing current across the sarcolemma into the cell, the longitudinal spread of electrotonic current is reduced.

Longitudinal resistance can be increased by the closing of channels formed by connexon molecules in the intercalated discs. This response to acidosis and elevated cytosolic calcium (Chapter 19) probably plays a role in the genesis of arrhythmias in diseased hearts. Although longitudinal resistance also reflects the conduction properties of the extracellular space, this probably changes little in response to physiological stimuli. However, fibrosis in the failing heart, by increasing extracellular resistance, may slow conduction and so contribute to the reentrant arrhythmias commonly responsible for sudden cardiac death in these patients (Chapter 25).

> The normally slow conduction in the SA and AV nodes is due in part to their small diameter, which is readily explained because of the high internal resistance in a small fiber. This effect, which slows conduction because it reduces longitudinal current flow, is magnified by the fact that SA and AV nodal cells contain few gap junctions, which also contributes to a high internal resistance that slows conduction.

The effects of the four determinants of conduction velocity described above can be compared to a row of falling dominoes (Fig. 21.3). Increasing the height of the dominoes, like an increase in action potential amplitude, increases the speed at which the "impulse" is transmitted because each domino reaches further ahead as it falls. Similarly, if the velocity at which each domino falls is increased (e.g., by putting the dominoes on the planet Jupiter), propagation of the impulse along the row of falling dominoes is increased in a manner similar to increasing the rate of depolarization of the heart. If each domino was tipped slightly, so as to reduce the energy needed to make it fall, the decreased mechanical threshold, like a decreased electrical threshold, would increase the velocity of propagation. Finally, placing the row of dominoes in a vacuum, like reducing the longitudinal resistance, would increase conduction velocity by accelerating their rate of fall. Although a bit fanciful, this analogy may prove useful in understanding the important relationships

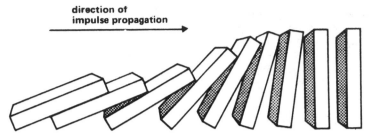

FIG. 21.3. A row of dominoes falling from left to right creates an "impulse" whose propagation is accelerated when the height of the dominoes is increased, the velocity at which each domino falls is increased, the inertia needed to tip each domino is decreased, or the resistance encountered by each falling domino is decreased.

between the currents in an electric cable and the determinants of conduction velocity in the heart.

Control of Conduction Velocity in the Heart

Three of the major determinants of conduction velocity listed in Table 21.2 (p. 529) reflect the inward currents responsible for the upstroke of the action potential; these currents, in turn, are determined by the molecular properties of the ion channels described in Chapter 18. In the working cells of the atria and ventricles and the rapidly conducting cells of the His-Purkinje system, a major determinant of conduction velocity is the rate and extent of sodium channel opening during the upstroke (phase 1) of the action potential. In the slowly conducting cells of the SA and AV nodes, on the other hand, conduction velocity reflects the much slower opening of calcium channels. Modification of these inward currents by drugs and neurotransmitters, either directly or indirectly, will therefore have important effects on conduction velocity. Because slowing of conduction is a common cause of clinical arrhythmias (see below), interventions that inhibit the opening of channels that carry inward current can have important arrhythmogenic effects.

Refractoriness, which is due to inactivation of the ion channels that carry depolarizing current, represents one of the most important determinants of conduction velocity. As discussed in Chapter 19, refractoriness can be caused by partial membrane depolarization prior to stimulation (Figs. 19.5 and 19.6), or prematurity that does not allow complete recovery of sodium (or calcium) channels after a previous action potential (Fig. 19.10). Inactivation of depolarizing currents in refractory cells, by reducing both the amplitude and rate of rise of the action potential, slows conduction and so can play a central role in the genesis of cardiac arrhythmias (see below).

Decremental Conduction

The influence of local factors, such as the type and state of the ion channels that carry inward currents, on conduction velocity accounts for the important property of decremental conduction. This term, which is self-explanatory, defines the phenomena that occur when a rapidly propagated action potential enters a region of the heart in which conduction velocity becomes slowed. Decremental (slow) conduction is seen, for example, when an impulse is propagated into a region of the ventricles in which disease has impaired the opening of the fast sodium channels. As noted above, this slows conduction by reducing the amplitude and rate of rise of the action potential (Fig. 21.4). As a result, these changes in local electrophysiological properties slow the propagation of a wave of depolarization that enters a region of decremental conduction.

Regions of slow conduction commonly occur in abnormal hearts, notably in areas in which the cells are partially depolarized. This can occur when the sodium pump is inhibited; for example in cells that are chronically energy-starved. Of greater pathophysiologic importance is the depolarization caused by a rise in extracellular potassium, which occurs immediately after a coronary artery occlusion (Chapter 24). Depolarization of the ischemic myocardium in these patients reflects a fall in the ratio $[K^+]_i/[K^+]_o$, which reduces the Nernst potential for potassium; the major determinant of resting potential in the heart (Eq. 19.1). As resting depolarization partially inactivates both sodium and calcium channels (Chapter 18), both action potential amplitude and the rate of depolarization are decreased, which slows conduction.

Decremental conduction is a normal property of the SA and AV nodes. This is because these more primitive regions of the heart are, as discussed above, charac-

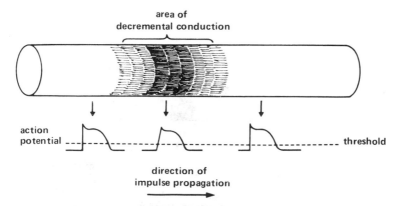

FIG. 21.4. Effects of decremental conduction on the amplitude and rate of rise of the action potential. When an impulse transmitted from left to right in a strand of cardiac muscle (*top*) encounters a region of decremental conduction (*shaded*), the action potential (*bottom*) becomes smaller and more slowly rising. If the impulse is transmitted through the region of decremental conduction into normal tissue (*right*), a normal action potential is once again generated, although its arrival is delayed.

terized by small and slowly rising action potentials, a relative paucity of gap junctions, and small fiber diameter.

When an impulse emerges from an area of decremental conduction into an area where local properties provide for the genesis of large action potentials, conduction velocity returns to normal (Fig. 21.4). This can occur, for example, when an impulse that is propagated slowly through a depressed, ischemic region returns to normally perfused myocardium. Similar heterogeneities of impulse propagation commonly occur around a scarred region of the heart. This behavior is also seen in the normal heart, when an impulse that has been slowed during passage through the AV node reaches the AV bundle, where conduction velocity again becomes rapid.

In some instances, the ability to generate a propagated action potential in a region of decremental conduction may be so depressed as to render the action potential too small to serve as an effective stimulus to the excitable tissue ahead (Fig. 21.5). Under these conditions, because the impulse cannot be transmitted through the area of decremental conduction, conduction is said to be *blocked*.

Clinically, block is seen most commonly in the AV node, where *AV block* occurs when the normal decremental conduction is increased by drugs or disease. Not all AV block is abnormal; for example, athletes with high resting vagal tone often exhibit minor—and clinically insignificant—AV block at rest. Impulse propagation can also be blocked within the SA node (*SA block*), or in the AV bundle (which is another cause of *AV block*) (Table 21.1). Localized block of impulse propagation can also occur in one of the bundle branches and the more distal fascicles of the His-Purkinje system, which cause the *bundle branch blocks* and *fascicular blocks* discussed in Chapter 20.

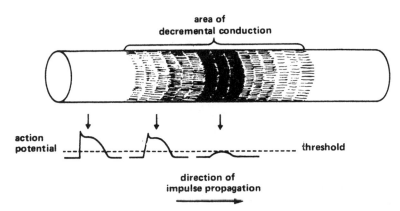

FIG. 21.5. Conduction block in a strand of cardiac muscle containing a region of marked decremental conduction. If the action potential generated in an area of marked decremental conduction (*dark shading*) is unable to bring the normal tissue ahead of the impulse (*right*) to its threshold, impulse transmission is blocked.

Unidirectional Block

Unidirectional block is extremely important as it explains several features of the failure of impulse conduction in regions where conduction is slowed (Chapter 22), and can play a critical role in the genesis of reentrant arrhythmias that commonly lead to the appearance of premature systoles and tachycardias (Chapter 23).

The term *unidirectional block* means what it implies: block of impulse conduction, but in only one direction. As is also true for decremental conduction, unidirectional block can be normal as it represents the usual pattern of conduction through the AV node, where antegrade (forward) conduction from atria to ventricles is usually more rapid than retrograde (backward) conduction from ventricles to atria. Unidirectional block also occurs in the diseased myocardium, for example in ischemic or scarred areas of the atria, ventricles, or His-Purkinje system. In both settings, unidirectional block can be the substrate for important arrhythmias.

A simple model of unidirectional block is produced by compressing a strand of myocardial tissue with a wedge-shaped wooden block (Fig. 21.6), which causes an asymmetrically distributed disturbance of cellular function. This is readily understood as the greater the compression, the greater is the depression of conduction. Asymmetrically depressed conduction, which is common in diseased hearts, often sets the stage for the appearance of unidirectional block. In the series of diagrams shown in Fig. 21.6–21.9, this is manifest as failure of conduction only in the retrograde direction (defined in these figures as conduction from right to left) and not in the antegrade direction (left to right). The appearance of unidirectional block after mild compression of the strand of muscle (Fig. 21.6B) means that the injury that blocked retrograde conduction still allowed antegrade conduction to persist; however, as shown below, antegrade conduction is not normal because it is slowed. If

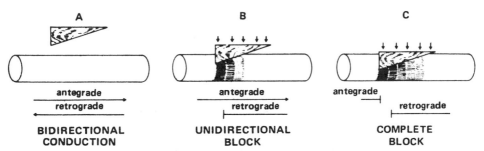

FIG. 21.6. Unidirectional block produced by compression of a strand of cardiac muscle by a wedge-shaped wooden block (*darker shading* indicates a greater degree of injury). *A:* Bidirectional conduction occurs in the normal, uncompressed tissue. *B:* Unidirectional block is produced by moderate compression of the strand, which allows conduction to proceed from left to right (defined here as conduction in the antegrade direction) but not from right to left (retrograde block). *C:* More severe compression of the strand causes conduction in both directions to be blocked.

the compression is increased, the greater severity of injury can cause complete block in which conduction is blocked in both directions (Fig. 21.6C).

The mechanism responsible for the unidirectional block illustrated in Fig. 21.6B can be understood by plotting the ability of impulses generated along the strand to initiate regenerative action potentials. This ability to stimulate resting tissue ahead of the wave of propagation is depicted on the ordinate of Fig. 21.7, where depression of the ability to conduct, like the extent of compression by the wooden wedge, is seen to be asymmetrically distributed. In the uncompressed regions of the tissue, from 0 to 2 cm and from 8 to 10 cm, the normal action potential has been arbitrarily given the ability to activate resting tissue up to 2 cm ahead. Between 2 and 3 cm, under the point of the wedge (Fig. 21.6) the tissue is so badly damaged as to have completely lost the ability to initiate a propagated action potential. However, in the less severely depressed tissue between 3 and 8 cm, action potentials can propagate but, depending on the degree of compression, only abnormally short distances.

If, in the strand depicted in Figs. 21.6 and 21.7, an action potential is initiated at 0 cm, it proceeds in an antegrade direction (Fig. 21.8). As the impulse arises normally in the uncompressed tissue, it is conducted electrotonically across the severely depressed area of the fiber that is unable to generate a propagated impulse. This is shown by the arrow (*a*) which, because it is able to generate an action potential 2 cm ahead, allows the normal tissue just to the left of the completely depressed area to initiate an action potential in tissue 2 cm further to the right, at 4 cm (Fig. 21.8). While the tissue at 4 cm is depressed, it is able to depolarize the

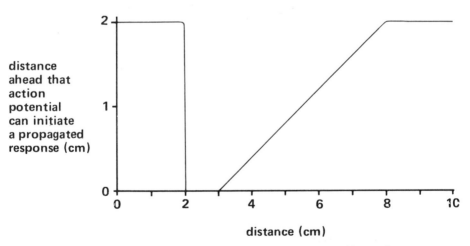

FIG. 21.7. Asymmetrically distributed decremental conduction caused by moderate compression as shown in Fig. 21.6. The distance ahead that an impulse can be propagated (*ordinate*) is plotted as a function of the distance along the strand of cardiac muscle (*abscissa*). Normal tissue (at 0–2 and 8–10 cm) can activate resting muscle up to 2 cm ahead. The ability of the tissue at 2 to 3 cm to initiate a propagated action potential is completely lost, and is depressed from 3 to 8 cm. This figure is used to explain unidirectional block in Figs. 21.8 and 21.9.

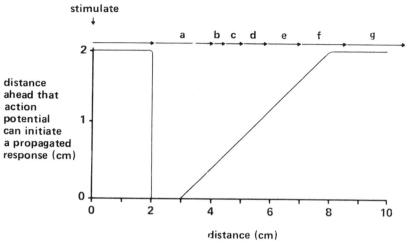

FIG. 21.8. Antegrade conduction in the strand of cardiac muscle in Fig. 21.7. An impulse entering from the left is able to cross the region where the ability to initiate a propagated action potential is completely lost, although the passage of the impulse in the antegrade direction (left to right) is delayed. Discussed in text.

tissue a short distance (0.4 cm) ahead, at 4.4 cm (arrow *b*); here the action potential is less depressed and so conducts 0.6 cm to the right, reaching the tissue at 5.0 cm (arrow *c*). At 5.0 cm the ability to conduct is still less depressed, so that as the impulse is propagated to the right, it emerges from the depressed area.

As each arrow in Figs. 21.8 and 21.9 can be viewed as a brief time interval, shorter arrows represent slowed conduction; in other words, conduction velocity is proportional to the lengths of the arrows. It is apparent, therefore, that antegrade conduction, after being slowed in the depressed area, gains speed as it emerges in the normal tissue at the right. Thus, although the antegrade impulse is able to cross the completely depressed area, it emerges as a normally propagated action potential (at 8 cm) only after a delay.

If retrograde condition is initiated in the above example by stimulating the tissue at 10 cm, rather than at 0 cm, the conduction abnormalities arising from the asymmetrical disturbance of conduction are quite different from those seen when conduction proceeds in the antegrade direction (Fig. 21.9). When the impulse reaches 8 cm, it encounters the depressed area and conduction begins to slow. At 8 cm, the impulse is still conducted normally to the left, and so depolarizes the tissue 2 cm ahead, at 6 cm (arrow *a'*) where action potentials can propagate only 1.2 cm. Thus, the next area to be depolarized is at the tip of the arrow *b'*, at 4.8 cm where the tissue is depressed still further. The impulse arising at 4.8 cm conducts only 0.8 cm, to reach the tissue at 4 cm (arrow *c'*). The impulse arising at 4.0 cm (arrow *d'*) conducts less effectively so that arrow *d'* is even shorter. This decreasing effectiveness of impulse propagation continues, each action potential propagating less and less further ahead until the impulse reaches the completely depressed area (3 cm),

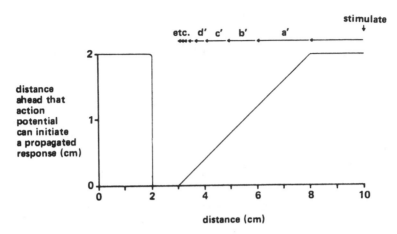

FIG. 21.9. Retrograde block in the strand of cardiac muscle in Fig. 21.7. An impulse entering from the right encounters progressively increasing decremental conduction that renders the impulse progressively less able to initiate an action potential that can depolarize the normal tissue to the left. When the impulse enters the severely depressed tissue (from 2 to 3 cm), retrograde conduction (right to left) is blocked. Discussed in text.

where action potentials are so depressed that they have completely lost the ability to initiate a conducted impulse. Because the impulse can no longer be propagated, retrograde conduction is blocked.

Unidirectional block arising from mechanisms similar to that shown in Figs. 21.6–21.9 is, in fact, commonly encountered in diseased hearts. Asymmetrical depression of conduction can occur in any bundle of myocardial tissue that sustains an injury that asymmetrically depresses any of the determinants of conduction velocity discussed above. These include an asymmetrical reduction in action potential amplitude or rate of depolarization; both of the latter can, in turn, be caused by asymmetrically distributed refractoriness or resting depolarization (see above). Asymmetrically distributed fibrosis, which slows conduction by increasing longitudinal resistance, can also cause unidirectional block, as can an uneven reduction in the number of open gap junction channels. Similarly, an asymmetrically distributed increase in threshold can cause unidirectional block. (The perceptive reader should, by this point, realize that this list simply recapitulates the determinants of conduction velocity discussed earlier in this chapter and summarized in Table 21.2.) In summary, any anatomical or electrophysiological inhomogeneity, singly or together, that produces an asymmetrically distributed abnormality of conduction, can give rise to unidirectional block.

The consequences of decremental conduction and unidirectional block are not confined to the bradyarrhythmias associated with failure of impulse conduction. In addition, as discussed next, unidirectional block is a major cause of reentry, which leads to abnormal impulse formation. Thus, these abnormalities also cause premature systoles and sustained tachyarrhythmias, including the severe disorganization of impulse propagation that leads to atrial and ventricular fibrillation.

TABLE 21.2. *Determinants of conduction velocity*

Variable	Structural and functional basis
Rate of action potential depolarization	Rate of onset and magnitude of sodium or calcium channel openings in the plasma membrane
Action potential amplitude	Magnitude of inward currents through open plasma membrane sodium or calcium channels
Threshold	Ability of sodium or calcium channels in the plasma membrane to open in response to depolarization
Electrical resistances	
Longitudinal resistances	
Extracellular	Volume and conductivity of extracellular fluid
Intracellular	Number of open connexon oligomers in the intercalated discs
Transverse resistance	Plasma membrane conductivity and capacitance

MECHANISMS RESPONSIBLE FOR PREMATURE SYSTOLES AND TACHYARRHYTHMIAS

There are several different types of tachyarrhythmia. A single early beat is usually called a *premature systole*, whereas a sustained run of premature systoles, when regular, is called a *tachycardia*. Very rapid, but generally regular, depolarization of the atria or ventricles is called *flutter*, whereas complete disorganization of depolarization, where there is no effective pumping, is *fibrillation*.

Not all tachycardias increase heart rates to above 100. For example, abnormal acceleration of a ventricular pacemaker to a rate of ~90 is also considered to be a tachycardia. Because these "slow ventricular tachycardias" do not have the same ominous prognosis of more rapid ventricular tachycardias, they are usually referred to as "accelerated idioventricular rhythms," reserving the term "ventricular tachycardia" for the more rapid ventricular beating which is much more dangerous.

As noted at the beginning of this chapter, the mechanisms responsible for premature systoles and tachyarrhythmias are not the opposite of those that cause the bradyarrhythmias. However, most definitions of the tachyarrhythmias center on their clinical features, rather than their pathophysiology. This is not hard to understand because it is difficult, and often impossible, to determine the pathophysiology of a clinical arrhythmia.

At least five different mechanisms account for most of the tachyarrhythmias (Table 21.3). These can occur singly, but often appear in various combinations.

Two older terms, which can reflect more than one of the mechanisms listed in Table 21.3, are "echo beat" and "reentry." Neither is a primary cause of premature beats and tachyarrhythmias; instead, both are abnormalities that can result from several of the mechanisms listed in the table.

TABLE 21.3. *Mechanisms for tachyarrhythmias*

Accelerated pacemaker activity
Triggered depolarizations
Early
Late
Abnormal conduction (decremental conduction and unidirectional block)
Inhomogeneous action potential characteristics
Depolarization: phase 0
Refractoriness and repolarization: action potential duration and
repolarization: phases 1, 2, and 3
Resting potential: phase 4
Abnormal conducting structures
Dual pathways in the AV node
Abnormal accessory pathways

Abnormal Pacemaker Activity

The most easily understood of the mechanisms that give rise to premature systoles and tachycardias is the accelerated discharge of a pacemaker cell, or group of cells. This mechanism is the usual cause of *sinus tachycardia* (Chapter 22), and can also occur in pacemaker cells "below" the dominant SA node pacemaker. Accelerated pacemaker activity can arise from any of the influences that increase the rate of firing of a pacemaker cell (Chapter 19). The single early discharge of a "lower" pacemaker gives rise to a premature systole; if the accelerated discharge is repetitive, it can cause a tachycardia.

Triggered Depolarizations

Early and late afterdepolarizations can lead to triggered depolarizations in the atria or ventricles that cause both premature systoles and sustained tachyarrhythmias (Fig. 19.11). Although little is known of the cause of the early afterdepolarizations, late afterdepolarizations are generated by oscillatory calcium release from the sarcoplasmic reticulum in the calcium-overloaded myocardium (Chapter 19). Triggered depolarizations are also caused by drugs that prolong the action potential, and can produce a characteristic ventricular tachycardia called "torsades de pointes" (Chapter 23). Unlike tachycardias due to accelerated pacemaker activity, which tend to remain regular, those caused by triggered depolarizations readily disorganize and so can lead to fibrillation (Chapter 23). They also differ from those caused by most of the other mechanisms listed in Table 21.3 in that they often become more severe when the heart is paced rapidly, whereas most other tachyarrhythmias are suppressed by rapid electrical stimulation (overdrive suppression, see Chapter 23).

Abnormal Conduction (Decremental Conduction and Unidirectional Block)

The importance of orderly impulse propagation in the heart has been emphasized at many points in this text. It is apparent that disorganization of the wave of depolarization that spreads over the heart, and especially the ventricle, is the "enemy" of efficient cardiac contraction. Mechanical efficiency is lost when one part of the heart contracts or relaxes "out of step," much as would occur if the rowers of a Greek trireme became disorganized. Moreover, conduction disorders in the heart tend to worsen spontaneously, and so are a major cause of sudden cardiac death. Most important are the terrible consequences that follow when spread of the wave of depolarization over the heart becomes completely disorganized; if this occurs in the ventricles, the resulting cessation of effective contraction is a common cause of cardiac arrest. The detrimental consequences of atrial fibrillation are less severe; although this arrhythmia results in loss of the ability of the atria to serve as a primer pump (Chapter 15), it is rarely lethal.

Conduction abnormalities caused by decremental (slow) conduction and unidirectional block probably represent the most important cause of premature systoles and tachycardias. This mechanism is readily demonstrated in experimental preparations, where a single impulse entering a region of decremental conduction can emerge as two or more impulses; these extra impulses are sometimes called echoes, and the process responsible for this phenomenon referred to as reentry.

A model for reentrant excitation, similar to one proposed almost 50 years ago by Schmitt and Erlanger, is shown in Fig. 21.10a. This model, which is based on the anatomy of a junction between a Purkinje fiber and the ventricular myocardium, is equally applicable to the situation in a bundle of conducting or working myocardial fibers (compare Fig. 21.10b with Fig. 19.17). In both models, the substrate for reentry is provided by an area of decremental conduction (unshaded area) that has the two properties discussed above: slow conduction and unidirectional block. In view of the ease with which an asymmetrically distributed region of decremental conduction can create these two properties (see above), they are commonly found in diseased hearts and when the heart comes under the influence of a variety of drugs.

Premature systoles are readily initiated in regions of the heart that satisfy the conditions shown in Fig. 21.10. The arrhythmia begins when an approaching wave of depolarization encounters the proximal end of the area of decremental conduction (A in Fig. 21.10), where antegrade conduction is blocked. Propagation of the impulse through other, normally conducting, areas of the functional syncytium of the heart can conduct the impulse around the area of decremental conduction, to reach a point distal to the depressed area. Starting at this distal point, the impulse enters the depressed area in a retrograde direction (B) and, because the unidirectional block is only in the antegrade direction, the impulse is propagated through the area of decremental conduction. Because conduction is slowed (Fig. 21.8), return of the retrograde impulse to the proximal end of the depressed area is delayed (A). If retrograde conduction is sufficiently slow to allow the proximal tissues to recover their excitability, the retrograde impulse can depolarize (reenter) the normal tissue proximal to the depressed area. The second impulse that is generated in the proximal region of the myocardium, sometimes called an echo beat, represents a premature systole.

This process can become repetitive if the premature systole returns to point B in Fig. 21.10 and produces a second reentrant premature systole. Although this mechanism can generate runs of premature systoles and sustained tachycardias, the first

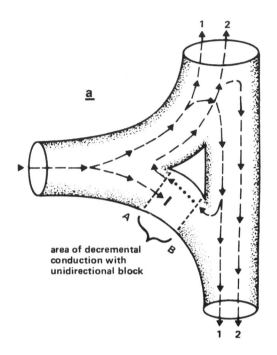

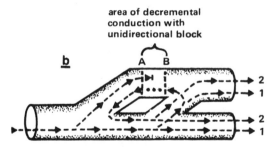

FIG. 21.10. Reentry at the point of impingement of a Purkinje fiber on the ventricular myocardium (*a*) and within a strand of cardiac muscle (*b*). In both situations a region of decremental conduction with unidirectional block (*A-B*) prevents antegrade conduction of the normal impulse (1) but allows this impulse to propagate slowly through the depressed region in the retrograde direction (*dotted line*). After a delay, the retrograde impulse reenters the myocardium proximal to the region of decremental conduction; if this occurs after the tissue proximal to the depressed area has recovered from the first impulse, the retrograde impulse can initiate a premature systole (2).

passage of the retrograde impulse often increases the refractoriness of the depressed area. When this occurs, conduction can be blocked in both directions, so that if the unidirectional block becomes complete block, retrograde conduction can no longer occur and the reentrant arrhythmia is terminated.

Ionic Basis for Slow Conduction in the Genesis of Arrhythmias

There is little doubt that the common occurrence of asymmetrical injury provides the substrate for unidirectional block in the diseased heart. However, there has been some question as to how the sodium channel opening could be slowed so as to cause sufficient delay in impulse propagation through a small area of decremental conduction to allow proximal regions to regain their excitability. In some animal models, for example, it was necessary to postulate conduction velocities as low as 1% of normal, which raised questions as to whether such weak sodium currents would be able to be conducted at all.

At one time it was suggested that severely depressed sodium-dependent action potentials might not be able to produce the extremely low conduction velocities calculated in reentrant circuits, but instead that the more slowly conducting calcium currents discussed in Chapter 19 played a major role in clinical arrhythmias. Although initially attractive, this hypothesis has had to be abandoned because most ventricular tachyarrhythmias do not respond to calcium channel blocking drugs. Instead, drugs whose major actions are on sodium channels generally terminate most reentrant arrhythmias (although not without frequent, and sometimes disastrous clinical side effects). These data indicate that most reentrant arrhythmias are, in fact, due to slow conduction involving severely depressed sodium channels, rather than to calcium-dependent action potentials.

Summation and Inhibition

Two phenomena related to the conduction abnormalities discussed in the preceding subsection are described at this point as they explain some fascinating features of the premature systoles that occur singly and repetitively in the clinical ECG. The setting for both summation and inhibition, like the reentry mechanisms described above, is provided by depressed regions of the heart that exhibit decremental conduction.

Summation

If two impulses arrive simultaneously at a branch in a depressed bundle of myocardial cells, the two weak action potentials can be summated to generate an action potential in the branch (Fig. 21.11a). If, on the other hand, either impulse enters alone (Fig. 21.11b,c), the depressed tissue at the branch point may not be able to

SUMMATION

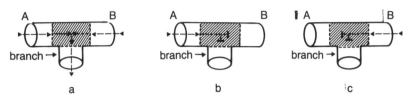

FIG. 21.11. Summation. The simultaneous arrival of impulses from opposite directions (*A* and *B*) in a region of decremental conduction (*cross-hatched*) near a branch initiates a propagated action potential in the branch (*a*). However, when only one impulse enters the area of decremental conduction, it is not propagated into the branch (*b, c*). Successful propagation into the branch thus requires summation of impulses entering the region of decremental conduction.

initiate a propagated action potential in the branch. Even though the simultaneous arrival of the two impulses is summated to propagate an impulse into the branch, the depressed conduction can delay the emergence of the impulse from the branch. If the delay is sufficient to allow other regions of the heart to recover from the initial wave of depolarization, the delayed summated impulse could reenter these regions so as to produce an echo. In this manner, summation represents a special type of reentry that can cause premature systoles.

Inhibition

The area of slow conduction at the branch point described above can also give rise to a phenomenon called inhibition, in which prior activation of the area proximal to the branch by a nonpropagated impulse blocks conduction of a stronger

INHIBITION

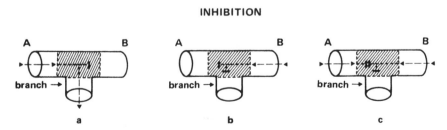

FIG. 21.12. Inhibition. An impulse entering from one side (*A*) of a region of decremental conduction (*cross-hatched*) near a branch is able to initiate a propagated action potential in the branch (*a*). However, an impulse entering the region of decremental conduction from the other direction (*B*) is blocked (*b*). The arrival of the weaker impulse (from *B*) in the region of decremental conduction immediately before the arrival of the stronger impulse (from *A*) can block (inhibit) the ability of the latter to activate the branch (*c*).

impulse into the branch. This phenomenon occurs when a strong impulse that enters a region of unidirectional block from one side is propagated into a branch (Fig. 21.12a), whereas a weaker impulse entering from the other side is blocked (Fig. 21.12b). If the weaker impulse enters the region of unidirectional block before the stronger impulse, it can, by generating nonconducted action potentials, block conduction of the latter. (This is an example of "concealed conduction," discussed further in Chapter 23.) The inhibitory effect of the weaker impulse is readily understood as arising from the refractoriness left behind after it depolarizes the depressed myocardium opposite the branch.

Inhomogeneous Action Potential Characteristics

Because of the importance of homogeneous activation in synchronizing the pumping of the heart, slowing or disorganization of the spread of the wave of depolarization through the myocardium can cause inhomogeneities that reduce cardiac efficiency and may lead to premature systoles or a tachyarrhythmia. Disorganized activation, in turn, can be caused by localized abnormalities in virtually any property of the cardiac action potential.

Inhomogeneous Action Potential Depolarization (Phase 0)

The importance of homogeneous depolarization in the rapid and organized depolarization of the heart has been emphasized throughout this chapter. The key role played by the rate of rise and amplitude of the action potential in determining conduction velocity explains why normal sodium and calcium channel opening is essential for normal conduction throughout the heart (see above).

Inhomogeneous Refractoriness and Repolarization: Action Potential Duration and Repolarization (Phases 1, 2, and 3)

Inhomogeneity of refractoriness and repolarization can arise from local abnormalities in the many repolarizing currents described in Chapter 19. As such abnormalities can depress and disorder the time- and voltage-dependent reactivation of sodium and calcium channels, electrical inhomogeneities and disorganized refractoriness represent important causes of arrhythmias.

There are two general mechanisms by which abnormalities in the ion currents that repolarize the heart can lead to arrhythmias. The first, as mentioned above, is incomplete reactivation of the sodium and calcium channels that carry the inward ion currents responsible for depolarization (phase 1) of the action potential (see above). The influence of repolarization on impulse conduction arises simply because incomplete reactivation of the channels that carry inward currents is a major cause of decremental conduction.

The second mechanism by which inhomogeneities of repolarization can produce premature systoles and tachyarrhythmias arises from the electrotonic spread of currents between regions of the heart that recover at different times. Thus, if one region of the heart repolarizes before an adjacent area following the passage of a single wave of depolarization, the tissue that has remained depolarized can reexcite the regions that have regained their excitablity. As shown in Fig. 21.13, a region with abnormally shortened action potentials can be reexcited by currents propagated from surrounding depolarized tissue that has not recovered prematurely. A similar situation can arise where the action potentials in one region of the heart are abnormally prolonged.

The ability of a number of common pathological conditions, notably regional ischemia, either to shorten or lengthen refractoriness and action potential duration makes this an important arrhythmogenic mechanism. Inhomogeneities of repolarization also account for some of the "proarrhythmic" effects of antiarrhythmic drugs. The latter, which represent unfortunately common side effects of many antiarrhythmic drugs, are readily explained by their ability to magnify inhomogeneities in refractoriness and repolarization that are so common in diseased, scarred hearts.

Inhomogeneous Resting Potential (Phase 4)

Partial depolarization of a region of the heart, like early repolarization, may lead to the electrotonic spread of currents that can give rise to premature systoles and tachyarrhythmias. One example of this mechanism is shown in Fig. 21.14, where currents arising in a depolarized region of the heart can excite the surrounding, normal, tissue.

This mechanism may account for some of the proarrhythmic effects of drugs that block the inward (anomalously) rectifying potassium channels that are open during diastole. Also important is the role of regional depolarization in causing sudden death in patients immediately after a coronary artery occlusion. As discussed in

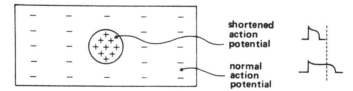

FIG. 21.13. Inhomogeneity of repolarization. The diagram represents potentials outside the cells in a region of the myocardium at a time, toward the end of an action potential (*vertical dashed line*, at *right*) when repolarization is inhomogeneous. If the cells at the center have repolarized because of abnormal shortening of their action potential duration, while the normal cells are still depolarized (action potentials at right), this inhomogeneity can allow the cells with the shorter action potential to be reexcited by the surrounding normal tissue, thereby causing a premature systole.

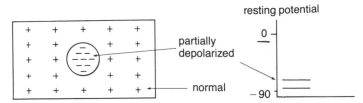

FIG. 21.14. Inhomogeneity of depolarization. The diagram represents potentials outside the cells in a region of resting myocardium in which the cells at the center are partially depolarized; this situation is commonly encountered in acute myocardial ischemia. The differences in resting potential may allow the normal tissue to be reexcited by the depolarized tissue, thereby causing a premature systole.

Chapter 24, the rapid loss of potassium from ischemic myocardial cells reduces the Nernst potential for potassium, which is of course the major determinant of resting potential (Chapter 19). Diastolic electrotonic currents from tissues depolarized by regional ischemia probably account for the common occurrence of sudden death in the first minutes after a myocardial infarction.

Abnormal Conducting Structures

The abnormal structures diagrammed in Fig. 20.4, which can give rise to electrical short circuits between the atria and ventricles, along with the dual conducting pathways in the AV node, represent the most common cause of the supraventricular tachycardias described in Chapter 23. As these pathways transmit impulses rapidly between the atria and ventricles, they give rise to *reciprocal rhythms*. The two most common causes of these reciprocal rhythms thus represent special types of reentry between the atria and ventricles.

Dual Pathways in the AV Node

It is now clear that in many patients, the AV node is divided longitudinally into parallel, and independent, conducting pathways (Fig. 21.15). If these pathways conduct at different speeds and have action potentials of different durations, antegrade impulses (from atria to ventricles) can be propagated in one pathway, and then return in a retrograde direction in the other. This gives rise to a reciprocating rhythm that represents the most common cause of the supraventricular tachycardias described in Chapter 23.

The tachycardias that arise in the dual AV nodal pathways shown in Fig. 21.15 are generally triggered by a premature atrial systole, which causes a wave of depolarization to arrive at the upper end of the AV node before it has fully recovered from the preceding (normal) sinus beat. As the action potentials in the slower pathway are generally both smaller and briefer than those in the faster pathway, a pre-

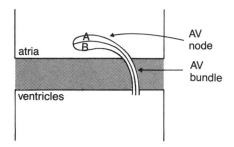

FIG. 21.15. Dual conduction in the AV node. Two parallel pathways (*A* and *B*) can conduct impulses independently within the AV node.

mature wave of depolarization can arrive at the upper end of the AV node at a time when the first pathway is still refractory, but the slow pathway has recovered its excitability (Fig. 21.16). This allows the premature impulse to propagate through the slow pathway in the antegrade direction, from the atria toward the ventricles, and then return in a retrograde direction via the fast pathway. Persistence of this reciprocal rhythm can generate a sustained tachycardia.

The alert reader should, at this point, have observed that Fig. 21.16 is not much different from Fig. 21.10, and that the combination of unidirectional block and slow

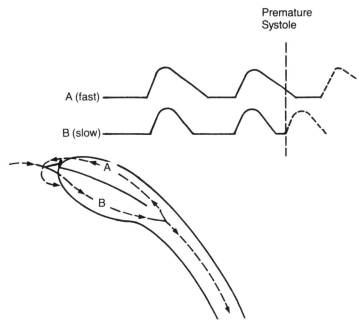

FIG. 21.16. Arrival of a premature depolarization at the atrial end of the two AV nodal pathways shown in Fig. 21.15 can, if only the slow pathway has repolarized (action potentials above), be propagated in an antegrade direction through the slow pathway (*B*) and in the retrograde direction via the fast pathway (*A*).

conduction in the AV node reflects inhomogeneities not unlike those depicted in Fig. 21.13. This example thus provides a clear example of the overlap in the arrhythmogenic mechanisms discussed in this chapter. The mechanisms depicted in both Fig. 21.10 and 21.16 depend on unidirectional block and slow conduction. In the tachycardias that arise from dual conducting pathways in the AV node, unidirectional block restricts antegrade conduction to the slow pathway, whereas slow conduction delays the return of the retrograde impulse to the atrial end of the slowly conducting pathway until the latter has regained its excitability.

Tachycardias that arise from dual pathways in the AV node are often terminated by mechanisms that inhibit the calcium channels responsible for conduction in this structure. Reciprocal rhythms within the AV node can thus be blocked by vagal stimulation (e.g., induced by carotid sinus massage), which often "breaks" a paroxysmal supraventricular tachycardia. Administration of adenosine, a purinergic agonist that, like vagal stimulation, activates G_i (the inhibitory G protein discussed in Chapter 12), has proved almost ideal for treating these arrhythmias because of its very short half-life. Another approach, which takes advantage of the dependence of these arrhythmias on calcium channels, is to administer a calcium channel blocker or β-adrenergic blocker, both of which inhibit the calcium currents responsible for impulse conduction in the AV node.

Accessory Pathways: Preexcitation (The Wolff-Parkinson-White Syndrome)

An *accessory pathway* (Chapter 20) is generally a strand of atrial myocardium that, by bridging the central fibrous body, provides an electrical short circuit for impulse transmission between the atria and ventricles. As the cells in accessory pathways generate sodium channel-dependent action potentials, they conduct more rapidly than the AV node. For this reason, when normal impulses in the atria are conducted down an accessory pathway, they arrive prematurely at an abnormal site in the ventricles (the actual site depends on the location of the accessory pathway which can be virtually anywhere along the AV junction).

The characteristic electrocardiographic abnormality caused by a functional accessory pathway is called preexcitation, or the Wolff-Parkinson-White syndrome (WPW) after the three cardiologists who first described this abnormality. The abnormal ECG in preexcitation (Fig. 21.17) is simply a reflection of the pathophysiology described in the preceding paragraph. Premature depolarization of the ventricles, which is due to the fact that the accessory pathway conducts more rapidly than the AV node, explains the shortened P-R interval (<0.12 sec), whereas the abnormal early deflection of the QRS (called a *delta wave*) occurs because the ventricles are not activated initially via the two bundle branches. Preexcitation is discussed at this point because it is a variant of the arrhythmogenic mechanism caused by dual pathways in the AV node, and so generates supraventricular tachycardias by a mechanism similar to that discussed above.

The special type of reciprocal beating in patients with preexcitation involves the AV node and the accessory pathway (Fig. 21.18). These reciprocal rhythms could

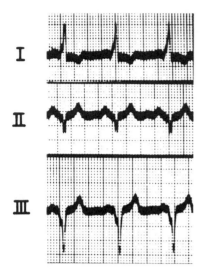

FIG. 21.17. Preexcitation (Wolff-Parkinson-White syndrome). The P-R interval is abnormally short (0.11 sec), and the QRS complexes are widened (to 0.14 sec) by the presence of delta waves. The latter cause the slurring of the beginning of the R wave in lead I and of the beginning of the QS complex in lead III. Note that the T wave is abnormally discordant from the QRS. (From Katz and Pick, 1956.)

arise when an impulse entering the ventricles by way of the AV node is conducted back to the atria via the accessory pathway, or conversely, when an impulse reaches the ventricles via the accessory pathway and returns to the atria by way of the AV node. The latter is, however, much less common because the tachycardias in patients with preexcitation, like those involving dual conduction in the AV node, are generally initiated when an atrial premature systole reaches the ventricle via only one of the two pathways. As accessory pathways generally contain atrial cells that are depolarized by sodium currents and have longer refractory periods than those in the AV node, they are analogous to the fast pathway described in Fig. 21.16. Thus, an atrial premature systole can be conducted from atria to ventricles down the slow pathway (the AV node) and return to the atria via the accessory pathway (Fig. 21.18). This explains why most supraventricular tachycardias in patients with preexcitation, which are usually initiated by an atrial premature systole, involve antegrade conduction through the AV node and retrograde conduction through the accessory pathway.

> This mechanism also accounts for the puzzling fact that delta waves generally disappear when patients with preexcitation develop supraventricular tachycardias. Unlike the situation during normal sinus rhythm, when antegrade conduction down an accessory pathway causes a short P-R interval and delta wave (Fig. 21.17), the tachycardias begin and are sustained by unidirectional antegrade block caused by the long refractory period of the accessory pathway.

The fact that conduction through an accessory pathway involves sodium channels has two important clinical implications. The first is that these channels conduct impulses rapidly from the atria to the ventricles. Thus, patients with preexcitation who develop atrial fibrillation, which itself is rarely a lethal arrhythmia (Chapter 23), are at risk of sudden death because fast conduction of the disorganized atrial

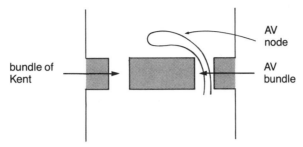

FIG. 21.18. An accessory pathway, or bundle of Kent, along with the AV bundle, provides two conduction pathways linking the atria and ventricles. The accessory pathway, usually a strand of atrial tissue that conducts rapidly across the nonconducting fibrous skeleton of the heart (*shaded*) between the atria and ventricles, activates an abnormal site in the ventricles. Rapid conduction through the accessory pathway shortens the P-R interval, whereas the abnormal site of ventricular activation explains the delta wave in Fig. 21.17.

impulses into the ventricles by way of an accessory pathway can cause ventricular fibrillation. This is especially likely if the action potentials in the accessory pathway are abbreviated by sympathetic stimulation, which as discussed in Chapter 19 opens the channels that carry i_{to} and, by an indirect effect produced by their action on calcium channels, increase outward currents through calcium-activated potassium channels.

The second implication of fast channel conduction in accessory pathways is that arrhythmias which involve these structures generally respond to drugs that selectively block sodium channels. In view of the hazards of conduction down an accessory pathway (see above), treatment is often begun with one of these drugs and not a calcium channel blocker. This is because the latter, although able to block the other limb of the reciprocal rhythm in the AV node, also lowers blood pressure and so can trigger the sympathetic responses that shorten accessory pathway refractoriness. The latter hazard is avoided by the β-blockers, which are not vasodilators and which directly inhibit sympathetic stimulation of the heart. Because of the risk of sudden cardiac death, some patients with rapid conduction through an accessory pathway are candidates for surgery or ablation therapy to destroy the accessory AV conduction pathway.

The other abnormal conduction pathways depicted in Fig. 20.4, notably the Mahaim fibers, have also been suggested to participate in the pathogenesis of clinical arrhythmias. However, their role is generally less clear than that of the accessory pathways described above.

Circus Movements and Their Interruption

Reentry is often viewed as a "circus movement," which was described in the early part of this century. Using a ring of excitable tissue (a jellyfish mantle), A. G. Mayer created a unidirectional block by briefly and gently clamping a small part of

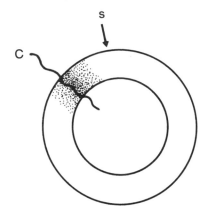

FIG. 21.19. Establishment of a circus movement when a ring of excitable tissue is lightly clamped (C) and then stimulated at one side of the clamp (s). Because counterclockwise conduction is transiently (unidirectionally) blocked by the clamp, the impulse propagates only in the clockwise direction. Removal of the clamp before the impulse reaches the area of block allows the latter to continue its travel in a clockwise direction around the ring.

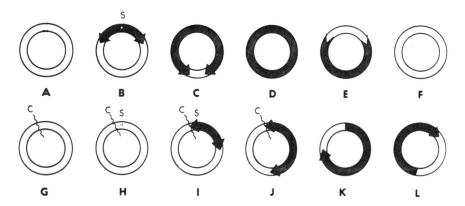

FIG. 21.20. Importance of unidirectional block in establishing the circus movement described in Fig. 21.19. Application of a stimulus to a ring of excitable tissue (*unshaded*) in the absence of block (*upper row*) depolarizes the ring in both directions (*B*) so that the mutual cancellation of the two impulses (*C*) depolarizes the entire ring (*D*) and does not establish a circus movement. If, however, unidirectional block is created by the clamp described in Fig. 21.19 (*lower row*), stimulation initiates a wave of depolarization that propagates only in a clockwise direction (*K*). If the block is removed, the wave of depolarization can continue its circuit of the ring (*L*). (Reprinted with permission of Macmillan Publishing Company from "The Pathophysiological Basis and Effects of Cardiac Arrythmias." In Katz LN, Silber EN, *Heart Disease*. Copyright 1975, Macmillan Publishing Company.)

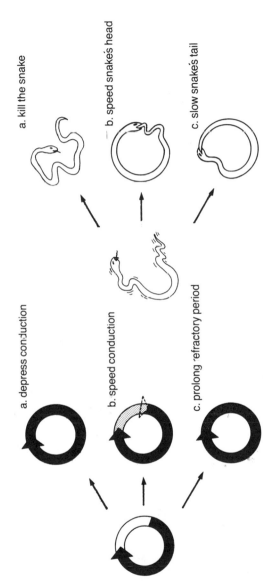

a. kill the snake

b. speed snakes head

c. slow snakes tail

a. depress conduction

b. speed conduction

c. prolong refractory period

FIG. 21.21. Three ways by which a circus movement can be terminated. *Left:* A circus movement (as in panel *K* of Fig. 21.20) can be stopped if conduction is completely blocked (*a*), if conduction is accelerated so that the front of the impulse reaches the previously cepolarized tissue (*b*), or if the refractory period is prolonged so the front of the impulse encounters tissue that can no longer be excited (*c*). *Right:* These three mechanisms can be viewed in terms of a snake traveling in a circle. The snake stops if it is killed (*a*), if it reaches ahead so as to bite its tail (*b*), or if its tail lags behind so as to be bitten by the advancing head (*c*).

the ring (Fig. 21.19). When the excitable ring was stimulated, the resulting wave of depolarization could propagate in only one direction (clockwise in the example shown in Fig. 21.19 because counterclockwise conduction was blocked by the clamp). If the clamp was removed before the impulse returned to the site of local block from the clockwise conduction, the impulse was able to continue its clockwise travel around the ring (Fig. 21.20). Such a circus movement could go around and around the ring until conduction deteriorated to the point that the circulating waves died out. The circus movement could also be stopped if conduction was accelerated or refractoriness prolonged, which allows the front of the conducted impulse to "catch up" with the refractory state left behind after the previous circuit of the impulse.

This model by G. R. Mines, applied to the heart, helps us to understand three approaches to antiarrhythmic therapy (Fig. 21.21). The first is simply to depress conduction by inactivating the channels that carry inward depolarizing currents, for example by administering a drug that inhibits channel opening throughout the ring (Fig. 21.21a). Second, one can do just the opposite and give a drug that accelerates conduction in the hope that this will allow the wave of depolarization to "catch up" with the regions in which the channels carrying depolarizing current have not had time to be reactivated after the prior passage of the wave front (Fig. 21.21b). The third approach is to give a drug that, by inhibiting repolarizing currents, prolongs the refractory period so as to cause the front of the wave of depolarization to be snuffed out when it encounters a region that cannot be excited (Fig. 21.21c).

An analogy that may help the reader understand these principles of antiarrhythmic drug actions is to consider the impulse traveling around the circular pathway as a snake that, if its head catches up with its tail, bites itself and dies. According to this rather homely analogy, depressing conduction is like killing the snake, whereas speeding the forward motion of the head of the snake or holding its tail in place allows the snake to bite itself and so terminate its movements.

Although the circus movement is a useful aid to understanding how therapy can terminate a reentrant circuit, this paradigm has been largely replaced by the classification of antiarrhythmic drugs described in Chapter 23.

BIBLIOGRAPHY

This is a vast topic, and is covered in many textbooks of electrophysiology, electrocardiography, and clinical electrophysiology. A classic that describes principles that remain relevant, from which many of the ECGs in this text have been reproduced is:
Katz LN, Pick A. (1956). *Clinical electrocardiography. Part I: The Arrhythmias.* Philadelphia: Lea & Febiger.
More modern discussions can be found in:
Fozzard HA, Arnsdorf MF. (1986). Cardiac electrophysiology. In: Fozzard H, Haber E, Katz A, Jennings R, Morgan HE, eds. *The heart and cardiovascular system.* New York: Raven Press; 1–30.

Josephson ME, Wellens HJJ. (1984). *Tachycardias: mechanisms, diagnosis, treatment.* Philadelphia: Lea & Febiger.

22

The Arrhythmias

II. Conduction Abnormalities and Block

This chapter, which along with Chapter 23 focuses on clinical arrhythmias, is intended to illustrate some applications of the principles set forth in Chapters 18 to 21. Chapters 22 and 23 do not, therefore, provide a systematic description of the arrhythmias. Instead, these clinical examples review important properties of cardiac ion channels (Chapter 18), the currents that they generate (Chapter 19), their manifestation at the body surface (Chapter 20), and the mechanisms by which abnormalities disorder the rate and rhythm of the heart (Chapter 21).

Chapter 22 focuses on the bradyarrhythmias, although for ease in presentation, the focus is not too sharp; for example, all abnormal sinus rhythms are described. Chapter 23 deals mainly with premature systoles and tachyarrhythmias, although, as stressed in Chapter 21, the mechanisms responsible for abnormally slow rhythms and abnormally rapid rhythms are often the same. The reader must, therefore, not be distressed if the boundaries between these two chapters become blurred: nature in her wisdom designed it that way!

ARRHYTHMIAS DUE TO ABNORMALITIES OF THE SINUS NODE

The normal heart rate, which by convention (and for ease of ECG interpretation) is 60 to 100, reflects the frequency of depolarization of the sinoatrial (SA) node pacemaker (Chapter 20). Heart rates greater than 100 that originate in the SA node are designated *sinus tachycardia*, whereas heart rates less than 60 that reflect slowing of the SA node pacemaker represent *sinus bradycardia*. Because of the sensitivity of the SA node to autonomic influences, most clinical examples of sinus tachycardia and sinus bradycardia are due to altered autonomic activity, rather than to primary disorders of the SA node pacemaker.

Sinus Tachycardia

The electrocardiographic characteristic of sinus tachycardia (Fig. 22.1) is a heart rate greater than 100 that is initiated by normal P waves; because the tachycardia originates in the SA node, atrial depolarization is normal. Other features of a sinus tachycardia include a normal P-R interval and normal QRS complexes, which reflect the fact that the ventricles are depolarized via the normal conduction pathway through the atrioventricular (AV) node, AV bundle, and His-Purkinje system.

The P-R interval in sinus tachycardia can be prolonged, especially if the rate is extremely rapid, because of refractoriness in the AV node (see below). Conduction through one of the bundle branches, which as noted in Chapter 19 have very long refractory periods, can also be blocked when the rate of a sinus tachycardia is extremely rapid or the bundle branches are abnormal (*aberrant conduction*, see Chapter 23).

Tachycardias in which the P-R interval is abnormally shortened, even when normal QRS complexes are preceded by P waves, are not usually sinus tachycardias. This is because the short P-R interval tells us that the impulse has not encountered the normal delay in the AV node. Thus, such arrhythmias either result from preexcitation (Chapter 21), or the tachycardia has originated in the AV node and so is a *junctional*, not a sinus, tachycardia (Chapter 23).

Pathophysiology of Sinus Tachycardia

Sinus tachycardia is not usually a sign of heart disease because increased sympathetic tone, by far the most common cause of this arrhythmia, is part of the normal response to physical exercise and emotional stress. Sinus tachycardia is also commonly caused by metabolic and endocrine abnormalities, including fever and ane-

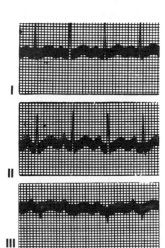

FIG. 22.1. Sinus tachycardia. The rates of atrial and ventricular beating are 125 (P waves and QRS complexes occur every 0.48 sec), and each QRS complex is preceded by a normal P wave with a normal P-R interval of 0.16 sec. (From Katz and Pick, 1956.)

mia. Although resting sinus tachycardia is among the signs of heart failure, it is not, in fact, a common presenting complaint in patients with cardiac disease.

Sympathetic Stimulation

Sympathetic stimulation of the sinus pacemaker is mediated by the binding of the β-adrenergic agonists to their receptors, which increases heart rate by mechanisms that are mediated by both direct and indirect effects of activated G_s (Chapter 12). Pacemaker activity is accelerated by the ability of activated G_s to increase the two inward currents i_f and i_{Ca}, described in Chapter 19. The direct effects include interactions between G_s and the channels responsible for i_f and i_{Ca} that occur within the plasma membrane itself. The indirect effects are mediated by the increased synthesis of cyclic AMP when adenylyl cyclase is stimulated by the activated α-subunit of G_s (Fig. 12.3).

Hyperthyroidism

Thyroid hormone accelerates the sinus pacemaker by several mechanisms, including effects on both the β-adrenergic receptors and the G proteins. These are discussed below, when we consider how hypothyroidism causes sinus bradycardia and SA block.

Fever

The increased heart rate caused by fever is due partly to the physical effects of elevated temperature, which accelerate conformational changes in the ion channels that depolarize the SA node, and partly to chemical mediators of inflammation released into the blood stream. The importance of the latter explains why accelerated heart rate is not always proportional to the degree of fever.

Sinus Bradycardia

Sinus bradycardia, by definition, occurs when heart rates under the control of the SA node pacemaker are less than 60. The ECG in sinus bradycardia shows the slow heart rate in which normal P waves are followed by normal QRS complexes after a normal P-R interval (Fig. 22.2).

Pathophysiology of Sinus Bradycardia

As was true for sinus tachycardia, altered autonomic tone is the most common cause of sinus bradycardia. In this case, of course, increased parasympathetic (va-

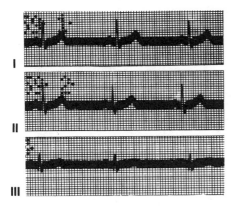

FIG. 22.2. Sinus bradycardia. The rates of atrial and ventricular beating are 54 (P waves and QRS complexes occur every 1.1 sec), and each QRS complex is preceded by a normal P wave with a normal P-R interval of 0.17 sec. (From Katz and Pick, 1956.)

gal) tone and decreased sympathetic tone slow the sinus pacemaker. The parasympathetic nervous system has the greater tonic influence on the resting heart; as noted in Chapter 19, this may be due partly to the greater inhibitory potency of G_i than G_s on i_f. This normal tonic parasympathetic influence is attenuated by aging and amplified by conditioning, the latter explains the sinus bradycardia that characterizes the "athlete's heart" in trained individuals.

Parasympathetic Stimulation (Acetylcholine) and Adenosine

Many clinical examples of sinus bradycardia result from excessive parasympathetic (vagal) tone, especially in younger patients. Chronic slowing of the sinus pacemaker, as already mentioned, is regularly seen in the "athlete's heart," whereas sudden and severe sinus bradycardia can occur abruptly in vasovagal syncope, the old-fashioned "swoon."

Parasympathetic slowing of the sinus pacemaker is mediated by changes in at least three different ion channels (Pappano and Mubagwa, 1991; Table 22.1); these changes are initiated when acetylcholine binds to cardiac M_2 muscarinic receptors. Similar effects are produced when adenosine binds to cardiac A_1 purinergic receptors (Chapter 12).

The first mechanism by which these agonists cause sinus bradycardia is by hyperpolarizing the SA node, which occurs when either acetylcholine or adenosine acti-

TABLE 22.1. *Mechanisms by which acetylcholine and adenosine may slow the sinus node pacemaker*

Ion current	Change	Result
$i_{K.Ach}$	Increase	Increased resting potential
i_f	Decrease	Slowed diastolic depolarization
i_{Ca}	Decrease	Decreased depolarizing currents

vates a resting *potassium current*, $i_{K.Ach}$, in the SA node. The effects of both M_2 and A_1 receptors on $i_{K.Ach}$ appear to be mediated by an inhibitory G_i that can be activated when either acetylcholine or adenosine binds to its receptor. The ligand-receptor complex, by activating this G protein, opens channels that carry the potassium current $i_{K.Ach}$ (Chapter 19). This brings resting potential closer to the Nernst potential for potassium. The ability of $i_{K.Ach}$ to hyperpolarize the resting cell reflects the fact that diastolic potentials in the SA node are considerably lower than E_K (Chapter 19).

The second ion channel that slows the SA node in response to acetylcholine and adenosine carries the inward *pacemaker current* i_f. This pacemaker current is inhibited both by a direct effect of G_i and an indirect effect that occurs when G_i inhibits cyclic AMP production (Chapter 12). The decrease in cyclic AMP concentration also attenuates the *calcium current* i_{Ca} by reducing the probability of calcium channel opening (Fig. 18.9). The resulting inhibition of i_{Ca}, by reducing the major inward current that depolarizes the SA node, also contributes to the SA block sometimes caused by vagal stimulation (see below).

Additional causes of sinus bradycardia are discussed below, when we examine the mechanisms that can lead to SA block.

Sinus Arrhythmia and Wandering Pacemaker

Variations in heart rate that accompany the respiratory cycle represent a *respiratory sinus arrhythmia*, which is readily apparent in most normal young individuals. Cyclic changes in sinus rate unrelated to respiration are also seen; these are called "nonrespiratory sinus arrhythmia." The electrocardiographic manifestations of sinus arrhythmia are cyclic alterations in the rate of the P waves, which, like the P-R interval and QRS complex, are normal (Fig. 22.3).

Respiratory sinus arrhythmia is caused by changes in the delicate balance between tonic sympathetic and parasympathetic influences on the SA node. Acceleration of heart rate during inspiration is due to decreased vagal tone and increased sympathetic tone, whereas increased vagal tone and decreased sympathetic tone slow the SA node during expiration. These changes in autonomic tone are attributed to stimuli arising from stretch receptors in the lung and the chest wall.

Respiratory variations in QRS morphology can also occur when movements of the diaphragm change the position of the heart in the chest. These slight shifts in the mean QRS vector are most evident in transitional complexes, usually in lead III or aVL which are at right angles to the midrange of normal QRS axis between $+30°$ and $+60°$ (Chapter 20). These mechanical variations in QRS axis can be increased dramatically in patients with a large pericardial effusion, where respiration causes the heart to swing back and forth like a pendulum in the distended, fluid-filled pericardium.

Respiratory sinus arrhythmia is not only a normal finding, but is also a sign of a healthy heart. Clocklike regularity of the heartbeat, which indicates that normal control by the autonomic nervous system has been lost, is one of the earliest mani-

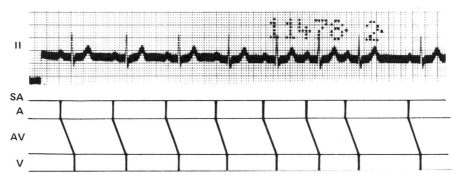

FIG. 22.3. Sinus arrhythmia. The rates of atrial and ventricular beating vary, but each QRS complex is preceded by a P wave with a normal P-R interval of 0.19 sec. (The variations in the shape of the P wave suggest a "wandering" pacemaker site in the SA node.) This arrhythmia is diagrammed in a "Lewis diagram," in which the top line (SA) represents the SA node, the upper space (A) the atria, the middle space (AV) the AV node and His-Purkinje system, and the lower space (V) the ventricles. Each beat begins in the SA node and is conducted normally through the atria, AV node, and ventricles as depicted by the lines that are read from top to bottom. (ECG from Katz and Pick, 1956.)

festations of heart failure. Sinus arrhythmias also tend to disappear with advancing age. Thus, a marked respiratory sinus arrhythmia, like the heightened vagal tone that slows the heart of the trained athlete, is a sign of good health!

Another common arrhythmia in normal individuals is the *wandering pacemaker*, which is characterized by cyclic changes in P wave morphology that are sometimes accompanied by slight variations in both cycle length (heart rate) and P-R interval. This arrhythmia, which like sinus arrhythmia may be related to respiration (Fig. 22.3), is probably caused by a shifting site of pacemaker activity within the SA node.

> Although a wandering pacemaker is seen in healthy individuals, the mechanisms responsible for this minor arrhythmia can be magnified in patients with chronic pulmonary disease, acute pulmonary embolism, and pneumonia, where reflexes arising in the lungs may also be responsible for a more serious arrhythmia called *multifocal atrial tachycardia* (Chapter 23). This tachyarrhythmia, in some ways, resembles a marked exaggeration of the wandering pacemaker.

The Lewis (Ladder) Diagram

Impulse conduction during complex arrhythmias can be conveniently depicted by drawing the passage of the wave of depolarization through the heart using a Lewis (or ladder) diagram; the former term recognizes Sir Thomas Lewis, one of the pioneers in the study of the ECG. The Lewis diagram, as illustrated for the sinus arrhythmia shown in Fig. 22.3, consists of four parallel lines delimiting three spaces; the horizontal axis, time, is read from left to right. The top line represents the SA node, whereas the space between the top two lines depicts the passage of the wave of depolarization through the atria. The wider space between the middle lines is used to diagram depolarization of the AV node, and the lower space indicates ventricular depolarization.

Each normal sinus beat begins at the top line (SA node), passes rapidly across the top space (atria), more slowly through the middle space (AV node), and again rapidly across the lower space (ventricles). The downward angle of the line drawn on the Lewis diagram thus represents the speed of impulse propagation. In a sinus arrhythmia, the speed of impulse propagation through the atria, AV node, and ventricles remains normal, the only change being in the interval between the impulses arising in the SA node. Hence as shown in Fig. 22.3, the abnormality consists of cyclic variations in the frequency with which the SA node (top line) initiates impulses that are then transmitted normally through the atria (top space), AV node (middle space), and ventricles (lower space).

Sinoatrial Block

Inhibited pacemaker discharge in the SA node is not the only cause of slowed P waves in the ECG because, as noted in Chapter 21, bradyarrhythmias can also be caused by block of conduction of pacemaker impulses out of the SA node into the atria. Thus, apparent slowing of the SA node pacemaker also occurs if some of the impulses arising in the SA node fail to be propagated into the atria, an abnormality called *SA block*.

Because depolarization of the SA node pacemaker cannot be recorded at the body surface, the distinction between sinus bradycardia and SA block is ordinarily made using indirect criteria. For example, while sinus bradycardias tend to be regular, SA block often causes irregular atrial rhythms. Certain patterns of irregular atrial beating that favor the diagnosis of SA block, such as dropped (absent) P waves and group beating, are similar to patterns seen in the AV blocks described below. The differential diagnosis between sinus bradycardia and SA block can be difficult, and may require intracardiac measurement of sinoatrial conduction time (see below). However, as the mechanisms that produce both arrhythmias are similar, it is rarely necessary to embark on these complex studies.

Sinoatrial Conduction Time

The time that elapses between firing of an SA node pacemaker and the beginning of atrial depolarization, the *sinoatrial conduction time*, cannot be measured from body surface electrodes. SA node depolarization can be recorded directly when intracardiac electrodes are placed over the SA node, but as this is difficult, such direct measurements are not practical for routine use. Indirect methods have been developed to estimate sinoatrial conduction time, but these also require intracardiac stimulation. Although not used routinely, two of the latter are described below (Fig.

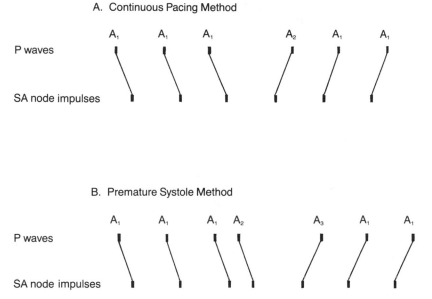

FIG. 22.4. Calculation of sinoatrial conduction time. *A*: Continuous pacing method,where the atria are paced at a cycle length (A_1–A_1) approximating that of the SA node pacemaker. The first spontaneous P wave after the pacemaker is turned off (A_2) is delayed. This delay, which reflects the time required for the impulse to travel between the atria and the SA node, is twice the sinoatrial conduction time. *B*: Premature stimulation method where an atrial premature stimulus "resets" the SA node pacemaker. Prolongation of the interval between the premature P wave (A_2) and the first P wave propagated from the reset SA node (A_3), relative to the normal cycle length (A_1–A_1), is due to conduction of the premature P wave into and out of the SA node. Thus the sinoatrial conduction time is half the difference between the normal cycle (A_1–A_1) and the cycle containing this delay (A_2–A_3).

22.4) to illustrate the clinical application of several principles outlined in Chapters 20 and 21.

Continuous Pacing Method

If the atria are paced at a rate approximating that of the SA node pacemaker, and the pacer abruptly turned off, the first atrial depolarization initiated by the SA node pacemaker appears after a delay (Fig. 22.4A). If the electronic pacemaker had exactly tracked the intrinsic rate of the SA node pacemaker, the latter should begin to fire at the same rate and timing as the electronic pacemaker. Thus, the late appearance of the fourth P wave (A_2) in Fig. 22.4A reflects a delay in propagation of the wave of depolarization between the atria and the SA node pacemaker. The delay, in fact, represents the time required for the last paced atrial depolarization to reach the SA node, *plus* the time required for the first spontaneous sinus depolarization to be propagated back out to generate the first sinus P wave. This delay, which is readily measured as the difference between the paced cycle and the first long cycle after atrial pacing had been ended, is twice the sinoatrial conduction time assuming that conduction velocities into and out of the SA node are the same.

Premature Stimulation Method

If, during a sinus rhythm, a premature stimulus is delivered to the atria after the end of the atrial refractory period, it will initiate a wave of depolarization that, when it is conducted into the SA node, "resets" the SA node pacemaker (Fig. 22.4B). Return of the impulse generated by the newly reset SA node depolarization will, however, be delayed because of the time required for the premature stimulus to be conducted into the SA node, and for the reset action potential to be conducted back out again to the atria. Assuming that conduction into and out of the SA node are the same, the sinoatrial conduction time will be half the difference between the normal cycle $(A_1–A_1)$ and the cycle containing this delay $(A_2–A_3)$.

Pathophysiology of Sinoatrial Block

As noted above, sinus bradycardia and SA block are commonly found together as both pacemaker discharge and conduction in the SA node are influenced by i_{Ca} (Chapter 19). Although i_{Ca} contributes only one of the depolarizing currents responsible for pacemaker activity, it is the major current that generates the upstroke of the slowly conducting wave of depolarization in the SA node.

Autonomic Influences

The influences of sympathetic and parasympathetic stimulation on i_{Ca} have already been discussed in this chapter. The same effects of G_s and G_i that modify the rate of pacemaker discharge also modify conduction through the sinus node.

Thyroid Abnormalities

Hypothyroidism, in addition to slowing the sinus pacemaker (see above), inhibits SA conduction. This effect is probably due in part to reduction in the number of cardiac β-adrenergic receptors (desensitization, see Chapter 12), and to increased synthesis of G_i (Levine et al., 1990), that together reduce cyclic AMP levels in the cells of the SA node.

Hyperkalemia

The effects of elevated extracellular K^+ concentration are due mainly to the depolarizing effects caused by the reduced potassium gradient $([K^+]_i/[K^+]_o)$ across the plasma membrane. As noted in Chapter 19, a decrease in this ratio lowers the Nernst potential for potassium in the resting heart. Because depolarization inactivates the channels that carry the inward currents that depolarize the heart (i_{Ca} in the SA node), reduced extracellular potassium slows conduction; as a result, severe hyperkalemia can produce SA block or even atrial standstill. Other effects of hyperkalemia, to produce tachyarrhythmias, are discussed in Chapter 23.

> Hyperkalemia can cause an unusual form of SA block in which impulse conduction from the SA node to the atria is blocked, but impulses are still conducted along special pathways (perhaps the SA ring bundles, whose existence is questioned in Chapter 20!) to depolarize the AV node and ventricles. This means that there can be a sinus rhythm without P waves.

Drug Effects

Among the many drugs that can cause both sinus bradycardia and SA block, the most easily understood are the *calcium channel blockers* and the β-*blockers*. The former bind directly to the calcium channels, where they inhibit i_{Ca} by the complex effects on channel state described in Chapter 18. The β-blockers inhibit calcium channel opening by preventing the β-adrenergic agonists from binding to their receptors (Chapter 12), which prevents the activation of G_s.

The *cardiac glycosides*, like hyperkalemia (see above) inhibit action potential propagation because sodium pump inhibition depolarizes resting myocardial cells. In addition to inhibiting the sodium pump in heart cells, these drugs have an important effect on the central nervous system that increases vagal tone. This central parasympathetic effect slows pacemaker discharge in the SA node and produces SA block by inhibiting calcium channel opening in the SA node (see above).

Most *antiarrhythmic drugs* can depress SA node conduction by a nonspecific effect to inhibit channel opening. These complex actions, most of which arise from the "detergent effect" described in Chapter 2, are discussed in Chapter 23.

Pathological Conditions

SA block, along with sinus bradycardia, is a hallmark of a common condition in the elderly, the *sick sinus syndrome* (or *bradycardia-tachycardia syndrome*). In addition to sinus bradycardia and SA block, this syndrome is frequently associated with AV block and supraventricular tachycardias. The latter are readily explained by the ability of depressed conduction to provide a substrate for reentrant arrhythmias (Chapter 21).

Surprisingly little is known of the pathophysiology of this common condition. *Occlusion of the SA node artery*, a branch of the right coronary artery that usually runs through the SA node, may cause SA block in some of these patients, whereas fibrosis, calcification, or degeneration of nodal cells (especially in the AV node) contributes to the conduction abnormality in others. However, in most patients the cause of this condition is not understood. The association of the sick sinus syndrome with aging suggests that synthesis of abnormal channel proteins, by processes analogous to those seen in the myosin heavy chains of the rat heart (Chapter 14), may play a role in the pathogenesis of this common condition.

ARRHYTHMIAS DUE TO ABNORMALITIES IN ATRIOVENTRICULAR CONDUCTION

Physiological slowing of impulse propagation through the AV node, which accounts for the normally long P-R interval of 0.12 to 0.20 sec, allows the atria to serve as a primer pump (Chapter 15). Because the slow conduction that is responsible for this delay is associated with a low safety factor (Chapter 18), exaggeration of the normally slow AV nodal conduction, which gives rise to AV dissociation or AV block, is common.

The role of dual pathways in the AV node in the pathogenesis of the supraventricular tachycardias is described in Chapter 21, and pathophysiological features of these tachycardias are discussed in Chapter 23. At this point we discuss the more obvious manifestation of depressed AV conduction, which is, of course, atrioventricular (AV) block.

Atrioventricular Block

Atrioventricular block should really be looked upon as two distinct arrhythmias, both of which inhibit conduction through the tissues that provide the only electrical connection between the atria and ventricles (Chapter 20). In fact, AV conduction can be impaired in two regions, the AV node and His-Purkinje system (AV bundle and bundle branches), where depolarization is effected by calcium and sodium currents, respectively. Not only do the inward currents in these two cell types depend on different ion channels, but quite different mechanisms are usually responsible for conduction abnormalities in these two regions of the heart. However, block in the AV node and block in the AV bundle or bundle branches cause similar—but not always identical—ECG changes. Because conduction abnormalities in these two regions of the heart have different causes and prognosis, the clinical management of AV block must be tailored to the specific pathophysiology in each patient. For this reason, it is necessary to understand the differences between depressed conduction of the calcium-dependent impulses generated in the AV node and the block arising more distally in the His-Purkinje system, where conduction depends on sodium currents.

Dissociation Versus Block

Although the terms *AV dissociation* and *AV block* are often used interchangeably, there is some justification for retaining an old convention that distinguishes between "normal" and "abnormal" failure of AV conduction. According to this convention, *dissociation* refers to all conditions in which AV conduction is delayed, or where impulses fail to be transmitted from the atria to the ventricles. In contrast, the term *block* is reserved for those conditions in which AV dissociation is caused by *abnormal* AV conduction. For example, normal individuals who develop a supraventricular tachycardia at rates above 200 often exhibit *AV dissociation* due simply to the normally low safety factor in the AV node. However, the appearance of AV dissociation at a normal heart rate represents *AV block* because it implies that AV conduction is abnormal.

Severity of Atrioventricular Block

Three degrees of AV block are recognized clinically. *First-degree AV block*, the mildest, is simply an abnormal delay in AV conduction that prolongs the P-R interval. *Second-degree AV block* is more severe in that it is associated with interruption, as well as delay, of conduction in which some, but not all, of the P waves fail to produce QRS complexes, which means that the more severely depressed AV conduction still allows some atrial impulses to excite the ventricles. In *third-degree AV block*, all impulses that enter the AV node are blocked; as noted above, all electrical connection between the atria and the ventricles is severed in the AV node, AV bundle, bundle branches or in the His-Purkinje system.

First-Degree Atrioventricular Block

First-degree AV block is readily identified on the ECG as prolongation of the P-R interval where all P waves are followed by QRS complexes (Fig. 22.5). By itself, this abnormality has little effect on the pumping action of the heart; its clinical significance is due to the fact that first-degree AV block can be a warning of the possible development of a more severe form of AV block.

Second-Degree Atrioventricular Block

Second-degree AV block is defined as the failure of some atrial impulses to depolarize the ventricles. The most important electrocardiographic feature of second-degree AV block is that some, but not all, P waves fail to initiate a QRS complex. The P-R interval is usually prolonged but, for reasons explained below, this is not always seen. In typical second-degree AV block, all ventricular depolarizations are initiated by impulses propagated through the AV node, so that all QRS complexes are preceded by a P wave; however, because some atrial impulses fail to reach the ventricles, not all P waves are followed by a QRS complex. This, of course, means that there are more P waves than QRS complexes. If every other P wave is blocked, the ratio between P waves and QRS complexes is 2:1, so that the resulting abnormality is called 2:1 AV block (Fig. 22.6). Other ratios between P waves and QRS complexes are often seen in second-degree AV block. The ECG in

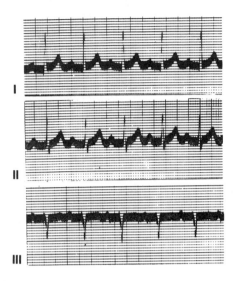

FIG. 22.5. First-degree AV block. Atrial and ventricular rates are both ~90, which is normal. Although each P wave is followed by a QRS complex, the P-R interval is abnormally prolonged to 0.26 sec, demonstrating an abnormal degree of block in the AV node. (From Katz and Pick, 1956.)

Fig. 22.7, where every fourth P wave has not been conducted to the ventricles, is an example of 4:3 AV block. Analysis of the ECG in Fig. 22.7, which is aided by a Lewis diagram, shows that every fourth impulse reaching the AV node from the atria has been blocked; thus, every fourth beat in the pulse of this patient is also "dropped."

The relationships between changes in the P-R interval and blocked P waves (i.e., those that are not followed by QRS complexes) serve as the basis for a very important classification of second-degree AV block. This classification (discussed below)

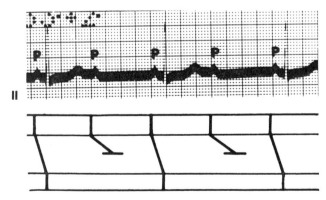

FIG. 22.6. Second-degree AV block with 2:1 AV conduction. There are twice as many P waves (P) as QRS complexes in this record, indicating that every second P wave is blocked. In the Lewis diagram (*below*) every other impulse is depicted as being blocked in the AV node (*short horizontal lines*). (ECG from Katz and Pick, 1956.)

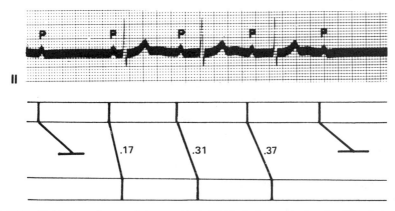

FIG. 22.7. Mobitz type I second-degree (4:3) AV block demonstrating the Wenckebach phenomenon. There are four P waves (P) for every three QRS complexes. In the Lewis diagram (*below*) it can be seen that the P-R interval (*numbers on diagram*) is shortest after the dropped beat. The P-R interval then increases, but by decreasing increments, until the next dropped beat. At the same time the R-P intervals shorten, from 0.79 sec after the first QRS complex to 0.69 sec after the second and third QRS complexes. This ECG demonstrates Mobitz type I AV block. (ECG from Katz and Pick, 1956.)

is useful in distinguishing block in the AV node from the more dangerous form of second-degree AV block caused by depressed conduction through the AV bundle and bundle branches.

The Wenckebach Phenomenon

An important feature in some patients with second-degree AV block, seen most commonly when the block is in the AV node, is progressive lengthening of the P-R interval before the dropped beat. Progressive P-R prolongation leading up to a non-conducted P wave, where the P-R interval has in effect become infinite, is called the *Wenckebach phenomenon*, after one of the pioneers in the analysis of the clinical arrhythmias. The Wenckebach phenomenon is seen in Fig. 22.7, where the first P-R interval after the initial nonconducted P wave (at the left of the tracing) is 0.17 sec. The following two P-R intervals are 0.31 and 0.37 sec, while the fourth P wave in the cycle is blocked, which means that the atrial impulse was not conducted to the ventricles.

An additional feature of the Wenckebach phenomenon, called *group beating*, is a slight acceleration of ventricular beating during each sequence of increasing P-R intervals. Group beating occurs because the P-R intervals characteristically increase by decreasing increments during each sequence that ends with a nonconducted P wave. This is seen in Fig. 22.7, where the P-R interval increases by increments of 0.14 sec (0.31 sec for the second P-R interval *minus* 0.17 sec for the first), and 0.06 sec (0.37 sec for the third P-R interval *minus* 0.31 sec for the second). When these decreasing increments are added to a constant atrial cycle length, the intervals between QRS complexes must also decrease. This results in a slight increase in heart rate which is referred to as group beating.

There are two possible explanations for the progressive prolongation of the P-R interval that characterizes the Wenckebach phenomenon: increasing depression of the AV node due to repeated impulse transmission, and increasing prematurity of the P waves relative to the preceding cardiac cycles. Both can be understood by referring to our friends the snakes, depicted in Fig. 21.22.

The first explanation of progressive P-R prolongation is easily understood. Each time an impulse propagates through a depressed AV node (or AV bundle), it inactivates a fraction of the calcium (or sodium) channels so that, with repeated depolarization, conduction slows progressively. The increasing depression of AV conduction further prolongs the P-R interval until, when too few channels open to generate a propagated action potential, conduction fails altogether and a P wave is blocked. The resulting pause allows the calcium (or sodium) channels to recover, so that the cycle starts again. This first explanation is thus similar to wearing out the snake discussed in Chapter 21.

The second explanation for the Wenckebach phenomenon emphasizes shortening of the R-P interval (the interval between the QRS and the P wave that follows), which occurs because progressive slowing of AV conduction moves succeeding P waves closer to the preceding cardiac cycle. In other words, the increasing P-R interval shortens the R-P interval. Shortening of the R-P interval, in turn, brings the atrial impulses closer to the relative refractory period of the already-depressed AV conduction system. Eventually, an atrial impulse reaches the AV node (or AV bundle) so early during the relative refractory period that the calcium (or sodium) channels have not had enough time to recover from their participation in the preceding action potential; as a result, they are not able to generate a propagated action potential. Most evidence now favors this second explanation, which would occur if each time the snake in Fig. 21.22 made a circle, it came closer to its tail.

It is an interesting historical footnote that the features of second-degree block that have made Wenckebach's name a part of the terminology of clinical cardiology (and sadly even a verb, as in: "The patient was Wenckebaching") were based on bedside analyses rather than the ECG. In fact, Wenckebach made his observations in 1899 by analyzing the timing of the waves in the carotid and jugular venous pulse!

Mobitz I and II Second-Degree AV Block

The fact that not all cases of second-degree AV block exhibit the Wenckebach phenomenon serves as the basis for the important distinction between Mobitz I and Mobitz II second-degree AV block, which is quite useful in identifying the site where AV conduction is blocked (Zipes, 1979).

Mobitz I block describes those patients in whom progressive prolongation of the P-R interval (the Wenckebach phenomenon) precedes the dropped beat; thus, the ECG shown in Fig. 22.7 is an example of Mobitz I block. Less frequently, the dropped beat in second-degree AV block is not heralded by P-R prolongation; for example, in the 3:2 AV block shown in Fig. 22.8 the P-R interval has not become longer before the dropped beat. Because the Wenckebach phenomenon is absent, this is an example of the rarer Mobitz II second-degree AV block. A quick way to make this distinction is to compare the P-R intervals just before and immediately following the nonconducted P waves; if these are the same, you are probably dealing with Mobitz II block.

The clinical importance of the distinction between these two types of second-degree AV block arises because Mobitz II block often forewarns of the sudden appearance of third-degree AV block in the His-Purkinje system, whereas Mobitz I block usually arises from a more benign form of block in the AV node. This difference reflects the fact that Mobitz I block in the AV node generally reflects a reversible physiological or pharmacological abnormality such as excessive vagal activity or a drug that inhibits calcium channel opening (see below). In contrast, the association of Mobitz II block with anatomic lesions in the His-Purkinje system means that this form of second degree AV block is less likely to be due to, or alleviated by, changing autonomic influences. Mobitz II block, which can be viewed as appearing when AV conduction "hangs by a thread," can progress suddenly, often without warning, to third-degree (complete) AV block. If severe AV block develops in a patient with block in the His-Purkinje system, drug therapy is generally ineffective, so that to maintain the heart beat systole in these patients, the ventricles must usually be stimulated directly with an electronic pacemaker. For this reason, the appearance of Mobitz II block is generally viewed as an indication for a permanent electrical pacemaker.

The reason that the P-R interval is not always prolonged in Mobitz II block (it is normal in Fig. 22.8) is the high safety factor of the His-Purkinje fibers in the AV bundle, which can allow even a small bundle of tissue to propagate a wave of depolarization. Although the large and rapidly rising action potentials can preserve conduction

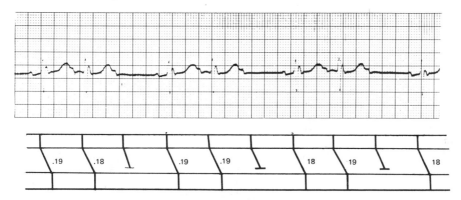

FIG. 22.8. Mobitz type II second-degree (3:2) AV block. The P-R interval is constant at 0.18–0.19 sec (*numbers in Lewis diagram, below*), and neither decreases after the nonconducted P waves nor increases prior to the dropped beats. The QRS complexes are wide (0.14 sec) due to a bundle branch block.

in a damaged AV bundle, further destruction of even a small portion of the damaged bundle can cause conduction to fail completely.

As already emphasized, Mobitz I second-degree AV block is relatively benign because it commonly arises from reversible depression of the calcium channels in the AV node. If progression occurs, it is often gradual (e.g., 4:3 block progressing to 3:2, then to 2:1 block); but more importantly, improvement can be expected if a physiological or pharmacological cause for depression of the AV node is identified and appropriately treated. For example, in patients with acute inferior or posterior myocardial infarction, in whom transient Mobitz I AV block is often caused when the von Bezold-Jarisch reflex increases vagal tone, AV conduction can usually be improved by pharmacological therapy. Because the automatic responsiveness of the calcium channels in the AV node is preserved, these patients generally respond to a muscarinic receptor blocker like atropine (sympathetic stimulation can cause dangerous side effects in these patients).

Intracardiac Electrograms in Atrioventricular Block

Although the distinction between Mobitz types I and II AV block can often be made with a reasonable degree of probability by careful analysis of the ECG, not all patients with second-degree AV block in the AV node exhibit the Wenckebach phenomenon and, conversely, typical Wenckebach periods are sometimes seen where the block is more distal in the His-Purkinje system. Furthermore, in patients with 2:1 AV block, where Wenckebach periods are not possible, electrocardiographic criteria cannot identify the probable site of the conduction disturbance. In such cases, an intracardiac electrogram can be obtained to distinguish between block within the AV node and the more dangerous His-Purkinje block. The site of AV block can readily be defined by timing the H deflection recorded from an electrode catheter over the AV bundle (see Chapter 20). When AV block results from conduction abnormalities in the AV node, the A-H interval is prolonged and the

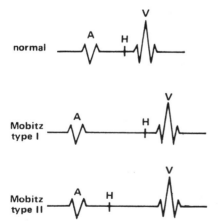

FIG. 22.9. Intracardiac electrograms. *Top*: Normal. *Middle*: Mobitz type I AV block showing a normal H-V interval and a prolonged A-H interval indicative of block within the AV node. *Bottom*: Mobitz type II AV block, showing a normal A-H interval and a prolonged H-V interval indicative of block distal to the AV node.

H-V interval is normal, whereas in AV block caused by a more distal lesion in the conduction system, the delay is between H and V (Fig. 22.9). These are sometimes called *supra-His* and *infra-His* block, respectively. Intracardiac recordings can also be helpful in identifying the site of block in patients with third-degree AV block (see below).

Bifascicular and Trifascicular Block

The practice of viewing the left bundle branch as dividing into two fascicles (Chapter 20), and the right bundle branch as a third fascicle, has given rise to several terms that define abnormalities of both intraventricular and atrioventricular conduction. As long as at least one of these three fascicles is able to conduct a wave of depolarization, AV conduction is preserved, although the QRS complex is abnormal. Terminology in this area, although complex, is rational (Table 22.2).

In *fascicular* block involving either fascicle of the left bundle branch, abnormal impulse propagation over the left ventricle shifts the QRS axis, but neither the P-R interval nor the QRS is prolonged (Chapter 20). Block of one of the two fascicles of the left bundle branch does not delay either AV or intraventricular conduction because parts of both bundle branches continue to conduct from the AV node to both ventricles. Block of the right bundle branch, as described in Chapter 20, prolongs the QRS but also does not interfere with AV conduction. The QRS axis can be

TABLE 22.2. *The fascicular blocks*

Conduction path blocked	Remaining pathways	ECG abnormality
Fascicular block		
Left anterior fascicle	Right bundle branch + left posterior fascicle	Left axis deviation
Left posterior fascicle	Right bundle branch + left anterior fascicle	Right axis deviation
Right bundle branch	Left anterior and posterior fascicles (left bundle branch)	RBBB
Bifascicular block		
Left anterior + left posterior fascicles (left bundle branch)	Right bundle branch	LBBB
Left anterior fascicle + right bundle branch	Left posterior fascicle	RBBB + left axis deviation
Left posterior fascicle + right bundle branch	Left anterior fascicle	RBBB + right axis deviation
Trifascicular block		
Left anterior + left posterior fascicles (left bundle branch) + right bundle branch	None	Third-degree AV block

LBBB, left bundle branch block; RBBB, right bundle branch block.

normal in right bundle branch block because left ventricular depolarization, which normally dominates the ECG, is not affected by the conduction abnormality.

Bifascicular block, which results from interruption of any two of these three fascicles, prolongs the QRS complex and can shift the QRS axis as listed in Table 22.2. As long as one of the three fascicles is still able to conduct impulses from the AV node into the ventricles, AV conduction is preserved.

In *trifascicular block*, sometimes referred to as *bilateral bundle branch block*, conduction through all three fascicles linking the AV node to the ventricles is abnormal; for this reason, trifascicular block delays or interrupts AV conduction.

> The diagnosis of trifascicular block is suggested when a patient with bifascicular block, which does not itself alter AV conduction, develops a prolonged P-R interval or higher degree of AV block. However, to establish this diagnosis usually requires analysis of intracardiac electrograms.

Block of atrioventricular conduction may also occur because of interruption of the more distal branches of the His-Purkinje system. Called *arborization block*, this condition is, for most practical purposes, indistinguishable from trifascicular block.

Third-Degree AV Block

Third-degree AV block, also called *complete AV block* or simply *heart block*, occurs when all conducting pathways between the atria and ventricles are interrupted so that the atria and ventricles beat independently of each other. The ECG in third-degree AV block is characterized by P waves and QRS complexes that bear no constant relationship to each other (Fig. 22.10). The P waves in complete heart block, which usually remain under the control of the SA nodal pacemaker, are therefore usually regular. The ventricular rate, however, is almost always slower than that of the atria because intrinsic pacemakers become slower as they move to lower sites (Table 20.1).

The clinical state of the patient with third-degree AV block depends mainly on the rate of the lower pacemaker that initiates ventricular beating. If the latter maintains a reasonable rate, as is common in congenital heart block, the patient can be asymptomatic, although there will be some functional impairment because the atrial "primer pump" is lost. Very slow heart rates reduce cardiac output (Fig. 16.7), whereas complete failure of lower pacemakers, in which the ventricles cease to beat, causes *asystolic cardiac arrest*. The development of third-degree AV block is therefore a common cause of sudden cardiac death. Patients with intermittent third-degree AV block often experience episodes of syncope if several seconds elapse between the onset of complete heart block and the initiation of pacemaker activity in the ventricles. Repeated syncope in such patients, first noted to be associated with a slow pulse 2,500 years ago by Hippocrates, is often called the Stokes-Adams syndrome.

The site of the subsidiary pacemaker that controls ventricular systole in a patient with third-degree AV block can generally be identified by the configuration of the QRS complex. Impulses generated by pacemakers above the bifurcation of the bun-

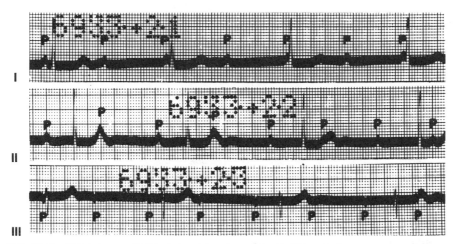

FIG. 22.10. Third-degree AV block (complete heart block). Although the appearance is superficially that of 2:1 AV block, careful examination of all leads demonstrates lack of a constant relationship between the P waves, which come at a basic rate of 78 (P), and the QRS complexes, which are regular at a rate of 36. Thus the atria and ventricles are beating independently. The QRS duration is normal (0.07 sec), which suggests that the ventricles are activated by a pacemaker above the bifurcation of the bundle of His. (From Katz and Pick, 1956.)

dle of His are conducted normally into the two ventricles so that ventricular depolarization follows the same path as it did before the onset of the third-degree AV block; this explains the narrow (normal) QRS complex in Fig. 22.10. In contrast, QRS complexes that are generated by a pacemaker in either ventricle are prolonged and bizarre (Fig. 22.11) because activation of the two ventricles via the rapidly conducting His-Purkinje system is no longer synchronous. As noted in Chapter 20, lower pacemakers also tend to be slower.

The location of a third-degree AV block can be determined most accurately by obtaining intracardiac electrograms. If *A* deflections are not followed by *H*, the block is presumed to be in the AV node, whereas *A* deflections that are followed by *H* but not *V* deflections probably represent a block below the bundle of His.

Normal QRS complexes are commonly seen in congenital third-degree AV block because the subsidiary pacemakers in these patients are often high in the AV bundle; as might be expected from this anatomical location, ventricular rates are only modestly slowed and generally respond to autonomic neurotransmitters. However, when third-degree AV block develops in an older individual, especially when the cause is disease in the His-Purkinje system (see below), the ventricles are usually depolarized by a pacemaker located below the bifurcation of the bundle of His. As these pacemakers tend to be slow and not responsive to autonomic influences, treatment with an electronic pacemaker is generally indicated.

The prolonged, bizarre QRS complexes generated by pacemakers located below the bifurcation of the bundle of His (Fig. 22.11) resemble those seen in patients with a bundle branch block (Chapter 20) because in both settings, the ventricles are not

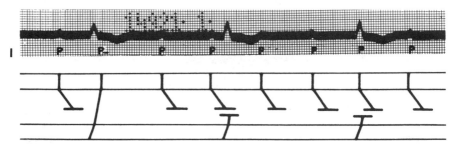

FIG. 22.11. Third-degree AV block (complete heart block). The P waves (P) appear at a rate of 73 (with one exception, see below), but have no fixed relationship to the three prolonged (0.14 sec) QRS complexes. The latter, which are regular at a rate of 27, are depicted by *lines* in the Lewis diagram that should be read upward from the *bottom* (ventricles). The diagnosis of third-degree AV block is made because there is no fixed relationship between P waves and the QRS complexes; the latter are prolonged because the ventricles are activated by impulses arising below the bifurcation of the bundle of His. The second P wave (P–) is an atrial "capture," caused by retrograde conduction of a ventricular impulse through the AV node. The appearance of this premature P wave indicates that the AV block is unidirectional with the unusual feature that complete block is in the antegrade direction. (ECG from Katz and Pick, 1956.)

depolarized synchronously. Thus, the QRS morphology in the ECG cannot distinguish between third-degree AV block where ventricular activation is initiated by a pacemaker below the bifurcation of the bundle of His, and bundle branch block, where the wave of depolarization that initiates ventricular systole, although transmitted normally through the AV node and AV bundle, is disordered in its conduction through the distal His-Purkinje system. In these patients, other criteria must be used to make this distinction.

Pathophysiology of Atrioventricular Block

As emphasized above, from a clinical standpoint there are really two types of AV block: in the AV node and in the His-Purkinje system. Although each can be first degree, second degree, or third degree, the pathophysiology of depressed AV conduction depends in large part on the properties of the tissue at the site of the block. Block in the AV node is usually functional, whereas block in the more distal His-Purkinje system most commonly arises from anatomical lesions of the AV bundle or bundle branches.

Block in the AV Node

As conduction in the AV node, like that in the SA node, depends on i_{Ca}, the causes of AV nodal block are generally similar to those for SA block described earlier in this chapter. Thus, block in the AV node can be caused by any intervention that inhibits calcium channel opening. These include *parasympathetic (vagal) stimulation* and *adenosine*, which have both direct and indirect effects, mediated by G_i, to inhibit calcium channel opening. First-degree AV block, and even mild forms of Mobitz I second-degree AV block, are sometimes seen in trained individuals who have high resting parasympathetic tone; that this does not reflect disease of the AV node is apparent during exercise, when these athletes conduct very rapid sinus rates through their AV node. As mentioned above, reflex AV block can also be caused by the von Bezold-Jarisch reflex in patients who suffer acute inferior or posterior myocardial infarction.

The β-*blockers*, which have both direct and indirect effects that result from reduced levels of the activated α-subunit of G_s, can cause or exacerbate AV block. Other drugs that cause sinus bradycardia and SA block (see above) also depress conduction in the AV node; these obviously include the *calcium channel blockers* that, as described in Chapter 18, act directly to inhibit calcium channel opening. The *cardiac glycosides* can impair AV conduction by depolarizing resting cells in both the AV node and AV bundle, and by a central effect that augments vagal tone (see above). Most antiarrhythmic drugs have non-specific effects that can depress conduction in the AV node (and AV bundle, see below) as can *hyperkalemia*, which reduces resting potential in both the AV node and His-Purkinje system. Block in the AV node can also be caused by *hypothyroidism*, which inhibits i_{Ca} by desensitizing the β-adrenergic receptors and increasing G_i (see above).

Depressed conduction in the AV node contributes to the AV block commonly seen in patients with the *sick sinus syndrome*, but block in these patients can also be caused by lesions in the His-Purkinje system (see below).

An important cause of functional AV block (AV dissociation) is the *refractoriness* left behind after an impulse penetrates this structure. This mechanism, which as noted above provides the preferred explanation for the Wenckebach phenomenon, is a common cause of P-R prolongation after a premature systole depolarizes the AV node, and accounts for AV dissociation at rapid heart rates.

Block in the AV Bundle and Distal His-Purkinje System

As noted earlier in this chapter, block below the AV node is usually caused by anatomical lesions; functional block can also occur in the cells of the His-Purkinje system, but this is not a regular finding as it is in patients where the block is in the AV node. As heightened parasympathetic tone is not a common cause of distal AV block, muscarinic blockers like atropine are usually ineffective in treating this condition. The nonspecific "detergent" effects of most antiarrhythmic drugs can depress conduction in all regions of the heart, including the AV bundle and distal His-Purkinje cells (Chapter 2).

Because of the extensive collateral circulation in the interventricular septum, AV block due to infarction of the His-Purkinje system is uncommon in patients who have sustained an acute myocardial infarction; when this occurs, there has usually been devastating damage to the left ventricle caused by multiple coronary artery occlusions. For this reason, the appearance of anatomical AV block in or below the AV bundle in a patient with acute myocardial infarction (usually manifest as Mobitz II second-degree or third-degree block) is a very bad prognostic sign, not so much because of the risk of third-degree AV block (which, although real, is readily prevented by the prophylactic insertion of an electronic pacemaker), but mainly because it is a marker for severe left ventricular damage.

From a clinical standpoint, the most common causes of block in or below the AV bundle are two degenerative diseases. The first, *Lenegre's disease*, is spontaneous degeneration of the His-Purkinje cells in and below the AV bundle, which are replaced by fibrous tissue. The other, *Lev's disease*, occurs when the more proximal regions of the His-Purkinje system are invaded by fibrous tissue; this commonly occurs in the elderly as the result of fibrosis of the connective tissue skeleton of the heart (the central fibrous body) and when calcification of the mitral and aortic valves extends to the upper part of the interventricular septum.

In the next chapter, when we turn our attention to the tachyarrhythmias, we will see how many of the mechanisms involved in the pathophysiology of the bradyarrhythmias described in the present chapter can also accelerate the heart by disorganizing the depolarization of the atria and ventricles.

REFERENCES

Katz LN, Pick A. (1956). *Clinical electrocardiography. Part I: The arrhythmias*. Philadelphia: Lea & Febiger.
Levine MA, Feldman AM, Robishaw JD, Ladenson PW, Ahn TG, Moroney JF, Smallwood PM. (1990). Influence of thyroid hormone status on expression of genes encoding G protein subunits in the rat heart. *J Biol Chem* 265:3553–3560.
Pappano AJ, Mubagwa K. (1991). Actions of muscarinic agents and adenosine on the heart. In: Fozzard H, Haber E, Katz A, Jennings R, Morgan HE, eds. *The heart and cardiovascular system*, 2nd ed. New York: Raven Press; In Press
Zipes DP. (1979). Second degree atrioventricular block. *Circulation* 60:465–472.

BIBLIOGRAPHY

As for Chapter 21, the reader who wishes to read further about these topics is referred to the many excellent textbooks of electrophysiology, electrocardiography, and clinical electrophysiology. Recent texts include:
Chung EK. (1989). *Principles of cardiac arrhythmias*, 4th ed. Baltimore: Williams and Wilkins.
Mandel WJ, ed. (1987). *Cardiac arrhythmias. Their mechanisms, diagnosis, and management*. Philadelphia: JB Lippincott.

23

The Arrhythmias

III. Premature Systoles, Tachycardias, Flutter, and Fibrillation

It has already been emphasized that the mechanisms responsible for the bradyarrhythmias discussed in Chapter 22 are not simply the opposite of those that lead to the tachyarrhythmias described in the present chapter. The fact that premature systoles, tachycardia, flutter, and fibrillation are caused by the same abnormalities that impair conduction (Chapter 21) explains many of the problems encountered in attempts to treat the tachyarrhythmias described at the end of this chapter.

The organization of this chapter is simple. We begin by describing several common clinical arrhythmias; as in Chapter 22, these provide examples of how the abnormalities in ion channels and ionic currents disorder the rate and rhythm of the heart. Subsequently, key principles of antiarrhythmic therapy are reviewed in terms of their ability to produce both desirable and undesirable effects on cardiac rhythm.

PREMATURE SYSTOLES

Premature systoles, which can be generated in any region of the heart, are often called *extrasystoles* or *ectopic beats*; however, both of these terms are sometimes misnomers. Many premature systoles are not "extra" in that they replace a beat of the atria or ventricles, rather than adding to the number of such beats. Nor do premature systoles always arise from "ectopic" sites as certain classes of premature systoles originate within the normal conduction pathway, although they do so in an abnormal way. It is true by definition, however, that premature systoles occur when regions of the myocardium are activated before they can be depolarized by the normal impulse conducted from the SA node.

The different types of premature systoles are usually named according to their presumed site of origin. Premature depolarization of the atria or ventricles is readily recognized by the early appearance of a P wave or QRS complex; however, much skill is often needed to determine the actual sites where other premature systoles are initiated. This is because depolarization of many important structures does not generate potential differences large enough to be recorded at the body surface (Fig. 20.9).

Atrial Premature Systoles

The typical electrocardiographic appearance of an atrial premature systole is the early occurrence of an abnormal P wave followed by a normal[1] QRS complex. The P-R interval after an atrial premature systole is not abnormally short, i.e., it is greater than 0.12 sec (Fig. 23.1). As premature atrial systoles often reach the atrioventricular (AV) node during its refractory period, the next P-R interval may be prolonged. In fact, some atrial premature systoles arise so early that they reach the AV node during its absolute refractory period; as a result, the impulse is blocked and no QRS complex follows. A premature P wave that is not followed by a QRS complex is generally referred to as a "blocked" atrial premature systole.

The QRS complex following a "typical" atrial premature systole is normal for the simple reason that the early impulse arising in the atria depolarizes the ventricles by the normal pathway. However, premature systoles arising in the atria, or anywhere in the AV junction above the bifurcation of the bundle of His, can be blocked in one of the bundle branches, which gives rise to an abnormality in the QRS complex called "aberrant conduction" (see below).

The atrial premature systole responsible for the fourth P wave in Fig. 23.1 illustrates the three typical features of this abnormality. First, the premature P wave follows the preceding P wave by an interval considerably shorter than the normal sinus interval, so that it is premature. Second, the contour of the early P wave differs from the remainder of the P waves in that it is smaller and narrower. Third, the P-R interval following the premature P wave is 0.16 sec and so is not abnormally shortened.

Aberrant Conduction

As noted above, not all QRS complexes that follow atrial premature systoles are normal in contour, even though the impulse approaches the ventricles by way of the normal conduction pathway via the AV node. In some cases, the QRS is distorted when the wave of depolarization conducted from the atrial premature systole is blocked in one of the bundle branches. The appearance of an abnormal QRS com-

---

[1]The term *normal*, used in this chapter to describe the electrocardiographic manifestations of premature excitation, means "like the P waves or QRS complexes of the basic ECG." Obviously, in patients whose ECG shows an abnormality such as ventricular hypertrophy or bundle branch block, the abnormality should also appear in the beats described here as normal.

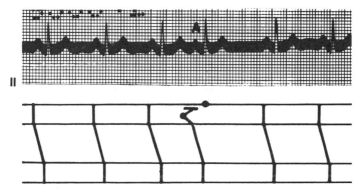

FIG. 23.1. Atrial premature systole. The fourth P wave (*A*) is premature, differs in contour from the other (sinus) P waves, and is followed by a normal QRS complex after a normal P-R interval. The interval between the two sinus P waves immediately before and after the premature systole is exactly twice the normal sinus interval, indicating that the premature systole did not penetrate the SA node and reset its timing. The *dot* on the *upper line* of the Lewis diagram (*below*) indicates the timing of a sinus impulse that did not activate the atria because its transmission into the atria was blocked by the premature systole. (ECG from Katz and Pick, 1956.)

plex after an atrial premature systole is seen in Fig. 23.2, where the fourth QRS complex is prolonged and different in contour (bizarre) compared to those in the remainder of the record. This QRS complex was initiated by an atrial premature systole whose premature P wave has been superimposed on the T wave following the preceding QRS complex, which is apparent when this T wave is compared with the other T waves in this record.

The abnormal contour of the fourth QRS complex in Fig. 23.2, which should have been conducted normally through the AV node and AV bundle, is due to a well-recognized conduction abnormality within the ventricles. The QRS abnormality, which is not unusual after very early premature systoles, occurs because the premature impulse is blocked in one of the bundle branches that did not have time to recover from the preceding beat. This abnormality, called "aberrant conduction," is depicted schematically in Fig. 23.3, which shows how the short interval between the third and fourth QRS complexes causes the premature impulse to arrive during the absolute refractory period in one of the bundle branches.

The fact that the site of the block in aberrant conduction is in the His-Purkinje system is not surprising as action potential duration, and thus refractoriness, is longest in this region of the heart (Chapter 19). Because the abnormalities in aberrant QRS complexes usually alter the terminal, rather than initial deflections, they are similar to the QRS abnormalities seen in bundle branch block. As aberrancy is usually due to block in the right bundle branch, the pattern most commonly resembles right bundle branch block.

The QRS abnormalities in aberrant conduction not only resemble those of bundle branch block, but because the two ventricles are not depolarized simultaneously, they also resemble the abnormal QRS complex caused by ventricular premature systoles

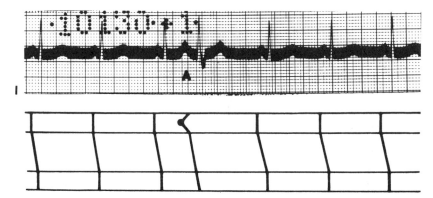

FIG. 23.2. Atrial premature systole with aberrant ventricular conduction. The fourth P wave (A) is premature and is superimposed on the T wave of the preceding ventricular beat, which explains the peaking of this T wave. The QRS complex caused by the premature P wave is abnormal, being prolonged to 0.12 sec and containing a small, broad S wave not seen in the normal QRS complexes. This abnormal QRS complex has been conducted aberrantly because, although it was initiated by a premature P wave, conduction through the ventricles was not normal. The interval between the sinus P waves immediately before and after the premature QRS complex is significantly less than twice the normal sinus interval, which indicates that the premature P wave penetrated the SA node where it advanced the timing of the following series of sinus beats. (ECG from Katz and Pick, 1956.)

(see below). Accurate interpretation of the mechanism responsible for a premature abnormal QRS complex can therefore be difficult, and sometimes impossible. In the example shown in Fig. 23.2, the premature P wave superimposed on the preceding T wave establishes the diagnosis of atrial premature systole with aberrant ventricular conduction.

Resetting of the Sinus Node by a Premature Systole

The atria often cannot be activated by the sinus impulse that follows an atrial premature systole (Figs. 22.1 and 22.2) because this sinus impulse is blocked when it reaches the atria during its refractory period. When this occurs, the subsequent sequence ("timetable") of sinus P waves may or may not be altered by the premature systole. The timetable of the subsequent P waves will be reset if an atrial premature systole is propagated back into the sinoatrial (SA) node (Fig. 23.4). On the other hand, if the wave of depolarization initiated by premature activation of the atria is not conducted into the pacemaker region of the SA node, subsequent sinus P waves appear after a compensatory pause (see below).

The atrial premature systole in Fig. 23.2 has reset the SA node because the first normal P wave following the atrial premature systole appeared sooner than would be expected if the SA node had maintained its normal timetable. This can be determined with a calipers by simply projecting ahead the timing of the P waves before the atrial premature systole. It is apparent that the premature systole shifted ahead the entire sequence of subsequent sinus beats.

A

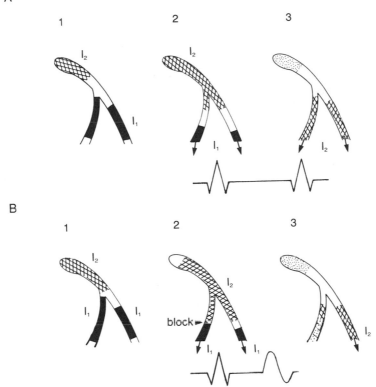

B

FIG. 23.3. Mechanism for aberrant conduction. *A.* Series of normal impulses penetrating the AV conduction system. *A1:* The first impulse (*shaded*) has penetrated both bundle branches, whereas the second impulse (*cross-hatched*) is still in the AV node. *A2:* The first impulse has entered the ventricles to give rise to the first normalf QRS complex, whereas the second impulse has entered the two bundle branches. *A3:* The second impulse has entered the ventricles to generate the second normal QRS; a third impulse (*dotted*) has entered the AV node. *B:* Similar to *A* except that the second impulse is premature and follows shortly after the first impulse (*B1*). Subsequently, the second impulse encounters the normally long refractory period in the right bundle branch (*B2*) where it is blocked (*B3*). Because the ventricles are depolarized only by the impulse conducted through the left bundle branch, the QRS complex is prolonged and bizarre.

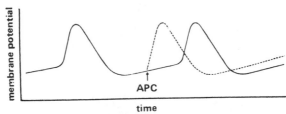

FIG. 23.4. Mechanism by which a premature systole that penetrates the SA node resets the sinus pacemaker. The action potential of a pacemaker cell in the SA node illustrates the normal sinus interval (*solid line*). The entry of an impulse conducted from an atrial premature systole (APC) causes early depolarization of the pacemaker cell (*dotted line*), thereby advancing the timing of the following series of action potentials.

Junctional Premature Systoles

Premature depolarization of either the AV node or AV bundle above the bifurcation of the bundle of His gives rise to a *junctional premature systole* that can include a premature QRS complex, a premature P wave, or both. The contour of the premature QRS complex, unless it is so early as to be aberrant, is normal because the ventricles are depolarized via the normal pathway; however, the P waves associated with junctional premature systoles are abnormal both in timing and in contour (see below).

Because the AV node and bundle lie in the conduction pathway that links the atria and ventricles, junctional premature impulses can proceed in the antegrade direction to activate the ventricles, the retrograde direction to activate the atria, or both (Fig. 23.5). The relationship between the antegrade QRS complex initiated by a junctional premature systole and the accompanying retrograde P wave (described below) is variable for reasons that are readily understood. Impulses that depolarize the atria before the ventricles generate a P wave before the premature QRS complex (Fig. 23.5A). However, the P-R interval in a junctional premature systole is abnormally short, < 0.12 sec.

A P-R interval > 0.12 sec implies that the impulse had encountered the normal delay in traversing the AV node, which indicates that the premature systole originated in the atria; thus, the correct diagnosis would be an atrial premature systole as described above.

If retrograde conduction is slower than antegrade conduction, the P wave produced by a junctional premature systole comes after the QRS complex (Fig. 23.5B), whereas P waves generated by junctional impulses that reach both structures at the same time are buried in the QRS complex and so are not seen (Fig. 23.5C). In some patients, conduction of a junctional premature systole is in only one direction, so that only a retrograde P wave or antegrade QRS is seen.

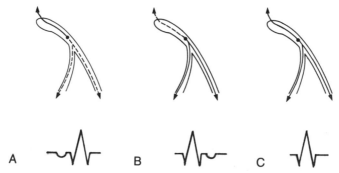

FIG. 23.5. Junctional premature systoles are conducted retrograde into the atria and antegrade into the ventricles. Depending on the time required for the impulse to reach these two structures, the retrograde P wave can precede (*A*), follow (*B*), or be buried in (*C*) the normal QRS complex.

Junctional premature systoles were once classified according to the relative timing of the retrograde P waves and QRS complexes. When a retrograde P wave preceded the QRS complex by < 0.12 sec, the beat was called an "upper nodal" beat; where a P wave and QRS complex were presumed to have occurred at the same time, the beat was a "middle nodal" beat; and when a retrograde P wave followed the QRS complex, the beat was a "lower nodal" beat. These terms are now obsolete because the relationship between the QRS complexes and the P waves associated with a junctional premature systole is probably determined more by the relative rates of antegrade and retrograde conduction than by the site in the AV junction where the premature systole originated.

Retrograde P Waves

When a junctional premature systole activates the atria, the resulting P wave has an abnormal frontal plane vector because the atria are depolarized in a retrograde direction by the impulse that has entered from below, instead of from above. The normal P wave vector (Fig. 23.6) is directed inferiorly and to the left because atrial depolarization normally begins in the SA node, which is located superiorly in the right atrial-superior vena caval junction. In contrast, the wave of depolarization initiated by retrograde conduction from a junctional premature systole enters the atria from the AV node, which lies at the inferior border of the right atrium near the top of the interventricular septum. As the latter generates a vector that is directed superiorly, and often to the right, retrograde P waves are inverted in lead II.

The characteristic appearance of the retrograde P wave is shown in Fig. 23.7, where an inverted P wave precedes the fourth QRS complex, which is normal in contour. The short P-R interval (0.08 sec), which is diagnostic of a junctional premature systole, is due to the fact that both the P wave and the QRS complex arise from a single wave of depolarization in the AV junction that reaches the atria just before it enters the ventricles (see Fig. 23.5A). The term *P-R interval* is therefore a misnomer as the impulse has not traveled from atria (P) to ventricles (QRS).

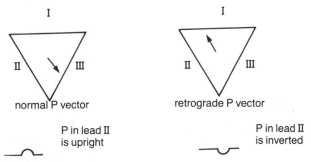

FIG. 23.6. Normal and retrograde P wave vectors. The normal P vector in the frontal plane is directed to the left and inferiorly, inscribing an upright deflection in lead II (*left*). Retrograde P vectors, on the other hand, are directed superiorly, and often to the right, so that they inscribe an inverted deflection in lead II (*right*).

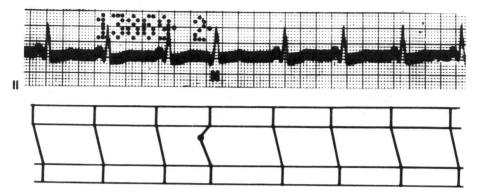

FIG. 23.7. Junctional premature systole with retrograde P wave in lead II. The fourth QRS complex is normal in contour, but is premature and preceded by an abnormal, inverted P wave. The P-R interval in this premature systole is 0.08 sec, which meets the criteria for a junctional premature systole. The inverted P wave preceding the premature systole was conducted from the same junctional focus that produced the premature QRS complex (shown in the Lewis diagram), and is a typical retrograde P wave in this lead II. (ECG from Katz and Pick, 1956.)

Compensatory Pause and Interpolation

Two different patterns associated with junctional premature systoles are shown in Fig. 23.8. Both premature QRS complexes meet the criteria of junctional premature systoles because their contour is similar to that of the remainder of the ventricular complexes in this record. Neither is associated with a P wave, the P wave that notches the T wave following the second premature QRS is the next sinus P wave as it comes exactly "on schedule." The relationships between these premature QRS complexes and the underlying sinus rhythm, however, differ. The second junctional premature systole (the sixth QRS complex) is the more typical as it is followed by a pause that ends when the *second* sinus impulse after the premature systole captures the ventricles (shown in the Lewis diagram below Fig. 23.8). In contrast, the first premature QRS complex, because it appears earlier, allows the next sinus P wave (superimposed on the T wave of the premature QRS complex) to generate a normal QRS complex (the third from the right).

The different effects of the two premature systoles in Fig. 23.8 illustrate two phenomena associated with premature systoles that do not reset (depolarize) the sinus pacemaker. The pause between the second premature QRS complex and the subsequent sinus beat (the seventh in Fig. 23.8) occurs because the sinus beat that originated shortly after the premature systole is blocked. This pause is called a *compensatory pause* as it allows the subsequent train of normal sinus impulses to resume its scheduled control of the heart. This is readily demonstrated by the fact that the interval between the two QRS complexes enclosing the junctional premature systole is exactly twice that between the normal sinus beats in this ECG, which means that the timetable of the SA node was not reset by the premature systole.

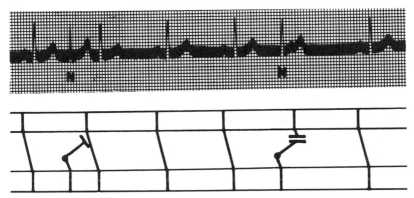

FIG. 23.8. Two junctional premature systoles. The second and sixth QRS complexes (N), which are premature, normal in contour, and not preceded by a P wave, meet the criteria for junctional premature systoles. The first junctional premature systole, which produces the second QRS complex, does not interfere with either the initiation or conduction of the following sinus beat and so is *interpolated*. (The sinus P wave preceding the third QRS complex falls on the T wave of the junctional premature systole, which is abnormally tall.) The second junctional premature systole, which produces the sixth QRS complex, follows the preceding QRS complex by a longer interval than the first junctional premature systole. This has allowed the premature impulse to propagate through the AV node into the atria, where it has prevented the next sinus beat from reaching the ventricles (shown in the Lewis diagram by *short horizontal lines*). The final QRS complex in this strip thus follows a *compensatory pause*. (ECG from Katz and Pick, 1956.)

The term *compensatory pause* is in some ways a misnomer as the pause does not really compensate for anything, except to allow the sinus beats to remain on the timetable they would have followed had there not been a premature systole.

The first junctional premature systole in Fig. 23.8, which produces the second QRS complex, comes earlier and so does not block conduction of the following sinus P wave into the ventricles. This is thus a true "extrasystole," which is *interpolated* because it has been inserted into the normal sequence of sinus cycles. The next P wave, which is superimposed on the T wave of the premature systole, is a sinus beat that is conducted "on schedule" into the ventricles where it gives rise to the third QRS complex.

Ventricular Premature Systoles

Premature impulses arising below the bifurcation of the bundle of His generate abnormal QRS complexes because the ventricles are depolarized via an abnormal pathway. Thus, prolonged and bizarre premature QRS complexes not preceded by P waves are usually ventricular premature systoles (Fig. 23.9). The QRS contour is altered because the impulse, instead of being conducted simultaneously into both ventricles, spreads over an abnormal pathway from the ventricle in which the impulse originated, into the opposite ventricle (Fig. 23.10). The abnormally long path-

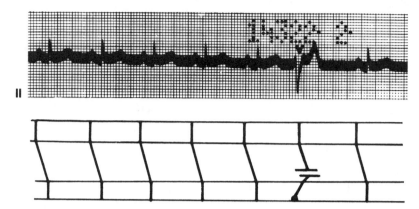

FIG. 23.9. Ventricular premature systole. The sixth QRS complex (V), which is premature and not preceded by a P wave, is prolonged and bizarre compared to the normal QRS complexes in this record. These are the criteria for a ventricular premature systole. This premature systole is followed by a compensatory pause because the next sinus P wave (which is "buried" in the QRS of the ventricular premature systole) is blocked, as shown in the Lewis diagram. (ECG from Katz and Pick, 1956.)

way and the fact that conduction through ventricular myocardium is slower than in the His-Purkinje system (Chapter 20) account for the long duration of the QRS.

> The asynchrony of ventricular activation that prolongs the QRS in a ventricular premature systole is similar to that which causes the QRS abnormalities in bundle branch block and aberrant conduction. In all of these abnormalities, ventricular activation loses its normal synchronization. In bundle branch block and aberrancy, synchrony is lost because the wave of depolarization is delayed in its passage to one of the ventricles, whereas in a ventricular premature systole synchrony is lost because the ventricle in which the impulse originated prematurely is activated before the opposite ventricle.

The ventricular premature systole shown in Fig. 23.9 is followed by a compensatory pause because the premature impulse was not conducted to the atria and so

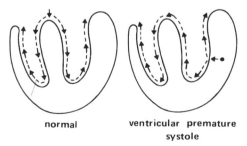

normal   ventricular premature
                      systole

FIG. 23.10. Normal conduction pathway followed by an impulse that depolarizes the ventricles simultaneously via the AV bundle and bundle branches (*left*), and the abnormal conduction pathway followed by an impulse arising in the left ventricle (*right*). The loss of synchrony, greater length of the path of depolarization, and slow conduction through ventricular myocardium contribute to the prolongation of QRS that characterizes ventricular premature systoles.

could not reset the timing of the SA node pacemaker. (The sinus P wave that followed the last normal beat before the premature systole is not seen as it is "buried" in the much larger premature QRS complex.) Ventricular premature systoles can also be interpolated. In some patients, retrograde conduction of a ventricular premature systole occurs when the impulse traverses the AV node to reach the atria; when this occurs, a retrograde P wave follows the premature QRS complex.

Fusion Beats

When ventricular premature systoles appear late during diastole, the wave of depolarization that originates in the ventricles may occur at the same time as the normal wave of depolarization is initiated by the next sinus impulse. When this occurs, the ventricles are depolarized simultaneously from two directions: from "below" by the premature ventricular impulse, and from "above" by the sinus impulse conducted via the AV node. A QRS complex initiated by two independent waves of depolarization, called a *fusion beat*, is seen in Fig. 23.11, where the fifth QRS complex is midway in contour between the normal QRS complexes that make up the majority of the ventricular beats in this record, and the ventricular premature systoles that initiate the first and ninth QRS complexes. The fifth QRS is a fusion beat because, as shown in the Lewis diagram, the impulse arising in the sinus node enters the ventricles shortly after the beginning of the ventricular premature systole, and so lessens the QRS abnormality. Recognition of fusion beats is of considerable importance in the diagnosis of ventricular tachycardias (see below).

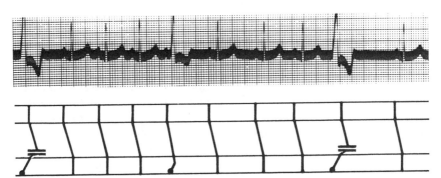

FIG. 23.11. Ventricular premature systoles showing a fusion beat. The first and ninth QRS complexes, which are premature, not initiated by P waves, and prolonged and bizarre, are typical ventricular premature systoles. The fifth QRS complex is also premature but is less prolonged and less bizarre than the other QRS complexes. The P-R interval preceding this QRS complex is 0.10 sec, so it can be deduced that the later portions of the QRS complex are initiated by the sinus impulse propagated normally into the ventricles by way of the AV bundle and bundle branches. However, the initial portion of this QRS complex is abnormal, its upstroke being slurred as is that of the other two "typical" ventricular premature systoles. This fifth premature systole thus represents a fusion beat that combines the features of both the normal and abnormal QRS complexes. The dual origin of the fusion beat is shown in the lower space (ventricles) of Lewis diagram. (ECG from Katz and Pick, 1956.)

The abnormal QRS complexes seen in patients with preexcitation (Wolff-Parkinson-White syndrome) are a special form of fusion beat; in this case, fusion is between the normal impulse that enters the ventricles normally via the AV bundle and bundle branches, and the wave of depolarization that begins at an abnormal site in the ventricles at the end of the accessory pathway.

"Complexity" of Ventricular Premature Systoles

The prognostic implications of ventricular premature systoles correlate with both their frequency and their "complexity." In general, more *frequent* ventricular premature systoles are more serious. As described below, when we discuss ventricular tachycardia, *repetitive* ventricular premature systoles are more dangerous than single ones. Similarly, *bigeminy*, where every other QRS is a ventricular premature systole, is more likely to herald a life-threatening ventricular arrhythmia. *Multifocal* ventricular premature systoles (having different QRS morphologies) are more complex than unifocal (single morphology), whereas very early ventricular premature systoles, that fall on the T wave of the preceding cycle (the *R on T phenomenon*) can, in some settings, be the most ominous of all.

TACHYCARDIAS

Tachycardia, defined as sustained, more-or-less regular, rhythms at rates greater than 100, can arise in any part of the heart. These arrhythmias, which can be caused by a number of mechanisms (Chapter 21), give rise to characteristic electrocardiographic features, and often have distinctive physiological properties. The common tachycardias described in the following pages have been selected to illustrate important pathophysiological abnormalities; the reader who wishes a more rigorous treatment of the diagnostic features of these arrhythmias is referred to the many clinical textbooks that deal with this subject.

Tachycardias are generally subdivided into two groups: *supraventricular*, which originate above the ventricles, and *ventricular*. Supraventricular tachycardias are generally the more benign, and include all rapid beating initiated by abnormalities of the SA node, atria, and AV junction. The more dangerous ventricular tachycardias arise from sites below the bifurcation of the bundle of His.

Sinus Tachycardia

The pathophysiology and electrocardiographic features of the tachycardias caused by acceleration of the normal SA node pacemaker are described at the beginning of Chapter 22. As the ECG in sinus tachycardia contains normal QRS complexes that follow normal P waves after a normal P-R interval (Fig. 22.1), the only ECG abnormality is the accelerated rate.

Sinus tachycardias generally occur when the sinus pacemaker is accelerated by extrinsic influences, usually sympathetic overactivity, that develop over several seconds, or more slowly. Thus the onset of a sinus tachycardia is typically gradual, and not sudden. As the SA node remains under autonomic control, sinus tachycardias are characteristically slowed by vagal stimulation. The heart rates in sinus tachycardia can exceed 200, but are usually less than 140. All of these features, especially their slow onset and termination and their response to vagal stimulation, distinguish this common—and usually benign—supraventricular arrhythmia from the more serious tachycardias that result from disorders intrinsic to the heart.

Supraventricular Tachycardias

The classification of the nonsinus tachycardias arising above the bifurcation of the bundle of His is difficult (Table 23.1). The older terms "atrial" and "junctional" tachycardia, were based almost entirely on electrocardiographic criteria, mainly P-wave morphology and the relationship between P waves and QRS complexes. Although still meaningful they are far less useful than newer classifications based on mechanism. This is because the advent of clinical electrophysiological testing has shown that different types of supraventricular tachycardia, which require different management, cannot always be distinguished by examination of the body surface ECG.

TABLE 23.1. *Supraventricular tachycardias*

| Tachycardia | Classified according to P-wave morphology and the P-R interval | | |
	P Waves	P-R interval	Onset and termination
Sinus	Normal	Normal or prolonged	Gradual
Atrial	Abnormal	Normal or prolonged	Paroxysmal
Junctional	Retrograde	Short or absent	Paroxysmal

| Tachycardia | Classified according to mechanism | |
	Mechanism	Prevalence
Sinus node reentry	SA node *reentry*	Uncommon
Automatic atrial tachycardia	Ectopic atrial *pacemaker*	Uncommon
Atrial reentry	Atrial *reentry*	Uncommon
Automatic AV junctional tachycardia	Ectopic His-bundle *pacemaker*	Uncommon
AV nodal reentry	*Reentry* involving dual pathways in the AV node	$\sim\frac{2}{3}$ of all supraventricular tachycardias
Bypass tract reentry	*Reentry* involving the AV node and a bypass tract	$\sim\frac{1}{5}$ of all supraventricular tachycardias

Traditional Classification Based on P-Wave Morphology and the P-R Interval

The two most important types of supraventricular tachycardia that can be distinguished on the basis of P-wave morphology and P-R interval are atrial and junctional tachycardia. Both differ from sinus tachycardia because P-wave morphology is not normal and because they often start and stop suddenly (see below).

Atrial tachycardia is characterized by abnormal P waves that are followed by normal QRS complexes after a normal (or slightly prolonged) P-R interval, so that atrial tachycardias resemble a run of atrial premature systoles. In many patients with atrial tachycardia, however, P waves are difficult to identify. Furthermore, as described later in this chapter, the QRS complexes in atrial tachycardia can be abnormal due to aberrant conduction. For these reasons, the clearly recognizable pattern of atrial tachycardia seen in Fig. 23.12 is not always apparent.

Junctional tachycardia (Figs. 23.13), like junctional premature systoles, is defined on the basis of the timing and appearance of atrial activation. P waves, when discernible, are retrograde and can precede or follow the QRS complex. The QRS complexes in a junctional tachycardia are normal unless conduction is aberrant.

"Modern" Classified Based on Mechanism

A more useful classification of supraventricular tachycardias is based on the mechanism responsible for the tachycardia. Unfortunately, however, mechanisms are not always apparent on the body surface ECG, which until recently was the only tool available to the clinician who must treat these patients. Today's "gold standard," therefore, is the invasive electrophysiological study that uses data obtained from stimulating and recording electrodes placed in the heart.

Table 23.1 describes six different mechanisms that can give rise to a supraventricular tachycardia; four represent *reentry* in different regions of the heart above

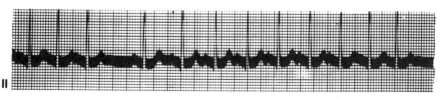

FIG. 23.12. Paroxysmal atrial tachycardia. Following the third QRS complex, which represents the final beat of a paroxysm of the tachycardia, a sinus beat produces the fourth QRS complex. Immediately afterward, another paroxysm of atrial tachycardia is initiated by a premature P wave, which is narrower than the preceding sinus P wave. The P-R interval in this beat is normal, so that the fifth cycle resembles an atrial premature systole. This is followed by seven similar complexes that gradually accelerate from a rate of ~110 to ~140; because of this "warming up," the later P waves become superimposed on the T waves of the preceding cycle. (ECG from Katz and Pick, 1956.)

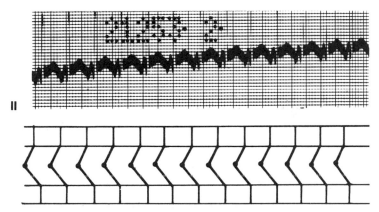

FIG. 23.13. Junctional tachycardia. The rapid tachycardia (rate ~170) exhibits narrow QRS complexes that are preceded by inverted P waves, which in this lead II are retrograde. The short P-R interval (0.08 sec) establishes the diagnosis of a junctional tachycardia in which the atria are depolarized slightly ahead of the ventricles as shown on the Lewis diagram, *below*. (ECG from Katz and Pick, 1956.)

the ventricles, the other two, often referred to as "automatic," are due to accelerated *pacemaker discharge*. As noted in the table, most supraventricular tachycardias are due to AV node reentry involving the dual pathways discussed in Chapter 21, and reentry using an accessory pathway.

Sinus Node Reentry

This uncommon arrhythmia differs from sinus tachycardia because it is generated by a reentrant circuit in the SA node, rather than depolarization of a pacemaker. Although SA node reentry gives rise to normal P waves, this arrhythmia is distinguished from sinus tachycardia because it is often paroxysmal and can be terminated when an electrical stimulus interrupts the reentrant circuit.

Automatic Atrial Tachycardia

Automatic atrial tachycardias, like the atrial reentrant tachycardias described below, generate abnormal P waves followed by a normal P-R interval. As noted earlier, the P-R interval may be prolonged by AV dissociation at rapid heart rates, which can be as high as 200. Unlike reentrant atrial tachycardias (see below), the onset and termination of an automatic atrial tachycardia is usually not sudden; for this reason, automatic atrial tachycardia is also called *nonparoxysmal atrial tachycardias*. The accelerated pacemaker rate in an automatic atrial tachycardia, in contrast to most reentrant arrhythmias, is not regularly triggered by a premature systole,

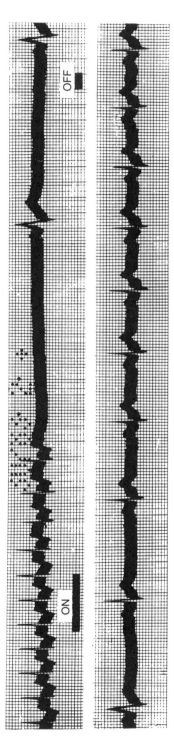

FIG. 23.14. Termination of supraventricular tachycardia by carotid sinus massage. The strip begins with a supraventricular tachycardia at a rate of ~190. The horizontal bar (ON) marks the onset of carotid sinus massage, which causes some slowing of the tachycardia before it stops abruptly. After a pause of more than 3 sec ("standstill"), three prolonged QRS complexes are seen; as these are preceded by P waves after a P-R interval of 0.13 sec, they probably represent junctional "escape" beats. This means that, because there are no sinus impulses, a slow pacemaker below the bifurcation of the bundle of His has fired to initiate these three cycles. After release of the carotid sinus massage (*horizontal bar* labeled OFF), this escape mechanism is replaced by a slowly acelerating sinus mechanism with a P-R interval of 0.18 sec. (ECG from Katz and Pick, 1956.)

so that the first P wave when this arrhythmia begins is similar to the subsequent P waves during the tachycardia.

Automatic atrial tachycardias, which represent only a fraction of the clinical supraventricular tachycardias, may be related to the more severe *multifocal atrial tachycardia* in which P wave morphology and P-R intervals vary with no apparent pattern. These chaotic supraventricular arrhythmias are often seen in patients with severe pulmonary disease, and may herald the appearance of atrial flutter and fibrillation (see below).

Atrial Reentry

Atrial reentry, like other reentrant arrhythmias, is generally triggered by a premature systole and, because it starts and stops suddenly, is paroxysmal. Rates are usually ~140. The reentrant circuit in this uncommon arrhythmia can be terminated by electrical stimuli applied to the atria, but unlike the reentrant tachycardias that utilize a pathway in the AV node, where conduction involves calcium channels, reentrant atrial tachycardias are not usually influenced by vagal stimulation and drugs that block i_{Ca}.

Automatic AV Junctional Tachycardia

Automatic AV junctional tachycardias are due to an accelerated pacemaker in the AV junction, most often in the His bundle. The rates of this arrhythmia, sometimes called "accelerated junctional rhythm," can be as low as 50 to 60; this terminology is confusing because, although the absolute rate is not rapid, it *is* faster than normal for a junctional pacemaker. P waves, when seen, are retrograde (see above). Like the automatic atrial tachycardias described above, automatic AV junctional tachycardias are usually nonparoxysmal and can be slowed by vagal stimulation. Unlike the reentrant tachycardias in which the arrhythmia depends on calcium channel-dependent conduction pathways in the AV node, automatic AV junctional tachycardias are not terminated by vagal stimulation or adenosine.

Automatic AV junctional tachycardias are commonly produced by digitalis, and their rates commonly accelerate as the dose of cardiac glycosides is increased. When slow (<50 to 60), this tachycardia is not necessarily a sign of an excessive dose of digitalis. However, automatic AV junctional tachycardias at rapid rates, often accompanied by blocked P waves due to depressed conduction into the atria via the AV node (inaccurately referred to in the past as "paroxysmal atrial tachycardia with block") is evidence of digitalis toxicity.

AV Nodal Reentry

The most common cause of supraventricular tachycardia is the reciprocal rhythm that utilizes dual pathways in the AV node described in Chapter 21. P waves often cannot be made out in this arrhythmia because they are either buried in the QRS complexes, or are absent because the atria are not part of the reentrant circuit. When P waves are seen, the P-R interval is usually longer then the R-P interval because antegrade conduction of the reciprocal rhythm is typically via the slower of the two pathways in the AV node (Chapter 21).

Like the other reentrant tachycardias, AV nodal reentry is usually paroxysmal and triggered by a premature systole. Because of the role of i_{Ca} in maintaining this arrhythmia, the reentrant circuit can be interrupted by vagal stimulation and adenosine, as well as by calcium channel blockers and β-blockers.

Accessory Pathway

Supraventricular tachycardias that involve an accessory pathway, like AV nodal reentry, are paroxysmal and generally initiated by a premature systole. Because the antegrade limb of the reentrant circuit usually depends on calcium-dependent conduction through the AV node, accessory pathway reentry can be terminated by vagal stimulation, adenosine, calcium channel blockers, and β-blockers (Chapter 21). Retrograde conduction, from ventricles to atria, is usually via sodium-dependent depolarization in the accessory pathway, so that when P waves are generated by the tachycardia, they are retrograde and occur during or shortly after the QRS complexes.

General Features of Supraventricular Tachycardias

As noted in Table 23.1, most supraventricular tachycardias arise from a reentrant circuit that, because it is either conducting or not conducting, means that these arrhythmias are generally true paroxysmal supraventricular tachycardias (PSVT). [An older term, *paroxysmal atrial tachycardia* (PAT) is obsolete because it refers to one of the less common mechanisms that cause these arrhythmias.] Regular supraventricular tachycardias are rarely dangerous unless coexistent heart disease, or another abnormality, has seriously reduced cardiac reserve. In children, however, their rates can be extremely high and AV conduction can allow rapid ventricular beating, so that these tachycardias can be quite serious, and sometimes fatal. Accessory pathway reentry, as noted in Chapter 21, is also dangerous in patients with atrial fibrillation.

Most supraventricular tachycardias are very regular, although "warming up" often occurs at their onset (Fig. 23.12). Their rates, which depend on the mechanism, usually range between 140 and 200, although they may be as low as 100 or as high as 250. The arrhythmias may last a few seconds or up to several days.

The abrupt termination of a paroxysmal supraventricular tachycardia by vagal stimulation caused by carotid sinus massage is shown in Fig. 23.14. Although slowing prior to cessation of the tachycardia is characteristic, the heart rate during a supraventricular tachycardia is less responsive to vagal stimulation than is that of a sinus tachycardia. This is apparent in Fig. 23.14, where powerful vagal stimulation that has only a minimal effect on the rate of the tachycardia eventually stops it altogether.

The abrupt cessation of the tachycardia in Fig. 23.14 is followed by a long pause; more than 3 sec elapse before a QRS follows the termination of the tachycardia. The first three beats after the end of the tachycardia have arisen in junctional tissue below the bifurcation of the bundle of His, which explains the widened QRS complexes and shortened P-R intervals. Marked depression of the SA node by acetylcholine (Chapter 22), along with overdrive suppression (see below), accounts for the long pause prior to the reestablishment of sinus rhythm. (Today this tachycardia would be treated with adenosine, which, as noted in Chapter 12, works by a mechanism similar to vagal stimulation but is safer because of its shorter half-life.)

Most reentrant supraventricular tachycardias are readily terminated by brief, externally applied direct current shocks, called *electrical cardioversion*. The mechanism by which cardioversion terminates these arrhythmias is not entirely clear, however. Although it is often taught that the electrical current depolarizes all of the cells and so resynchronizes reentrant circuits, tachycardias often continue for a few beats after the shock before "breaking." It may be that the electrical discharge causes potassium to leak from the massively stimulated heart cells, which by depolarizing parts of the reentrant circuit, increases the block so as to terminate the arrhythmia.

Overdrive Suppression

Normal pacemaker activity is often slow to take over the heartbeat following the termination of a tachycardia (Fig. 23.14), whether spontaneously or after cardioversion. Spontaneous pacemaker discharge can also be suppressed experimentally by rapid electrical stimulation of the heart. This phenomenon, called overdrive suppression, is caused largely by outward currents generated by the electrogenic sodium pump (Chapter 10), which is activated when rapid stimulation increases intracellular Na^+ concentration. The repolarizing currents generated when three intracellular sodium ions are exchanged for two extracellular potassium ions slow the sinus pacemaker by counterbalancing the inward currents i_f and i_{Ca} (Chapter 19).

Ventricular Tachycardia

Tachycardias in which the QRS complexes are widened (>0.12 sec) and bear no fixed relationship to P waves are most often ventricular in origin (Fig. 23.15). They are more ominous than the corresponding paroxysmal supraventricular tachycardias and can herald the advent of ventricular fibrillation (see below).

Supraventricular tachycardias can also have wide QRS complexes, due mainly to preexisting bundle branch block or aberrant conduction, but even so they are more benign than ventricular tachycardia. Difficulties in distinguishing between supraventricular tachycardias with prolonged QRS complexes and ventricular tachycardias has led to the growing use of the term *wide QRS tachycardia*. The value of this

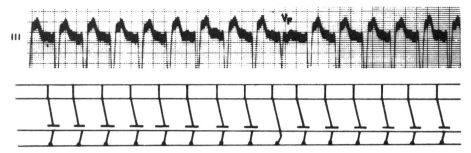

FIG. 23.15. Ventricular tachycardia. All but one of the QRS complexes, which appear at a rate of ~120, are prolonged (0.16 sec). The P waves have no fixed relationship to the QRS complexes so that the salient criteria for the diagnosis of ventricular tachycardia are met. In the tenth beat (labeled V_F), the P wave falls ~0.16 sec before the QRS. The resulting QRS, which is narrowed (0.11 sec) is called a fusion beat because the ventricles are depolarized both by the focus in the ventricles and the impulse arising in the atria. The presence of a fusion beat confirms the diagnosis of ventricular tachycardia. (ECG from Katz and Pick, 1956.)

term is that it neither implies a mechanism nor forces a course of treatment, but instead makes it clear that more data are needed to make the critical differential diagnosis between supraventricular and ventricular tachycardia.

Ventricular tachycardias have rates similar to most supraventricular tachycardias, although the rhythm in ventricular tachycardia is often slightly irregular, in contrast to the more regular rhythm of a paroxysmal supraventricular tachycardia. Most rapid ventricular tachycardias are due to reentry (see below), but do not respond to vagal stimulation because the entire reentrant circuit utilizes sodium-dependent action potentials in the distal His-Purkinje system and ventricles. For this reason, vagal stimulation rarely breaks a ventricular tachycardia.

The finding of a fusion beat can sometimes establish the diagnosis of ventricular tachycardia. In the ECG shown in Fig. 23.15, the QRS complex labeled V_F, which is narrower and less bizarre than the other QRS complexes in this record, is a fusion beat. It is preceded by a P wave with a P-R interval of 0.16 sec, so that its timing is consistent with a beat that is initiated partly by the impulse arriving from the atria by way of the AV node and partly by the abnormal focus in the ventricles. The electrocardiographic distinction between ventricular tachycardia and supraventricular tachycardia with persistent aberrant conduction or intraventricular (bundle branch) block can be suggested by QRS morphologies in various leads and by such clinical "lore" as the useful aphorism that any wide QRS tachycardia in a patient with coronary disease should be considered as a ventricular tachycardia until proved otherwise. In many cases, it is necessary to carry out a formal intracardiac electrophysiological study to make this clinically important differential diagnosis.

Single ventricular premature systoles (Fig. 23.9) are usually benign, but "runs" of ventricular tachycardia (Fig. 23.15) can be dangerous and may herald sudden cardiac death. Not surprisingly, two ventricular premature systoles in a row (a *couplet*) is more ominous than two isolated ventricular premature systoles; more serious

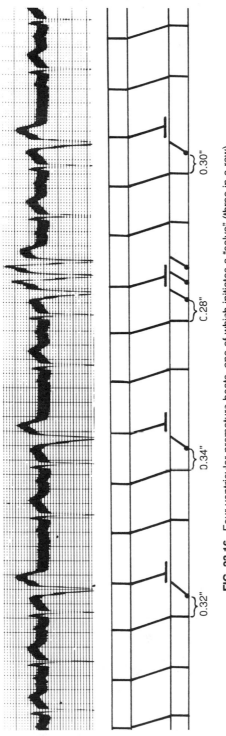

FIG. 23.16. Four ventricular premature beats, one of which initiates a "salvo" (three in a row). The coupling interval between the premature QRS and the preceding normal QRS (numbers at the *bottom* of the strip) is shortest before the ventricular premature systole that initiates the salvo. This is an example of the "R on T" phenomenon in which an early premature systole that falls during the vulnerable period of the preceding QRS init ates repetitive firing. (ECG from Katz and Pick, 1956.)

0.32"   0.34"   C.28"   0.30"

are three ventricular premature systoles in a row (a *salvo* or triplet) as shown in Fig. 23.16. More than three in a row is generally defined as ventricular tachycardia; when these occur as brief (<30 sec) episodes that terminate spontaneously, they are referred to as *nonsustained ventricular tachycardia*. When a ventricular tachycardia lasts longer than 30 sec, it is usually referred to as *sustained ventricular tachycardia*.

> Not all ventricular tachycardias give rise to the uniform QRS complexes shown in Fig. 23.15. As in the case of the ventricular premature systoles, *polymorphic ventricular tachycardia* has a more ominous prognosis than *monomorphic ventricular tachycardia*. One special type of polymorphic ventricular tachycardia in which QRS morphology gradually alternates between upward- and downward-directed complexes, called "torsades de pointes" (twisting of the points), has attracted considerable attention partly because of the striking appearance and mellifluous French name, but mainly because this pattern is a marker for underlying mechanisms caused by repolarization abnormalities (the "long Q-T syndromes") that require special therapy.

Pathophysiology of Ventricular Tachycardias

The majority of ventricular tachycardias are reentrant arrhythmias; however, as noted in Chapter 21, there are many different causes for reentry. The complexity of the underlying mechanisms, their variability at different times in a given patient, and the often unpredictable response to therapy, have cast a pall over the empirical use of antiarrhythmic drugs to prevent lethal ventricular arrhythmias. As discussed below, this gloomy prospect has recently been heightened by the demonstration that antiarrhythmic drugs often have "proarrhythmic" effects that can increase mortality when these drugs are administered to inadequately evaluated patients.

Parasystole

The main exception to the generalization that ventricular tachycardia is a reentrant arrhythmia is *parasystole*, which is a slow "automatic" ventricular rhythm that arises from pacemaker activity in the ventricles. The QRS complex in a parasystole, as in the more rapid reentrant ventricular tachycardias, is prolonged and bizarre, but unlike the reentrant ventricular tachycardias, which can be associated with horrendous mortality, parasystolic rhythms are generally benign and do not require treatment.

The rates of discharge of a parasystolic pacemaker are much slower than a reentrant ventricular tachycardia. Parasystolic rates can be as slow as 30; when they range between 60 and 80 the rhythm is often referred to as an *accelerated idioventricular rhythm* or *slow ventricular tachycardia*.

> Parasystolic rhythms range from very simple to very complex. In its simplest form, the regular discharge of a parasystolic pacemaker in the ventricles competes with cycles that are initiated by the sinus pacemaker. When this occurs, two types of QRS complex appear at different regular rates: the normal sinus beats, which normally are narrow

and preceded by a P wave; and a slow sequence of ventricular premature systoles that, when a long rhythm strip is examined, are regular in timing. Because the parasystolic focus continues to fire during the refractory period of a sinus QRS, not all parasystolic impulses are able to capture the ventricles. However, sinus impulses cannot enter and reset a typical parasystolic focus, so that once the parasystolic interval has been identified, a prolonged, bizarre QRS complex should appear "on schedule," whenever the parasystole fires at a time that the ventricles are not refractory from the sinus beats.

Many years ago my father likened a parasystolic focus to a wicked knight in a castle who raided the surrounding villages on a strict schedule, unless his exit from the castle was blocked when the king's men (the sinus QRS) were in the vicinity. Because the king's men could not enter the castle, the knight was able to maintain his strict schedule of raids.

In recent years, the timing of some parasystolic pacemakers has been shown to be quite complex in that electrotonic influences caused by depolarization of the myocardium surrounding a parasystolic focus can either accelerate or delay the discharge of the parasystolic pacemaker (Jalife and Moe, 1981). The effects of the electrotonic spread of currents initiated by sinus beats on the parasystolic pacemaker can be remarkably, but predictably, variable so as to produce a veritable exotic garden of patterns of ventricular premature systoles.

The Vulnerable Period

Although most ventricular premature systoles cause only a single ectopic beat, some can trigger ventricular fibrillation. This lethal arrhythmia can begin when a ventricular premature systole falls on the T wave of the preceding cycle, which is the *vulnerable period* of ventricular repolarization. The correlation between the ability of a ventricular premature systole to induce repetitive ventricular depolarization and the degree of its prematurity is seen in Fig. 23.16, where among four ventricular premature systoles only the third initiates a brief salvo. This premature systole follows the onset of the preceding sinus QRS complex by 280 msec, whereas the other ventricular premature systoles, which do not initiate repetitive firing, occur 300 to 340 msec after the preceding sinus beat. This tendency of very early ventricular premature systoles ("R" on "T") to induce ventricular tachycardia and fibrillation (see below) identifies a period of ventricular repolarization, immediately following the peak of the T wave, called the vulnerable period (Fig. 23.17). Premature stimulation during the vulnerable period tends to initiate a repetitive ventricular response, and may cause a lethal ventricular arrhythmia. Even small electrical currents applied to the ventricles during the vulnerable period can induce ventricular tachycardia or ventricular fibrillation because the *ventricular fibrillation threshold* reaches its nadir at or near the peak of the T wave.

Vulnerability is due largely to the fact that impulses reaching the ventricles are most easily disorganized during the relative refractory period, which coincides with the end of the T wave. Earlier stimulation of the ventricles, during the S-T segment, finds the ventricular myocardium in its absolute refractory period, and so unable to

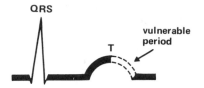

FIG. 23.17. Timing of the vulnerable period (*unshaded*) during the middle and terminal portions of the T wave on the ECG.

generate a propagated wave of depolarization. Stimuli that arrive later, after the end of the T wave, find the ventricles fully recovered and so able to respond with large, rapidly rising action potentials that, because they generate a wave of depolarization that conducts rapidly throughout the ventricles, do not tend to become disorganized (Chapter 21). However, stimuli that reach the ventricles during the vulnerable period find sodium channels that have recovered only partially, and unevenly, from the preceding depolarization. For this reason, the ventricles do not respond with a full-sized action potential, but instead generate small slow-rising responses that propagate slowly and exhibit the characteristics of decremental conduction that provide the substrate for reentrant arrhythmias (Chapter 21).

> Although the vulnerable period occurs at about the same time as the supernormal period, these two phenomena are not directly related. Supernormality is due to a fall in threshold that, while facilitating the response to a weak stimulus, does not disorganize conduction.

FLUTTER AND FIBRILLATION

Two special tachyarrhythmias can occur in either the atria or ventricles. Very rapid depolarization at regular rates exceeding 200 to 300 is called *flutter*, whereas total disorganization of depolarization at even faster rates is *fibrillation*. As described below, both are reentrant arrhythmias that effectively end the pumping of the involved chamber. Atrial flutter and fibrillation, in addition to abolishing the atrial primer pump (Chapter 15), accelerate ventricular rate and so can impair filling. Ventricular flutter and fibrillation, because they do not allow the ventricles to pump blood, are lethal arrhythmias.

> Although the hemodynamic consequences of atrial flutter and fibrillation can be minor, especially when ventricular rate can be controlled in patients with a normal heart, both arrhythmias are dangerous because clots tend to form in the static pool of blood in the fluttering or fibrillating atria. These clots readily break off and travel as *emboli* from the right atrium to a pulmonary artery, or from the left atrium to a peripheral artery. This can lead to disaster, especially when an embolus blocks a cerebral artery and causes a stroke.

Atrial Flutter and Fibrillation

Very rapid activation of the atria occurs in *atrial flutter*, where the atrial rate is rapid and the rhythm extremely regular, and *atrial fibrillation*, in which the atrial rhythm is irregular. These atrial arrhythmias sometimes change back and forth, and intermediate rhythms may be seen; the latter are sometimes called "impure atrial flutter."

Atrial Flutter

Atrial flutter can be viewed as a very rapid atrial reentry (see above) whose rates are between 250 and 350, and usually very close to 300. Ventricular rates, however, are almost always slower, due to AV dissociation. Atrial depolarization in atrial flutter often gives rise to a "sawtooth" pattern, called *F waves*, which replace the normal P waves (Fig. 23.18). QRS complexes are normal unless there is aberrant conduction or coexistent bundle branch block.

Although the ECG in atrial flutter shows what appears to be organized atrial activity, the fluttering atria usually generate little or no pressure. The jugular venous pulse in patients with atrial flutter commonly shows rapid oscillations, rather like vibrations, instead of the forceful *a* wave seen in sinus rhythm.

The fact that not all F waves are conducted to the ventricles in most patients with atrial flutter is due to AV dissociation caused by the normal low safety factory in the AV node (Chapter 18). The flutter rate is usually a multiple of the ventricular rate; for example, Fig. 23.18 shows 4:1 AV dissociation (one QRS complex per four F waves) where F waves appear at a rate of ~250 and regular QRS complexes are seen at a rate of ~62.

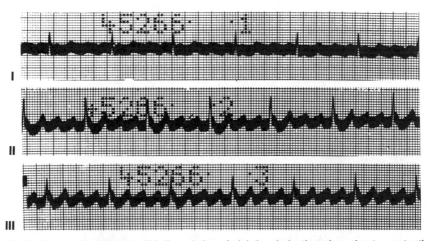

FIG. 23.18. Atrial flutter with 4:1 AV dissociation. Atrial depolarization gives rise to sawtooth undulations of the baseline, which are regular at a rate of ~250. Because of 4:1 AV dissociation, ventricular rate is exactly one-fourth that of the atria. (ECG from Katz and Pick, 1956.)

The flutter rate in Fig. 23.18 is slower than usually seen in this clinical arrhythmia. This can be explained by atrial hypertrophy, which is also responsible for the large amplitude of the F waves.

The normal low safety factor in the AV node protects patients with rapid atrial rhythms from the impaired ventricular filling that would result from shortened diastole at very rapid ventricular rates. Thus, the inability of the AV node to conduct all impulses from the fluttering atria into the ventricles is an example of the "protective" role of the normally precarious conduction in the AV node.

Pathophysiology of Atrial Flutter

Most examples of atrial flutter are due to a reentrant circuit that is confined to the atria, most likely a wave of depolarization that goes round an round one or both atria (Olshansky et al., 1990). Because the reentrant circuit is maintained by cells that are depolarized via sodium channels, interventions like vagal stimulation and drugs that inhibit i_{Ca} are ineffective in treating this arrhythmia. This statement must be qualified, however, because drugs that inhibit AV conduction are very useful in slowing the "ventricular response" in atrial flutter by increasing the extent of AV dissociation. Carotid sinus massage (vagal stimulation) has little or no effect on the atrial flutter rate, but often increases the degree of AV dissociation. For example, in atrial flutter with 2:1 AV dissociation, where the atrial rate is typically 300 and the ventricular rate 150, increased vagal activity can increase AV dissociation to 4:1, so as to slow the ventricular rate to 75.

Atrial Fibrillation

In atrial fibrillation, which is much more common than atrial flutter, atrial rates exceed 400 and, most important, the rhythm is completely irregular. As a result, the fibrillating atria do not contract in an organized manner, but instead resemble a bag of worms in which the disorganized atrial contraction is ineffective in raising intra-atrial pressure. As in atrial flutter, ventricular rates are much less than those of the atria; but unlike atrial flutter, the ventricular rhythm is usually irregularly irregular. The P waves in atrial fibrillation are replaced by undulations in the baseline, often called *f waves*, that are irregular in amplitude and frequency (Fig. 23.19). Although the timing of the QRS complexes is irregular, their contour is normal unless other abnormalities, such as bundle branch block or ventricular hypertrophy, modify ventricular depolarization.

Although the irregular ventricular rhythm in atrial fibrillation is due in part to the irregular arrival of atrial impulses at the upper end of the AV node, another mechanism is usually responsible for the marked variations in R-R interval seen in these patients. In fact, variations in the refractory period of the AV node, rather than the irregular atrial depolarization, is the major cause of ventricular irregularity in atrial fibrillation. This is apparent on close examination of the ECG shown in Fig. 23.19.

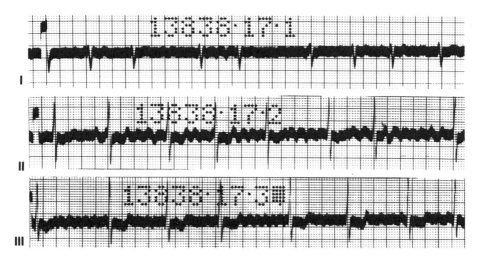

FIG. 23.19. Atrial fibrillation. The rapid, disorganized atrial activity causes the irregular undulations of the baseline (f waves) that appear at intervals of 130 to 170 msec. QRS complexes are irregularly irregular, with R-R intervals ranging between 560 and 1,160 msec, which corresponds to an average ventricular rate of ~75. The large variations in R-R interval cannot be explained simply by variations in the timing of the arrival of f waves at the AV node, but in addition reflect large variations in its refractory period caused by concealed conduction. The narrow QRS complexes in this patient show right-axis deviation. (ECG from Katz and Pick, 1956.)

If the refractory period in the AV node was constant at 500 msec, refractoriness in the AV node would allow the ventricles to be depolarized at a maximal rate of 120. Yet R-R intervals almost as long as 1,200 msec are seen in Fig. 23.19, even though intervals between f waves average ~150 msec. As the refractory period of the AV node can be no more than ~550 msec, the shortest R-R interval in Fig. 23.19, random variations in the arrival of atrial impulses at the upper end of the AV node are not the major cause of the markedly irregular cycle length. Instead, the irregular appearance of the QRS complexes is due to marked variations in the refractory period of the AV node.

Concealed Conduction

The evidence just discussed raises yet another question: What causes the large variations in the length of the refractory period in the AV node? The answer lies in a phenomenon called "concealed conduction," which occurs when an impulse enters a region of the heart but is not conducted through this region, the only effect of such a wave of depolarization being to block conduction of the subsequent impulse (Fig. 21.12). In other words, concealed conduction occurs when an impulse that cannot traverse a structure prolongs its refractory period and so blocks the next impulse.

A simple example of concealed conduction is diagrammed in Fig. 23.20. During a sinus rhythm at a rate of 75, where the interval between successive beats is 800

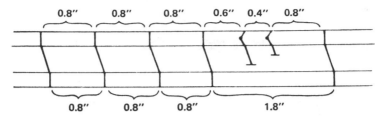

FIG. 23.20. Concealed conduction in the AV node. The arrival of a pair of atrial premature systoles (the fifth and sixth *vertical lines* in the *upper space* of this Lewis diagram) causes an 1,800-msec pause in ventricular beating (*lower space*). The AV node and ventricles, however, are able to conduct at intervals of at least 800 msec as demonstrated by the normally conducted sinus impulses at a rate of 75 in the initial portion of this diagram. Failure of the second atrial premature systole to be conducted through the AV node is therefore due to prolonged refractoriness in the AV node caused by the first atrial premature systole.

msec, a pair of blocked atrial premature systoles at intervals of 600 and 400 msec, respectively, cause a long pause in ventricular beating because neither atrial premature systole is conducted through the AV node. The failure of the first premature systole to be conducted is readily understood because it arrives during the refractory period left behind by the preceding normal systole. Failure of conduction of the second atrial premature systole, which arrives at the AV node a full second after passage of the last sinus beat, is more complex. The block cannot be attributed to the normal refractoriness in the AV node caused by the last conducted sinus beat because the AV node was clearly able to transmit impulses at 800 msec intervals during the sinus rhythm. This means that the first blocked atrial premature systole must have prolonged the refractory period in the AV node so as to block the second atrial premature systole. Thus, the first atrial premature systole exhibits concealed conduction; it is *conducted* into the AV node because it has blocked the subsequent impulse. But its conduction is *concealed* because this impulse is not transmitted through the AV node to initiate a QRS complex.

Concealed conduction is readily demonstrated in the student laboratory when an isolated heart preparation (e.g., turtle heart) is impaled with fine copper wires and arranged so that electrical stimuli well above threshold can be administered by depressing a switch. At slow frequencies of stimulation, each depression of the switch is followed by a ventricular contraction. If the rate of stimulation is gradually increased, the heart initially contracts in response to each stimulus, but at higher rates the response becomes irregular owing to second-degree block in the depressed tissue around the copper wires which, like the AV node, represents a region of depressed conduction. A further increase in stimulation frequency can lead to "standstill," where no contractions occur in response to stimuli that are rapidly delivered to the depressed myocardium. That standstill is not due to irreversible damage to the heart is readily shown by stopping the stimulation for a few seconds, after which a single stimulus again causes a contraction. Conduction fails at the high rates of stimulation because each stimulus produces only a local response in the depressed areas around the copper wires. These local responses, which are not conducted into the remainder of the heart, prolong the refractory period in the tissue around the wire, and so prevent subsequent impulses from activating the heart. In other words, cardiac standstill is attributable to repetitive concealed conduction.

Pathophysiology of Atrial Flutter and Fibrillation

Between the early 1930s and the 1950s, electrophysiologists attempting to explain the mechanism of atrial flutter and fibrillation were divided into two camps: those who believed that these arrhythmias arose from single or multiple ectopic foci, and those who attributed atrial flutter and fibrillation to circus movements in the atria.

The *ectopic focus* proponents postulated that atrial flutter arose from a single rapidly discharging focus in the atria, and that atrial fibrillation was produced by multiple foci discharging at different rapid rates. The advocates of this explanation showed that application of an irritant to a single point in the atria of the open-chested dog could initiate rapid atrial beating that exhibited the electrocardiographic features of atrial flutter, whereas multiple points of irritation produced a more rapid, irregular arrhythmia that resembled atrial fibrillation.

The proponents of the *circus movement* explanation for these atrial arrhythmias based their theory on Mayer and Mines' studies of the ring of excitable tissue (Chapter 21), which gave credence to the view that atrial flutter resulted from a large circus movement that passed around the atria. Large circus movements were documented in the fluttering atria of open-chested anesthetized dogs by slow-motion cinematography. The proponents of this theory argued that atrial fibrillation was caused by a multiplicity of disorganized circus movements, which today are referred to as reentrant pathways.

The controversy between the circus movement and ectopic focus explanations for atrial flutter and fibrillation has virtually disappeared as these once mutually exclusive explanations really represent different ways of looking at the same phenomena. The distinction between a reentrant circuit and an ectopic focus is blurred because an ectopic focus can be produced by a reentry mechanism in a tiny area of the myocardium; for this reason, the difference between multiple ectopic foci and disorganized reentrant pathways has become largely one of semantics.

The disorder that allows a wave of depolarization to wander over the fluttering or fibrillating atria (or ventricles) depends on sustained reentry. As illustrated by our friend the snake (Fig. 21.22), this is facilitated not only by depressed conduction and a short refractory period, but also a large mass of myocardial tissue. These considerations explain the increased incidence and difficulty of restoring and maintaining sinus rhythm after cardioversion of atrial fibrillation in patients with dilated atria. Depressed conduction in hypertrophied atria also tends to disorganize the front of depolarization, that is, to break it up into multiple reentry pathways. These concepts also provide a basis for understanding the pathophysiology of atrial flutter, where a large circus movement is maintained when large atrial size or slow conduction establishes a long pathway that permits the tail of the snake to continue to slip away from its head. The tendency for a wave of depolarization to continue to go around the atria as a giant reentry mechanism is, of course, facilitated by the normally short atrial refractory period (Chapter 19).

> An experiment that illustrates the importance of hypertrophy in the pathogenesis of fibrillation was described in 1914 by Garrey, who noted that fibrillation was difficult to produce in a small heart, like that of the cat, but hard to avoid in a large heart, such as that of a cow. These observations led Garrey to postulate that the maintenance of fibrillation required a large mass of myocardium. To test this hypothesis, Garrey isolated a large heart, caused it to fibrillate, and then cut it into smaller and smaller pieces. As the mass of fibrillating tissue became progressively smaller, the pieces eventually ceased to fibrillate, but instead either beat synchronously or else stopped contracting altogether.

Ventricular Flutter and Fibrillation

Both flutter and fibrillation can occur in the ventricles, but unlike the corresponding atrial arrhythmias, which can persist for years, ventricular flutter and fibrillation are lethal arrhythmias. This is simply because disorganized ventricular contraction stops the circulation.

The ECG in ventricular flutter (Fig. 23.21), which often resembles a sine wave, may result from a large circus movement that circles the ventricles. In ventricular fibrillation, where chaotic oscillations of the baseline replace the QRS complex (Fig. 23.22), no effective ventricular contraction takes place.

As in the case of atrial flutter and fibrillation, the corresponding ventricular arrhythmias are caused by reentry. The most effective treatment is electrical cardioversion, which today can be effected by an implantable electronic defibrillator. Although it is obvious that these arrhythmias are best prevented, drug therapy, as pointed out below, is often neither safe nor effective.

ANTIARRHYTHMIC DRUGS

The principles by which membrane-active drugs can be used to treat and prevent arrhythmias are complex, and often the subject of texts larger than this. At this point, therefore, our discussion of this subject is limited to a few major features of these drugs that illustrate salient principles of the pathophysiology of arrhythmias.

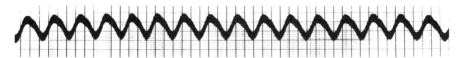

FIG. 23.21. Ventricular flutter. The electrical activity of the ventricles is manifest as broad oscillations of the baseline that resemble sine waves in which neither QRS complexes nor T waves can be made out. Atrial activity is not seen. (ECG from Katz and Pick, 1956.)

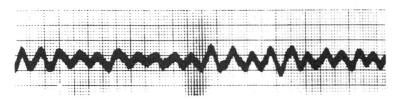

FIG. 23.22. Ventricular fibrillation. This lethal arrhythmia causes the rapid, chaotic undulations in the baseline that reflect total disorganization of ventricular depolarization. (ECG from Katz and Pick, 1956.)

Three mechanisms of antiarrhythmic therapy that were described in Chapter 21 and illustrated in Fig. 21.22 are: (a) depress conduction by inactivating inward currents, (b) accelerate conduction so as to cause an abnormal wave of depolarization to lose its ability to conduct when it "catches up" with the refractory period left behind by the preceding impulse, and (c) prolong the refractory period so as to block conduction of the following abnormal wave of depolarization. The second of these mechanisms is best accomplished by effective treatment of the condition that caused the arrhythmia. The first and third mechanisms, inhibition of depolarizing and repolarizing currents, are the basis for the actions of essentially all antiarrhythmic drugs.

Classification of Antiarrhythmic Drugs

The classification of antiarrhythmic drugs is reminiscent of a library in which books are catalogued according to size and the order in which they were received. In fact, the author wrote the first edition of this text in a university where the main library was said to be organized in this manner, which meant that only the librarians could use the stacks. The situation is not too different in the case of the antiarrhythmic drugs, where the unsatisfactory classification means that treatment of potentially lethal arrhythmias is best left to the expert (who also brings to the patient a growing array of electrical devices and ablation procedures that are beyond the scope of this discussion).

The most widely accepted classification of the antirrhythmic drugs (Table 23.2) was proposed many years ago by Vaughan Williams. Examination of Table 23.2 demonstrates that the different classes are not, in fact, congruent. Although reminiscent of the library mentioned above, this terminology has become a part of the daily language of those who care for patients with tachyarrhythmias.

Class I Agents

All of the Class I antiarrhythmic drugs block sodium channels, but they differ in subtle, yet important ways that have led to their separation into three subclasses.

TABLE 23.2. *Classification of the antiarrhythmic drugs*

Class	Mechanism of action	Examples
I. Sodium channel blockade		
IA	Moderate/marked inhibition of i_{Na}; prolongs refractoriness and repolarization	Quinidine, procainamide, disopyramide
IB	Mild/moderate inhibition of i_{Na}; may shorten refractoriness and repolarization	Lidocaine, diphenylhydantoin, mexilitine, tocainide
IC	Marked inhibition of i_{Na}; some prolongation of refractoriness; little effect on repolarization	Encainide, flecainide, propafenone, ethmozine
II. β-adrenergic blockade Inhibits i_{Ca}		Propanolol, metoprolol, atenolol, esmolol, timolol
III. Prolong action potential Prolongs refractoriness and repolarization; little effect on depolarization		Amiodarone, bretylium, sotalol
IV. Calcium channel blockade Inhibits i_{Ca}		Verapamil, diltiazem, nifedipine, nicardipine

Class IA Agents

The major drugs in this class (quinidine, procainamide, disopyramide) have moderate effects to depress sodium channels, and thus to slow conduction in the atria, ventricles, and His-Purkinje system. They have additional effects that prolong the action potential and so increase refractoriness.

Class IB Agents

These drugs have less inhibitory effect on the sodium channels of the resting cell, but as noted below, can be more potent inhibitors of sodium-dependent conduction when the cells are depolarized. The major drugs in this class (lidocaine, diphenylhydantoin, mexilitine, tocainide) can shorten the action potential, which is a major difference from class IA drugs.

Class IC Agents

The members of this class of antiarrhythmic drugs (encainide, flecainide, propafenone, ethmozine) exert potent and long-lasting effects to inhibit sodium channel opening, but have less effect on refractoriness. Although quite effective in preventing the nonlethal ventricular premature systoles that are markers of an increased risk of sudden death, some Class IC drugs were found to cause a severalfold increase in sudden cardiac death in some patients (CAST Investigators, 1989).

Class II Agents

This class of drugs is made up of the β-adrenergic blockers, which inhibit i_{Ca} by the effects discussed in Chapters 12 and 18.

Class III Agents

These drugs (amiodarone, bretylium, sotalol) can have remarkably effective anti-arrhythmic actions. Although all prolong the cardiac action potential, their mechanisms of action at a molecular level remain poorly understood.

Class IV Agents

Like the Class II drugs, the Class IV agents (verapamil, diltiazem, nifedipine, nicardipine) inhibit calcium channel opening. As pointed out in Chapter 18, calcium channel blockade by these two classes of drugs is effected by quite different mechanisms. Although the ultimate targets of the Class II and Class IV drugs are molecules that carry i_{Ca}, they are quite different clinically. The β-blockers (Class II) act by preventing the activation of G_s, which reduces both the interaction of the latter with the calcium channels and adenylyl cyclase (Chapter 12), whereas the calcium channel blockers (Class IV) interact directly with specific states of the channel (Chapter 18). As the calcium channel blockers, but not the β-blockers, are potent vasodilators, their ability to lower blood pressure triggers reflexes that increase sympathetic stimulation of the heart.

The Modulated Receptor Hypothesis

Important and dynamic changes in the ion channels are the key to understanding the basis for the different actions of the three subtypes of the Class I agents on the sodium channels, as well as more subtle differences between members of each subclass. Although all Class I agents inhibit i_{Na}, the potency of their effects is affected by time- and voltage-dependent changes in the state of the channel that allow the various Class I agents to interact differently with their three major states (Chapter 18). These effects are systematized by the *modulated receptor hypothesis*, which considers an ion channel to be a receptor that is modulated by membrane voltage, by time-dependent changes in channel conformation, and by the drugs themselves.

As discussed in Chapter 18, there is evidence that voltage-dependent ion channels exist in at least three functional states: open, closed (resting), and closed (inactivated). The time- and voltage-dependent properties of the transitions between these states, which are summarized in Table 23.3, indicate the complexity of the determinants of these transitions. It is now clear that membrane-active drugs can have

TABLE 23.3. *Time- and voltage-dependent transitions between the major states of an ion channel*

Opening	
Voltage dependent:	Rate and extent depend on E_m in the resting cell
Time dependent:	Rate and extent depend on the time the channel has remained at a given potential
Closing	
Voltage dependent:	Rate and extent depend on E_m at the peak of the action potential
Time dependent:	Rate and extent depend on the rate of depolarization
Reactivation	
Voltage dependent:	Rate and extent depend on E_m during repolarization
Time dependent:	Rate and extent depend on the duration of the depolarized state of the membrane

specific interactions with each of these states. In some cases, a single drug can have opposite effects on two states of the channel, as evidenced by the ability of the dihydropyridine calcium channel blockers to both activate and inhibit calcium channel opening, and at the same time (Chapter 18). Drug effects on an ion channel thus include at least three reversible reactions that involve the association and dissociation of complexes between the drug and at least three states of the channel, each of which has different kinetics.

The states of an ion channel, both free and bound to an antiarrhythmic drug, are diagrammed in Fig. 23.23, which characterizes the interactions of the drug with the different channel states according to the modulated receptor hypothesis. The most important of these interactions is, of course, the ability of the drug to block ion flux through the channel.

In addition to interacting differently with each of the three states of an ion channel, antiarrhythmic drugs alter the rates of the transitions of the channel between its three functional states. As channel opening and closing are, themselves, determined by probability functions, it is no surprise that this has become an almost impossibly difficult subject. Although the kinetic approach summarized in Fig. 23.23 is useful in analyzing the different effects of various antiarrhythmic drugs, an extended discussion of this valuable model is beyond the scope of this text. For this reason, the following narrative has been simplified in an attempt to lead the reader through a limited number of the important features of this hypothesis.

The many variables described in Fig. 23.23 can be simplified because two of the transitions of sodium channels are rapid: *closed (resting)* ↔ *open*, and *open* ↔ *closed (inactivated)*. For this reason, our discussion focuses on the slowest of the transitions: *closed (inactivated)* ↔ *closed (resting)*. The most important result of this transition is dissipation of the refractory state of the channel, which can be described as *closed (inactivated)* → *closed (resting)*. Comparison of two commonly used drugs, quinidine (Class IA) and lidocaine (Class IB) is especially illuminating (Chen and Gettes, 1976), so that the following discussion focuses on the time- and voltage-dependent interactions of these two drugs with the *closed (inactivated)* state of the sodium channel, where closure of the h gate has caused this channel to

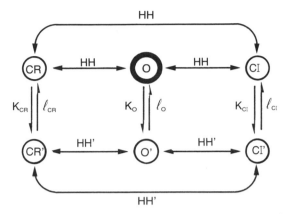

FIG. 23.23. The modulated receptor hypothesis. The three states of an ion channel on the *upper line* [CR: *closed (resting)*, O: *open*, CI: *closed (inactivated)*] undergo transitions that are determined by Hodgkin-Huxley (HH) kinetics. A channel blocking drug can bind to the channel in each of the three states, giving rise to three new inactive states (CR', O', and CI') which correspond to the three states of the unbound channel. The kinetics of the association and dissociation of the drug with each of these three states are defined by three association constants (k_{CR}, k_O, and k_{CI}) and dissociation of the drug by three dissociation constants (l_{CR}, l_O, and l_{CI}). The transitions between the three drug-bound states of the channel also exhibit Hodgkin-Huxley kinetics (HH'), although the rate constants are different because of the presence of the drug. Note that of all six channel states, the ion can cross the membrane only when the channel is in the free, open state (O).

become refractory (Chapter 18). Key to this discussion is that sodium channel opening is a major determinant of conduction velocity in the ventricles.

The voltage-dependence of the rate of the action potential upstroke illustrated in Fig. 23.24, provides an approximate quantification of the effects of membrane potential on sodium channel opening (see Fig. 19.5). The decline in dV/dt_{max} as membrane potential falls from -90 to -60 mV is due largely to the voltage-dependent inactivation of i_{Na} that occurs when the h gates close in the sodium channels of a depolarized membrane. Quinidine, which causes a proportionate reduction in dV/dt_{max} at all levels of E_m, does not shift the voltage-dependence of inactivation, whereas lidocaine has a proportionately greater effect to inhibit sodium channel opening when the cell is depolarized. This means that lidocaine is more effective in blocking sodium channels in depolarized cells, which explains why it is more useful than quinidine in suppressing arrhythmias in patients immediately following an acute myocardial infarction, when the heart contains large depolarized areas (Chapter 24).

In addition to their different voltage-dependent effects on the *closed (inactivated)* sodium channel, quinidine and lidocaine have different effects during the time-dependent transition: *closed (inactivated)* → *closed (resting)*. As shown in Fig. 23.25, the inhibitory effects of quinidine on dV/dt_{max} are similar throughout reactivation, whereas lidocaine, whose effects are greatest on the *closed (inactive)* chan-

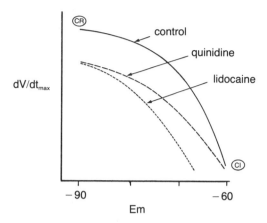

FIG. 23.24. Effects of quinidine and lidocaine on the voltage-dependent reactivation of sodium channels. The rate of depolarization (dV/dt_{max}), an index of the extent of sodium channel opening, is plotted as a function of resting membrane potential (E_m). The fraction of sodium channels inhibited by quinidine is similar at all levels of membrane potential, whereas the inhibitory potency of lidocaine is markedly increased when the call is depolarized. The labels CR and CI indicate when the channels are in the *closed (resting)* and *closed (inactivated)* states, respectively.

nel immediately after the preceding cycle, is a much more potent inhibitor of reactivation at rapid heart rates. This accounts for another feature of lidocaine's clinical action: it is quite effective in abolishing isolated premature systoles.

The increased potency of lidocaine during the relative refractory period (Fig. 23.25) explains why this drug is not particularly effective in treating atrial arrhythmias. Because atrial action potentials are shorter than those in the ventricles and His-Purkinje

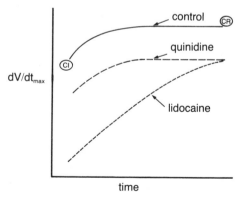

FIG. 23.25. Effects of quinidine and lidocaine on the time-dependent reactivation of sodium channels. The rate of depolarization (dV/dt_{max}) is plotted as a function of the time elapsed after the prior action potential. The fraction of sodium channels inhibited by quinidine is similar at all times during the relative refractory period, whereas the inhibitory potency of lidocaine is markedly increased early during the refractory period. The labels CR and CI indicate when the channels are in the *closed (resting)* and *closed (inactivated)* states, respectively.

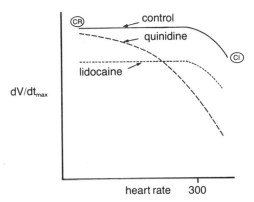

FIG. 23.26. Effects of quinidine and lidocaine on the rate of depolarization (dV/dt_{max}) at different heart rates. The fraction of sodium channels inhibited by quinidine is increased markedly at rapid heart rates, whereas the effect of heart rate on the potency of lidocaine is much less. The labels CR and CI indicate when the channels are in the *closed (resting)* and *closed (inactivated)* states, respectively.

system (Chapter 19), at rapid heart rates the time-dependent potentiation of the effects of lidocaine is greater in the ventricle than in the atria. In other words, the response of the ventricles to lidocaine is heightened because their longer action potential maintains a larger fraction of the sodium channels in the lidocaine-sensitive *closed (inactivated)* state.

A third difference between quinidine and lidocaine explains the clinical observation that the Class IA drugs are more effective than the Class IB drugs in slowing established tachyarrhythmias, notably atrial flutter and fibrillation. As shown in Fig. 23.26, quinidine is a more effective inhibitor of dV/dt_{max} at rapid heart rates than is lidocaine. At first glance, this appears to contradict the data in Fig. 23.25, which show that lidocaine is the more effective blocker during short cycles. However, action potential duration is not the major cause of the differences shown in Fig. 23.26; instead, the effects of quinidine are markedly increased at rapid heart rates ("use dependence"; see below) because quinidine dissociates from the inactivated channel much more slowly than lidocaine. This difference is not apparent after a single premature systole (Fig. 23.25) because the inhibitory effect of quinidine "accumulates" slowly during repeated cycles at the rapid heart rates.

Use-Dependence

The increasing inhibitory effect of a drug on an ion channel after it has passed through the normal transitions of *closed (resting)* → *open* → *closed (inactivated)* is called *use-dependence*. This important property of many antiarrhythmic drugs means that all of the electrophysiological consequences of channel inhibition are increased at rapid heart rates.

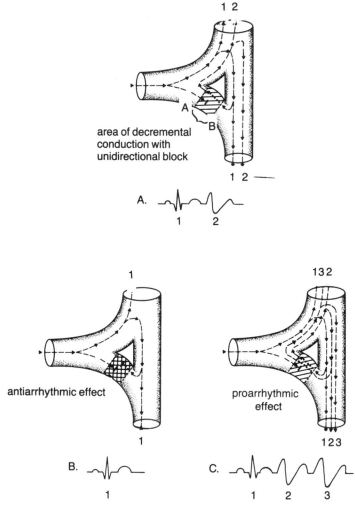

FIG. 23.27. Antiarrhythmic and proarrhythmic effects in a reentrant circuit involving a depressed region of the heart where decremental conduction and unidirectional block have established a reentrant circuit that generated a single premature systole (*A*), as shown in Fig, 21.10. If the major effect of an antiarrhythmic drug is to cause further impairment of conduction in the region of decremental conduction and unidirectional block (*B*), the reentrant circuit becomes completely blocked and the arrhythmia diasappears (antiarrhythmic effect). However, if the drug slows conduction elsewhere in the reentrant circuit so as to allow sufficient time for the depressed region to recover its ability to propagate additional retrograde impulses (*C*), the first premature systole can be followed by additional premature systoles (proarrhythmic effect). The latter can slow impulse conduction elsewhere in the myocardium, which can give rise to additional premature systoles. The result can further disorganize the spread of depolarization and so cause ventricular fibrillation.

In the case of the calcium channel blockers, especially verapamil which is used to treat supraventricular tachycardias that depend on calcium channel conduction in the AV node (see above), the negative inotropic effect caused by i_{Ca} inhibition can be dangerous. Although administration of verapamil to a patient with a rapid supraventricular tachycardia usually blocks the reentrant circuit in the AV node and so breaks the arrhythmia, if verapamil does not break the tachycardia, enhancement of its negative inotropic effect at the rapid heart rate can precipitate acute heart failure. The hypotensive effect of this negative inotropic effect is made worse by the vasodilator effect of the calcium channel blocker, which also relaxes smooth muscle. The result can be one of the many vicious cycles that occur in heart failure; in this case, the fall in blood pressure reduces coronary flow and adds ischemia to the woes of the weakened heart. Unless these pathophysiological mechanisms are understood and appropriately anticipated and treated, they can kill a patient.

Proarrhythmic Effects of the Antiarrhythmic Drugs

There are two major limitations in the clinical use of antirrhythmic drugs. First, although these drugs are often viewed as more or less specific (Table 23.2), most—especially the Class I and Class III drugs—can have a variety of serious side effects. Some make patients ill by affecting other organs, but others lead to the second, and most serious limitation to their clinical use: their ability to worsen arrhythmias; that is, these drugs can be *proarrhythmic*.

A number of complex mechanisms account for the proarrhythmic actions of most antiarrhythmic drugs. The mechanism illustrated in Fig. 23.27 should suffice to alert the reader to the dangers that accompany the use of any drug that, by depressing impulse conduction or prolonging the refractory period in the heart, has the potential to exacerbate reentry. These dangers are especially great in patients whose arrhythmias complicate conditions that have damaged the myocardium, notably patients with ischemic heart disease (Chapter 24) or heart failure (Chapter 25). The simple model shown in Fig. 23.27, which shows how an antiarrhythmic drug can either terminate or worsen reentry, illustrates but one of many proarrhythmic mechanisms that limit the clinical value of these drugs.

At this point we turn our attention to two major causes of cardiac disability: ischemic heart disease and heart failure. Like the preceding discussion, the following chapters demonstrate the extent to which an understanding of pathophysiology, which in turn depends on knowledge of *cell* biochemistry and *gene* regulations, as well as *organ* physiology, is essential for the management of the cardiac patient.

REFERENCES

The Cardiac Arrhythmia Suppression Trial (CAST) Investigators. (1989). Preliminary report: effect of encainide and flecainide on mortality in a randomized trial of arrhythmia suppression after myocardial infarction. *N Engl J Med* 321:406–412.

Chen C-M, Gettes LS. (1976). Combined effects of rate, membrane potential, and drugs on maximum rate of rise (V_{max}) of action potential upstroke of guinea pig papillary muscle. *Circ Res* 38:464–469.

Garrey WE. (1914). The nature of fibrillary contraction of the heart. Its relation to tissue mass and form. *Am J Physiol* 33:397–414.

Jalife J, Moe GK. (1981). Excitation, conduction, and reflection of impulses in isolated bovine and canine cardiac Purkinje fibers. *Circ Res* 49:233–247.

Katz LN, Pick A. (1956). *Clinical electrocardiography. Part I: The arrhythmias*. Philadelphia: Lea & Febiger.

Olshansky B, Okumura K, Hess PG, Waldo AL. (1990). Demonstration of an area of slow conduction in human atrial flutter. *J Am Coll Cardiol* 16:1639–1648.

BIBLIOGRAPHY

Akhtar M. (1990). Clinical spectrum of ventricular tachycardia. *Circulation* 82:1561–1573.

Hondeghem L, Katzung BG. (1977). Time- and voltage-dependent interaction of antiarrhythmic drugs with cardiac sodium channels. *Biochim Biophys Acta* 472:373–398.

Langendorf R. (1948). Concealed A-V conduction: the effect of blocked impulses on the formation and conduction of subsequent impulses. *Am Heart J* 35:542–552.

Zipes DP. (1988). Genesis of cardiac arrhythmias: electrophysiological considerations. In: Braunwald E, ed. *Heart disease*, 3rd ed. Philadelphia: WB Saunders; 581–620 (Chapter 20).

Zipes DP. (1988). Specific arrhythmias: diagnosis and treatment. In: Braunwald E, ed. *Heart disease*, 3rd ed. Philadelphia: WB Saunders; 658–716 (Chapter 22).

See also Bibliography to Chapters 21 and 22.

24

The Ischemic Heart

Rapid and sustained energy consumption by the working heart, which can only be met by the efficient pathways of oxidative phosphorylation (Chapter 5), carry a price; this is the dependence of the heart on an uninterrupted supply of substrates, mainly oxygen, that cannot be stored in the myocardium. For this reason, the heart cannot tolerate prolonged ischemia, and obstruction of a coronary artery is rapidly followed by cell death. Although this chapter focuses on the heart's response to ischemia, it must be emphasized that this approach really misses the point, for *the heart is the victim and not the perpetrator in the pathogenesis of ischemic heart disease*.

Ischemic heart disease arises from disease of the coronary arteries and not of the myocardium, so that the other names for this condition, coronary heart disease and arteriosclerotic heart disease, are more appropriate. These terms highlight the underlying pathogenic processes that are the subject of the newly emerging field of vascular biology, which describes the mechanisms that lead to coronary artery occlusion. The pathophysiology of atherosclerosis, the chronic obstructive disease of the coronary arteries, and the subsequent thrombotic processes that are the most common cause of acute myocardial infarction are beyond the scope of this text. However, as we examine the myocardial response to interrupted coronary flow, it must be kept in mind that the real problem arises in the vessel wall and the interactions between the endothelium of the diseased coronary artery and such blood elements as the platelet and macrophage which, along with blood coagulation, are central to the pathophysiology of ischemic heart disease.

The immediate sequelae of coronary occlusion are twofold: the initial loss of contractile function and arrhythmias, and the subsequent death of ischemic myocardial cells that represents an acute myocardial infarction. This review of pathophysiological mechanisms illustrates how disordered normal cardiac function described in earlier chapters can explain the abnormalities that appear in the ischemic heart. Our initial focus is on the events during the first minutes following coronary occlusion, after which we discuss the possible causes of myocardial cell death when ischemia is prolonged.

As recently as the 1960s, there were few explanations for any of the consequences of interrupted coronary flow, whereas today there seem to be too many. This is because, as is so often true in science, there are no simple explanations. Metabolic and cellular control are remarkably complex, so that obvious answers, although attractive, usually turn out to be oversimplifications. So much for Ockham's razor (Chapter 4).

There are two immediate detrimental effects of myocardial ischemia: impaired pump function and lethal arrhythmias. The major consequence of prolonged ischemia is cell death. Although the early pump failure and acute arrhythmias share common origins, the pathophysiologic processes involved in each are different because interrupted coronary flow has special actions on excitation-contraction coupling and the contractile process, and on the origin and propagation of the wave of depolarization that activates the heart.

EARLY ABNORMALITIES IN THE ISCHEMIC HEART

The heart, like the rest of the known universe, is subject to the laws of thermodynamics; for this reason, the heart cannot perform mechanical work without a corresponding expenditure of chemical energy (Chapter 3). As the heart has no significant store of oxygen, it might seem that the pathogenesis of depressed contraction is due simply to a state of energy starvation caused by cessation of oxidative phosphorylation. This logical conclusion is, however, incorrect because, as emphasized at many points in earlier chapters, chemistry and physiology are so tightly integrated that function is impaired well before the state of energy starvation becomes severe in the ischemic heart.

The major hemodynamic consequences of coronary occlusion arise from abnormalities involving the left ventricle, and the extent of left ventricular damage is a major determinant of the clinical course in most patients following coronary occlusion. As discussed in Chapter 25, left heart failure reduces both cardiac output and blood pressure, while at the same time causing symptoms of breathlessness when the ability of the left ventricle to accept blood from the pulmonary veins is impaired. Infarction of the right ventricle, which is less common, is more difficult to detect and to quantify. As the ECG is dominated by depolarization of the left ventricle (Chapter 20), the electrocardiographic criteria for right ventricular infarction are less reliable than those for infarction of the left ventricle. The hemodynamic consequences of right ventricular infarction are not easily recognized; even though blood accumulates in the great veins and systemic venous pressure is elevated, similar abnormalities are seen when a severely damaged left ventricle cannot pump blood out of the lungs; the resulting rise in pulmonary artery pressure can impair ejection even by a normal right ventricle. For these reasons, the diagnosis of right ventricular infarction often requires bedside catheterization, which shows right ventricular failure without evidence of severe left ventricular failure.

Ischemia and Hypoxia

Although most of the important effects of ischemia are due to oxygen lack (see below), ischemia and hypoxia have different effects on the myocardium. This is because coronary occlusion, in addition to halting the delivery of oxygen to the heart, prevents the removal of important metabolites and reduces intramyocardial pressure. Important metabolites that accumulate in the ischemic heart include *protons* (H^+) and *lactate*, which inhibit glycolysis at a time when myocardial cells still contain significant amounts of glycogen; *phosphate*, which along with protons exerts a direct negative inotropic effect; and *potassium*, which contributes to the genesis of arrhythmias. In part because the hypoxic heart continues to metabolize glycogen, as well as any glucose delivered in the coronary inflow, the effects of hypoxia are less devastating than those of ischemia.

It is of interest that the hearts of some turtles can function anaerobically for indefinite periods of time. This is possible because circulatory demands are limited when this reptile assumes a torpid state while lying at the bottom of a cool pond.

Anaerobic ATP Production

Because of the very high affinity of the cytochromes for oxygen, the cells of the ischemic myocardium are either aerobic or anaerobic. Thus, when the heart is deprived of its supply of oxygen, myocardial cells continue to consume their limited supply until, generally after less than a minute, oxygen tension falls sharply and the cells enter an anaerobic state in which no further oxidative phosphorylation is possible. The cessation of oxidative metabolism after coronary occlusion accelerates anaerobic adenosine triphosphate (ATP) production by both *humoral* and *biochemical* mechanisms (Chapter 4).

Humoral Stimuli

Glycogen breakdown and glycolysis are accelerated by increased cellular adenosine 3', 5'-cyclic monophosphate (cyclic AMP) levels that are part of the sympathetic response to the pain and impaired pump function seen in patients with acute myocardial infarction. Sympathetic stimulation also increases the carrier-mediated entry of glucose. Cyclic AMP accelerates the conversion of phosphorylase from the inactive *b* form to the more active *a* form, and inhibits glycogen synthetase (Fig. 4.7). Glycolysis is also accelerated because cyclic AMP activates 6-phosphofructo-2-kinase, which catalyzes the production of fructose, 2,6-bisphosphate that directly stimulates the rate-limiting phosphofructokinase reaction (Chapter 4).

Biochemical Stimuli

Anaerobic ATP production in the ischemic heart is accelerated by several biochemical reactions that increase glycolytic rate. Perhaps the most important is release of the inhibitory effects of ATP and glucose-6-phosphate, which in the normal heart maintain glycolysis at a low rate. A fall in myocardial contents of these two metabolites also accelerates the hexokinase and phosphofructokinase reactions, as well as the breakdown of glycogen, by increasing that activity of phosphorylase *b* (Chapter 4). Many of these effects are amplified by increased cellular levels of adenosine diphosphate (ADP), adenosine monophosphate (AMP), and P_i, products of ATP hydrolysis that accumulate when oxidative ATP production ceases. (Increased concentrations of ADP and P_i also reduce the free energy released when ATP is hydrolyzed.)

The increased rate of anaerobic glycolysis in the ischemic heart is transient, and eventually ceases largely because of the accumulation of reduced nicotinamide-adenine dinucleotide (NADH) and lack of oxidized nicotinamide-adenine dinucleotide (NAD), which inhibit glycolysis at the step where glyceraldehyde-3-phosphate is reduced (Fig. 4.1). In addition, acidosis in the ischemic heart (see below) inhibits several steps in glycolysis, notably the rate-limiting reaction catalyzed by phosphofructokinase. The interested reader may wish to review Chapters 4 and 5 in order to reexamine these key regulatory steps to define how they might be altered as the result of a decrease in the oxidative resynthesis of ATP.

Early Pump Failure

Interruption of coronary flow to a portion of the mammalian heart is followed almost immediately by a marked depression of contractility, systole being abbreviated within a few seconds. Although the myocardium can still develop tension, within a minute following coronary occlusion the ischemic portion of the ventricle bulges outward during each systole, because it is unable to overcome the intraventricular pressure generated by the normally perfused myocardium. As noted below, relaxation and filling are also depressed very soon after coronary flow is interrupted.

In analyzing the early pump failure of the ischemic myocardium, it is useful to recall the "four cases" defined by Aristotle. The *efficient cause* initiates the processes that depress mechanical function in the ischemic myocardium, whereas the *formal* and *material causes* represent the actual changes in the calcium cycle and interactions between the contractile proteins that impair both ejection and filling. The *final cause* is the end, or purpose, of these phenomena in the ischemic myocardium.

Efficient Cause of Impaired Contractility

At least three efficient causes now appear to contribute to the rapidly developing inotropic and lusitropic abnormalities in the ischemic heart; one is mechanical, the others biochemical. Together, these mechanisms initiate the changes that depress systolic function and inhibit relaxation in the ischemic myocardium.

The Garden Hose Effect

The first of these efficient causes is the mechanical effect that occurs when the distending effect of the coronary arterial perfusion pressure is lost following coronary artery occlusion (Vogel et al., 1982). The "garden hose effect" (Chapter 16), which normally enhances contractile performance by stretching the heart's sarcomeres (Starling's law of the heart), if thus attenuated when coronary artery occlusion moves the sarcomeres in the ischemic myocardium down their length-tension curve, sarcomere shortening reduces contractile performance. In this way, the decreased perfusion pressure causes an immediate fall in contractility, which explains why the initial negative inotropic effect of ischemia precedes measurable changes in the biochemical variables described below.
biochemical variables described below.

Substrate Deprivation

The second efficient cause of the early pump failure of the ischemic heart is metabolic: the absence of substrates, of which oxygen is by far the most important. Within a minute after the blood supply to the heart is interrupted, intramyocardial oxygen tension falls to extremely low levels because, as noted in Chapter 3, the heart has virtually no stores of oxygen. In contrast, considerable quantities of glycogen persist long after the ischemic myocardium has ceased its effective contraction, and the myocardial content of fats can actually increase when blood supply is interrupted.

Metabolite Accumulation

The third efficient cause of the early pump failure of the ischemic heart is related to the many compounds that accumulate under these conditions. Most important of these metabolites are protons and phosphate, which accumulate inside the ischemic cells, and potassium, whose major effects are due to accumulation of this cation in the extracellular space. Other compounds, notably fatty acids and their derivatives and free radicals, also accumulate in the ischemic heart; however, they appear to play a more important role in the irreversible changes that occur later, after prolonged ischemia (see below).

Protons. The major source of the protons that accumulate in the ischemic heart is the hydrolysis of high-energy phosphate compounds, which release large amounts of inorganic phosphate, a weak acid that liberates hydrogen ions. However, intracellular acidification is reduced initially because the creatine released by the hydrolysis of phosphocreatine is a weak base that absorbs protons. Another source of protons is glycolysis, in which the weak acid lactate is formed from glucose. The reactions involved in these proton shifts represent a difficult and complex subject, but while experts disagree as to what produces protons and how (Gevers, 1977; Seelye, 1980; Wilkie, 1979) there is no question that the ischemic heart becomes acidotic (Cobbe and Poole-Wilson, 1980; Jacobus et al., 1982).

Protons have two major effects in the ischemic heart. The first is to inhibit glycolysis through several enzyme reactions that are sensitive to acidosis, notably the rate-limiting phosphofructokinase reaction (Chapter 4). Acidosis also inhibits reactions that are initiated by calcium binding to a number of its physiological binding proteins because protons displace calcium from anionic binding sites. The ability of acidosis to inhibit the interactions between actin and myosin, which occurs when protons bind to troponin I (Chapter 14), probably plays an important role in the negative inotropic effect of ischemia.

Inorganic Phosphate. The hydrolysis of both ATP and phosphocreatine in the ischemic heart liberates large amounts of phosphate that reduce the calcium sensitivity of the cardiac contractile proteins and so can contribute to the loss of which contractility in the ischemic heart. Because phosphate, along with lactate, readily crosses the plasma membrane, these anions rapidly leave the ischemic heart accompanied by the major intracellular cation, which is potassium. This is probably the major cause for the rapid loss of potassium by ischemic myocardial cells (see below).

Potassium. Within a few seconds after a coronary artery is occluded, potassium begins to pour out of the ischemic myocardial cells. This loss of intracellular potassium begins so soon and is so rapid that it cannot be attributed to inhibition of the sodium pump. The fact that the cell becomes depolarized at the same time that large amounts of potassium are crossing the plasma membrane means that this cation is not carrying an outward current, which can only be explained if the potassium leaving the cell is accompanied by an anion. The best explanation for rapid potassium efflux in the ischemic heart is that this cation flux is secondary to the efflux of lactate and phosphate anions described above.

The most important effects of the potassium that accumulates in the extracellular space of the ischemic heart are related to membrane depolarization (see below), which inactivates the channels that carry inward currents (Chapter 19). Because this depresses conduction, potassium loss leads to arrhythmias. The depressed excitability in depolarized ischemic cells contributes to loss of mechanical function in two ways: by reducing the number of contracting myofibers, and by causing inhomogeneities of both contraction and relaxation that impair ventricular ejection and filling.

Fatty Acids and Their Derivatives. Long-chain fatty acids and their acyl derivatives with coenzyme A (CoA) and carnitine, along with lysophosphatides, accumulate in the ischemic heart. These amphipathic compounds are formed by phospholipase action and by interrupted β-oxidation in the ischemic heart; the latter causes the long-chain fatty acyl derivatives, which are reaction intermediates, to accumulate. Initial data indicated that large amounts of these amphipathic molecules, which can exert detergent-like effects that alter membrane structure and function (Chapter 2), appear in the ischemic heart. However, subsequent measurements (Shaikh and Downar, 1981; van der Vusse et al., 1985) raise questions as to whether enough of these substances accumulate in the ischemic myocardium to play an important pathophysiological role in altering function or in causing irreversible cell damage.

Free Radicals. Although free radicals may contribute to the functional abnormalities that appear rapidly in the ischemic heart, they are more commonly assumed to play an important role in the pathogenesis of the irreversible changes that occur later; for this reason, this topic is considered below.

Formal and Material Causes

Impaired Contractility

The negative inotropic response in experimental models of ischemia follows a complex time course; as depicted in Fig. 24.1 a small and rapid fall in contractility that occurs immediately after interruption of coronary flow is followed by a more gradual decline. The initial negative inotropic effect precedes the major fall in ATP content, inorganic phosphate accumulation (which mirrors the fall in phosphocreatine), and a fall in pH (Jacobus et al., 1982) not shown in Fig. 24.1. These findings indicate that the early decline in contractility is not metabolic, but instead is caused by the *mechanical* decrease in sarcomere length when coronary perfusion pressure is reduced (the "garden hose effect").

The subsequent decrease in contractility, which is *biochemical*, has many causes. These include the fall in ATP level, which would reduce the allosteric effects described in earlier chapters (Table 24.1), as well as the rise in inorganic phosphate and decreased pH discussed above. Attenuation of the allosteric effects of ATP, which accelerate calcium entry through plasma membrane calcium channels and calcium release via intracellular calcium channels, probably contributes to the negative inotropic effect of ischemia. Attenuation of the other effects shown in Table 24.1 probably plays a more important role in the lusitropic effects of coronary occlusion (see below).

The negative inotropic effects of acidosis and phosphate, which desensitize the calcium-binding site on troponin C, are due to a requirement for higher cytosolic Ca^{2+} concentrations to produce the same degree of activation of the cross-bridge cycle (Fig. 24.2).

Loss of intracellular potassium was once believed to contribute to the fall in myocardial contractility in the ischemic myocardium; however, cytosolic potassium does not

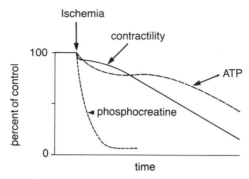

FIG. 24.1. Time courses of the decline in contractility (*solid line*) and decreased contents of ATP (*dashed line*) and phosphocreatine (*dotted line*) after the onset of ischemia (*arrow*). The increased content of inorganic phosphate (not shown) follows a time course similar to the fall in phosphocreatine. Curves are based on the data of Williamson (1966).

play a direct role in regulating myocardial contractility (Chapter 14). As excitability is only minimally impaired at a time when mechanical function is severely depressed, loss of potassium is probably not an important cause of the depressed mechanical performance during the early phases of ischemia.

Impaired Relaxation

Relaxation abnormalities can be extremely important in the initial response to ischemia, where depressed lusitropy can be the first functional change to appear after coronary artery occlusion. The mechanisms responsible for the negative lusitropic effects in the ischemic heart are even more complex than those that depress contractility.

TABLE 24.1. *Effects of diminished allosteric effects of ATP on the regulation of myocardial contraction and relaxation*

Process	Immediate consequence	Mechanical effect
Actin-myosin interactions	Loss of "plasticizing" effect; reduced dissociation of thick and thin filaments	Negative lusitropic; contracture (rigor)
Plasma membrane calcium channels	Reduced Ca influx into the cytosol	Negative inotropic
Plasma membrane calcium pump	Reduced Ca efflux from the cytosol, increased intracellular Ca	Negative lusitropic; contracture
Plasma membrane sodium pump	Reduced Na efflux; increased intracellular Na; increased Ca influx and decreased Ca efflux by Na-Ca exchange; increased cytosolic Ca	Negative lusitropic; contracture
Sarcoplasmic reticulum calcium channels	Reduced Ca release during systole; reduced Ca binding to contractile proteins	Negative inotropic
Sarcoplasmic reticulum calcium pump	Reduced Ca transport during diastole; failure to remove Ca from contractile proteins	Negative lusitropic; contracture

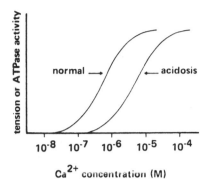

FIG. 24.2. The calcium-sensitivity of the contractile proteins is reduced in the acidotic heart, so that higher than normal levels of calcium are needed to achieve a given extent of actin-myosin interaction. A similar shift in calcium sensitivity is caused by elevated cytosolic levels of inorganic phosphate.

As discussed in Chapter 11, the balance among the calcium fluxes that relax the heart and those that deliver calcium to the cytosol to initiate systole is precarious, and favors contraction (Table 11.2). It is not surprising, therefore, that relaxation is sensitive to small changes in cellular energetics. Even so, in the initial phases of ischemia, ATP levels do not fall to levels sufficiently low to attenuate either their substrate or allosteric effects in a manner that explains the impairment of relaxation. Thus, measured ATP contents do not provide an obvious explanation for the rapid impairment of filling that occurs in the ischemic heart.

One possible explanation of the early impairment of relaxation is loss of one or more of the allosteric effects listed in Table 24.1 in one or another small "compartment" in the ischemic myocardial cells. This could occur without a measurable fall in ATP content because of the difference between *concentration*, which is the amount of a substance per unit volume in a defined region of the myocardial cell, and *content*, which describes the amount of substance present per unit weight of a tissue sample. Metabolic reactions, of course, depend on substrate and metabolite concentrations in the areas where the reactions take place. However, because measurements of high-energy phosphate levels in the ischemic heart are contents, they cannot rule out larger changes in a small, but critical compartment. There is no assurance, for example, that the ATP content of a biopsy specimen provides an accurate index of ATP concentration in the intracellular compartment that contains the sarcoplasmic reticulum. Furthermore, measurements of ATP content in a biopsy specimen may not provide a valid index of the ability of the energy-producing mechanisms to deliver high-energy phosphate at a time of rapid ATP utilization. This caution is especially important because slight changes in ATP concentration are often amplified, as occurs in the regulation of phosphofructokinase (Chapter 4).

Supply Ischemia and Demand Ischemia.

The severity of the relaxation abnormalities in the ischemic myocardium is influenced not only by the imbalance between energy supply and demand, but also by the side of the balance that is modified. If energy demands are increased in the heart of an animal in which a coronary artery has been partially occluded (*"demand ischemia"*), contracture develops rapidly in the ischemic myocardium. If, on the other hand, a coronary artery is *totally* occluded (*"supply ischemia"*), the picture is dominated by the loss of contractility and the negative lusitropic effects are milder and develop more slowly (Monomura et al., 1985). These differences cannot be attributed to different rates of ATP depletion, although pH is much lower in *supply ischemia*. The greater degree of acidosis in the hearts with the less severe lusitropic abnormality could reflect an effect of the reduced energy demands caused by the negative inotropic effect of protons (see above). Alternatively, the preservation of relaxation in the acidotic *supply ischemia* could be a marker for a high rate of glycolytic ATP production, which might sustain calcium transport by the sarcoplasmic reticulum because ATP produced by glycolysis appears to be more effective in maintaining the function of ion pumps than ATP produced in the mitochondria.

Final Cause of Impaired Contractility

Depressed myocardial contractility after a coronary occlusion, although obviously harmful to the body as a whole, has distinct advantages to an ischemic region in the heart. By reducing mechanical activity, the most costly of the ATP-utilizing functions, the early pump failure of the ischemic heart probably conserves chemical energy for reactions that are important in the preservation of myocardial integrity, and so could delay the appearance of necrosis. Rapid inhibition of excitation-contraction coupling also prevents continued mechanical activity from depleting the ischemic myocardium of its high-energy phosphate stores, and so could also delay the appearance of rigor. As the initial depression of contractility in the ischemic heart is reversible, the ischemic regions of the heart may be protected when they curtail their contribution to the pumping action of the heart, even though this compensatory mechanism impairs overall cardiac performance.

> Brief episodes of reversible ischemia actually delay the appearance of cell death during a subsequent, prolonged period of ischemia. The mechanism for this protective effect is not clear, but may be due to negative inotropic effects or a "stress response" caused by the "conditioning" ischemia.

INFARCT SIZE REDUCTION

Negative inotropic agents such as the β-blockers and calcium channel blockers, when administered before the heart of an experimental animal is made ischemic, slow the appearance of irreversible myocardial damage. This protective effect is most likely due to the energy-sparing effects associated with the reduction in contractility. Although once advocated as a means to limit infarct size in patients after coronary artery occlusion, there are at least three important problems in the clinical application of this approach. First, there is little or no important "border zone" around an infarct because, as noted in Chapter 1, the small coronary arteries are true end-arteries. Second, delivery of any form of therapy to a region of the heart with no blood supply is difficult, and for all practical purposes, impossible. Finally, and most important, as noted at the beginning of this chapter, the problem in acute myocardial infarction arises in the coronary arteries and not in the heart muscle. Thus, the ischemic myocardium will inevitably die unless coronary flow is reestablished.

> This limitation does not apply to the situation during open heart surgery, where *cardioplegic solutions* that slow cardiac energy utilization have been found to prolong the time that the surgeon can repair an arrested, unperfused heart. In this setting, of course, the operating team has excellent control of the substances that reach the myocardium via the coronary circulation.

The impracticality of limiting infarct size in a region of the heart supplied by a totally occluded coronary artery, other than by reestablishing perfusion, does not mean that negative inotropic agents are not useful in situations where coronary flow is reduced, rather than completely interrupted. In fact, β-blocker therapy is of proven value not only in reducing symptoms in patients with stable angina pectoris, but also in patients after an acute myocardial infarction, where these drugs clearly reduce mortality. Calcium channel blockers, although also of benefit in relieving the symptoms of stable angina, appear to be of less value in patients who have had an acute myocardial infarction. These differences, which may reflect the ability of the calcium channel blockers but not the β-blockers to cause reflex sympathetic stimulation, are discussed in Chapter 25.

JEOPARDIZED MYOCARDIUM AND ISCHEMIA AT A DISTANCE

Although the normal human coronary arteries are true end-arteries, extensive collaterals develop in the large epicardial arteries in patients with chronic ischemic heart disease. As these collateral vessels make it possible for more than one major coronary artery to supply a given region of the heart, occlusion of one artery may reduce, but not totally interrupt, the blood supply to a region of *jeopardized myocardium*. This is shown diagrammatically in Fig. 24.3A, where collateral vessels that have formed between a partially occluded left circumflex coronary artery and a normal right coronary artery have provided a dual blood supply to the region of the left ventricle supplied by the diseased circumflex.

Occlusion of an artery that supplies both its normal distribution and the area normally perfused by another partially occluded artery causes infarction of the former, but only makes the latter ischemic. Because the new ischemia is outside the usual distribution of this artery, it is referred to as *ischemia at a distance* (see below).

STABLE AND UNSTABLE ANGINA PECTORIS; ACUTE MYOCARDIAL INFARCTION

Coronary artery occlusion gives rise to a discomfort that, although the symptom varies among different patients, is called *angina pectoris* (literally strangling in the

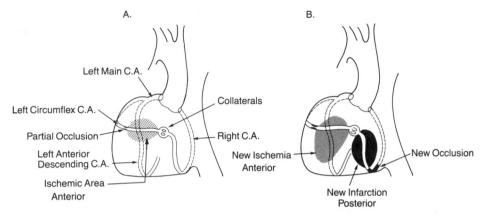

FIG. 24.3. Posterior view of the heart where partial occlusion of the left circumflex coronary artery has led to the formation of collateral vessels linking the occluded artery to a normal right coronary artery (*A*). The anterior wall of the left ventricle normally supplied by the partially occluded circumflex can become ischemic (*shaded*) if the energy demands of the heart are increased. Total occlusion of the right coronary artery (*B*) has two important effects on the heart: the posterior area that it normally supplies will be infarcted (*solid area*) if there is insufficient collateral flow to maintain viability. In addition, the anterior area in the distribution of the circumflex that had depended on the dual blood supply (*diagonal shading*) develops a jeopardized circulation because it has lost a significant portion of its blood supply. The latter is an example of "ischemia at a distance."

chest). Because angina is a visceral pain, it is poorly localized; although usually in the left chest, the discomfort can radiate to the inner arm, neck, or jaw, and may even be felt at the site of an old injury such as a scar on the upper back or the socket of a lost tooth. Angina is classically a heaviness or squeezing, but because of its visceral origin, can be an ache or like indigestion. In fact, about a quarter of patients who experience a myocardial infarction either deny or are not aware of angina; this is often called "silent infarction."

Stable Angina

Patients who have stable occlusive disease in the coronary arteries, with or without collaterals as shown in Fig. 24.3A often experience *stable angina pectoris*. This clinical syndrome is characterized by angina that is worse when myocardial oxygen demand is increased, for example by exertion. The basis for this symptom pattern is obvious; increased oxygen demand in a heart where oxygen delivery cannot be adequately increased causes the myocardial cells to become anaerobic. The pattern of angina can remain stable for years, and may decrease in severity because of the growth of collateral vessels.

Vasospastic Angina

Angina that is not caused by increased energy demands, notably "rest angina," is presumed to be caused by coronary vasospasm. This form of angina, also called "variant angina" or "Prinzmetal's angina," can be very dangerous because, unlike the much more common "demand" angina described above, this is a "supply" angina that cannot be relieved simply by rest.

Unstable Angina

Unstable angina is an anginal syndrome in which the symptoms are increasing in frequency or severity, or where the amount of exertion needed to provoke symptoms is decreasing. This importance of the instability is readily understood; it indicates that the extent of coronary artery obstruction is increasing. The hazards of serious arrhythmias are especially high in patients with unstable angina because, as discussed below, the depolarizing effects of ischemia wax and wane.

Myocardial Infarction

In its simplest presentation, an acute myocardial infarction represents the death of heart muscle caused by a coronary artery occlusion. The extent and complications of the infarction depend on the amount of the left ventricle that is infarcted and, as discussed below, the location of the infarction. When collaterals are extensive a new occlusion may only increase the severity of an anginal syndrome.

Any intervention that increases coronary blood flow or reduces the energy demands in a partially ischemic region of the ventricle will reduce the extent of the energy deficit and so can relieve symptoms in patients with ischemic heart disease. However, as already emphasized, myocardium supplied by a totally occluded coronary artery is doomed to die unless the tissue is reperfused.

Ischemia at a Distance

In the situation shown in Fig. 24.3B, occlusion of the right coronary artery causes infarction of the posterior wall of the left ventricle when collateral flow cannot deliver an effective blood supply to the bed of the occluded right coronary artery. However, as shown in Fig. 24.3B, right coronary occlusion has also caused a new problem: increased ischemia in the region normally supplied by the circumflex, which has been deprived of its collateral flow. This situation is called "ischemia at a distance" because the right coronary occlusion has not only infarcted the myocardium that this vessel normally supplies, but has also increased the severity of the ischemia in a distant region of the left ventricle—that is supplied by the partially occluded circumflex.

Electrocardiographic Localization of a Myocardial Infarction

The electrocardiographic leads that "face" an area of the left ventricle that has been infarcted provide criteria for localizing the infarct (Table 24.2). Such a lead is identified by the presence of abnormal Q waves and the ST segment shifts described below. Although the electrocardiographic criteria for localization of an infarct often correlate poorly with its pathological location, the terms listed in Table 24.2 are part of the daily language of the cardiologist. The most important distinction is between the *anterior* and *inferoposterior* infarctions, which differ clinically because the latter are commonly associated with important reflex bradyarrhythmias (see below).

ARRHYTHMIAS IN THE ISCHEMIC HEART

Approximately half the deaths caused by ischemic heart disease result from disordered cardiac rate and rhythm. In some cases lethal arrhythmias represent a terminal event in patients whose clinical course is complicated by severe and progressive heart failure, whereas other patients with minimal cardiac damage die suddenly in the first minutes to hours after the onset of an acute myocardial infarction. In the following section we first discuss the dynamic mechanisms responsible for the different types of arrhythmia that arise in the acutely ischemic heart, after which we turn our attention to the arrhythmias seen in patients with chronic coronary disease.

The vast majority of the sudden deaths in patients who have sustained an acute myocardial infarction are due to lethal arrhythmias; a small number are caused by cardiac rupture. The importance of prevention or rapid treatment of ischemic cardiac arrest arises from the well-known fact that even a small infarct can cause a lethal arrhythmia; in such cases, prevention of the arrhythmia would allow the patient to recover and often to live many healthy and productive years. In fact, the

TABLE 24.2. *Electrocardiographic localization of myocardial infarctions*

Localization	Leads in which abnormal Q waves are found
Anterior	
Anteroseptal	V_1, V_2
Anterior	V_2, V_3, V_4
Anterolateral	I, aVL, (V_4), V_5, V_6
Extensive anterior	I, aVL, V_1–V_6
Inferoposterior	
Inferior	II, III, aVF
Posterior	R in V_1[a]
Inferolateral	II, III, aVF, (V_5), V_6
Posterolateral	R in V_1[a], (V_5), V_6
Inferoposterior	R in V_1[a], II, III, aVF

[a]An abnormal R in V_1 is a "Q wave equivalent" because a lead placed at the back of the left chest wall would record a (downward) Q wave in a patient with a posterior infarction. Thus, the abnormal (upward) R waves recorded in this anterior chest lead are really upside down Q waves.

average life expectancy of a patient who survives a small myocardial infarction, which was about 12 years in the late 1960s (based on mortality data from control patients in large clinical trials) is likely to be a 15 to 20 years today.

Electrophysiological Abnormalities in Acute Myocardial Infarction

The two most important causes of lethal arrhythmias in patients with an acute myocardial infarction are ventricular fibrillation and complete heart block with asystolic cardiac arrest. The former, which is more common, is also more complex.

The Injury Current

Among the mechanisms that cause ischemic arrhythmias is the injury current, which arises from resting depolarization in ischemic myocardial cells. The injury current is thus associated with slow conduction, and gives rise to potential differences that participate in the pathogenesis of some of the early arrhythmias described below. Injury currents also give rise to important diagnostic features on the electrocardiogram of patients with different complications of coronary artery obstruction.

The major cause for depolarization of the ischemic heart is the rapid loss of potassium, as mentioned above. Leakage of potassium from an energy-starved cell, which is not electrogenic because it is accompanied by the efflux of lactate and phosphate, decreases the ratio $[K^+]_i/[K^+]_o$ and so depolarizes resting myocardium (Chapter 19); the depolarizing effect of reduced intracellular potassium is amplified when this cation cannot be washed out of the nonperfused extracellular space around the ischemic cells. The injury currents that flow between normal and ischemic regions of the resting heart not only give rise to arrhythmias, but also cause diagnostically important ST segment displacements in the ECG of patients with myocardial ischemia.

ST Segment Displacement

To understand the mechanisms by which injury currents displace the ST segment, it must be remembered that the clinical ECG has no zero (Chapter 20); instead, zero potential is assumed to be that inscribed during the TP segment (Fig. 24.4). Thus, injury currents that displace the TP segment are interpreted as causing opposite displacements of the ST segment.

ST Segment Elevation in Transmural Ischemia

The ST segments are elevated in the lead facing a region of transmural injury because the injury current established by the depolarized cells means that an electrode facing the injured cells is in an area of resting electronegativity. This diastolic

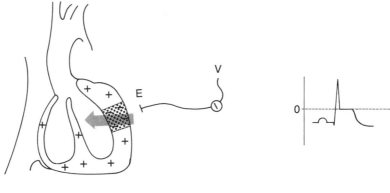

A. Transmural Ischemia

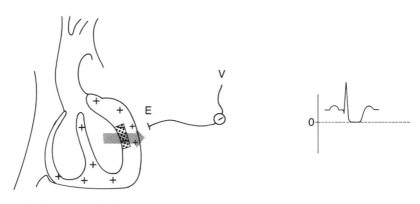

B. Subendocardial Ischemia

FIG. 24.4. Effects of the injury currents caused by transmural (*A*) and subendocardial (*B*) ischemia on an ECG recorded by an electrode (E) that records the potential difference between the surface of the ischemic region and a central terminal (V). The ischemic area is *shaded*, and surface potentials during diastole are shown. In transmural ischemia, the injury current in the ischemic cells causes an electrical vector during diastole that, because the recording electrode over the ischemic area is in an area of electronegativity, points away from the electrode. Because the injury potential is abolished during systole, when the normal myocardium is also depolarized, the resulting depression of the TP segment during diastole is "read" as ST segment elevation. In subendocardial ischemia, the injury current causes a diastolic electrical vector that, because the recording electrode is in an area of electropositivity, points toward the electrode; this elevates the TP segment during diastole, which is "read" as ST segment depression because the potential difference returns to zero during systole.

current depresses the TP segment, which is assumed to be the baseline of the ECG (Fig. 24.4A). The magnitude of this potential difference falls during systole, when the entire heart becomes depolarized, which elevates the ST segment relative to the TP segment. As the TP segment is assumed to record a zero potential difference during diastole, the decreased electronegativity during systole is interpreted as elevating the ST segment as shown in Fig. 24.4A.

> Other explanations for ST segment elevation in acute ischemia include potential differences that arise during the later phases of systole because of abbreviation of the action potential in the ischemic area. Another explanation is based on a delay in the conduction of depolarizing currents that, because they propagate slowly through the ischemic area, generate a wave of depolarization that inscribes an elevated ST segment when it approaches the electrode.

The return of elevated ST segments to baseline in a patient who has developed the pattern shown in Fig. 24.4A can have two meanings. The first is that the ischemia has gone away, as, for example, after the coronary artery has reopened, either spontaneously or in response to thrombolytic therapy. Although this interpretation is often correct, especially when ST segment abnormalities resolve quickly after only a brief period of ischemia, there is another equally valid explanation: the injury currents have gone away because the infarcted myocardium became "uncoupled" from the viable cells, as occurs when the gap junction channels close as the result of acidosis or calcium overload in the ischemic cells (Chapter 19). By abolishing the longitudinal currents required for impulse propagation (Fig. 21.1), closure of the connexon channels in a dying cell also resolves the ST segment abnormalities. For this reason, measurement of the extent of ST elevation, by "ST segment mapping," cannot define the true extent or severity of an infarct in a patient following coronary artery occlusion.

ST Segment Depression in Subendocardial Ischemia

Unlike the *transmural* ischemia described above, which causes ST elevation, *subendocardial* ischemia causes an exactly opposite shift in the ST segment. Subendocardial ischemia is common because energy starvation develop most rapidly in this layer of the left ventricle, where energy demands are high and the blood supply is precarious. In fact, subendocardial ischemia and ST depression are often seen in left ventricular hypertrophy (Fig. 20.39), even when the coronary arteries are normal, because the subendocardium is especially sensitive to demand ischemia (Chapter 25). ST segment depression develops in subendocardial ischemia because a layer of normal epicardium separates the partially depolarized ventricular endocardium from an electrode on the body surface, which means that during diastole, the latter is in an area of positivity (Fig. 24.4B). As a result the TP segment is elevated, which is read as ST depression.

The electrocardiographic difference between transmural and subendocardial ischemia is important clinically. Supply ischemia, as occurs following total interruption

of flow through a coronary artery supplying a large area of the left ventricle, typically causes ST elevation, whether the obstruction is due to a thrombosis in a
patient with acute myocardial infarction, or to coronary artery spasm in vasospastic
angina. In either setting, until the obstruction is removed—either by thrombolysis
or a coronary artery vasodilator—ischemia persists and ultimately leads to necrosis.
Demand ischemia, as occurs during a stress test, begins in the subendocardial regions
of the left ventricle and so causes ST depression; although ST elevation might occur
if continued exercise were to cause the ischemia to become transmural, stress tests
are stopped before this occurs, either by the patient because of severe chest pain or
by the physician who has obtained the information needed for diagnosis.

Abnormal Q Waves, Necrosis, and the "Window Potential"

The electrocardiographic "marker" for ventricular necrosis is the abnormal Q
wave. These initial downward QRS deflections appear in leads facing an infarction
because the normal wave of ventricular depolarization that should approach the
electrode is lost (Fig. 24.5). A useful way to understand the genesis of the abnormal
Q wave is to view the necrotic myocardium as a "window" that, because it cannot
generate a wave of depolarization (but can still conduct electricity) allows the electrode to see through the dead muscle into the cavity of the left ventricle. This is
reflected in the fact that an electrode placed in the left ventricular cavity normally
records only a downward deflection (a QS complex) because left ventricular depolarization begins in the endocardium, which causes all vectors to recede from its
cavity. The number of abnormal Q waves in a patient with an acute myocardial
infarction is a guide as to the extent of infarction.

> Abnormal Q waves are seen in other conditions—for example when viable myocar-
> dium has been replaced by scar tissue, as in a ventricular aneurysm, or when a tumor
> invades the wall of the ventricle.

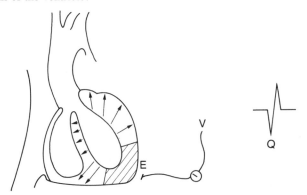

FIG. 24.5. An abnormal Q wave is recorded during the propagation of the wave of depolarization in a heart containing a region of transmural necrosis because depolarization of the noninfarcted myocardium gives rise to electrical vectors that point away from this area of the left
ventricle.

Viable epicardium can produce a small wave of depolarization that generates an R wave. This has also led to the clinical distinction between *Q wave infarction* and *non–Q wave infarction*. (The older terms *transmural* and *nontransmural* infarction have been abandoned because abnormal Q waves correlate imperfectly with the pathological extent of an infarct.) As might be expected, the immediate prognosis of a non–Q wave infarction is better than a Q wave infarction; however, the prognosis over 6 to 12 months is about the same, largely because the long-term course of the patient with ischemic heart disease is determined mainly by progression of the disease of the coronary arteries.

Tachyarrhythmias

The premature systoles and tachycardias that are seen in patients following an acute myocardial infarction arise from a number of pathyphysiological mechanisms. Clinical studies, as well as animal models, have defined at least three mechanisms that appear sequentially after an acute coronary artery occlusion. The first is membrane depolarization as described above, the second is accelerated pacemaker activity and triggered depolarizations, and the third, which gives rise to the late arrhythmias, is reentry in scarred, structurally abnormal regions of the infarcted myocardium. These distinctions are not always clear, and several mechanisms can operate together at any time to cause a tachyarrhythmia.

The First Phase: Depolarization

The depolarizing effect of the rapid loss of potassium from the ischemic myocardium reduces membrane potential, so that in the first minutes after a coronary artery becomes occluded, only a fraction of the sodium channels retain their ability to open. The result is the appearance of small, slowly conducting action potentials that represent the substrate for decremental conduction and reentrant arrhythmias.

Depolarization has additional arrhythmogenic effects; for example, potential differences between the ischemic regions of the heart and areas that still have a normal resting potential, in addition to causing ST segment elevation and depression, contribute to the inhomogeneity of depolarization discussed in Chapter 21 (Fig. 21.14).

Ischemic myocardial cells ultimately lose so much potassium as to cease either to initiate or propagate a sodium-dependent action potential; this is the mechanism for the abnormal Q waves described above. Thus, in accord with the motto "dead men tell no tales," such cells lose their ability to conduct in reentrant circuits. However, cells can remain persistently ischemic in an area where the circulation is jeopardized, as occurs in "ischemia at a distance" (Fig. 24.3), and so may continue to generate arrhythmias. Thus, although the hazard of a lethal arrhythmia rapidly wanes after a completed infarction, the risk of sudden death remains high in patients who continue to experience intermittent ischemia.

It was once postulated that the slow responses in ischemic regions of the heart were due to calcium-dependent action potentials, which conduct less rapidly and are less sensitive to inactivation by membrane depolarization than the fast sodium currents (Table 19.2). However, an important role for i_{Ca} in arrhythmogenesis now appears to be unlikely, and the calcium channel blockers have little or no ability to prevent sudden cardiac death in patients with ischemic heart disease. There is one exception: patients with vasospastic angina, where the ability of these drugs to prevent coronary vasoconstriction explains both their antianginal and antiarrhythmic efficacy.

Mechanisms besides depolarization contribute to the appearance of arrhythmias in the first hours after a coronary occlusion. These include changes in action potential duration, both shortening and prolongation, that give rise to inhomogeneities of repolarization that can cause reentry by the electrotonic mechanism shown in Fig. 21.13. The ability of inhomogeneities of refractoriness to disorganize the wave of depolarization as it spreads over the ventricles is also of importance in the pathogenesis of premature systoles and tachycardias. The effect of acidosis to close gap junction channels in the intercalated disc (Chapter 19), by increasing internal resistance, also slows conduction (Chapter 21).

The Second Phase: Reperfusion

Many of the arrhythmias that appear in patients 18 to 36 hours after an acute myocardial infarction are due to reperfusion, which reflects the dynamic nature of the coronary occlusion in most patients with acute myocardial infarction. In fact, the majority of the "infarct arteries," whose occlusion had caused the infarct, reopen spontaneously within less than a week.

The ventricular arrhythmias that appear 18 to 36 hours after an acute myocardial infarction are more like *automatic* (pacemaker-induced) *arrhythmias* than reentrant arrhythmias. In many cases, accelerated ventricular pacemakers are unmasked when the sinus rate slows in a sleeping patient; these may cause one or two brief runs of an *idioventricular rhythm*. These automatic rhythms, usually having rates between 60 and 100, are clinically benign and so resemble a parasystole (Chapter 23) rather than the earlier reentrant ventricular premature systoles that can herald sudden cardiac death. A second mechanism that causes these arrhythmias, and which is probably also responsible for alarming arrhythmias seen when coronary reperfusion is effected by thrombolytic therapy, is *triggered activity* caused by delayed afterdepolarizations. As noted in Chapter 19, these arrhythmias are caused by inward currents that appear in the calcium overloaded myocardium; the reason that they are seen during reperfusion is discussed below when we examine the role of calcium overload as a possible cause for myocardial cell death after coronary reperfusion.

The Third Phase: Arrhythmias in Chronic Ischemic Heart Disease

Acute depolarization and reperfusion play little role in the genesis of arrhythmias in patients who have a healed myocardial infarction. Cells are no longer acidotic, potassium efflux stops, and calcium overload ends when the cells either become necrotic or recover from the metabolic injuries associated with the acute phases described above. However, yet another group of pathophysiological mechanisms generate the most prevalent of the arrhythmias seen in patients with ischemic heart disease.

That early and late arrhythmias are due to entirely different mechanisms became apparent many years ago when it was found that patients successfully resuscitated after experiencing ventricular fibrillation in the first hours after a myocardial infarction had little or no increased risk of a late arrhythmic death. Instead, the hazards of late sudden death were predicted most accurately by the finding of complex ventricular premature systoles, and especially runs of sustained ventricular tachycardia, which are markers for an increased risk of sudden cardiac death.

Both the nonlethal premature systoles and the more serious ventricular tachycardias generally arise from reentrant mechanisms that are caused by decremental conduction. The substrate for these reentrant arrhythmias is provided by slow, sodium channel-dependent conduction in scarred regions of the left ventricle, in which bundles of viable ventricular myocardial fibers, most often in the endocardium, are surrounded by dense connective tissue. The resulting susceptibility to reentrant arrhythmias is exacerbated by hypertrophy of noninfarcted regions of the left ventricle, which increases the path length of the reentrant circuits. Heart failure is an important predictor of sudden cardiac death because, as noted in Chapter 23, large hearts are prone to fibrillate. This relationship is even stronger when scarring slows conduction and increases the length of the path that must be followed by a wave of depolarization as it spreads over the ventricles. Hypertrophy may also be accompanied by alterations in membrane architecture and ion channel structure that slow conduction (Chapter 25).

The arrhythmogenic impact of hypertrophy is apparent in several clinical studies that show that the risk of sudden cardiac death is increased to about the same extent by complex ventricular premature systoles and heart failure; when both are present, the increased risks are additive.

Slow conduction due to scarring and hypertrophy, rather than episodes of transient ischemia, is the most important cause of arrhythmias in patients with chronic stable angina and healed infarction. In unstable angina, as noted above, episodic ischemic greatly increases the hazards of sudden death because of the repeated appearance of the depolarization and repolarization abnormalities described above.

Atrial arrhythmias can occur in patients with ischemic heart disease, but these are less common because atrial ischemia and infarction are infrequent. Atrial fibrillation caused by atrial dilatation in patients with severe left ventricular failure is an ominous sign because it identifies patients with a poor prognosis due to progressive heart failure.

The finding of frequent and complex ventricular arrhythmias in a patient with chronic ischemic heart disease, which indicates that there is a high risk of a lethal arrhythmia, is associated with late potentials caused by abnormal persistence of electrical activity in the damaged ventricle. These long-lasting depolarizations persist when impulses continue to be propagated well after the end of the QRS complex in the normal regions of the ventricles. Late potentials, although not detectable by standard electrocardiography, can be identified when a large number of cardiac cycles are averaged and analyzed on a signal-averaged ECG.

Bradyarrhythmias: Sinus Bradycardia and AV Block

The distinction between functional and anatomical causes for the bradyarrhythmias (Chapter 22) is especially important in patients who have had an acute myocardial infarction. This is because the functional bradyarrhythmias are generally transient and do not correlate with the extent of left ventricular damage, whereas structural atrioventricular (AV) block caused by infarction of the AV conducting system generally accompanies large infarcts and so heralds a poor prognosis.

Functional (Reflex) Bradyarrhythmias

Functional abnormalities of the sinoatrial (SA) and AV nodes are common in patients with infarction of the inferior or posterior regions of the left ventricle, which contain receptors for the von Bezold-Jarisch reflex. When activated, these receptors trigger a powerful parasympathetic reflex that slows the sinus node pacemaker and depresses calcium-dependent conduction in the AV node; the accompanying vagal effect on peripheral resistance vessels also causes hypotension, and a visceral response causes nausea and vomiting. In spite of the fact that patients who manifest this syndrome generally appear to be at death's door in the early hours after the infarction, the reflex response is soon ended and the patient, who may have had only a small infarction, can go on to make an excellent recovery. The treatment is, of course, dictated by the cause; since the problem is a parasympathetic reflex, both the sinus slowing and AV block generally respond to the muscarinic antagonist atropine. If an electrical pacemaker is required, it is usually needed only temporarily.

The identification of AV block due to reflex parasympathetic depression of i_{Ca} in the AV node, as discussed in Chapter 22, depends on such findings as the Wenckebach phenomenon and responsiveness to atropine.

Bradyarrhythmias Caused by Structural Abnormalities

Sinus bradycardia and SA block may accompany atrial infarction in patients with inferoposterior infarctions because the SA node artery is a branch of the right coronary artery that supplies this region of the ventricle. Bradycardias due to sinus node ischemia, which is usually transient, are less common than the reflex depression described above.

Structural damage of the AV conduction system is generally seen in patients with large infarctions, most commonly anterior infarction (Table 24.2). Such infarctions are usually due to multiple coronary artery occlusions because the interventricular septum receives its blood supply from both the left anterior descending coronary artery and the posterior descending coronary artery; the latter may originate from the circumflex, but in about 90% of patients is derived from the right coronary (Chapter 1). As noted in Chapter 22, structural AV block gives rise to Mobitz II second-degree AV block which, because the risk of subsequent permanent third-degree AV block is high, is generally an indication for the insertion of a permanent pacemaker.

The poor prognosis in patients with structural damage to the AV conduction system usually arises not from failure of conduction, which can be avoided by prophylactic pacemaker implantation, but from heart failure. This also applies to patients who develop bundle branch block in the setting of an acute anterior infarction; some studies have found that almost half of such patients do not survive the initial infarction because the conduction abnormality is a marker for the multivessel coronary artery disease that causes severe left ventricular failure.

CELL DEATH IN THE ISCHEMIC HEART

Myocardial cell death (necrosis) begins after 15 to 40 min of total ischemia in experimental animals; after about 6 hours, few viable cells remain. Necrosis begins in the endocardium, where energy requirements are greatest, and spreads outward through the wall of the left ventricle toward the epicardium. However, this timetable does not apply to all patients who have sustained an acute myocardial infarction, for several reasons. In the first place, the onset of a myocardial infarction is often "stuttering" rather than sudden, due to dynamic changes in the occlusive process in the coronary artery in which both platelet plugs and thrombi form and lyse spontaneously. In addition, many patients with ischemic heart disease, especially older patients who have had a previous myocardial infarction, develop an extensive collateral circulation, so that the occlusion of a vessel may diminish rather than halt the flow of arterial blood to a given region of the left ventricle (Fig. 24.3).

In addition to its lethal effects on cardiac myocytes, ischemia damages the capillary endothelium. This leads to endothelial swelling that can prevent capillary reperfusion even when the occlusion of the large epicardial artery that was initially responsible for the ischemic damage is relieved. The result has been called the "no-reflow" phenomenon.

Ischemic myocardial cells can die in either of two ways, depending on whether the heart has been reperfused. Regions that have not been reperfused develop a pale, acellular infarct that has sometimes been called *mummification*. As leukocytes cannot gain access to the necrotic tissue in an area supplied by an occluded coronary artery, the myocardial cells autolyze in this type of infarction. A much more violent process takes place when irreversibly damaged ischemic cells are reperfused. Under these conditions, uncontrolled calcium entry, probably due both to membrane damage and to sodium/calcium exchange (see below) causes the cells to literally tear themselves apart. Restoration of blood flow thus leads to a *hemorrhagic infarct* in which inflammatory cells, with all of their catabolic products (lipases, proteases, free radicals), destroy the hypercontracted myocardial cells. However, it appears that remodeling is improved by reperfusion as it seems to result in a stronger scar that, because it allows less ventricular dilatation, reduces wall tension and is energy-sparing (Chapter 16).

Mechanisms of Ischemic Damage and Cell Death

One of the most important unanswered questions in cardiology is the mechanism of ischemic cell death. This question has assumed an almost philosophical meaning because, although it is clear when a cell has actually died, identifying the "point of no return" is quite difficult. The definition of irreversible cell injury, like irreversibility in a terminally ill patient in whom one system fails after another, may never be unequivocal.

Membrane Damage

There is universal agreement that during prolonged ischemia, the plasma membrane rapidly loses its ability to function as a barrier that maintains a normal intracellular environment. This leads to the leakage of key intracellular substances, such as cytosolic enzymes that when they appear in the circulating blood are markers of irreversible cellular injury. There are several possible causes for membrane damage in cells that have undergone prolonged ischemia; at this time, however, no one mechanism has been generally accepted as providing a unique answer to the riddle of the pathogenesis of ischemic cell death. It is likely that, as in the case of the early pump failure of the ischemic heart, there are several explanations.

Phospholipase and Protease Attack

Although probably contributing to the late membrane damage in necrotic cells, activation of cellular lipolytic and proteolytic enzymes does not appear to play a major role in the early processes that lead to plasmalemmal disruption in ischemic cells.

Free Radicals

Free radicals are molecules that, because they contain an unpaired electron, are extremely reactive. These include the superoxide radical $O_2^-\cdot$ (the dot identifies the unpaired electron) and the reactive hydroxyl radical (OH·). Hydrogen peroxide, although not itself a free radical, forms reactive compounds in reactions that are catalyzed by Fe^{2+} and Fe^{3+}. Hydrogen peroxide also reacts with the superoxide radical, to produce even more reactive free radicals.

There are several potential sources of free radicals in the ischemic myocardium. Paradoxically, free radicals are generated by the respiratory chain in the ischemic heart, when the electron carriers described in Fig. 5.9 become reduced. Another source is ATP, which when hydrolyzed initially forms ADP, two moles of which are then reconverted to ATP and AMP in the reaction catalyzed by adenylyl kinase (myokinase). The AMP formed in this reaction is rapidly converted to adenosine which is irreversibly deaminated to yield inosine and hypoxanthine (Fig. 24.6). The latter is converted to xanthine in a reaction that produces superoxide radicals as by-products.

> The importance of this reaction has recently been questioned because xanthine oxidase, the key enzyme in this mechanism for free radical formation, is present in very low amounts in the human heart, where ischemic damage can be quite severe.

Free radicals are also formed during the breakdown of catecholamines and the metabolism of arachidonic acid, as well as by products of phospholipase action. Free radicals can also be "imported" into reperfused infarcts by neutrophils.

In spite of a large number of careful studies, the role of free radicals, whether generated by chemical reactions involving ischemic myocardial cells or brought in by neutrophils, in the pathogenesis of ischemic cell death remains controversial (Lucchesi et al., 1989; Reimer et al., 1989).

Detergent Effects of Lipids

As noted earlier in this chapter, amphipathic compounds are formed in the ischemic myocardium; these include long-chain fatty acyl carnitines and fatty acyl CoA, and lysophosphatides formed by the action of phospholipase 2 on membrane phospholipids (Chapter 2). High concentrations of these compounds can damage membranes, but it is not certain that the concentrations reached in the ischemic heart are sufficiently high to play an important role in causing membrane damage.

Osmotic Effects

Large amounts of small molecules appear in the cytosol of myocardial cells during the early phases of ischemia; for example, ATP is rapidly hydrolyzed to ADP and P_i, phosphocreatine is degraded to creatine and P_i, glycogen breaks down to form glucose-1-phosphate, and glucose is metabolized to form a variety of trioses as well as lactate. Together, these have been suggested to give rise to an osmotic overload that, by causing cell swelling, physically ruptures the plasma membrane.

Calcium Overload

Excessive calcium entry occurs in irreversibly damaged cells when this cation can no longer be excluded by an injured plasma membrane. Because calcium is a pow-

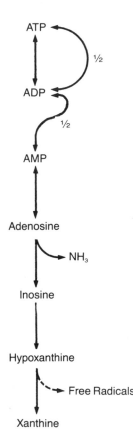

ATP

½

ADP

½

AMP

Adenosine

→ NH₃

Inosine

Hypoxanthine

→ Free Radicals

Xanthine

FIG. 24.6. Hydrolysis of ATP leads eventually to the production of inosine by the irreversible deamination of adenosine. Free radicals are generated as by-products of the conversion of hypoxanthine to xanthine in a reaction catalyzed by xanthine oxidase.

erful intracellular messenger, when allowed uncontrolled access to the binding sites on the troponin complex, calcium activates the contractile proteins to such an extent that the cell literally tears itself apart. This situation is most dramatic after reperfusion of irreversibly damaged cells, where calcium entry leads to the appearance of contracture bands. Thus, *contraction band necrosis*, which refers to the hypercontracted state of necrotic cells, is seen in infarcted cells that have been reperfused.

Calcium accumulation in the mitochondria of the ischemic heart, which probably reflects the activity of the ATP-dependent calcium pump found in the inner membrane, is a marker for the less dramatic calcium overload seen when ischemic tissue is not reperfused. Although the low calcium affinity of the mitochondria calcium pump makes it unlikely that this transport system plays an important role in physiological excitation-contraction coupling (Chapter 11), these structures can serve as a buffer in situations of calcium overload. Unfortunately, the cell pays a price for this protective mechanism because elevated intramitochondrial calcium inhibits oxidative phosphorylation (Chapter 5).

Although calcium overload causes cell disruption, it is still not clear whether uncontrolled calcium entry is the cause of the cell death, or is, instead, a marker for irreversible damage to the plasma membrane.

Sodium/Calcium Exchange

Dynamic changes in calcium fluxes can lead to calcium overload even when the membrane is not irreversibly damaged. The most readily understood of these functional abnormalities is excessive calcium entry via the sodium/calcium exchanger (Chapter 10). This can occur during reperfusion of cells that had been maintained in an energy-starved state for long periods of time, which allows sodium to accumulate in the cell because of sodium pump inhibition (the latter is attributable to decreased allosteric stimulation of the Na-K-ATPase caused by a modest decline in ATP levels as described above). Under these conditions, other regulated ion fluxes, notably the sodium/calcium exchanger, are also inhibited. If coronary flow is restored to such a cell, ATP levels quickly increase, which activates the sodium/calcium exchanger at a time that large amounts of calcium are delivered to the cell via the now-reopened coronary circulation. These conditions can lead to uncontrolled calcium entry.

Although this scenario is not universally accepted as being relevant to ischemic necrosis, it provides one explanation for another even more puzzling phenomenon: the *calcium paradox*. In this phenomenon, restoration of normal calcium concentration to the medium surrounding a cell that had been exposed for a long time to very low extracellular calcium also leads to contracture and cell death. The mechanism for the calcium paradox is controversial, like that for ischemic cell death, and may also involve plasma membrane damage caused by prolonged exposure to the low calcium medium.

Stunning and Hibernation

Two terms have recently been popularized to describe prolonged hypofunctional states of the myocardium after it recovers from prolonged ischemia. *Stunning* is a period of depressed mechanical function that follows a brief period of ischemia, whereas *hibernation* refers to poorly functioning regions of the heart in patients with chronic ischemic heart disease that regain their ability to contract when coronary flow is reestablished following bypass surgery or angioplasty. The mechanisms responsible for these states, however, are not well understood.

Adenine nucleotide depletion has been postulated to account for stunning because, although rephosphorylation of ADP to form ATP is almost instantaneous when a viable ischemic myocardial cell is reperfused, the deamination of adenosine to form inosine is irreversible (Fig. 24.6). Thus, replacement of adenine nucleotides lost as the result of deamination following prolonged or repeated ischemia requires *de novo* adenine synthesis, which is a very slow process that can take several days.

A novel, and fascinating explanation for the persistence of sequelae of ischemic damage in reperfused cells is that ischemic stress initiates changes in protein composition that persist for days, or even weeks. Altered gene expression may also explain characteristic, long-lasting, repolarization abnormalities called T wave "evolution," which are seen during the first few weeks following ischemia and acute myocardial infarction. As noted in Chapter 18, these long-lasting changes might be due to changes in the subunit composition of the highly plastic potassium channels of the heart.

At this point we have seen how the pathophysiology of the myocardial abnormalities in ischemic heart disease alter the function of the heart as an *organ* as the result of abnormalities in *cell biochemistry*. As suggested in the preceding paragraph, these problems in cardiovascular pathophysiology appear now to have entered the realm of the third paradigm: altered *gene* expression. This is clearly seen to be the case in the next chapter, where we turn our attention to the final topic in our text: heart failure.

REFERENCES

Cobbe SM, Poole-Wilson PA. (1980). The time of onset and severity of acidosis in myocardial ischemia. *J Mol Cell Cardiol* 12:745–760.

Gevers W. (1977). Generation of protons by metabolic processes in heart cells. *J Mol Cell Cardiol* 9:867–874.

Jacobus WE, Pores IH, Lucas SK, Weisfeldt ML, Flaherty JT. (1982). Intracellular acidosis and contractility in the normal and ischemic heart as examined by ^{31}P NMR. *J Moll Cell Cardiol* 14(Suppl 3): 13–20.

Lucchesi BR, Werns SW, Fantone JC. (1989). The role of the neutrophil and free radicals in ischemic myocardial injury. *J Mol Cell Cardiol* 21:1241–1251.

Monomura S-I, Ingwall JS, Parker JA, Shagian P, Ferguson JJ, Grossman W. (1985). The relationship of high energy phosphates, tissue pH, and regional blood flow to diastolic distensibility in the ischemic dog myocardium. *Circ Res* 57:822–835.

Reimer K, Murry CE, Richard VJ. (1989). The role of neutrophils and free radicals in the ischemic-reperfused heart: why the confusion and controversy? *J Mol Cell Cardiol* 21:1225–1239.

Seelye RN. (1980). Proton generation and control during anaerobic glycolysis in heart cells. *J Mol Cell Cardiol* 12:1483–1486.

Shaikh NA, Downar E. (1981). Time course of changes in porcine myocardial phospholipid levels during ischemia. A reassessment of the lysolipid hypothesis. *Circ Res* 49:316–325.

Van der Vusse GJ, Roemen THM, Reneman RS. (1985). The content of non-esterified fatty acids in rat myocardial tissue. A comparison between the Dole and Folch extraction procedures. *J Mol Cell Cardiol* 17:527–531.

Vogel WM, Apstein CS, Briggs LL, Gaasch WH, Ahn J. (1982). Acute alterations in left ventricular diastolic chamber stiffness. Role of the "erectile" effect of coronary arterial pressure and flow in normal and damaged hearts. *Circ Res* 51:465–476.

Wilkie DR. (1979). Generation of protons by metabolic processes other than glycolysis in muscle cells. A critical view. *J Mol Cell Cardiol* 11:325–330.

Williamson JR. (1966). Glycolytic control mechanisms. II. Kinetics of intermediate changes during the aerobic-anoxic transition in perfused rat heart. *J Biol Chem* 241:5026–5036.

BIBLIOGRAPHY

Gettes LS. (1986). Effect of ischemia on cardiac electrophysiology. In: Fozzard H, Haber E, Katz A, Jennings R, Morgan HE, eds. *The heart and cardiovascular system*. New York: Raven Press; 1317–1341.

Hazen SL, Gross RW. (1991). Principles of membrane biochemistry and their application to the pathophysiology of cardiovascular disease. In Fozzard H, Haber E, Katz A, Jennings R, Morgan HE, eds. *The heart and cardiovascular system*, 2nd ed. New York: Raven Press, in press.

Katz AM, Messineo FC. (1981). Lipid-membrane interactions and the pathogenesis of ischemic damage in the myocardium *Circ Res* 48:1–16.

Katz AM, Reuter H. (1979). Cellular calcium and cardiac cell death. *Am J Cardiol* 44:188–190.

Kléber AG. (1983). Resting membrane potential, extracellular potassium activity, and intracellular sodium activity during global ischemia in isolated perfused guinea pig hearts. *Circ Res* 52:442–450.

Liedtke AJ. (1981). Alterations of carbohydrate and lipid metabolism in the acutely ischemic heart. *Prog Cardiovasc Dis* 23:321–336.

McCord JM. (1985). Oxygen-derived free radicals in postischemic tissue injury. *N Engl J Med* 312:159–163.

Opie LH. (1976). Effects of regional ischemia on metabolism of glucose and fatty acids. Relative rates of aerobic and anaerobic energy production during myocardial infarction and comparison with effects of anoxia. *Circ Res* 38(Suppl I):I–52–I–68.

Reimer KA, Jennings RB. (1986). Myocardial ischemia, hypoxia, and infarction. In: Fozzard H, Haber E, Katz A, Jennings R, Morgan HE, eds. *The heart and cardiovascular system*. New York: Raven Press, 1133–1201.

See also Bibliography to Chapters 4 and 5.

25

Heart Failure

Heart failure has many definitions, which reflect the evolution of our understanding of this important condition in terms of the three paradigms discussed in Chapter 14 (Table 14.1) (Katz, 1989, 1990a). In the early part of this century, heart failure was defined in terms of the first paradigm of *organ physiology*, which highlighted the interplay between the abnormal heart and the circulation whose needs it cannot satisfy. These early definitions, however, tended to draw attention away from the heart to focus on circulatory abnormalities that, although devastating to the patient, are complications rather than causes of heart failure. In the 1960s, identification of abnormal contractility and energetics in the failing heart shifted emphasis from these hemodynamic changes to the second paradigm of *cell biochemistry*. According to this paradigm, the major problem in heart failure is depressed contractility and impaired relaxation. However, since the mid-1980s, it has become clear that these biochemical and biophysical abnormalities can themselves be secondary to even more fundamental abnormalities in *gene expression* in the failing heart. The molecular alterations described by the third paradigm not only contribute to the circulatory and cellular abnormalities in the patient with heart failure, but probably account for what now appears to be the major problem in the patient with heart failure: a terrible prognosis due to accelerated deterioration of overloaded myocardial cells.

> The signs and symptoms of heart failure are, of course, the immediate concern to those who care for these patients. However, efforts to slow the rapid deterioration of the failing heart are also an important objective of therapy because the average life expectancy of the usual patient with mild to moderate symptoms is only about 5 years, whereas in severe heart failure average survival is less than a year.

As details regarding the abnormalities in gene expression in the failing heart are only now coming into focus, the following definition must suffice: *Heart failure is a clinical syndrome in which impaired cardiac pumping decreases ejection and impedes venous return. These hemodynamic abnormalities are generally complicated by depressed myocardial contractility and relaxation, which reflect biochemical and biophysical disorders in the myocardial cells. The latter, in turn, are due partly to molecular abnormalities that not only impair the heart's performance, but also accelerate the deterioration of the myocardium and hasten myocardial cell death.*

ORGAN AND CIRCULATORY PHYSIOLOGY

The first of the paradigms that describe the causes and therapy of heart failure views this condition in terms of depressed pump function and altered circulatory dynamics. The latter include abnormalities of salt and water metabolism that lead to fluid retention and vasoconstriction, which are circulatory consequences of reduced cardiac performance that can now be managed with effective diuretics and several classes of vasodilators. As the renal and peripheral aspects of the pathophysiology of heart failure are reviewed in standard textbooks of medicine and cardiology, they are not considered further in this text.

Hemodynamics of Heart Failure

The hemodynamic abnormalities in patients with heart failure are conceptually simple because, like any pump (Fig. 25.1), the heart has only two ways to fail: reduced ejection of blood under pressure into the aorta and pulmonary artery (*forward* or *inotropic* failure) and inadequate emptying of the venous reservoirs (*backward* or *lusitropic* failure). As the primary abnormality often arises in either the right or left ventricle, there are actually four types of heart failure (Table 25.1). However, because blood flows in a circle, none of these occurs in pure form. In forward failure, where the ventricle empties poorly, filling is also reduced, and conversely, in backward failure, where filling is reduced, the ventricle cannot eject a normal stroke volume. Furthermore, when the right ventricle fails, the resulting increase in systemic venous pressure and decreased ejection of blood into the pulmonary artery reduce the output of the left ventricle (Fig. 25.2). In left ventricular failure, increased pulmonary venous pressure impedes the flow of blood out of the

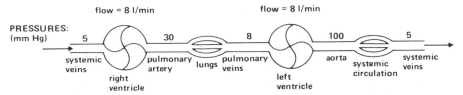

FIG. 25.1. The normal circulation. Reading from left to right, the systemic veins empty into the right ventricle, which pumps blood through the pulmonary artery to the lungs. Blood returns via the pulmonary veins to the left ventricle from which it is pumped into the systemic circulation via the aorta. Efflux from the systemic circulation returns to the right ventricle via the systemic veins. As the blood moves continuously in a circle, the outputs of the two ventricles are equal, the normal cardiac output (*above*) being approximately 8 liters/min. Normal mean pressures are approximately 5 mm Hg in the systemic veins, 30 mm Hg in the pulmonary artery, 8 mm Hg in the pulmonary veins, and 100 mm Hg in the aorta.

TABLE 25.1. *Four types of heart failure*

Site of failure	Backward failure	Forward failure
Right heart failure	Increased systemic venous pressure	Reduced ejection into pulmonary artery
Left heart failure	Increased pulmonary venous pressure	Reduced ejection into aorta

lungs and so increases pulmonary capillary pressure. Because this elevated pressure is transmitted across the pulmonary circulation, the resulting rise in pulmonary arterial pressure can impair right ventricular ejection (Fig. 25.3).

The fact that the outputs of both ventricles must, over any period of time, be equal, diminishes the heuristic value of the dichotomy between "backward failure" (Fig. 25.4) and "forward failure" (Fig. 25.5). Furthermore, the circulatory responses to impaired pump function can exacerbate either of these problems—as can therapy itself. These concepts remain useful, however, as backward failure describes the signs and symptoms caused by a rise in pulmonary or systemic venous pressure, whereas forward failure highlights the consequences of reduced ejection by either ventricle, that is, a fall in cardiac output.

Because systemic reflexes have developed so as to maintain the perfusion of vital organs, notably the brain and the heart, vasoconstriction generally protects blood pressure at the expense of cardiac output. As a result, in most patients with chronic heart failure, cardiac output is reduced to a greater extent than is blood pressure. Thus, hypotension is uncommon in chronic heart failure, and usually appears only in the late stages, when pump function has become severely impaired.

A "typical" example of heart failure, due to a primary abnormality in the left ventricle, and complicated by modest elevation of right heart pressures is shown in Fig. 25.6.

Overload and Heart Failure

Causes of heart failure include the poorly understood disorders of the myocardium and supporting tissues (cardiomyopathies), infarction due to coronary artery

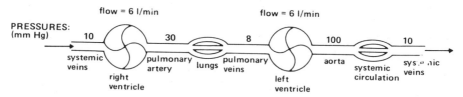

FIG. 25.2. "Right ventricular failure." Impaired pumping by the right ventricle causes the output of both ventricles to be reduced so that cardiac output falls, e.g., to 6 liters/min. Systemic venous pressure rises (e.g., to 10 mm Hg) because right ventricular end-diastolic pressure is increased, but circulatory reflexes tend to maintain mean pulmonary artery pressure and left ventricular end-diastolic pressure at virtually normal levels.

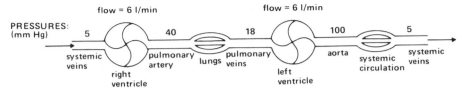

FIG. 25.3. "Left ventricular failure." Impaired pumping by the left ventricle causes the output of both ventricles to be reduced, i.e., cardiac output falls (e.g., to 6 liters/min). Pulmonary venous pressure rises (e.g., to 18 mm Hg) because left ventricular end-diastolic pressure is increased, but circulatory reflexes tend to maintain mean aortic pressure at a virtually normal level. The elevated pulmonary venous pressure is transmitted through the lungs, causing a slight rise in mean pulmonary artery pressure, e.g., to 40 mm Hg.

occlusive disease, and a variety of valvular and structural abnormalities. Common to virtually all of these conditions is a chronic increase in the load on whatever myocardial fibers are viable and active; as noted below, this overload plays an important role in the development of hypertrophy (see below). For complete discussions of the many causes of heart failure, the reader is referred to standard textbooks of medicine and cardiology.

Signs and Symptoms of Heart Failure

The clinical picture in heart failure consists of *signs*, the objective manifestations of depressed cardiac performance, and *symptoms*, which are abnormalities perceived by the patient. The most important signs and symptoms of right heart failure are caused by the increased systemic venous pressure, whereas those in left heart failure are related to the rise in pulmonary capillary pressure, which causes symptoms of breathlessness called dyspnea. In patients who suffer from right heart fail-

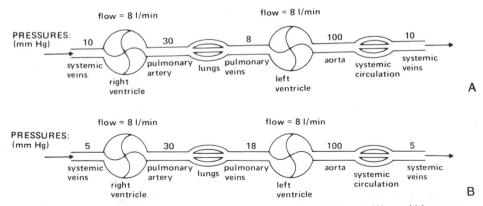

FIG. 25.4. "Backward failure." "Pure" backward failure of the right heart (A) would increase systemic venous pressure (e.g., to 10 mm Hg) without causing other abnormalities. "Pure" backward failure of the left heart (B) would increase pulmonary venous pressure (e.g., to 18 mm Hg) without causing other abnormalities.

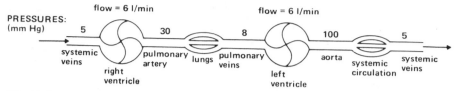

FIG. 25.5. "Forward failure." "Pure" forward failure of either ventricle would reduce cardiac output (e.g., to 6 liters/min) without causing other abnormalities.

ure, increased systemic venous pressure causes peripheral edema and, when severe, hepatic and renal insufficiency. Left heart failure, of course, increases the pressures in the pulmonary venous system, which impairs respiration. In both abnormalities, a fall in cardiac output usually causes fatigue.

Dyspnea (literally difficulty in breathing) in left heart failure is due partly to arterial hypoxia, caused when transudation of fluid around the pulmonary capillaries interferes with oxygen transport from the alveoli, and partly to decreased lung compliance that results when the excess fluid transudated from the pulmonary capillaries is transported back to the systemic venous system via distended lymphatic vessels in the lungs. In mild left heart failure, dyspnea occurs only during heavy exercise or extreme emotional stress; however, as the failure worsens, less exertion is needed to cause this symptom so that in very severe heart failure, this symptom is present at rest. When heart failure becomes more severe, so much fluid moves into the alveoli as to cause bubbling noises (rales) during respiration. In end-stage left heart failure, the fluid can be forced into the alveoli so as to fill the bronchial system; the result is *pulmonary edema*, in which severe dyspnea is accompanied by the production of frothy sputum. If this condition cannot be treated, the patient literally drowns.

In many patients, the progression described above is modified by reactive pulmonary vasoconstriction and obliteration of the small pulmonary arteries. The resulting decrease in pulmonary capillary pressure protects the lungs from edema, but because this response increases pulmonary artery pressure (pulmonary hypertension), elevated left ventricular filling pressure can lead to a chronic increase in pulmonary artery pressure that overloads the right ventricle. In this way, left heart failure can lead to right heart failure.

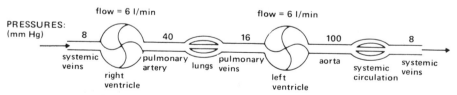

FIG. 25.6. Clinical heart failure. As encountered in most patients, heart failure is due to impaired pumping of the left ventricle. When moderately severe, heart failure is accompanied by a fall in cardiac output (e.g., to 6 liters/min), significant elevation of pulmonary venous pressure (e.g., to 16 mm Hg), modest elevation of mean pulmonary artery (e.g., to 40 mm Hg), and systemic venous (e.g., to 8 mm Hg) pressure, with no significant abnormality in mean aortic pressure.

Fatigue and reduced exercise capacity, among the most prominent symptoms in patients with heart failure, are often attributed to reduced perfusion of the skeletal muscles caused by the low cardiac output. However, it is now apparent that a skeletal muscle myopathy plays a major role in causing these often disabling symptoms (Wilson and Mancini, 1990). This skeletal myopathy may be due in part to chronic underperfusion of the muscles, but its biochemical features resemble those of disuse atrophy. This skeletal myopathy can improve when patients are encouraged to exercise, even when there is no other change in therapy.

Enlargement of the heart (cardiomegaly), one of the major signs of heart failure, is due initially to the operation of the Frank-Starling relationship. Subsequent remodeling of the muscular walls of the ventricles is a complex process that depends on the abnormality responsible for the heart failure. A pressure overload, such as occurs in hypertension or when the aortic valve orifice becomes narrowed (stenosis), causes the left ventricle to hypertrophy "inward" so as to reduce cavity volume (concentric hypertropy). This response is of considerable benefit as it reduces wall tension according to the law of Laplace (Chapter 16). In a volume overload, as occurs in aortic regurgitation, the hypertrophied ventricle dilates (eccentric hypertrophy) so as to accommodate the increased diastolic filling caused by the leaky valve.

Circulatory Failure, Heart Failure, and Myocardial Failure

It is important, both conceptually and clinically, to distinguish between three distinct pathophysiological mechanisms that can cause the signs and symptoms of heart failure. In *circulatory failure*, many of the clinical features described above can appear even when the heart is normal. For example, one can easily appreciate that intravenous infusion of large amounts of saline would increase both systemic and pulmonary venous pressure and so produce many of the signs and symptoms of backward failure. The unwary physician can be misled when such findings as peripheral edema, ascites (fluid in the peritoneal cavity), or pleural effusion appear in a patient with fluid retention due to renal or hepatic disease. The resulting signs could be erroneously attributed to heart failure; however, although the circulation is clearly abnormal, the primary problem is not in the heart.

Salt and water retention caused by abnormal renal function complicate the clinical picture in heart failure because a decrease in cardiac output initiates powerful neurohumoral reflexes that increase circulating blood volume. This compensatory mechanism, because it worsens the problems already caused by backward failure, represents one of the many vicious cycles that must be treated in these patients.

Heart failure, as already noted, represents any abnormality in the pumping action of the heart that reduces its ability to perform external work. The heart can fail even when the myocardium is normal, as occurs in valvular disease, after infarction, or in hypertension, so that only a minority of cases of heart failure begin as a cardiomyopathy where the heart muscle itself is abnormal (*myocardial failure*). However, because virtually all forms of heart failure overload the cells of the myocardium, they initiate both short-term and long-term changes in the walls of the heart that, as described later in this chapter, can cause a "cardiomyopathy of overload" (Katz, 1990a).

Short-Term and Long-Term Responses to Reduced Cardiac Output

Adjustments involving both the peripheral circulation and the myocardium allow the body to adapt to a decrease in cardiac work. Although the acute and chronic adjustments to reduced output share many features, the short-term adaptation to a sudden decrease in the work of the heart differs in important ways from the long-term adaptation to the sustained low-output state seen in congestive heart failure (Table 25.2).

In acute heart failure, initial compensation for the tendency for blood pressure to fall is effected by vasoconstriction, and after a few hours, also by salt and water retention. These compensatory responses maintain perfusion of essential organs, notably the brain and the heart that cannot survive prolonged reduction in blood flow, and so are vital to survival in acute low-output states. Diversion of blood to vital organs occurs when vasoconstriction in the skin and viscera helps to maintain

TABLE 25.2. *Short-term and long-term responses to impaired cardiac performance*

Response	Short-term effects (mainly adaptive) (hemorrhage, acute heart failure)	Long-term effects (mainly deleterious) (chronic heart failure)
SALT AND WATER RETENTION	Augments preload	Pulmonary congestion, anasarca
VASOCONSTRICTION	Maintains pressure for perfusion of vital organs (brain, heart)	Exacerbates pump dysfunction increases cardiac energy expenditure
SYMPATHETIC STIMULATION	Increases heart rate and ejection	Increases energy expenditure
Desensitization		Energy-sparing
HYPERTROPHY	Unloads individual muscle fibers	Deterioration and death of cardiac cells: Cardiomyopathy of overload
Capillary Deficit		Energy starvation
Mitochondrial Density	Increase; helps meet energy demands	Decrease; energy starvation
Appearance of Slow Myosin		Increases force integral, decreases shortening velocity and contractility; energy sparing
Prolonged Action Potential		Increases contractility and energy expenditure
Decreased Density of SR Calcium Pump Sites		Slows relaxation, possibly energy sparing
Increased Collagen	May reduce dilatation	Impairs relaxation

Modified from Katz (1990a).

blood pressure. These short-term circulatory responses, which are similar to those initiated by hemorrhage, are therefore important to survival in acute heart failure— for example, in cardiogenic shock complicating a large acute myocardial infarction.

In chronic low-output states, the same responses that initially aided survival in the patient with acute heart failure can become deleterious (Table 25.2). For example, vasoconstriction, although clearly useful for short-term survival, causes an increase in afterload that, when sustained, becomes detrimental. Similarly, salt and water retention by the kidney, by elevating venous pressure in both the lungs and peripheral circulation, worsens backward failure and so becomes a major cause of disability, and even of death.

Neurohumoral Response to the Low-Output State in Heart Failure

The short-term adjustments to a fall in cardiac output are mediated primarily by neurohumoral responses that act upon both the heart and peripheral vessels (Francis

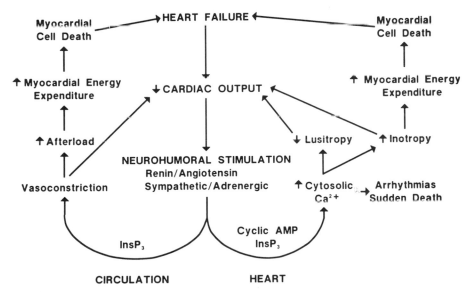

FIG. 25.7. The low-output state in congestive heart failure can accelerate cell death in the failing heart by stimulating the renin/angiotensin and sympathetic/adrenergic systems that act upon both the circulation (*left*) and the heart (*right*). Vasoconstriction increases afterload, which further decreases cardiac output; by increasing the work of the heart, the increased afterload may also accelerate myocardial cell death. In the heart, increased cyclic AMP and inositol-1,4,5-trisphosphate (InsP$_3$) promote calcium entry and so augment contractility; along with a chronotropic response (not shown) this inotropic response increases cardiac output and so is compensatory. However, the increased calcium that enters the cytosol can overload the systems that pump this ion out of the cell during diastole, and so can impair relaxation. Calcium overload may also induce arrhythmias and lead to sudden death. Because the inotropic and chronotropic responses to sympathetic/adrenergic stimulation increase myocardial energy expenditure, they might also accelerate cell death in the failing heart. Thus, initial adaptive responses of both the circulation and the heart to a chronic low-output state can, when they are sustained, have deleterious long-term effects in patients with congestive heart failure. (Modified from Katz, 1990a.)

et al., 1984). The interplay between important beneficial and harmful effects of renin/angiotensin and sympathetic/adrenergic stimulation are shown in Fig. 25.7, which summarizes key circulatory and cardiac adjustments to a fall in cardiac output. The left side of Fig. 25.7 depicts some of the consequences of sustained vaso-constriction, which by raising blood pressure ensures perfusion of the brain and heart when the work of the heart is reduced. However, the resulting increase in afterload further reduces cardiac output and, by increasing myocardial energy demands, may contribute to the deterioration of the failing heart.

Some of the cardiac responses to adenosine 3',5'- cyclic monophosphate (cyclic AMP) and inositol-1,4,5- trisphosphate, second messengers produced in response to neurohumoral stimulation of the heart (Chapter 12), are shown on the right side of Fig. 25.7. Probably the most important effect of these second messengers is to increase calcium entry into the cells of the heart. This causes an inotropic response, which along with the chronotropic response (not shown), helps to maintain cardiac output. However, increased cytosolic calcium also tends to overload the systems that pump calcium out of the cell during diastole, and so impairs relaxation. While sympathetic stimulation promotes relaxation in the normal heart by accelerating calcium uptake into the sarcoplasmic reticulum (Chapter 14), other abnormalities in the failing heart depress calcium uptake, and so lead to slowed, incomplete relaxation (see below).

Deleterious side effects of the positive inotropic and chronotropic effects of sympathetic/adrenergic stimulation also result from their ability to increase energy expenditure (Chapter 16). Like the increased afterload shown at the left of Fig. 25.7, this response may accelerate cell death in the chronically overloaded heart. Cellular calcium overload caused by neurohumoral stimulation may also cause triggered depolarizations that contribute to the arrhythmias commonly seen in patients with heart failure (Chapter 21). Thus, although the initial neurohumoral response to an acute fall in cardiac output is one of short-term benefit, the same responses, when sustained, have deleterious long-term effects on the failing heart.

Effects of Heart Failure on the Pressure-Volume Loop

Heart failure alters not only the interactions between the heart and the circulation, but also the interplay between the contractile (inotropic) and relaxation (lusitropic) properties of the heart. As already noted, the fact that the blood flows in a circle makes it impossible for either forward or backward failure to occur in "pure" form; instead, abnormalities of both filling and emptying usually coexist when the heart fails. The interplay between these two aspects of cardiac pumping, as well as that between the heart and the circulation, is seen in the pressure-volume loop (Chapter 16). This depiction of the cardiac cycle is constrained within boundaries that define the interactions between the heart and circulation at end-diastole and at end-systole (Fig. 16.16).

The combination of negative inotropic and lusitropic interventions, which com-

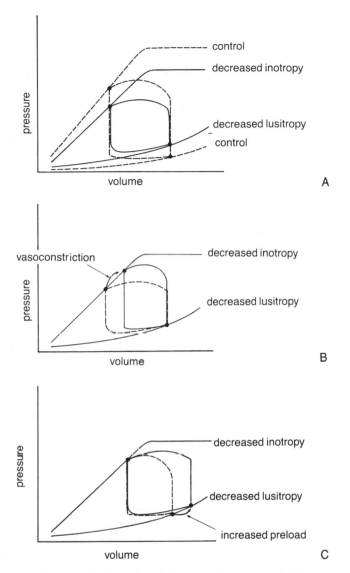

FIG. 25.8. Schematic diagrams of left ventricular pressure-volume loops. **A:** The combination of negative inotropic and lusitropic states, as commonly occurs in heart failure, "compresses" the pressure volume loop between the abnormal end-diastolic and end-systolic pressure-volume relationships. In this illustration, where stroke volume is assumed to remain constant, end-diastolic pressure is increased, and developed pressure is reduced. The control pressure-volume loop (Fig. 16.3 is shown as a *dashed line* between the control end-diastolic and end-systolic pressure-volume relationships, also represented by *dashed lines*. **B:** Effect of vasoconstriction on the pressure-volume loop shown in A. As shown by the *curved arrow*, vasoconstriction shifts the end-systolic point upward and to the right along the depressed end-systolic pressure volume loop. This circulatory adjustment returns blood pressure toward normal, but at the expense of a fall in stoke volume. **C:** Effect of increased preload (*curved arrow*) on the pressure-volume loop in heart failure. Elevation of filling pressure shifts the end-diastolic point upward and to the right along the abnormal end-diastolic pressure volume loop. Although this leads to a further increase in blood pressure, through the operation of Starling's law of the heart, it does so at the expense of both a rise in filling pressure and an increased end-diastolic volume.

monly occurs in heart failure, "compresses" the pressure volume loop as shown in Fig. 25.8A. In this example, which has been simplified in that stroke volume is assumed to remain constant, the decreased end-systolic pressure and increased end-diastolic pressure reduce the area within the loop, which means that the failing heart does less work. As noted below, two circulatory adjustments come into play. These are vasoconstriction and increased preload, both of which are mediated in part by the neurohumoral responses described above.

Vasoconstriction

One of the most important consequences of the neurohumoral response to a fall in cardiac work is peripheral vasoconstriction (Table 25.2), which shifts the end-systolic point of the pressure-volume loop upward and to the right along the depressed end-systolic pressure-volume relationship (Fig. 25.8B). This circulatory response, which does not modify contractility, increases afterload so as to maintain blood pressure. Increased afterload has only a minor effect to reduce the stroke volume of the normal heart, in which Starling's law of the heart readily adjusts the work capacity of the ventricle so as to meet the increased resistance to ejection (Chapter 15); however, because the failing ventricle is unable to sustain a normal stroke volume when afterload is increased (Fig. 25.9), vasoconstriction exacerbates forward failure and contributes to one of the vicious cycles depicted in Fig. 25.7.

Increased Preload

Because ejection is impaired in patients with heart failure, end-systolic volume increases: this leads to a rise in atrial pressure that increases cardiac work (Starling's law of the heart). The increased preload, which moves the end-diastolic point of the pressure-volume loop to the right along the abnormal end-diastolic pressure-volume

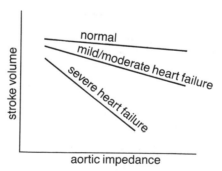

FIG. 25.9. Effect of changing afterload on stroke volume in a normal heart, and in moderate and severe left ventricular failure.

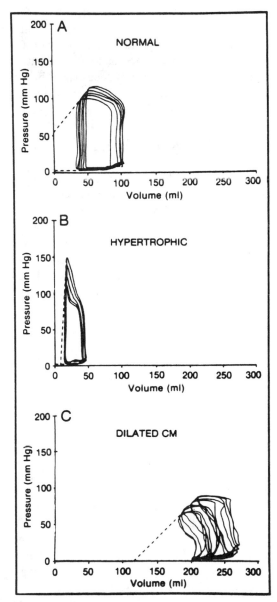

FIG. 25.10. Pressure-volume loops from three patients: **(A)** normal, **(B)** hypertension with hypertrophy, and **(C)** dilated cardiomyopathy. Each panel contains several loops; the ones to the right were obtained under resting conditions; those to the left reflect the effects of a decrease in venous return caused by inflation of a balloon in the inferior vena cava. (From Kass, 1988 with permission of *Heart Failure*.)

relationship (Fig. 25.8C), is also due to venoconstriction and fluid retention (Table 25.2). The resulting increase in cardiac work tends to return both stroke volume and blood pressure toward normal. Although alleviating forward failure, the elevated end-diastolic pressure impairs cardiac filling and so exacerbates backward failure. Furthermore, the enhanced contractile performance caused by dilatation of the ventricle, through the operation of the law of Laplace, increases wall tension and energy expenditure, and so decreases cardiac efficiency (Chapter 16).

Clinical Heart Failure as Seen on the Pressure-Volume Loop

Left ventricular pressure-volume loops obtained from three patients are shown in Fig. 25.10, which depicts a series of records obtained after venous return was abruptly reduced by inflation of a balloon in the inferior vena cava. The first series (Fig. 25.10A) is a control obtained in a patient with normal ventricular function. The middle panel (Fig. 25.10B) shows pressure-volume loops obtained in the same manner from a patient with chronic hypertension; here, hypertrophy has impaired left ventricular filling and so has shifted the loops to the reduced volumes that are characteristic of lusitropic heart failure (compare with Fig. 16.19). These loops also enclose an obviously reduced area, which reflects the decrease in stroke work caused by impaired filling of the hypertrophied left ventricle. The third example (Fig. 25.10C) shows the pressure-volume loops obtained from a patient with a congestive cardiomyopathy; here, marked depression of the end-systolic pressure-volume relationship has moved the loop to the right; that is, the ventricle has become dilated in this patient with inotropic heart failure (compare with Fig. 16.17).

BIOCHEMICAL AND BIOPHYSICAL ABNORMALITIES IN THE FAILING HEART

Up to this point, our discussion of heart failure has focused on the first of the three paradigms that describe the pathophysiology of heart failure. Although these circulatory responses to a decrease in the work of the heart play an important role in the pathophysiology of heart failure, this condition is now known to involve important abnormalities in the biochemistry and biophysics of the heart muscle itself. Even when pump performance is impaired by such structural disorders as a stenotic or leaky valve, or damage to a part of the left ventricle following myocardial infarction, the chronic hemodynamic overloading increases energy expenditure by the active myocardial cells. Chronic overloading, therefore, leads to biochemical and biophysical abnormalities in the myocardial cells that play an important role in the pathophysiology and prognosis of heart failure.

Energetics in the Failing Heart

An imbalance between energy production and energy utilization is among the most important of the biochemical changes in the failing heart. The most obvious cause for this imbalance is, of course, the overload itself, which increases the external work of the heart. Unfortunately, a number of changes in the hypertrophied heart limit the provision of the chemical energy needed to meet the increased rate of energy utilization. As a result, the failing heart is likely to be in a state of "energy starvation," due both to increased energy utilization and decreased high-energy phosphate production. This imbalance explains the finding that myocardial high-energy phosphate contents are decreased in both animal models of heart failure and in biopsies of hypertrophied, failing human hearts.

Structural Changes in the Chronically Overloaded Heart

Although hypertrophy causes the overloaded heart to enlarge, it is important to recognize that the failing heart is not simply an enlarged version of the normal heart. Architectural changes depend on both the nature and duration of the overload (Dalla-Volta et al., 1988). Pressure overload generally causes the walls of the heart to thicken so that, except in end-stage heart failure when these ventricles dilate (see below), the cavity of the ventricle becomes smaller (see Fig. 25.10B). In contrast, a volume overload causes the heart to dilate, a change that persists even when the heart is fully compensated.

Most important is that the cells of the hypertrophied heart begin to die in patients with severe, long-standing, heart failure. Because myocyte necrosis stimulates fibroblast proliferation, muscle is replaced by connective tissue (Linzbach, 1960; Fig. 25.11) and the failing heart begins to dilate, which according to the law of

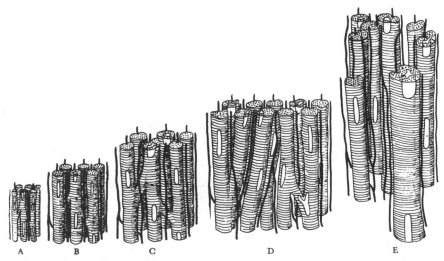

FIG. 25.11. Drawings of the morphology of a 15-gm infant heart (*A*), a 300-gm adult heart (*B*), a 500-gm heart of an athlete (*C*), a 650-gm pressure overloaded heart (*D*), and a 900-gm dilated, decompensated heart (E). (From Linzbach, 1960.)

Laplace, increases wall tension and so establishes a vicious cycle that further over-loads the cells of the failing heart. Enlargement and fibrosis also contribute to the propensity for arrhythmias in the failing heart (Chapter 21). Together, these detri-mental consequences of cardiac hypertrophy establish yet another vicious cycle in the patient with heart failure (Fig. 25.12).

Altered Blood Supply

A decrease in capillary density (Wearn, 1939–40) along with a relative deficit of mitochondria (see below) contribute to still another vicious cycle, caused by energy starvation, that contributes to the deterioration of the failing heart. Because the number of capillaries supplying the cells of the hypertrophied heart does not in-crease in proportion to its increased mass, intercapillary distance is increased and capillary density is decreased (Table 25.3). The decrease in coronary reserve is especially marked in the relatively underperfused subendocardial regions of the ven-tricle (Hoffman and Spaan, 1990), which accounts for the subendocardial ischemia, and even necrosis, that are often seen in the severely pressure-overloaded left ven-tricle.

Altered Proportions of Mitochondria and Myofibrils

An important change in the cellular composition of the chronically hypertrophied heart is an increased ratio of myofibrils to mitochondria, which means that more energy-consuming myofibrils must be supplied with ATP by relatively fewer mito-chondria (Table 25.3). The disproportionate increase in the content of contractile proteins relative to that of mitochondria is likely to exacerbate a state of energy starvation in the cells of the chronically failing heart.

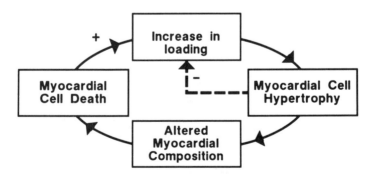

FIG. 25.12. Hypertrophy by increasing the number of contractile units in the overloaded heart, reduces the loading on each sarcomere and so is beneficial (−). However, hypertrophy also initiates myocardial changes that cause the cells of the failing heart to deteriorate and die, thereby establishing a vicious cycle that, by reducing the number of contractile units, increases the load on each surviving cell (+). (From Katz 1989.)

TABLE 25.3. *Changes in cardiac myocyte composition in the pressure-loaded rat ventricle*

Structure	Control heart	Overloaded heart	Percent change
Mitochondria (um³)*	2620	3510	+ 34
Myofibrils (um³)*	3770	6290	+ 67
Ratio *Mitochondria/Myofibrils*	0.69	0.56	− 23
Intercapillary Distance (um)	15.6	17.9	+ 15

*Expressed as volume of mitochondria or myofibrils per nucleus. Because the number of myocyte nuclei does not change significantly the overloaded heart, this denominator provides an index of the relative contents of these structures in the control and overloaded hearts. Data from Anversa et al. (1980).

Effects of Energy Depletion on Contraction and Relaxation

The ability of energy starvation to cause both systolic and diastolic dysfunction in the failing heart arises from mechanisms that are generally similar to those described in Chapter 24. In heart failure, the imbalance is like a "demand ischemia" (complicated by hypertrophy) that usually impairs filling more than it does ejection. For this reason, the once widely held view that inotropic drugs are "specific" therapy for patients with heart failure is no longer tenable. In fact, there is growing evidence that inotropic drugs accelerate the deterioration and exacerbate arrhythmias in the failing heart.

This caveat may not apply to the cardiac glycosides, which have important indirect vasodilator and negative chronotropic effects that may reduce cardiac energy expenditure in patients with heart failure.

Arrhythmogenic Mechanisms in the Hypertrophied Heart

Enlargement and fibrosis of the atria and ventricles increase the susceptibility of the failing heart to arrhythmias because these changes slow conduction and increase the path length followed by the cardiac impulse. As noted in Chapter 21, both of the latter represent substrates for the appearance of reentrant arrhythmias. This propensity for the development of arrhythmias is increased by calcium accumulation in the cells of the energy-starved heart (Chapter 24), which can initiate triggered activity (Chapter 21). Lowered resting potential, due to sodium pump inhibition caused by attenuation of the allosteric effect of adenosine triphosphate (ATP) (Chapter 10), can also slow conduction by inhibiting sodium channel opening and thereby decreasing the amplitude and rate of rise of the action potential. Acidosis and elevated intracellular calcium, by reducing the permeability of the gap junctions, increases internal resistance and so may contribute to the slowing of conduction (Chapter 21). These many arrhythmogenic mechanisms explain the fact that about half of the deaths in patients with heart failure are sudden.

ALTERED GENE EXPRESSION IN THE CHRONICALLY OVERLOADED, FAILING HEART

Our search for an understanding of the poor prognosis in patients with heart failure has, in the past few years, led us to the third paradigm in Table 14.1, which focuses on the role of altered gene expression in physiology and pathophysiology. It is becoming apparent that the appearance of abnormal proteins in the cells of the failing heart may represent an unwelcome side effect of the accelerated protein synthesis that allows the overloaded heart to hypertrophy. These changes, in fact, may play an important role in the accelerated myocardial deterioration that accounts for the dismal prognosis in patients with heart failure.

Hypertrophy of the cells of the overloaded heart, like the neurohumoral response to overload, has both beneficial and harmful consequences (Table 25.2). Although the initial changes in architecture and cellular composition contribute a remarkable adaptation of form to function (Katz and Katz, 1989) that helps the heart to meet an acute overload, long-standing hypertrophy is accompanied by abnormalities in gene expression that appear to accelerate the deterioration of this energy-starved organ (Fig. 25.12). The detrimental consequences of hypertrophy seem to represent a "price" that the overloaded heart must pay in order to accelerate protein synthesis. Stated simply, although the useful life of the normal human heart appears to be at least 80 to 100 years, synthesis of abnormal proteins during hypertrophy may lead to a "cardiomyopathy of overload" that reduces the life span of the hypertrophied heart to about 5 years.

Three Phases in the Response of the Heart to Overload

The heart's response to overload can be divided into three phases (Meerson, 1961) that have different functional and prognostic implications (Table 25.4). The sudden imposition of an overload leads to an initial phase of *acute heart failure* in which the functional reserves of the nonhypertrophied myocardium are overwhelmed. The resulting signs and symptoms of heart failure (see above) can improve spontaneously with the development of the second phase of *compensatory hyperfunction*, which appears when enlargement of the overloaded myocytes increases the heart's ability to meet the overload. However, because the cells of the overloaded heart deteriorate and die, the response ends in a final phase of *exhaustion, cell death*, and *fibrosis*, in which "wearing out" of the cells of the hypertrophied myocardium causes progressive heart failure.

These three phases are illustrated by the clinical course often seen in patients following a massive myocardial infarction. During the initial phase, in which the picture is dominated by acute heart failure, extensive left ventricular infarction generates excessive demands that exceed the functional reserves of the noninfarcted myocardium. This leads to an initial phase of acute heart failure that gradually abates when hypertrophy of the surviving myocardium heralds the transition to the second phase of compensatory hyperfunction. In this second phase, the enlarged cells in the noninfarcted myo-

TABLE 25.4. *Meerson's three stages of cardiac response to hemodynamic overloading of the left ventricle*

First short-term stage of acute heart failure
  Clinical: Left heart failure, pulmonary congestion.
  Pathological: Dilatation of the left ventricle.
  Histological: Swelling and separation of the myofibrils.
  Biochemical: Glycogen and ATP levels decreased, phosphocreatine level markedly decreased, lactate production slightly increased. Protein synthesis, RNA, and mitochondrial mass (especially the inner membranes) increased.
Second long-term stage of compensatory hyperfunction
  Clinical: Relief of symptoms.
  Pathological: Hypertrophy.
  Histological: Increased size of cardiac fibers, minimal fibrosis.
  Biochemical: Glycogen, ATP, phosphocreatine levels normal. Lactate production increased. Protein synthesis, RNA level normal, DNA level decreased. Myofibrillar mass increased relative to that of the mitochondrial mass.
Third long-term stage of progressive exhaustion, cell death, and fibrosis
  Clinical: Reappearance of heart failure.
  Pathological: Fibrous replacement of muscular tissue.
  Histological: Disproportionate appearance of connective tissue, fatty dystrophy; muscle cell nuclei become pyknotic.
  Biochemical: As in second stage, except decline in protein synthesis and marked decline in DNA levels.

cardium share the overload among an increased number of sarcomeres. Although this response initially alleviates the hemodynamic abnormalities, compensation is far from perfect because the hypertrophied myocardium is not normal muscle. For this reason, this adaptive response does not end well as the cells of the chronically overloaded, hypertrophied myocardium deteriorate and die, which leads to the typical downhill clinical course of end-stage congestive heart failure.

Physiological and Pathological Hypertrophy

The cardiac hypertrophy induced by exercise (physiological hypertrophy) differs fundamentally from the hypertrophic response to chronic overload (pathological hypertrophy) described above. Physiological hypertrophy is mainly, if not entirely, adaptive and does not appear to lead to the serious deleterious sequelae associated with pathological hypertrophy.

These two types of hypertrophy lead to different morphological (Fig. 25.11) and molecular changes in the myocardium. Best understood of the latter is the synthesis of different myosin heavy chain isoforms in the rat heart when hypertrophy is caused by swimming exercise, or by a chronic pressure overload. In exercise-induced hypertrophy, the fast α-myosin heavy chain is preferentially synthesized, whereas pathological hypertrophy favors the appearance of the slow β-isoform (the significance of these isoform shifts is discussed below). Additional molecular differences between these two types of hypertrophy are suggested by the finding that sarcoplasmic reticulum calcium transport is accelerated in physiological hypertrophy and slowed by pathological hypertrophy in the rat. In humans, as well, there is evidence that relaxation is accelerated in physiological hypertrophy (Granger et al., 1985).

The important distinction between physiological and pathological hypertrophy may reflect differences in the nature of the stimulus for cell growth, and the extent to which this stimulus is sustained. In aortic stenosis, for example, the mechanical abnormality that leads to pathological hypertrophy persists throughout the day and is even present during sleep. In contrast, exercise, the usual stimulus to physiological hypertrophy, is episodic and mediated largely by the sympathetic neurotransmitters. Elucidation of the mechanisms by which different causes of hypertrophy lead to different patterns of myocardial cell growth can be expected to provide important clues regarding the pathophysiology of heart failure.

Variability of the Hypertrophic Response to Overload

The hypertrophic response to overload exhibits a wide clinical spectrum (Fig. 25.13). At one end are patients in whom, without apparent stimulus, the heart undergoes inappropriate, and sometimes lethal, hypertrophy; this is, of course, the condition recognized as *hypertrophic cardiomyopathy*. At the other end of the spectrum are patients, notably the elderly, in whom severe and long-standing overload (for example, systemic hypertension) causes relatively little hypertrophy. Blunting of the hypertrophic response in the aged heart has been proposed as one cause for the high incidence of heart failure in the elderly, which has been supported by experimental evidence that aortic valve lesions cause less hypertrophy in aged than young rats (Isoyama et al., 1988).

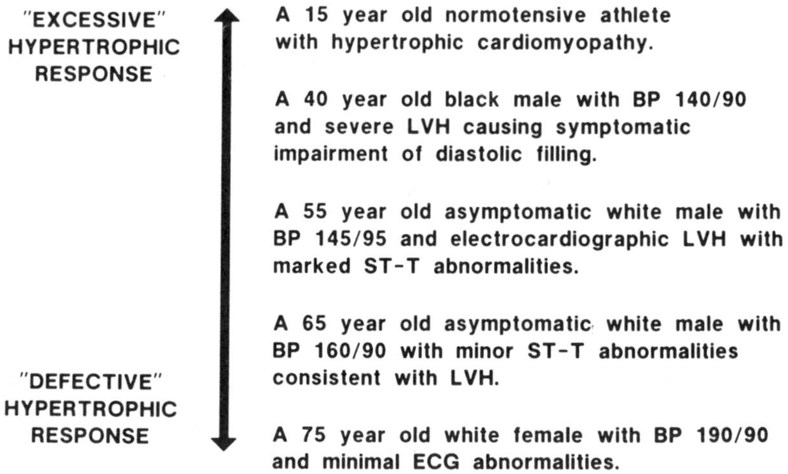

"EXCESSIVE" HYPERTROPHIC RESPONSE

A 15 year old normotensive athlete with hypertrophic cardiomyopathy.

A 40 year old black male with BP 140/90 and severe LVH causing symptomatic impairment of diastolic filling.

A 55 year old asymptomatic white male with BP 145/95 and electrocardiographic LVH with marked ST-T abnormalities.

A 65 year old asymptomatic white male with BP 160/90 with minor ST-T abnormalities consistent with LVH.

"DEFECTIVE" HYPERTROPHIC RESPONSE

A 75 year old white female with BP 190/90 and minimal ECG abnormalities.

FIG. 25.13. The hypertrophic response to overload varies markedly among individuals; this ranges from "excessive" hypertrophy in patients who suffer from hypertrophic cardiomyopathy (*top*), to a "defective" response that can be seen in the elderly, where a marked pressure overload causes relatively little hypertrophy (*bottom*).

Hypertrophic Cardiomyopathy

Recent studies of several families with inherited hypertrophic cardiomyopathy, which represents an inappropriate growth response in the myocardium, have demonstrated that this condition can be associated with a number of specific gene abnormalities. A single amino acid replacement in a ventricular myosin heavy chain encoded by a gene on chromosome 14 was associated with this cardiomyopathy in one family (Geisterfer-Lowrance et al., 1990), whereas in another family the abnormality was a crossover on this chromosome between the genes that encode the α- and β-myosin heavy chains (Tanigawa et al., 1990). In other families, however, the molecular abnormalities are encoded by genes on other chromosomes. These remarkable findings, like many major discoveries, raise far more questions than they answer. It is by no means clear why or how the synthesis of either of two quite different abnormal myosin heavy chains causes inappropriate hypertrophy rather than the dilated cardiomyopathy that might be expected if the myocardium had been weakened. This puzzle is made even more complicated by evidence that abnormalities involving other gene products also cause hypertrophic cardiomyopathy.

Adaptive Nature of Early Hypertrophy

By adding new sarcomeres to meet increased mechanical demands, hypertrophy reduces both total energy expenditure and the tension that must be developed by each sarcomere in the walls of the failing heart. Because energy utilization during systole is inversely proportional to wall tension (Chapter 16), hypertrophy increases myocardial efficiency and so has an energy-sparing effect.

Detrimental Effects of Chronic Hypertrophy

Hypertrophy, like the neurohumoral response in heart failure, represents an adaptation that is best suited for the short-term because when the stimulus to hypertrophy is sustained for months and years, important deleterious effects begin to appear. Several of these deleterious effects have already been discussed, notably abnormalities in architecture, blood supply, and ultrastructure that exacerbate energy-starvation in the overloaded heart. More recently, observed changes in the molecular composition of the chronically hypertrophied heart have begun to provide clues as to how the stimulus to cell growth, which was initially beneficial, can lead to myocardial cell death when the stimulus for cell growth is sustained (see below).

Initiation of Hypertrophy

The mechanisms that regulate cell growth, like all vital regulatory functions, are extremely complex. Thus, the stimulus by which overload initiates hypertrophy involves interactions among a number of control mechanisms that translate an increase in the work of the heart into a signal that increases cell growth (Cooper et al., 1989; Komuro et al., 1990; Morgan and Baker, 1991; Samuel et al., 1986).

Several possible mediators of the processes by which overload stimulates cell growth are listed in Table 25.5. As noted in the table, this list is almost certainly incomplete. Furthermore, many of the signals listed in Table 25.5 are known to interact, some initiating or regulating others. The difficulty in deciding what actually initiates hypertrophy is more like analyzing a Monet landscape than a Wagner opera. Key elements are interwoven throughout, so that the processes involved in hypertrophy, like the painting, lack a unique starting point. In fact, both the painting and hypertrophy succeed not because they have a unique beginning and an end, but instead because of effective interactions between the many elements that together express the artist's (and nature's) intentions. Elegant analogies notwithstand-

TABLE 25.5. *Possible mediators of the signal that initiates hypertrophy in the overloaded heart*

Cell deformation
  Stretch-activated ion channels
  Cytoskeletal rearrangements (microtubules, desmin)
Extracellular growth factors
  FGF (fibroblast growth factor)
  TGFβ (type β transforming growth factor)
Extracellular neurotransmitters and hormones
  α-adrenergic agonists
  β-adrenergic agonists
  Angiotensin II
  Thyroxine
  Insulin
  Growth hormone
  Glucocorticoids
Intracellular energy deficit
  Decreased high energy phosphates
    ATP, phosphocreatine
  Increased products of excessive energy utilization
    ADP, AMP, creatine
Intracellular second messengers
  Cyclic AMP, cyclic AMP-dependent protein kinases
  Calcium
  Inositol trisphosphate
  Diacylglycerol, protein kinase C
Cellular protooncogenes
  c-fos, c-myc, c-jun

This list is neither complete, nor does it imply that each of these possible mediators acts independently. In fact, there is every reason to believe that intricately interwoven interactions between these putative mediators of call growth are responsible for the remarkable plasticity of cell growth that adapts the heart's form to many different types of stimulus.

ing, of course, one or more signals must tell the systems that control cell growth that the myocardium has been overloaded. These are discussed briefly below.

Stretch Receptors

Among the many candidates for the mediator of the initial step in the hypertrophic response are a variety of stretch receptors that could initiate a signal when overload increases initial fiber length in the walls of the heart.

> The idea that stretch regulates cell growth is actually a remarkable concept because there are so many situations that stretch myocardial cells. Because Starling's law of the heart represents a simple hemodynamic mechanism that operates continually to adjust the output of the heart to the ever-changing needs of the circulation (Chapter 13), input from stretch receptors may be regulating cell growth in our hearts at all times!

The existence of stretch receptors in the heart has been known for decades. The ability of stretch to increase the rate of the sinoatrial (SA) node pacemaker explains the long-recognized heart rate response to increased venous return often referred to as the Bainbridge reflex. As noted in Chapter 1, stretch also releases atrial granules that contain atrial natriuretic factor. A number of ion channels are modified by stretch (Morris, 1990); these include sodium and calcium channels, which are activated, and potassium channels, which are inhibited. Together, these mediate a depolarizing effect of stretch that, in addition to accelerating pacemaker activity, may constitute one of the initial stimuli to cell growth.

> Effects of cell deformation on cell growth may also be mediated by structural rearrangements involving cytoskeletal structures such as the microtubules, actin and de smin. However, evidence defining a role for these mediators is limited at this time.

Extracellular Growth Factors

A number of peptide growth factors may play a role in the response of the heart to overload (Schneider and Parker, 1990). Among the most prominent are the *acidic* and *basic fibroblast growth factors* (aFGF and bFGF, respectively) and *type β transforming growth factors* (TGFβ). All are widely distributed in the cells of the heart, although their roles in the growth response to overload remain incompletely understood. Both of the FGFs and TGFβ (along with many other peptide growth factors) not only control the overall rate of cell growth, but also influence the protein isoforms that are synthesized. These growth factors, for example, can determine the relative expression of muscle-specific genes that encode the proteins found in adult muscle, as opposed to the genes that encode the homologous proteins found in more undifferentiated tissues. Both bFGF and TGFβ, which stimulate the overall rate of cell growth, increase the synthesis of fetal isoforms of muscle proteins at the same time that they inhibit the expression of the adult muscle-specific genes. This preferential expression of fetal proteins may contribute to the accelerated deterioration of the overloaded hypertrophied heart (see below).

The response of the heart to most peptide growth factors begins when these ligands bind to specific plasmalemmal receptors. The ligand-receptor complex, in turn, modifies cell function by stimulating a variety of tyrosine kinases that phosphorylate tyrosine residues in a number of proteins. These signaling cascades are mediated by the G-proteins discussed in Chapter 12, which themselves have complex effects on cell growth that may arise from interactions with other plasma membrane proteins, such as calcium channels, or when they modulate the synthesis of intracellular messengers such as cyclic AMP, diacylglycerol, and inositol phosphates.

Neurotransmitters and Hormones

The effects of the extracellular messengers to modify contractile and electrophysiological function have been discussed at several points in this text. Neurotransmitters and circulating hormones, including the α- and β-adrenergic agonists, peptide hormones like angiotensin II, thyroxine, and insulin, and even steroid hormones such as the glucocorticoids, also have important effects on cell growth and differentiation. These substances, which were initially viewed as modifying *organ* and *cell* function, thus have important effects on the rate and patterns of *gene* expression. In fact, these substances may have appeared early in evolution as growth regulators, and only later, with the evolution of eukaryotic cells and multicellular organisms did they assume their better known roles as physiological and biochemical regulators (Katz, 1990b).

Intracellular Energy Deficit

Decreased levels of high-energy phosphate compounds [adenosine triphosphate (ATP) and phosphocreatine] and a corresponding rise in their hydrolytic products [adenosine diphosphate (ADP), adenosine monophosphate (AMP), creatine] have been proposed to stimulate cell growth during the periods of excessive energy utilization that accompany hemodynamic overloading. However, the extent to which changes in cellular energetics represent a direct stimulus that accelerates cell growth is not known.

Intracellular Second Messengers

It is clear that the many intracellular messengers produced in the responses discussed above, including cyclic AMP, diacylglycerol, inositol phosphates, and calcium, play a role in stimulating cell growth. These substances, through effects that are generally mediated by their ability to activate protein kinases, regulate both the overall rate and specific products of protein synthesis. Their role in the integrated response to overload is, however, not well understood.

Cellular Proto-Oncogenes

The cellular proto-oncogenes constitute an extremely complex system that plays a central role in regulating growth and differentiation of the heart. In recent years, increasing attention has been directed to their role in mediating the processes by which overload leads to hypertrophy (Bugaisky and Zak, 1986; Izumo et al., 1988; Simpson, 1989). Whatever the initiating signal, the growth response to hemodynamic overloading appears to involve increased expression of *c-fos, c-myc,* and *c-jun,* proto-oncogenes that encode short-lived nuclear proteins which promote and regulate cell proliferation and differentiation at a transcriptional level. This response is accompanied by the appearance of the heat-shock protein *HSP 70,* one of a family of proteins initially noted to increase when cells are exposed to elevated temperature, and which may help to maintain the structure of damaged proteins. These responses of the overloaded heart resemble the early mitogenic responses to a variety of stimuli in other cell types, and may be part of a general adaptive response to stress.

Abnormal Gene Expression in the Hypertrophied Heart

The cells of the adult heart normally synthesize protein at a very slow rate, so that it should not be surprising that the hypertrophic response to overload involves substantial modification of the systems that regulate protein synthesis. These modifications not only induce an overall acceleration of protein synthesis, but also modify specific patterns of gene expression. These resulting changes in the protein composition of the hypertrophied heart can be explained by at least two different mechanisms: expression of abnormal members of the multigene families that encode important myocardial cell proteins (Emerson and Bernstein, 1987; Swynghedauw, 1986), and alternative splicing, which allows the information contained in a single gene, through variations in transcription of genomic DNA into messenger RNA, to encode different protein isoforms (Breitbart et al., 1987).

The functional and prognostic significance of most of the many molecular changes that accompany the accelerated growth of the hypertrophied heart remain shrouded in mystery. With the notable exception of the preferential synthesis of the slow myosin heavy chain isoform described below, it is not clear how—or even if—abnormal gene expression influences the long-term course of patients with congestive heart failure.

Alterations in Myosin

The most extensively characterized of the molecular changes known to occur in both clinical and experimental heart failure involve the heavy chains of myosin. In the rat ventricle, chronic pressure overload cause the α (V1) myosin heavy chain, which determines a high myosin adenosine triphosphatase (ATPase) activity and rapid shortening velocity, to be replaced by the slow β (V3) myosin heavy chain (Chapter 14). This isoform shift, by slowing cross-bridge cycling, reduces myocardial contractility. From the standpoint of the circulation, this is obviously detrimental. However, the preferential synthesis of slow myosin facilitates ejection and improves the mechanical efficiency of the overloaded heart (Hamrell and Alpert, 1986). Thus, although expression of slow myosin gene in the failing rat heart has a negative inotropic effect, it is also energy-sparing.

> In the human ventricle, only a slow myosin isoform is normally synthesized, so that the isoform shift described above cannot occur. However, overload does cause myosin isoform shifts in human atria, where a decreased proportion of fast (α) atrial myosin heavy chain parallels left atrial hypertension and enlargement (Mercadier et al., 1987; Tsuchimochi et al., 1984).

Other abnormal protein isoforms appear in the hypertrophied heart, but in most cases the functional significance of these alterations in gene expression is not clear. Synthesis of an abnormal troponin T isoform may, like that of the slow myosin heavy chain, depress contractility by reducing the rate of actin-myosin turnover.

Synthesis of Fetal Myocardial Protein Isoforms in the Hypertrophied Heart

At the same time that the cells of the adult myocardium increase their rate of protein synthesis in response to an overload, they preferentially express genes that encode the fetal isoforms of several myocardial proteins. This probably reflects the fact that adult cardiac myocytes are terminally differentiated cells that have lost not only the ability to divide, but also the capacity for rapid protein synthesis. Thus, in resuming their earlier capacity for rapid growth in response to overload, the cells of the adult myocardium also increase the expression of the genes that had encoded protein isoforms present during fetal life.

Reversion to a cellular composition seen earlier in ontogeny may contribute to the central problem in heart failure: that whereas the normal human heart can function for 80 to 100 years, chronic overload leads to the appearance of abnormal heart muscle that deteriorates rapidly—as noted above, the average life expectancy of a patient with even mild to moderate heart failure is only about 5 years. It is tempting to postulate that the appearance of fetal protein isoforms in the response to chronic overload might contribute to the deterioration of the failing heart, but data to establish such a causal link are lacking.

Temporal and Spatial Heterogeneities in the Appearance of Altered Protein Isoforms in the Overloaded Heart

Hypertrophy of the overloaded heart is not simply an overall stimulation of muscle growth; instead, altered protein isoforms appear at different times, and in different places. In the initial response to overload, for example, the appearance of the slow myosin isoform and the fetal isoform of actin follow different time courses (Izumo et al., 1987). Even more dramatic, the abnormal isoforms of myosin and actin appear in different locations in the overloaded rat heart (Bugaisky et al., 1990; Schiaffino et al., 1989). The newly synthesized β-myosin heavy chains appear first in the subendocardial regions of the left ventricle and around blood vessels, whereas the fetal isoform of actin appears more uniformly throughout the overloaded myocardium (Fig. 25.14). The distribution of β-myosin heavy chain messenger RNA

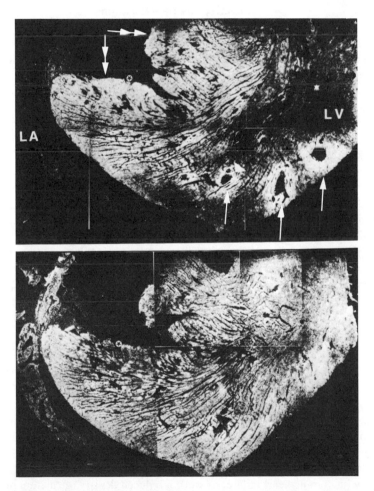

FIG. 25.14. Serial, nonconsecutive sections of a rat heart hybridized with riboprobes to β-myosin heavy chains (*above*) and α-skeletal actin (*below*) 2 days after aortic constriction. In the left ventricle (LV), the "slow" myosin isoform initially appears around blood vessels (*single arrows*) and in the subendocardial regions (*double arrows*), but is virtually absent in the left atrium (LA) and ventricular midwall. In contrast, the skeletal isoform of actin is distributed more homogeneously in both the left ventricle and left atrium. (Modified from Schiaffino et al., 1989, with permission of the American Heart Association, Inc.)

shown in Fig. 25.14 may reflect mechanical heterogeneities in the pressure-overloaded heart, such as the higher tension in the subendocardium and around blood vessels, but it is also possible that the genes that regulate the synthesis of these abnormal proteins are controlled by different growth factors. For example, the initial appearance of the slow myosin isoform in the subendocardium and around blood vessels might reflect the initiation of the synthesis of this isoform by growth factors released from endothelial and endocardial cells.

Connective Tissue Alterations

Alterations in the connective tissue matrix of the hypertrophied heart probably play an as yet incompletely understood role in the myocardial abnormalities commonly encountered in patients with congestive heart failure. These alterations include not only an increased collagen content, but also changes in the specific types of collagen molecules synthesized in the overloaded heart. For example, the collagen initially synthesized in response to overload is the "softer" embryonic type III collagen, which also appears in wounds shortly after injury; but when the overload becomes chronic, much of this collagen is replaced by type I collagen, associated with scar tissue, that has higher tensile strength (Weber et al., 1988).

Proliferation of collagen probably serves an adaptive role in the initial response to overload, where its ability to increase wall stiffness can reduce dilatation and, as a consequence of the law of Laplace, lessen wall tension in the overloaded heart (Table 25.2). However, proliferation of the extracellular matrix after sustained overloading may eventually impair filling and so contribute to the prominent lusitropic abnormalities in patients with heart failure. Excessive growth of connective tissue may also injure myocardial cells and, by effects that slow impulse conduction, be arrhythmogenic.

Abnormal Membrane Assembly

Changes in cell membrane architecture, as well as the preferential synthesis of abnormal protein isoforms, contribute to the important functional changes in the hypertrophied, failing heart. Altered membrane assembly has been noted in the sarcoplasmic reticulum of the overloaded rat heart, where slowed calcium uptake is due in part to a reduced concentration of calcium pump ATPase molecules in this internal membrane, rather than the expression of an altered isoform of this large molecule (De la Bastie et al., 1990; Komuro et al., 1989; Nagai et al., 1989). In patients with chronic heart failure, as well, a reduced density of calcium pump sites in the sarcoplasmic reticulum also contributes to the slowed relaxation (Mercadier et al., 1990).

Other membrane abnormalities may also contribute to the increased diastolic stiffness in the failing heart. These include spontaneous recycling of calcium in the sarcoplasmic reticulum during diastole (Lakatta, 1989), abnormalities in the sodium/calcium exchanger (Hanf et al., 1988; Wagner et al., 1989), and alterations in plasmalemmal ion channels described below.

Electrophysiological Abnormalities

Arrhythmias, which are responsible for almost half of the deaths in patients with congestive heart failure, are due in part to cardiac enlargement and fibrosis, which prolong and disorganize the spread of the wave of depolarization over the failing heart (see above). In addition to these structural abnormalities, there is growing evidence that molecular changes in plasma membrane ion channels also play a role in the pathogenesis of the arrhythmias seen in patients with heart failure.

Prolongation of the action potential is among the most prominent electrophysiological abnormalities in hypertrophied myocardial cells (Ten Eick and Bassett, 1989). This abnormality, which may contribute to inhomogeneities of repolarization that favor reentry (Chapter 21), may be due in part to delayed inactivation of L-type calcium channels (Keung, 1989) or attenuation of one or more of the outward potassium currents that cause repolarization. It is not clear at this time if the number of calcium channels, which can be estimated by measuring the binding sites for the dihydropyridine calcium channel blockers, is altered in the hypertrophied heart (Ferrante and Triggle, 1990). Data regarding possible molecular abnormalities of individual channel proteins are not yet available.

Abnormal Autonomic Responsiveness

Sympathetic drive is increased in patients with heart failure (Bristow et al., 1985; Feldman and Bristow, 1990), but the cells of the failing heart lose their ability to respond to the β-adrenergic receptor agonists through the processes of desensitization (Chapter 12). Several molecular alterations contribute to this decreased sensitivity to sympathetic stimulation. Most important is a decreased number of functioning β-adrenergic receptors, which blunts the inotropic response of the failing heart to sympathetic stimulation. The major decrease is in the number of β_1-adrenergic receptors, β_2-receptors being relatively preserved. Although the response to β-adrenergic agonists is reduced, other classes of inotropic agents, notably the cardiac glycosides and calcium, can still elicit normal responses (Schmitz et al., 1987).

Desensitization of β-adrenergic receptors is likely to be both beneficial and deleterious in patients with heart failure. By reducing energy expenditure by the energy-starved myocardium, this adaptive response is beneficial; however, by reducing contractility and depressing the ability of the failing heart to increase its output in response to exercise, desensitization is also deleterious. The complexity of these effects has raised an as yet unresolved therapeutic question of whether β blockers or β agonists are appropriate therapy for these patients.

The immediate effect of β-blocker therapy would be to decrease contractility which, by exacerbating the low-output state in heart failure, would increase symptoms and can be dangerous, especially in patients with acute heart failure. However, long-term β-blocker therapy in chronic heart failure, if tolerated by the patient, would have significant theoretical advantages. One is a decrease in the energy demands of the resting heart, which could improve the state of this energy-starved organ. At the same time, the ability of the β-blockade to resensitize the heart's β-receptors (Chapter 12), could improve the response to exercise, when high concentrations of the β-adrenergic agonists would be available to displace the β-blockers from their binding to the receptors. Understanding of the appropriate role of these agents in the therapy of heart failure will require results of clinical trials not available at the time this chapter is written.

Alterations in the G-Proteins

Abnormalities in the G-proteins, like desensitization of the cardiac β-adrenergic receptors, blunt the response of the failing heart to sympathetic stimulation. There is now general agreement that the levels of G_s are reduced, whereas those of G_i are increased in the failing heart (Bristow et al., 1985; Insel and Ransnäs, 1988; Karliner and Scheinman, 1988; Neumann et al., 1988). The resulting decrease in the ratio of G_s to G_i, like β-adrenergic receptor desensitization, can have both beneficial and detrimental effects, as described above.

CONCLUSION

This chapter, which reviews our knowledge of the pathophysiology of heart failure in terms of the three paradigms discussed in Chapter 14 (Table 14.1) serves as a fitting conclusion for this text. We have seen how *organ physiology*, the first paradigm, describes heart failure in terms of abnormal pump function and altered circulatory dynamics (Chapter 16). Among the major consequences of reduced cardiac performance is the neurohumoral response that leads to salt and water retention and vasoconstriction, as well as increased adrenergic stimulation of the failing heart. *Cell biochemistry and biophysics*, the second paradigm, view heart failure in terms of altered myocardial cellular performance. These abnormalities include an energy deficit and depressed contractility and relaxation, which arise from altered interactions between the contractile proteins (Chapter 8) and altered calcium fluxes involved in excitation-contraction coupling (Chapter 14). *Altered gene expression*, the third paradigm, focuses on the appearance of abnormal proteins in the cells of the failing heart, notably the selective expression of fetal isoforms. These abnormalities, which may contribute to deterioration of the chronically failing heart, can be viewed as undesired side effects of the processes that allow the overloaded heart to hypertrophy by accelerating its rate of protein synthesis. These molecular changes may also explain the "cardiomyopathy of overload" that reduces the average life of the failing heart to only about 5 years, compared to the normal of 80 to 100 years.

Together, the abnormalities encountered in the patient with heart failure provide eloquent testimony to the importance of understanding the normal physiology of the heart in dealing with the clinical problems manifest in the pathophysiology of human disease.

REFERENCES

Anversa P, Olivetti G, Melissari M, Loud AV. (1980). Stereological measurement of cellular and sub-cellular hypertrophy and hyperplasia in the papillary muscle of adult rat. *J Mol Cell Cardiol* 12:781–795.

Breitbart RE, Andreadis A, Nadal-Ginard B. (1987). Alternative splicing: a ubiquitous mechanism for the generation of multiple protein isoforms from single genes. *Annu Rev Biochem* 56:467–495.

Bristow MR, Kantrowitz NE, Ginsburg R, Fowler MB. (1985). β-adrenergic function in heart muscle disease and heart failure. *J Mol Cell Cardiol* 17(Suppl 2):41–52.

Bugaisky L, Zak R. (1986). Biological mechanisms of hypertrophy In: Fozzard H, Haber E, Katz A, Jennings R, Morgan HE, eds. *The heart and cardiovascular system*. New York: Raven Press; 1491–1506.

Bugaisky LB, Anderson PG, Hall RS, Bishop SP. (1990). Differences in myosin isoform expression in the subepicardial and subendocardial myocardium during cardiac hypertrophy in the rat. *Circ Res* 66:1127–1132.

Cooper G, Kent RL, Mann DL. Load induction of cardiac hypertrophy. (1989). *J Mol Cell Cardiol* 21(Suppl 5):11–30.

Dalla-Volta S, Razzolini R, Scognamiglio R, Rubino A, Chioin R. (1988). Myocardial function in heart failure. *Cardiology* 75:8–18.

De la Bastie D, Levitsky D, Rappaport L, Mercadier J-J, Marotte F, Wisnewsky C, Brokovich V, Schwartz K, Lompre A-M. (1990). Function of the sarcoplasmic reticulum and expression of its Ca^{2+} ATPase gene in pressure-overloaded cardiac hypertrophy in the rat. *Circ Res* 66:554–564.

Emerson CP Jr, Bernstein SI. (1987). Molecular genetics of myosin. *Annu Rev Biochem* 56:695–726.

Feldman AM, Bristow MR. (1990). The β-adrenergic pathway in the failing human heart: implications for inotropic therapy. *Cardiology* 77 (Suppl 1):1–32.

Ferrante J, Triggle DJ. (1990). Drug-and disease-induced regulation of voltage-dependent calcium channels. *Pharmacol Rev* 42:29–44.

Francis GS, Goldsmith SR, Levine TB, Olivari MT, Cohn JN. (1984). The neurohumoral axis in congestive heart failure. *Ann Intern Med* 101:370–377.

Geisterfer-Lowrance AAT, Kass S, Tanigawa G, Vosberg H-P, McKenna W, Seidman CE, Seidman JG. (1990). A molecular basis for familial hypertrophic cardiomyopathy: a β cardiac myosin heavy chain gene missense mutation. *Cell* 62:999–1006.

Granger CB, Karimeddini MK, Smith VE, Shapiro HR, Katz AM, Riba AL. (1985). Rapid ventricular filling in left ventricular hypertrophy. I. Physiological hypertrophy. *J Am Coll Cardiol* 5:862–868.

Hamrell BB, Alpert NR. (1986). Cellular basis of the mechanical properties of hypertrophied myocardium. In: Fozzard H, Haber E, Katz AM, Jennings R, Morgan HE, eds. *The heart and cardiovascular system*. New York: Raven Press; 1507–1524.

Hanf R, Drubaix I, Marotte F, Lelievre LG. (1988). Rat cardiac hypertrophy. Altered sodium-calcium exchange activity in sarcolemmal vesicles. *FEBS Lett* 236:145–149.

Hoffman JEI, Spaan JAE. (1990). Pressure-flow relations in the coronary circulation. *Physiol Rev* 70:331–390.

Insel PA, Ransnäs LA. (1988). G proteins and cardiovascular disease. *Circulation* 78:1511–1513.

Isoyama S, Grossman W, Wei JY. (1988). Effect of age on myocardial adaptation to volume overload in the rat. *J Clin Invest* 81:1850–1857.

Izumo S, Lompré A-M, Matsuoka R, Koren G, Schwartz K, Nadal-Ginard B, Mahdavi V. (1987). Myosin heavy chain messenger RNA and protein isoform transitions during cardiac hypertrophy. *J Clin Invest* 79:970–977.

Izumo S, Nadal-Ginard B, Mahdavi V. (1988). Protooncogene induction and reprogramming of cardiac gene expression produced by pressure overload. *Proc Natl Acad Sci USA* 85:339–343.

Karliner JS, Scheinman M. (1988). Adenylate cyclase activity coupled to the stimulatory guanine nucleotide binding protein in patients having electrophysiologic studies and either structurally normal hearts or idiopathic myocardial disease. *Am J Cardiol* 62:1129–1130.

Kass DA. (1988). Evaluation of left-ventricular systolic function. *Heart Failure* 4:198–205.

Katz AM. (1989). Changing strategies in the management of congestive heart failure. *JACC* 13:512–523.

Katz AM. (1990a). Cardiomyopathy of overload. A major determinant of prognosis in congestive heart failure. *N Engl J Med* 322:100–110.

Katz AM. (1990b). Angiotensin II: hemodynamic regulator or growth factor? *J Mol Cell Cardiol* 22:739–747.

Katz AM, Katz PB. (1989). Homogeneity out of heterogeneity. *Circulation* 79:712–717.
Keung AC. (1989). Calcium current is increased in isolated adult myocytes from hypertrophied rat myocardium. *Circ Res* 64:753–763.
Komuro I, Kaida T, Shibazaki Y, Kurabayashi M, Katoh Y, Hoh E, Takaku F, Yazaki Y. (1990). Stretching cardiac myocytes stimulates protooncogene expression. *J Biol Chem* 265:3595–3598.
Komuro I, Kurabayashi M, Shibazaki Y, Takaku F, Yazaki Y. (1989). Molecular cloning and characterization of a $Ca^{2+} + Mg^{2+}$-dependent adenosine triphosphatase from rat cardiac sarcoplasmic reticulum. Regulation of its expression by pressure overload and developmental stage. *J Clin Invest* 83:1102–1108.
Lakatta E. (1989). Chaotic behavior of myocardial cells: possible implications regarding the pathophysiology of heart failure. *Perspect Biol Med* 32:421–433.
Linzbach AJ. (1960). Heart failure from the point of view of quantitative anatomy. *Am J Cardiol* 5:370–382.
Meerson FZ. (1961). On the mechanism of compensatory hyperfunction and insufficiency of the heart. *Cor et Vasa* 3:161–177.
Mercadier JJ, De La Bastie D, Menasche P, N'Guyen Van Cao A, Bouvenet P, Lorente P, Piwnica A, Slama R, Schwartz K. (1987). Alpha-myosin heavy chain isoform and atrial size in patients with various types of mitral valve dysfunction: a quantitative study. *J Am Coll Cardiol* 9:1024–1030.
Mercadier JJ, Lompre AM, Duc P, Boheler KR, Fraysse JB, Wisnewsky C, Allen PD, Kmoajda M, Schwartz K. (1990). Altered sarcoplasmic reticulum Ca^{2+}-ATPase gene expression in the human ventricle during end-stage heart failure. *J Clin Invest* 85:305–309.
Morgan HE, Baker KM. (1991). Cardiac hypertrophy. Mechanical, neural, and endocrine dependence. *Circulation* 83:13–25.
Morris CE. (1990). Mechanosensitive ion channels. *J Membr Biol* 113:93–107.
Nagai R, Zarain-Herzberg A, Brandl CJ, Fujii J, Tada M, MacLennan DH, Alpert NR, Periasamy M. (1989). Regulation of myocardial Ca^{2+} ATPase and phospholamban mRNA expression in response to pressure overload and thyroid hormone. *Proc Natl Acad Sci USA* 86:2966–2970.
Neumann J, Schmitz W, Scholz H, von Meyernick L, Döring V, Kalmar P. (1988). Increase in myocardial G_i-proteins in heart failure. *Lancet* 2:936–937.
Samuel JL, Marotte F, Delcayre C, Rappaport L. (1986). Microtubule reorganization is related to rate of heart myocyte hypertrophy in rat. *Am J Physiol* 251:H1118–H1125.
Schiaffino S, Samuel JL, Sassoon D, Lompre AM, Garner I, Marotte F, Buckingham M, Rappaport L, Schwartz K. (1989). Nonsynchronous accumulation of α-skeletal actin and β-myosin heavy chain mRNAs during early stages of pressure-overloaded-induced cardiac hypertrophy demonstrated by in situ hybridization. *Circ Res* 64:937–948.
Schmitz W, Scholz H, Erdmann E. (1987). Effects of α- and β-adrenergic agonists, phosphodiesterase inhibitors and adenosine on isolated human heart preparations. *Trends Pharmacol Sci* 8:447–450.
Schnieder MD, Parker TG. (1990). Cardiac myocytes as targets for the action of peptide growth factors. *Circulation* 81:1443–1456.
Simpson P. (1989). Proto-oncogenes and cardiac hypertrophy. *Annu Rev Physiol* 51:189–201.
Swynghedauw B. (1986). Developmental and functional adaptation of contractile proteins in cardiac and skeletal muscles. *Physiol Rev* 66:710–771.
Tanigawa G, Jarcho JA, Kass S, Solomon SD, Vosberg H-P, Seidman JG, Seidman CE. (1990). A molecular basis for familial hypertrophic cardiomyopathy: an α/β cardiac myosin heavy chain hybrid gene. *Cell* 62:999–1006.
Ten Eick RE, Bassett AL. (1989). Cardiac hypertrophy and altered cellular electrical activity of the myocardium. In: *Physiology and pathophysiology of the heart*, 2nd ed. Boston: Kluwer; 521–542.
Tsuchimochi H, Sugi M, Kuro-o M, Ueda S, Takaku F, Furuta S-i, Shirai T, Yazaki Y. (1984). Isozymic changes in myosin of human atrial myocardium induced by overload. Immunohistochemical study using monoclonal antibodies. *J Clin Invest* 74:662–665.
Wagner JA, Weisman HF, Snowman AM, Reynolds IJ, Weisfeldt ML, Snyder SH. (1989). Alterations in calcium antagonist receptors and sodium-calcium exchange in cardiomyopathic hamster tissues. *Circ Res* 65:205–214.
Wearn JT. (1939–40). Morphological and functional alterations of the coronary circulation. *Harvey Lect* 35:243–270.
Weber KT, Janicki JS, Schroff SG, Pick R, Chen RM, Bashey RI. (1988). Collagen remodeling of the pressure-overloaded, hypertrophied nonhuman primate myocardium. *Circ Res* 62:757–765.
Wilson JR, Mancini DM. (1990). The mechanism of exertional fatigue in heart failure. *Cardioscience* 1:3–6.

Subject Index